Praise for
Anatomy of Writing for Publication for Nurses,
Fifth Edition

"*This updated version of* Anatomy of Writing for Publication for Nurses *remains on the cutting edge of trends in publishing for nurses. Its comprehensiveness leaves no topic unaddressed. There is something for every nurse who wants to write or write better. The chapter on writing an EBPQI initiative is a highlight, as more nurses are engaged in this meaningful work to improve health and healthcare.*"

–Julee Briscoe Waldrop, DNP, FNP-C, PNP-C, EBP-C, CNE, FAANP, FAAN
Clinical Professor, Duke University School of Nursing
Editor-in-Chief, *The Journal for Nurse Practitioners*

"*I remember writing my first paper in my undergraduate nursing class. I wrote what I thought was a masterpiece . . . turns out my professor didn't think the same way that I did. How I wish I had Saver's 5th edition of* Anatomy of Writing for Publication for Nurses *to use as a reference. This book is a must for everyone. I highly recommend it as the go-to book for anyone writing for publication.*"

–Ernest J. Grant, PhD, DSc(h), RN, FAAN
Vice Dean – Diversity, Equity, Inclusion and Belonging
Duke University School of Nursing
Immediate Past President, American Nurses Association

"*An easy-to-read treasure trove of information and tips from seasoned editors and other experts, this book is an amazing resource for nurses at any career phase needing inspiration or direction to move a particular writing or presentation project forward or just wanting to better understand various formats for disseminating knowledge in our profession. I would also heartily recommend it to anyone mentoring nurse academics, clinicians, or practice leaders who are building portfolios of scholarship. An up-to-date gem of a book that deserves a wide audience.*"

–Sean Clarke, PhD, RN, FAAN
Ursula Springer Professor in Nursing Leadership and Executive Vice Dean
NYU Rory Meyers College of Nursing
Editor-in-Chief, *Nursing Outlook*

"*Cindy Saver's book should be a staple in everyone's resources. It is a practical, user-friendly guide and a fabulous resource that provides outstanding tips for publication success.*"

–Bernadette Mazurek Melnyk, PhD, APRN-CNP, FAANP, FNAP, FAAN
Vice President for Health Promotion and University Chief Wellness Officer
Helene Fuld Health Trust Professor of Evidence-Based Practice
Founder of the Helene Fuld Health Trust National Institute for
Evidence-Based Practice in Nursing and Healthcare
Former Dean, College of Nursing
Professor of Pediatrics & Psychiatry, College of Medicine
The Ohio State University

"This 5th edition is better than ever if that's even possible. With vital and relevant additions on AI in writing, using bias-free language, and updated industry terminology, this book remains the quintessential guide to writing for nurses whether novice or seasoned pro."

–Donna Cardillo, MA, RN, CSP, FAAN
The Inspiration Nurse, Author, Keynote Speaker
DonnaCardillo.com

"This book is a 'must-have' for aspiring nurse authors as well as those highly experienced in professional publication. It contains every aspect of advice that nursing editors want you to know and apply in all your writing endeavors. With Saver's text as your essential writing companion, you will have instant access to user-friendly, expertly crafted content that can help pave your way to publishing success. Hands down, it is my personal go-to reference!"

–Linda Laskowski-Jones, MS, APRN, ACNS-BC, CEN, NEA-BC, FAWM, FAAN
Editor-in-Chief, *Nursing2024: The Peer-Reviewed Journal of Clinical Excellence*
Health, Learning, Research & Practice, Lippincott/Wolters Kluwer

"Cynthia Saver has dedicated years of her career to enhancing the writing skills and publication potential of numerous nursing colleagues in all levels of education and experience. Her work has been reviewed and taken to heart by many, including those preparing to publish while earning a practice doctorate degree. The structure of her book, and the inclusion of dozens of talented colleagues, reinforces her ability and passion to elevate our profession. Buy this book. Read this book. Publish. We owe her a debt of gratitude for sharing the tips and instructions in this invaluable resource."

–David Campbell-O'Dell, DNP, APRN, FNP-BC, FAANP
Co-founder and CEO, Doctors of Nursing Practice, Inc.
Founder, The Academy of Doctoral Prepared Nurses

FIFTH EDITION

Anatomy of WRITING FOR PUBLICATION FOR NURSES

CYNTHIA SAVER, MS, RN

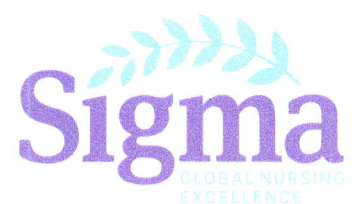

Copyright © 2024 by Cynthia Saver

All rights reserved. This book is protected by copyright. No part of it may be reproduced, stored in a retrieval system, or transmitted in any form or by any means, electronic, mechanical, photocopying, recording, or otherwise, without written permission from the publisher. Any trademarks, service marks, design rights, or similar rights that are mentioned, used, or cited in this book are the property of their respective owners. Their use here does not imply that you may use them for a similar or any other purpose.

This book is not intended to be a substitute for the medical advice of a licensed medical professional. The author and publisher have made every effort to ensure the accuracy of the information contained within at the time of its publication and shall have no liability or responsibility to any person or entity regarding any loss or damage incurred, or alleged to have incurred, directly or indirectly, by the information contained in this book. The author and publisher make no warranties, express or implied, with respect to its content, and no warranties may be created or extended by sales representatives or written sales materials. The author and publisher have no responsibility for the consistency or accuracy of URLs and content of third-party websites referenced in this book.

Sigma Theta Tau International Honor Society of Nursing (Sigma) is a nonprofit organization whose mission is developing nurse leaders anywhere to improve healthcare everywhere. Founded in 1922, Sigma has more than 135,000 active members in over 100 countries and territories. Members include practicing nurses, instructors, researchers, policymakers, entrepreneurs, and others. Sigma's more than 540 chapters are located at more than 700 institutions of higher education throughout Armenia, Australia, Botswana, Brazil, Canada, Chile, Colombia, Croatia, England, Eswatini, Finland, Ghana, Hong Kong, Ireland, Israel, Italy, Jamaica, Japan, Jordan, Kenya, Lebanon, Malawi, Mexico, the Netherlands, Nigeria, Pakistan, Philippines, Portugal, Puerto Rico, Scotland, Singapore, South Africa, South Korea, Sweden, Taiwan, Tanzania, Thailand, the United States, and Wales. Learn more at www.sigmanursing.org.

Sigma Theta Tau International
550 West North Street
Indianapolis, IN, USA 46202

To request a review copy for course adoption, order additional books, buy in bulk, or purchase for corporate use, contact Sigma Marketplace at 888.654.4968 (US/Canada toll-free), +1.317.687.2256 (International), or solutions@sigmamarketplace.org.

To request author information, or for speaker or other media requests, contact Sigma Marketing at 888.634.7575 (US/Canada toll-free) or +1.317.634.8171 (International).

ISBN: 9781646481804
EPUB ISBN: 9781646481811
PDF ISBN: 9781646481828

Library of Congress Control Number: 2024013936

Publisher: Dustin Sullivan
Acquisitions Editor: Emily Hatch
Development Editor: Jillmarie Leeper Sycamore
Cover Designer: Rebecca Batchelor
Interior Design/Page Layout: Kim Scott, Bumpy Design
Indexer: Larry D. Sweazy

Managing Editor: Carla Hall
Publications Specialist: Todd Lothery
Project Editor: Todd Lothery
Copy Editor: Erin Geile
Proofreader: Todd Lothery

To all my writing mentors over the years, my family (especially my mother, who introduced me to the pleasure of reading and writing), and Jackie, Terry, and David.

Acknowledgments

Thank you to my incredible team of contributors, most of whom have been with me through all five editions of this book. I am honored to be in such stellar company. The contributors bring a wonderful wealth of collective knowledge that reflects all the roles of publishing—author, editor, peer reviewer, designer, publisher—along with a strong commitment to help nurses share their expertise through publishing. I truly appreciate how they have generously shared their talents. I also appreciate the many others who read portions of the book and gave valuable feedback.

Thanks to Joan Borgatti for first linking anatomy to writing and to Patricia Dwyer Schull for her insightful comments and unfailing support.

Special thanks to the talented staff members at Sigma Theta Tau International, who always make authors look great: to Jill Sycamore and Erin Geile for their expert editing, Todd Lothery for proofreading, and Kim Scott for design and layout.

Publishing is truly a team effort!

About the Editor and Lead Author

Cynthia Saver, MS, RN, of CLS Development, is an award-winning author. She has more than five decades of experience in nursing, including more than four decades of publishing experience as a writer, editor, and senior vice president of editorial teams. Saver has written for many nursing publications, including *American Nurse Journal, American Journal of Nursing, AORN Journal, Journal of Nursing Regulation, Nurse Leader, Nursing Management, Nursing Spectrum, The Nurse Practitioner,* and *OR Manager,* to name a few. Her writing experience includes a 10-part writing for publication series for *AORN Journal,* research reports, case studies, interviews, clinical articles, and continuing education activities. She has written materials for nurses, physicians, pharmacists, social workers, physical therapists, occupational therapists, dentists, and other healthcare professionals.

Saver has worked with the top publishers as an author, editor, managing editor, and editorial director, including Editorial Director for *American Nurse Journal,* the official journal of the American Nurses Association, and Executive Vice President of Editorial for *Nursing Spectrum.* She was an invited reviewer for the *Publication Manual of the American Psychological Association* (7th ed., 2020). Saver's writing for publication program for nurses has received excellent reviews—and participants have published many articles. She received her master's degree in nursing from The Ohio State University, is an author-in-residence for *Nurse Author & Editor,* serves on the editorial board for *The Maryland Nurse,* and blogs for *American Nurse Journal* at The Writing Mind (https://www.myamericannurse.com/category/the-writing-mind).

About the Contributing Authors

Mary Alexander, MA, RN, CRNI, CAE, FAAN, is Chief Executive Officer Emerita at the Infusion Society (INS). She was named CEO of the INS and the Infusion Nurses Certification Corporation (INCC) in 1997 and served until her retirement in 2023. For 25 years as Editor of the *Journal of Infusion Nursing,* Alexander wrote bimonthly columns and had editorial responsibilities for *INSider,* the bimonthly membership newsletter. She is Editor of *Core Curriculum for Infusion Nursing* (5th ed.) and Editor-in-Chief of the INS textbook *Infusion Nursing: An Evidence-Based Approach.* Alexander's areas of expertise include infusion therapy with an emphasis on patient safety, practitioner competency, and standards development. Her clinical experience spans a variety of practice settings, including home care, alternative sites, and acute care settings.

Nancy J. Brent, JD, MS, RN, is a nurse attorney in private law practice. After practicing and teaching psychiatric nursing for more than 15 years, Brent graduated from Loyola University of Chicago School of Law in 1981. Her private practice is concentrated in professional licensure defense for nurses and other healthcare providers, consultation to nurses and school of nursing faculty, and educational programs in law and nursing practice for nurses and other healthcare groups. She has published extensively in the area of law and nursing practice. Brent is also the author of a legal blog at Nurse.com (https://www.nurse.com/blog/author/nbrent).

Christopher Burton, DPhil, RN, is Professor of Health Services Research, Health Foundation Improvement Science Fellow, Canterbury Christ Church University, Canterbury, Kent, England. Burton is a registered nurse with a special interest in supporting patients affected by stroke and long-term health conditions. As Professor of Health Services Research at Canterbury Christ Church University, he leads a programme of research and scholarship that seeks to close the gap between evidence, policy, and practice. He works with researchers across the globe to develop knowledge of "what works" in implementation and improvement and networks to embed this within educational programmes for nurses and other healthcare professionals.

Marianne Ditomassi, DNP, MBA, RN, NEA-BC, FAAN, is Executive Director of Nursing and Patient Care Services Operations and Magnet® Recognition at Massachusetts General Hospital (MGH). Ditomassi is the Chief of Staff for the Senior Vice President for Patient Care and Chief Nurse, who oversees the operations of nursing, therapy departments, and social services. Ditomassi's key areas of accountability include strategic planning, professional practice environment development and evaluation, recruitment and retention initiatives, business planning, fundraising, and communications. She also is the Magnet Program Director for MGH and coordinated MGH's initial Magnet designation journey in 2003 and subsequent Magnet redesignations in 2008, 2013, 2018, and 2023.

Susan Gennaro, PhD, RN, FAAN, is a Professor in the Connell School of Nursing at Boston College. She is an internationally renowned perinatal clinician and scholar whose research has improved healthcare for childbearing women and their families around the world. She is also the Editor of the *Journal of Nursing Scholarship*, which is read in more than 103 countries and whose mission is to advance knowledge to improve the health of the world's people. Gennaro has been active in supporting that mission by leading an understanding of how best to promote global dissemination of nursing scholarship.

Pamela J. Haylock, PhD, RN, FAAN, is a nurse educator and cancer survivorship consultant. Throughout her career, Haylock has held staff, advanced practice, management, nursing education, and consultation roles and is a past President of the Oncology Nursing Society. She contributes to professional and peer-reviewed literature as an author, editor, and manuscript reviewer, and by serving on professional journals' editorial boards. Her introduction to writing for general audiences was as coauthor of *Women's Cancers: How to Prevent Them, How to Treat Them, How to Beat Them* (with Kerry A. McGinn), followed by *Cancer Doesn't Have to Hurt* (with coauthor Carol P. Curtiss), and as editor and contributor for *Men's Cancers: How to Prevent Them, How to Treat Them, How to Beat Them*. Haylock was a team member and writer for the National Coalition for Cancer Survivorship's award-winning *Cancer Survival Toolbox*—audio instructional programs for survivors and family caregivers. In 2002, Haylock received the Distinguished Alumni Award for Service from the University of Iowa College of Nursing, and in 2008, she received a Distinguished Alumni Award for Service from the University of Iowa. She was inducted as a Fellow of the American Academy of Nursing in 2011.

Lisa Hopp, PhD, RN, FAAN, is Dean Emerita, Nursing, Purdue University Northwest; and Vice Dean, College of Nursing, Rosalind Franklin University of Medicine and Science, Chicago. She is internationally recognized for her work in evidence-based nursing practice. She has trained hundreds of faculty, advanced practice nurses, and library scientists in systematic review methodologies. Hopp is the founding director of the Indiana Center for Evidence Based Nursing, part of a global collaboration of JBI (formerly Joanna Briggs Institute) centers and groups that aim to improve healthcare outcomes through evidence-based healthcare. She continues to serve as a Deputy Director for a JBI Center of Excellence at Rosalind Franklin University of Medicine and Science. She has been an educator for more than 30 years, helping prepare future advanced practice and registered nurses.

Timothy Landers, PhD, RN, APRN-CNP, CIC, FAAN, is a nurse practitioner and infection prevention researcher. His research focuses on practical, evidence-based infection prevention strategies to address the most pressing problems in infectious disease prevention. He has written multiple guidelines on infection prevention using a One Health paradigm. Landers was an Associate Professor at The Ohio State University for 10 years, where he taught in the graduate programs, and has served as the Nurse Scientist at Nationwide Children's Hospital. He was a Fulbright Scholar in Ethiopia from 2017 to 2018. Landers was on the editorial board of the *American Journal of Infection Control*, and his scholarly work has been widely featured in the media and lay press. He has mentored students and nurses in writing and publishing for many years.

Fidelindo Lim, DNP, CCRN, FAAN, is a Clinical Associate Professor in the NYU Rory Meyers College of Nursing at New York University. He has worked as a critical care nurse for 18 years, and concurrently, since 1996, as a nursing faculty member. Lim has published more than 200 articles on an array of topics, including clinical practice, geriatrics, nursing education, LGBTQ+ health, reflective practice, preceptorship, men in nursing, nursing humanities, and Florence Nightingale. *American Nurse Journal*, the official journal of the American Nurses Association, designated him as a Nurse Influencer. Lim is a Fellow of the American Academy of Nursing. He holds a DNP from Northeastern University, a master of arts in nursing education from NYU, and a BSN from Far Eastern University in Manila, Philippines.

Deborah Lindell, DNP, MSN, RN, CNE, ANEF, FAAN, is a Professor in the Frances Payne Bolton School of Nursing at Case Western Reserve University, Cleveland, Ohio. For over 30 years, Lindell has been an educator and administrator in undergraduate and graduate nursing programs. Currently, she coordinates Frances Payne Bolton School of Nursing's schoolwide Curriculum Transformation Initiative. Lindell's clinical background is in community/public health nursing, and her scholarship concerns nursing theory, history, and education. Internationally, she has consulted and taught masters' level courses in Vietnam and China and was a Fulbright Scholar in Kenya from 2021 to 2022. Lindell was instrumental in the development and implementation of the National League for Nursing's Certified Nurse Educator (CNE) Program and served as Chair of the CNE Commission. She is a Fellow in the NLN's Academy of Nursing Education and in the American Academy of Nursing.

Kayla Little, MSN, APRN, AGCNS-BC, PCCN, is a Clinical Nurse Specialist who supports the cardiovascular medicine, heart and lung transplant, and vascular surgery stepdown nursing units within the Heart, Vascular, and Thoracic Institute at the Cleveland Clinic Main Campus. She earned a BSN from Walsh University and an MSN from Kent State University. Little has been published in *Critical Care Nurse Journal, American Nurse Journal,* and *Clinical Nurse Specialist Journal*. She was an invited reviewer for the *AACN Procedure Manual for Progressive and Critical Care* (8th ed., 2023) and a contributor to *Foundations of Clinical Nurse Specialist Practice* (4th ed.). Little was the recipient of the Rising Star Clinical Nurse Specialist of the Year Award in 2022 from the National Association of Clinical Nurse Specialists. Her passion for mentoring nurses and future Clinical Nurse Specialists led her to be the recipient of the Barbara Donaho Distinguished Leadership in Learning Award from Kent State University in 2023. Little values lifelong learning and professional citizenship. She is a column editor for the *Clinical Nurse Specialist Journal* and serves on the board of directors for the National Association of Clinical Nurse Specialists.

Tina M. Marrelli, MSN, MA, RN, FAAN, is President of Marrelli and Associates Inc., a consulting and publishing firm. She is the author of 13 best-selling and award-winning healthcare books, including *Handbook of Home Health Standards: Quality, Documentation, and Reimbursement* (6th ed.); *Nurse Manager's Survival Guide* (4th ed.); *Hospice & Palliative Care Handbook* (4th ed.); *Home Health Aide: Guidelines for Care – Instructor Manual* (3rd ed.); and *A Guide for Caregiving: What's Next? Planning for Safety, Quality, and Compassionate Care for Your Loved One and Yourself*. Marrelli has also authored apps to assist with care planning. She received her BSN degree from Duke University and has master's degrees in health administration and in nursing. Marrelli has worked at CMS on Medicare home care and hospice Part A policy and operations, been the editor of three peer-reviewed publications, and practiced as a visiting nurse and manager in home care and hospice.

Cheryl L. Mee, MSN, MBA, RN, FAAN, leads the editorial team for *American Nurse Journal*, the official journal of the American Nurses Association. She is an Adjunct Instructor at Frances Payne Bolton School of Nursing, Case Western Reserve University, Cleveland, Ohio, working with doctor of nursing practice students. Her past roles include Editor-in-Chief for *Nursing* and Vice President of Nursing and Health Professions Journals at Elsevier. Mee has written over 130 articles addressing the current, persistent, challenging problems confronting nurses delivering direct patient care. She is on the board of Americans for Native Americans, where she has worked to provide scholarships, NCLEX fees, and varied clinical experiences for Native American nursing students, as well as planning annual health screening programs assessing hundreds of Navajo elementary school children.

Patricia Gonce Morton, PhD, RN, ACNP-BC, FAAN, is Dean Emeritus, University of Utah College of Nursing, where she served as Dean and Professor and held the Louis Peery Endowed Presidential Chair. Before her deanship, Morton served in various administrative positions at the University of Maryland School of Nursing. An educator and scholar who is known for her work in critical care nursing and nursing education, Morton has written multiple editions of three textbooks, numerous book chapters, and over 60 journal articles. She has served on the editorial board of eight nursing journals and for seven years was the Editor of the journal *AACN Clinical Issues: Advanced Practice in Acute and Critical Care*, sponsored by the American Association of Critical-Care Nurses. Currently, Morton is Editor of the *Journal of Professional Nursing*, sponsored by the American Association of Colleges of Nursing. She also is an author-in-residence for *Nurse Author & Editor*. In recognition of her contributions to nursing and healthcare, Morton was inducted as a Fellow in the American Academy of Nursing in 1999.

Cindy L. Munro, PhD, RN, ANP-BC, FAAN, FAANP, is Dean and Professor at the University of Miami School of Nursing and Health Studies in Coral Gables, Florida. She has served as Coeditor of *American Journal of Critical Care* for more than 10 years. An experienced peer reviewer, she has published more than 200 articles and presented at many national and international conferences. Munro received a diploma from York Hospital School of Nursing, a BSN from Millersville University of Pennsylvania, and an MSN from the University of Delaware. She earned her

PhD in nursing and microbiology and immunology at Virginia Commonwealth University. Her NIH-funded research on oral care in critically ill adults has had an important effect on clinical practice. In 2016, Sigma Theta Tau International Honor Society of Nursing inducted Munro into its International Nurse Researcher Hall of Fame. She is an American Academy of Nursing Edge Runner.

Sandra M. Nettina, MSN, ANP-BC, is owner and founder of Prime Care House Calls in West Friendship, Maryland, and Editor of *The Lippincott Manual of Nursing Practice*. She attended the Sisters of Charity Hospital School of Nursing in Buffalo, New York; completed a bachelor's degree at Marymount College of Virginia; and received her MSN from the University of Pennsylvania, Philadelphia. As an adult nurse practitioner, Nettina's multidimensional career includes founding a nurse practitioner independent-house-calls practice; writing, editing, and reviewing for several publishing companies; providing leadership in her state nurse practitioner association; and volunteering for several health-related organizations.

Leslie H. Nicoll, PhD, MBA, RN, FAAN, is principal and owner of Maine Desk LLC and Editor-in-Chief of *CIN: Computers, Informatics, Nursing*. Nicoll has more than 43 years of experience in nursing and healthcare and has worked in clinical practice, research, and academia. She founded her own business, Maine Desk LLC, in 2001. Nicoll has been the Editor-in-Chief of *CIN: Computers, Informatics, Nursing* since 1995 and was the Editor-in-Chief of *Nurse Author & Editor* from 2014 to 2022. She served as Editor-in-Chief of *The Journal of Hospice and Palliative Nursing* for eight years (2001–2009). Nicoll is the author of more than 130 published professional articles, book chapters, and books, including *Writing in the Digital Age: Savvy Publishing for Healthcare Professionals*, coauthored with Peggy L. Chinn, and *The Editor's Handbook* (3rd ed.). She was the founding editor of *Perspectives on Nursing Theory*. In the non-nursing literature, she is the author of four "For Dummies" books, including *Kindle Paperwhite For Dummies*. Nicoll enjoys helping nurses and other healthcare professionals achieve their publication goals. She has done this through one-on-one support in her business as well as leading writing workshops for the National League for Nursing, a consortium of universities in Switzerland, and various colleges and schools of nursing in the United States. Nicoll became a Fellow in the American Academy of Nursing in 2014. She is active in INANE: The International Academy of Nursing Editors and received their leadership award for excellence in editorial publication in 2015.

Susanne J. Pavlovich-Danis, MSN, RN, APRN-C, CDCES, is Director of Clinical Continuing Education at TeamHealth Institute in Knoxville, Tennessee. She has 42 years of experience in nursing and healthcare in diverse clinical, academic, and consultant-based settings. As Director of Clinical Continuing Education at TeamHealth Institute, she currently oversees the Joint Accreditation for Interprofessional Continuing Education that includes the Accreditation Council for Continuing Medical Education (ACCME), the Accreditation Council for Pharmacy Education (ACPE), and the American Nurses Credentialing Center (ANCC). She serves in the chief editorial capacity for more than 600 annual continuing education activities nationwide for a multidisciplinary audience. She also maintains a private adult primary care practice in Plantation, Florida, and is a certified diabetes care and education specialist (CDCES). Pavlovich-Danis is an approved continuing nursing education provider for the Florida Board of Nursing. She has been published in the nursing literature more than 500 times since 1996 and lectured nationally and internationally.

Demetrius J. Porche, DNS, PhD, PCC, ANEF, FACHE, FAANP, FAAN, is Dean and Professor at the Louisiana State University Health Sciences Center School of Nursing in New Orleans. Porche is Chief Editor of the *American Journal of Men's Health* and was Associate Editor of the *Journal of the Association of Nurses in AIDS* for 10 years. He is a Virginia Henderson Fellow of Sigma Theta Tau International and a Society of Luther Christman Fellow for Contributions to Nursing by Men. He is also a Fellow in the National League for Nursing Nurse Educator Academy, the American Academy of Nursing, and the American Academy of Nurse Practitioners. He is board-certified in healthcare by the American College of Healthcare Executives. Porche is author of *Health Policy: Application for Nurses and Other Health Care Professionals* (2nd ed.) and *Epidemiology for the Advanced Practice Nurse: A Population Health Approach*. He has published many articles in peer-reviewed journals.

Jo Rycroft-Malone, OBE, PhD, MSc, BSc (Hons), RN, is Distinguished Professor, Executive Dean of Health & Medicine at Lancaster University, England. She has a nursing background and is a health services researcher who studies the processes and outcomes of evidence-informed service delivery in different health service contexts across the globe. Rycroft-Malone is also the Director of the National Institute for Health Research (NIHR) Health Services & Delivery Research Programme, which funds research to generate evidence to improve the quality, accessibility, and organisation of health and care services in the United Kingdom. She was the inaugural Editor of *Worldviews on Evidence-Based Nursing.*

Nadine Salmon, MSN, RN, NPD-BC, IBCLC, is a Curriculum Designer in the Acute Vertical at Relias, a leading provider of online continuing education for healthcare, senior care, and disability professionals. Salmon obtained her BSN in South Africa more than 30 years ago and has worked as an RN in South Africa, England, and the United States in various settings, including labor and delivery, postpartum, home health, and adult surgical units. She has an MSN with an emphasis in leadership in healthcare systems from Grand Canyon University. Salmon has served as an appraiser for the American Nurses Credentialing Center, is certified in nursing professional development, and is an international board-certified lactation consultant. She has been involved in creating nursing continuing education content and certification review courses for more than 20 years, and enjoys collaborating with subject matter expert writers, instructional designers, and quality assurance and education technicians in developing continuing education courses for nurses, physicians, and allied health professionals.

Patricia Dwyer Schull, MSN, BS, is President of MedVantage Publishing LLC. She has more than 30 years' experience in medical and nursing publishing. She has published, written, and edited many nursing journals, books, websites, and other healthcare publications. Her company offers publishing solutions that support and educate healthcare professionals, including developing and launching the award-winning publications *Nursing Spectrum* and *McGraw Hill Nurses Drug Handbook, American Nurse Journal* (official journal of the American Nurses Association), and *Journal of Nursing Regulation* (official journal of the National Council of State Boards of Nursing). Previously, Schull held executive management positions with Reed Elsevier (Springhouse Corporation) and Wolters Kluwer (Lippincott, Williams & Wilkins), where she was responsible for leading editorial, sales, marketing, and new product development of nursing publications. Before entering the publishing industry, she practiced as a registered nurse in direct patient care, hospital management, and staff education.

Stephanie J. Schulte, MLIS, is Professor, Assistant Vice President, Health Sciences, and Director, Health Sciences Library at The Ohio State University. She is a library director and faculty health sciences librarian who specializes in teaching students, faculty, and staff advanced skills to support evidence-based practice and research endeavors. Her research work currently focuses on librarians who work directly with basic or life scientists. Schulte teaches within the medical school curriculum as well as the biomedical sciences undergraduate program at The Ohio State University and leads a team of research and education librarians serving five health sciences colleges and a large academic medical center. She has been active in university governance, the Medical Library Association, and the Midwest Chapter of the Medical Library Association.

Rose O. Sherman, EdD, RN, NEA-BC, FAAN, is Emeritus Professor, Christine E. Lynn College of Nursing at Florida Atlantic University, and a faculty member of the Marian K. Shaughnessy Nursing Leadership Academy at Case Western Reserve University. Before becoming a faculty member, Sherman was a nurse leader with the Department of Veterans Affairs for 25 years. She edits a popular leadership blog (www.emergingrnleader.com) and is Editor-in-Chief of *Nurse Leader,* the official journal of the American Organization for Nursing Leadership. Sherman has extensive experience with both podium and poster presentations at professional conferences. She has also served as an abstract reviewer for numerous professional conferences at the state and national levels. Sherman is a Gallup-certified strengths coach and author of the books *The Nurse Leader Coach: Become the Boss No One Wants to Leave, The Nuts and Bolts of Nursing Leadership: Your Toolkit for Success,* and *A Team Approach to Nursing Care Delivery: Tactics for Working Better Together.*

Lorraine Steefel, DNP, RN, CTN-A, is Director of LTS Writing/Mentoring & Editorial Services for RNs and students. She is a professional writer and writing consultant who has presented webinars and writing for publication workshops to nurses across the country. Her experience includes teaching academic writing to all levels of nursing students, especially mentoring DNP students who are writing their capstone project papers and turning them into published articles. Steefel has been widely published in peer-reviewed journals, nursing magazines, and on websites. She served as the American Nurses Association representative to the Centers for Disease Control and Prevention (CDC) Work Group to update the CDC website on ME/CFS (myalgic encephalomyelitis/chronic fatigue syndrome). Her book *What Nurses Know…Chronic Fatigue Syndrome* was published by Demos Publishers in New York. Steefel is a member of the Research Roadmap for ME/CFS for the National Institutes of Health, which is creating webinars about the illness to identify research priorities to move the field forward. Steefel is the Associate Editor for Peer Review for *Creative Nursing: A Journal of Values, Issues, Experience & Collaboration*, published by Sage, and an editorial board member of the *Journal of Nursing Practice, Applications and Reviews of Research* (JNPARR), the official journal of the Philippine Nurses Association of America. She is a mentor for the Thomas Edison State University School of Nursing online nursing program.

Additional Book Resources

To download a sample chapter and other free book resources, visit the Sigma Repository at https://sigma.nursingrepository.org/handle/10755/23681 or scan the QR code below.

Facilitator Guide and Student Workbook Available

A facilitator guide and student workbook are available for purchase from Sigma Marketplace (SigmaMarketplace.org) and from other online retailers. Simply search for this book title with added keywords of "facilitator guide" or "student workbook" to purchase one or both. You can also email our Marketplace team for bulk orders at solutions@sigmamarketplace.org.

Special Note to Readers

Here at Sigma, we realize that language is constantly evolving. The meaning of a word often changes over time, some words become obsolete, and some terms that were once acceptable may become controversial or even offensive, depending on the context or circumstances. We have made every effort to make language choices that are inclusive and not offensive. Should you identify words in this book that you believe negatively impact a group or groups of people, please reach out to us at Publications@SigmaNursing.org.

Table of Contents

About the Editor and Lead Author vii
About the Contributing Authors vii
Foreword xv
Introduction xvii

Part I: A Primer on Writing and Publishing . . . 1

1. Anatomy of Writing 3
   Cynthia Saver

2. Finding, Refining, and Defining a Topic . . 25
   Patricia Dwyer Schull and Cynthia Saver

3. How to Select and Query a Publication . . 37
   Cynthia Saver

4. Finding and Documenting Sources 57
   Leslie H. Nicoll

5. Organizing the Article 73
   Kayla Little and Mary Alexander

6. Writing Skills Lab 89
   Cynthia Saver

7. All About Graphics 103
   Susanne J. Pavlovich-Danis

8. Submissions and Revisions 121
   Patricia Gonce Morton and Tina M. Marrelli

9. Writing a Peer Review 135
   Cindy L. Munro

10. Publishing for Global Authors 145
    Susan Gennaro

11. Legal and Ethical Issues 155
    Nancy J. Brent

12. Promoting Your Work 171
    Timothy Landers and Stephanie J. Schulte

Part II: Tips for Writing Different Types of Articles 185

13. Writing the Clinical Article 187
    Cheryl L. Mee and Fidelindo Lim

14. Writing the Research Report 199
    Patricia Gonce Morton

15. Writing the Review Article 215
    Lisa Hopp

16. Reporting the Quality Improvement or Evidence-Based Practice Project . . . 231
    Jo Rycroft-Malone and Christopher Burton

17. Writing for Presentations 241
    Rose O. Sherman

18. From Student Project or Dissertation to Publication 255
    Deborah Lindell and Lorraine Steefel

19. Writing a Continuing Professional Development Activity 267
    Nadine Salmon

20. Writing the Nursing Narrative 283
    Marianne Ditomassi

21. Think Outside the Journal: Alternative Publication Options 297
    Demetrius J. Porche

22. Writing a Book or Book Chapter 307
    Sandra M. Nettina

23. Writing for a General Audience 319
    Pamela J. Haylock

Part III: Appendices 331

A. Tips for Editing Checklist 333
B. Proofing Checklist 335
C. Publishing Terminology 337
D. Guidelines for Reporting Results 341
E. Statistical Abbreviations 345
F. What Editors and Writers Want 347
G. Publishing Advice From Editors 349

Index 353

Foreword

"I attribute my success to this—I never gave or took an excuse."
–Florence Nightingale

Most nurses know Florence Nightingale as the founder of "modern" nursing. She also was a scholar who wrote extensively about nursing, public health, health policy, women's issues, spirituality, and what we now understand to be health statistics. For her time, she was an exceedingly well-educated woman with a wide range of interests in human health and well-being, which remain the foundational foci of nursing science. Although her most well-known publication was *Notes on Nursing* (1859), she wrote more than 150 books, pamphlets, and essays. She wrote because she had something about which she was passionate and about which she thought others should know. These are the same reasons most of us write. Unlike us, however, Ms. Nightingale did her writing without a computer, without an online library, without any sort of easy access to extant writing about a particular topic, and, to our knowledge, without any particular instruction about how to write for publication.

Fortunately, we have help with publication writing in this fifth edition of *Anatomy of Writing for Publication for Nurses*. Edited by Cynthia Saver, an award-winning author and highly respected writing authority, the book includes chapters by some of nursing's most prolific and distinguished authors and editors. *Anatomy* covers a wide variety of topics associated with writing for publication, from determining a topic and finding references to writing the manuscript and revising as needed.

This comprehensive book contains chapters for specific types of papers—research reports, review articles, quality improvement projects, book chapters, and more. Readers will also learn how to write a peer review (a skill set equally important for writing good articles) and about legal and ethical issues in writing. This book benefits both newer authors (e.g., one chapter describes how to publish a school project) and more seasoned authors who want to refine their writing (e.g., one chapter provides detailed information on how to incorporate graphics and tables). There is also help for authors for whom English is not their primary language. *Anatomy*'s scope extends to after publication with a chapter on how to promote your published work—something that authors may overlook.

In keeping with publishing trends, you'll find information about using artificial intelligence (AI) software for writing. AI is a relatively new topic for most scholarly writers, and the AI landscape is ever-changing. This subject, and other emerging subjects, are nicely incorporated into the book's chapters.

Five years into my editor position at *Nursing Research*, I have read many papers (~3,000). It is a pleasure to read a well-written research report or research review and quite gratifying to see those papers through to publication. It is not so pleasurable to review papers that lack focus, are poorly written or referenced, or fail to follow journal guidelines. *Anatomy* will not help authors whose scientific premise or approach is weak. It will not help those who have not given due diligence to the work about which they are writing. However, *Anatomy* will help those authors who have quality work to report yet lack the specific skills or confidence to produce a publishable document. In fact, this very useful book will provide a handy reference for almost all writers.

Like Ms. Nightingale, many of us are passionate about our work. We have important ideas, research findings, discoveries, care improvements, or innovations that we need to communicate. The guidance provided in *Anatomy of Writing for Publication for Nurses* will help you transform your important ideas into publishable documents. Using the book will help you learn to write, just as prior editions have helped many other novice and experienced writers develop the skills they need to begin and continue writing. For those who want to improve their writing, this new edition will meet your needs.

–Rita Pickler, PhD, RN, FAAN
Editor, *Nursing Research*
The FloAnn Sours Easton Professor
of Child and Adolescent Health
Martha S. Pitzer Center for Women,
Children & Youth
The Ohio State University College of Nursing
Columbus, Ohio

Introduction

"I admire anybody who has the guts to write anything at all."
–E.B. White

Writing well is not the result of luck or innate talent. Writing is a skill you can learn, just as you learned nursing skills such as venipuncture and suctioning.

However, nurses often find it challenging to write. After all, as Margaret McClure says in *Words of Wisdom From Pivotal Nurse Leaders*, "One of nursing's biggest handicaps is that we are in a field where your basic practice requires that you never write in complete sentences" (Houser & Player, 2008, p. 70). *Anatomy of Writing for Publication for Nurses*, Fifth Edition, is designed to help you bridge the gap between incomplete sentences and a published manuscript. The book's contributors include the best and the brightest from publishing today. Many of the contributors have experience as editors of nursing journals, where their role is to decide which articles to accept for publication. These decision-makers share important insights that will enhance the likelihood your manuscript is accepted for publication.

You also can draw a wealth of knowledge from the many years of writing experience that the contributors bring to this book. These authors have a long history of success in having their work published; the important tips they share will set you on track to seeing your own work published.

Some might wonder why a new edition is needed, thinking that little changes in writing and publishing from year to year. Not true. Like any field, writing and publishing evolve over time. A simple example is artificial intelligence (AI). AI wasn't on most writers' and publishers' radars when the previous edition of this book was published in 2021 (or if it was, it was a tiny blip). Now the use (and misuse) of AI looms large, and information about its role is integrated into this new edition. (However, keep in mind that AI is developing at a rapid pace, so you'll want to keep alert for publishing trends in this area.)

Other developments include the increasing use of video and graphical abstracts, which enhance dissemination of your work, and the greater use of transformative agreements between publishers and consortia (discussed in Chapter 3), which also can lead to wider dissemination of your work.

Terminology evolves as well. For instance, the new term for continuing education for nurses is *nursing continuing professional development*, the preferred term for double-blind review is now *double-anonymous*, and *text recycling*, which addresses when you can reuse text without plagiarizing, is being used more commonly. This new edition also has more information on bias-free language, many new examples, and updated references.

How to Use This Book

Anatomy of Writing for Publication for Nurses is divided into two parts, both of which have been updated for this edition to include new topics and to provide further guidance.

Part I, "A Primer on Writing and Publishing," describes the basics of publishing, from generating a great idea and writing the article to revising your manuscript and sharing your work. This section is packed with information on how to bolster the chance that your manuscript will be accepted for publication.

Topics include how to query a journal; working with a writing team; the role of accountability partners; writing and submitting the manuscript; legal and ethical issues; and effective use of tables, figures, graphs, illustrations, and photos. If English is your second language, don't miss the chapter for global authors. Part I also includes a chapter on peer review, a great way to improve your own writing skills. Even if you don't plan to be a peer reviewer, understanding the reviewer's perspective will help you anticipate what comments reviewers might have about your manuscript.

Part I has been revised to include new topics and more information about preprints, graphical (or visual) abstracts, and plain language summaries. You'll also learn more about predatory and low-quality journals and how to avoid both. Be sure to read the chapter on promoting your work—authors often neglect this important step.

By the time you complete Part I, you'll have a solid understanding of the entire publishing process.

Part II, "Tips for Writing Different Types of Articles," is where you can apply what you learned in Part I. Each chapter takes you through writing a particular type of manuscript or article, including clinical articles, research reports, books, personal narratives, continuing education content, and writing for consumers. You can dip into the relevant chapter in Part II depending on your writing goals.

Part II has been revised to include more information on writing literature reviews and how to convert your student project or dissertation into an article. It also features two chapters that will help you craft an effective article based on your study. The first focuses on the research report and covers quantitative, qualitative, and mixed-methods studies. The second focuses on writing the review article, including systematic, scoping, and integrative reviews. You'll also find a chapter guiding you in how to write an article based on your quality improvement or evidence-based practice project.

In the back of the book, you'll find a wealth of resources, including checklists, a list of reporting guidelines that can help in organizing your article, a guide to publishing terminology, common statistical abbreviations, and useful advice from editors in the field.

I've given a snapshot of some of the changes from the previous edition, but you should also know that each chapter has been revised by the authors to ensure it conveys the best possible information.

Writing Can Be Fun

The contributors and I have forgone the traditional textbook style of writing for something that we hope is livelier and more approachable. This doesn't mean we don't take writing seriously. We do. Writing is a core nursing responsibility, right up there with being a patient advocate.

Our goal is to show you that even though writing effectively takes work, it is within every nurse's reach to do so—and you can have some fun while doing it.

Special Elements in This Book

In each chapter of *Anatomy of Writing for Publication for Nurses*, Fifth Edition, you'll find these features:

- **Opening quotes:** Quotes at the start of each chapter provide pithy words of wisdom related to the craft of writing.

- **What You'll Learn in This Chapter:** This provides an overview of what's to come.

- **Q&A sidebars:** Here you'll find answers to some common questions related to the chapter's topic.

- **Confidence Booster:** Lack of confidence can hold nurses back from sharing their wealth of knowledge. These special sections are designed to inspire you and to encourage you to break down that barrier.

- **Write Now!:** These exercises at the end of each chapter help you apply what you have learned.

A Call to Action

Remember: The best way to become a better writer is to write! Like any other skill, practice is a key component to success. I hope this book inspires you to take on writing as a lifetime practice.

I also hope you use *Anatomy of Writing for Publication for Nurses*, Fifth Edition, as a guide to getting your work published. Remember: You don't need any particular degree or certification to write—just the desire to share what you know or have experienced. In fact, we have an obligation to share our knowledge with other nurses, other healthcare professionals, and the public; in essence, we have a duty to disseminate.

Reference

Houser, B. P., & Player, K. N. (2008). *Words of wisdom from pivotal nurse leaders*. Sigma Theta Tau International.

Part I
A Primer on Writing and Publishing

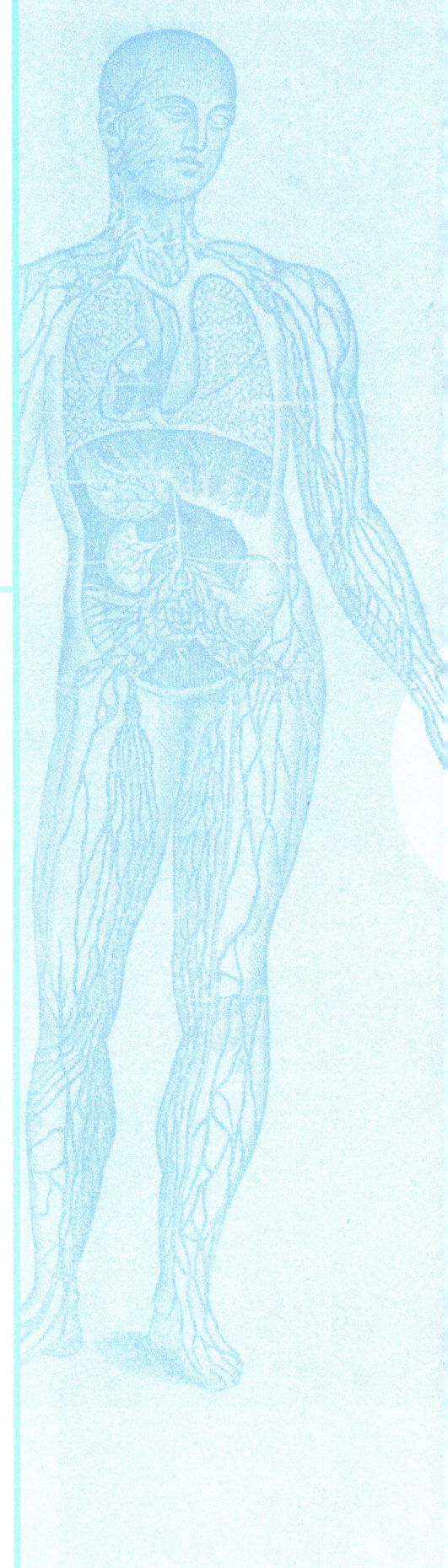

1	Anatomy of Writing	3
2	Finding, Refining, and Defining a Topic	25
3	How to Select and Query a Publication	37
4	Finding and Documenting Sources	57
5	Organizing the Article	73
6	Writing Skills Lab	89
7	All About Graphics	103
8	Submissions and Revisions	121
9	Writing a Peer Review	135
10	Publishing for Global Authors	145
11	Legal and Ethical Issues	155
12	Promoting Your Work	171

Anatomy of Writing

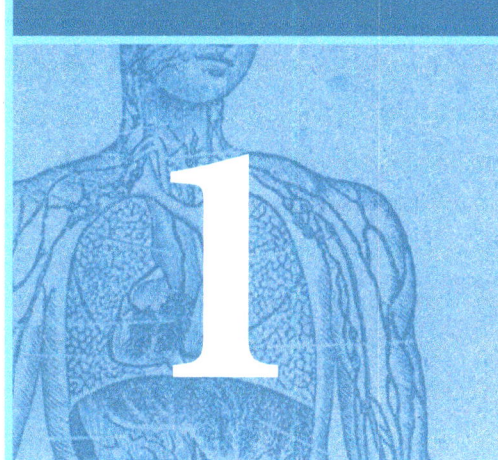

−Cynthia Saver, MS, RN

*"When asked, 'How do you write?'
I invariably answer, 'One word at a time.'"*
–Stephen King

WHAT YOU'LL LEARN IN THIS CHAPTER

- Writing something can be compared with anatomy: If you passed your anatomy course in nursing school, you can write for publication.

- Like nursing, publishing has a specific process that you can follow.

- Collaboration is just as important with your writing and publishing teams as it is with a healthcare team.

Writing is a skill. Like other nursing skills—such as starting an IV, suctioning a patient, or analyzing an ECG strip—writing can be learned. That doesn't mean you will necessarily become the next Toni Morrison or Malcolm Gladwell or be able to surpass your favorite nurse author, but you can become confident enough in your writing to achieve a variety of goals, from publishing your first journal article to contributing to your organization's newsletter.

Of course, nurses have different levels of expertise for different skills. For example, we learn how to insert an IV in nursing school, and for many of us, this becomes a daily part of our routine. However, you likely know of at least one nurse who is particularly adept at IV insertion. When you have a difficult "stick," you can rely on their advanced expertise, correct?

Writing can be the same way. Some might be much better at it than others, but every nurse can learn this basic skill. Learning how to write is your first step in becoming a published author. You also need to learn the ropes about how publishing works. This chapter gives you an overview of the writing, editing, and publishing process. Subsequent chapters give you many more details, but by the end of this chapter, the big picture of writing for publication should be in view.

Why Write?

Many articles have been written about why nurses should write. Although the most basic reason is to disseminate information, others find that writing can help them with job advancement, academic work, and sharing what works in practice. For example, a single nurse speaking in front of an audience about the latest treatment for sepsis might reach, at best, a few hundred nurses. But after your work is published as a journal article, a chapter in a book, a magazine article, or even a newsletter write-up, your contribution is much more widely available, particularly if your published piece is indexed in one of the large databases that researchers and clinicians search for information.

Writing gives you the opportunity to:

- Share information (e.g., an inspirational experience with a patient)
- Improve patient care (e.g., a program for reducing pressure injuries that improves outcomes)
- Promote yourself (e.g., tenure track for faculty, professional development ladder, getting your name known so you can speak at national meetings)
- Enhance your knowledge (e.g., a review article on patient handoff techniques that helps you explore a topic in-depth)
- Advance the profession (e.g., publishing in other disciplines' journals or online, coauthorship with people outside nursing, an innovative way of defining nursing outcomes)

As nurses we have a duty to disseminate—a duty embedded in the "Code for Ethics for Nurses With Interpretive Statements" (American Nurses Association [ANA], 2015). For instance, Provision 7.1 includes the statement: "All nurses must participate in the advancement of the profession through knowledge development, evaluation, *dissemination* [italics added], and application to practice" (p. 27).

We should take that duty just as seriously as we take our other responsibilities as nurses, from caring for patients to communicating with families and other healthcare professionals. If you want to help others, you need to write and share your knowledge. As Susan Gennaro, editor of the *Journal of Nursing Scholarship*, writes,

> I write because I hope that somewhere, someone is helped by a thought that I have had. I believe that I am only doing half a job if I do a project, conduct a study, or develop an insight if I don't communicate it to others in writing. (Gennaro, 2016b, p. 117)

Gennaro notes that dissemination has an ethical component when it comes to research (Gennaro, 2020). Researchers frequently tell participants that being part of a study will create knowledge that will help others. If you don't share your results, then you are not fulfilling that promise. The "Code of Ethics" weighs in on this too, with the statement: "Dissemination of research findings, regardless of results, is an essential part of respect for the participants" (ANA, 2015, p. 27). Now that you understand the importance of writing, you're ready to learn more about how to write and get published.

Anatomy of Writing

Like many skills that fall outside our comfort zone, writing can be intimidating. Coaches, mentors, and editors have heard it all:

- "I want to write, but I'm a terrible writer!"
- "I don't know where to start!"
- "I could never finish an article, a paper, or a book!"

None of these are true. If you passed anatomy and physiology in nursing school, you can write for publication. In fact, grounding writing in an anatomy analogy makes it easier to understand (see Figure 1.1).

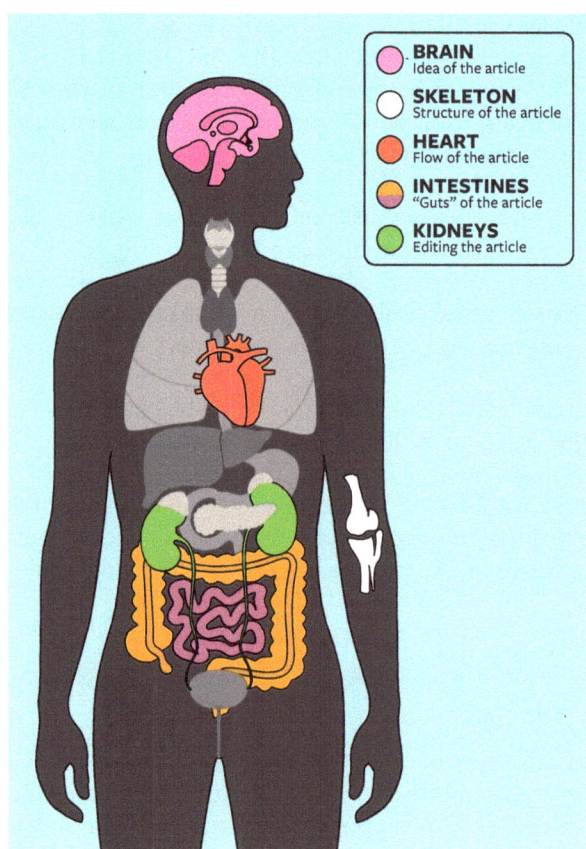

FIGURE 1.1 Think about writing in terms of parts of the body.

As you read this section, keep in mind that these basic principles are the same whether you're writing for online or in print (or both) or whether you're writing anything from a blog post to a book.

Brain

The brain is the idea for the article. (In this discussion, an "article" can include anything from a blog post to a book chapter.) Ideas are all around you. Perhaps the most challenging part for you is to take a broad idea (say, reducing readmissions) and narrow it down (how to reduce readmissions in newly diagnosed patients with diabetes).

Heart

The heart pumps the blood through the body, maintaining a constant flow. Like the heart, your article must have a flow to it so that the reader can easily read it. Remember that you never want to make the reader work to understand your message.

Flow is how your article moves from one point to the next: how your article is organized and how you lead your reader to your conclusion through a flow of information such as how to manage the patient receiving negative pressure wound therapy. Or, how you move your reader through your idea, opinion, column, or even heart-wrenching story. Different kinds of articles will have different types of flow; here are some examples:

- **Disease process** provides an overview of a disease. You likely remember this from nursing school: incidence, pathophysiology, assessment, diagnosis, treatment, and nursing care.
- **How-to articles** are well suited to quality improvement projects or clinical or career tips. For example, the authors of one article described how nurses can keep meetings productive (Shellenbarger & Chicca, 2020), and a team of nurses wrote about how to assess patients who have an altered level of consciousness (Hill et al., 2023).
- **Chronology articles** present information in a time-based format. A good example is preoperative, intraoperative, and postoperative care.
- **Case studies** are just what they sound like—clear descriptions of a patient's presentation, assessment, diagnosis, treatment, nursing care, and outcomes. A unique patient might present you the opportunity to write about an unusual experience, or you can use a case study as an example within a larger article.

You can incorporate one or more of these techniques into your article. For example, if you are writing an article on the latest surgical technique for a general nursing journal such as *Nursing* or *American Nurse Journal*, you might start with a case study to draw the reader in and then move to a chronological approach: preoperative, intraoperative, and postoperative care.

Skeleton

The skeleton, along with ligaments, muscle, and tendons, holds your body together. Your skeleton is the basic structure that applies to nearly every article—a beginning, a middle, and an end. This basic structure forms the bones of an *outline*, and it's an essential part of the writing process. As Silvia (2007, p. 79) notes, "People who write a lot outline a lot."

Just like you learned your skeletal anatomy, your outline will start out with the basics, becoming more complicated as you flesh out (no pun intended) your work. The beginning, middle, and end are critical to communicating your points to your audience.

The *beginning*, or introduction, sets the tone of the article, lets your reader know what is coming, and conveys why the information to follow is important. Editors in newspapers and magazines would call it a *lede*, and it's that opening line, image, or paragraph that sets a compelling scene. This is your chance to grab readers and draw them into your topic or story. Consider the first lines from a few notable books that you will probably recognize:

I am the invisible man.
–*Invisible Man* by Ralph Ellison (1995)

124 was spiteful.
–*Beloved* by Toni Morrison (2006)

Each of these opening lines draws in the reader, giving the promise of interesting things to come. You might think that you can't get the same impact from the beginning of a nonfiction article, but consider these first two sentences from "The Body's Most Embarrassing Organ is an Evolutionary Marvel," by Katherine J. Wu (2021):

To peer into the soul of a sea cucumber, don't look to its face; it doesn't have one. Gently turn that blobby body around, and gaze deep into its marvelous, multifunctional anus.

First sentences in healthcare publications can deliver startling information that draws the reader in, as is the case with these examples:

> Studies of clinical alarms have indicated that the vast majority are false (Nguyen et al., 2020, p. 15).

> Despite the well-known benefits of physical activity for older adults during hospitalization, it has repeatedly been found that they spend at least 80% of their acute care stay in bed (Resnick et al., 2023, p. 265).

Depending on the tone of your target publication and your audience, you can be creative with your beginning. Look at this example from an article on the role of nurses in firearm safety, published in *American Nurse Journal* (Lee et al., 2023):

> Theoretical debates about gun violence disappear within the realities of practice: the emergency department (ED) nurse supporting a family who's lost a loved one to suicide, the surgical team nurse collaborating to mend the violent impact of bullet wounds on the body, the school nurse grieving after a mass school shooting. Rising incidents of gun violence, including mass-casualty events across the country—some in healthcare settings—create cause for alarm and intensify the need to address firearm safety. (p. 12)

If the publication you are writing for is more scholarly in tone, you can still have strong beginnings, such as the start of this article on testing an evidence-based practice survey (Crawford et al., 2020), which was published in *Worldviews on Evidence-Based Nursing*:

> Consumers of 21st century health care expect that the care they receive is informed by evidence from scientific findings. Evidence-based practices (EBP) replace nonscientific, ritual laden, and traditionalistic practices with those that are based on the best available evidence ... (p. 118)

Think about what impressed you most about your topic, and keep in mind that you might have "buried" the lede after the first few paragraphs. Often authors need a "warm up" period before they get to the crux of the article. You might find you can delete these early paragraphs. Early on in your manuscript, include what the article will be about and why it's important for the reader to know the information.

The *middle*, or body, is the meat of the article. Stick to the topic at hand. Depending on what you're writing about, use one or more of the flow techniques listed earlier in this chapter. You can use paragraphs and subheads to keep yourself organized, breaking text into smaller pieces as necessary.

The Basics of IMRAD

The *IMRAD* (Introduction, Methods, Results, and Discussion) format is an example of an article structure (Gastel & Day, 2022; JAMA Network Editors, 2020; Silvia, 2015, 2019). It's typically used to present quantitative research, such as a research study comparing screening tools for delirium.

- **Introduction:** Why did you start? This section lets readers know why you did the research. It should include the importance of the topic, the research question(s), and why you approached the topic the way you did.

- **Methods:** What did you do? You should include the research protocol, patient or sample selection, interventions, and data analysis.

- **Results:** What did you find? This includes your findings with statistical details. Stick to the facts, with no discussion, and organize it from the most to the least important results.

- **Discussion:** What do the results mean? Include the answer to the research question(s), the supporting evidence, and the implications of the results. In essence, state the results within the context of your study and within the broader body of knowledge. It's here that you address what's important for the reader to take away from the study, the study limitations, and what additional research you recommend.

Q *How can I decide what structure will fit my article best?*

A Think about the publication you would like to submit to and review past articles to gain a sense of the types of structure used for different topics. In addition, consider the nature of the publication: A blog post will have a different structure than a journal article or even an article for a newsletter or nursing magazine.

The publication style will dictate some of your middle structure. Some magazines want small sections with other small, related sections—*sidebars* or *marginalia*—broken out. A book chapter might call for longer sections, more in-depth discussion of your topic, and fewer subheadings. Journal articles frequently use sidebars (along with tables, charts, and figures), to support text. For example, an article on enteral feeding complications might have a sidebar on how to avoid tubing misconnections.

The *end*, or conclusion, of the article is the last opportunity you have to make your point with the reader. Depending on the style of article, it might be a simple conclusion or summary of your research, or you could ask your readers to take a stand. To help write the conclusion, ask yourself: What is the most important idea or message that I want the reader to take away from what I wrote? If your article is reporting results of a study, be sure your conclusions relate to what you found in your study instead of generalizing beyond your findings (Gennaro, 2016a). Do not introduce new information.

The ending is just as important as the beginning when it comes to structure. Examples of endings include:

- A call to action (e.g., "Nurses can use this tool to quickly screen patients in the emergency department for psychiatric disorders.")
- A summary of key points (e.g., "Plan ahead, keep your cool, and remember to take a step-by-step approach to assessment.")

Ask yourself: What is the most important idea or message that I want the reader to take away from this article? Here is an example from an article on preventing pressure injuries (Ruhland et al., 2023):

> These case studies support the use of polyurethane foam dressings in addition to a standardized prevention bundle. Including staff training as part of the standardized prevention bundle is essential, especially when the training is carried out by wound and skin care nurse specialists.

Intestines

Intestines are the guts of the article, the important part that makes it function, including all the data and information (the *nutrients*) that you need to include. Involve your reader whenever possible.

A basic rule is to *show, not tell*. Here are some ways in which you can *show* the reader:

- **Use examples.** Examples are the most powerful way to engage your reader, yet they are often forgotten. In an article on developing personal resilience, Stephens (2019) provides examples to illustrate how nurses can use a tool for developing a plan for resilience. For instance, readers can take steps such as having a diverse network of peer support to address perspective, one of the four Ps of resilience.

- **Add anecdotes and case studies when appropriate.** People like reading about people and their experiences. You can use "stories" such as anecdotes and case studies, but be sure not to identify the patient.

- **Add graphics.** Use tables, figures, graphs, illustrations, and photographs, which are collectively referred to as *graphics*. Be sure your graphics are easy to understand. Graphics are a great way to reduce word count and engage the reader's eye. Some topics lend themselves to certain types of graphics. For example, articles related to wounds and dermatological conditions lend themselves to photographs. Just remember not to repeat in the text what you are showing in your graphic. (See Chapter 7 for more information about graphics.)

- **Create sidebars.** These short pieces of key or supplemental information are usually presented in a shaded box. For example, "The Basics of IMRAD" section earlier in this chapter is a sidebar. Another example is a list of key signs and symptoms of pulmonary edema. Sidebars help make your article more succinct because you do not need to repeat and explain the sidebar content in the text.

As you write, keep your intended audience in mind. A common piece of advice is to write the way you talk, but that isn't true in most cases. Instead, write to the readers of the publication. Adapt your approach to fit the reader the same way that you would teach how to suction differently whether your "audience" was a patient, a patient's family, or a new nurse. For example, your article for the *Journal of Nursing Scholarship* should be more formal in tone than your article for *Nursing*.

One way to write to your audience is to be alert to the "curse of knowledge," which refers to how hard it is for us to imagine what it's like for someone else not to know something we know (Pinker, 2015). For instance, you have cared for many patients receiving negative-pressure wound therapy, so it's second nature to you. It can be hard, therefore, for you to remember what it was like when you first started caring for these patients, which might result in your skipping over key details in an article on the topic.

Even if you were writing for experienced wound care nurses, you would still want to consider that readers don't have the same knowledge and background you do. Pinker's advice on this is helpful, "When in doubt, connect" (2015, p. 168). It's better to err on the side of providing too many connections than too few.

The best ways to ensure you have written your article at the right level is to first, be aware of the potential pitfalls, and second, have a few people in your target audience read your article before submission.

Kidneys

The human body can't live without functioning kidneys, and your article can't live and thrive without editing. Editing comes after you have given yourself permission to write freely, without spending time agonizing over every word, and then revised your work. Just as the kidneys filter out toxins and unnecessary electrolytes, editing is the chance for you to trim the fat from an article. Be on the lookout for unnecessary words and redundant sentences, thoughts, and ideas. Remember to keep your eyes open for places where a simple verb can replace a wordy phrase, for example, "examine" instead of "conduct an examination of" (Gastel, 2015). Cutting your own work can be painful, but it's necessary.

Be sure to check for overall organization by determining if one section flows into another, whether items in lists appear in logical order, and if the main point of each paragraph is clear (Gastel, 2015). See if you have missed any opportunities for presenting material as graphics, instead of a lengthy paragraph, to improve clarity.

It can be hard to edit your own work, but it's an essential part of effective writing. You might find an editing checklist like the one in Appendix A helpful.

Q *What are some more ways to self-edit my work?*

A Two items that you should always check for are *qualifiers* and *obvious statements*.

> Qualifiers such as "I believe..." or "We think..." make you sound unsure of yourself. As the author, your work implies that it is what you think or believe. You can also quickly eliminate obvious statements, such as, "The nursing shortage is a problem in today's society." If you make a statement that you think most people would know, such as, "Heart disease is the leading cause of death in the US," back it up with a few interesting statistics.

After you complete your first draft, share it with a few colleagues or readers you trust. No matter what their response, take their advice as it's intended—as constructive criticism. Even a comment that you feel is negative or unsupportive might be just what your writing needs. Most reviewers will truly want your writing to be the best it can be. And you would rather hear any criticism now, before your writing is published.

Here are some ways to make an outside review more useful:

- **Ask at least one expert on the topic to review your article.** Say that you are writing an article on post-intensive care syndrome with the goal of teaching progressive care unit nurses about this issue. One of your reviewers should be an expert in this area.

- **Ask someone who is not an expert but who represents your target audience for the article.** Now you turn to a progressive care nurse who is not an expert on post-intensive care syndrome. This is a great way to identify unclear areas. Remember that at this stage, you are too close to the article to be objective.

- **Select reviewers who will be honest and objective.** Your friend might be your best support, but perhaps not the best person to give you truly objective feedback.

- **Ask a good writer or editor to read your article.** For your article on post-intensive care syndrome, perhaps you contact a friend (in this case, friends are fine because you are asking only about grammar and style) who has had many articles published, or even your neighbor, who teaches English at the local community college. This type of review is a great way to identify awkward sentences and major grammar errors. This step is not essential, because journals have editing experts, but will make your copy "cleaner" and clearer, perhaps boosting your chance of acceptance.
- **Consider each person's input and then decide whether to follow the advice.** You do not have to follow everyone's suggestion, lest your article appear to be written by a committee. Think about the reason behind the suggestions—and then make thoughtful decisions.
- **Always thank your reviewers.** And, if your article is published, provide an online link to the finished product.

Q *How do I find people to review my article before I submit it for publication?*

A Network, network, network. Ask your friends and colleagues for ideas. For your expert reviewer, you might contact the author of several articles on the topic. These writers are usually passionate about their topic and may be willing to help conduct a review or refer you to someone else. Be considerate by sending a nearly final version, not a rough draft, for review.

Breaking Down Barriers

At this stage, you might be thinking that you understand the writing process, but you doubt your ability to produce the finished product. It can be hard to sit down and write. Consider ways to break down barriers to writing. Two common barriers are lack of confidence and lack of time.

Lack of Confidence

Lack of confidence often comes from two sources: self-doubt that you have something worthwhile to share, and discomfort with writing.

For too long, nurses have been passive in acknowledging their expertise. When nurses are praised for their expertise, they frequently say things like, "I was just doing my job," or, "It was no big deal." However, what we do *is* a big deal, and we have a responsibility to share it with others. Believe in your expertise.

Q *What should I do if I feel like I need to improve my basic writing skills?*

A Even professionals need an occasional tune-up when it comes to the basics of writing. Stephen King is well known for his fiction, but his classic text *On Writing: A Memoir of the Craft* contains a wealth of advice useful for authors who write nonfiction, too (King, 2010). Another classic text is *On Writing Well* (Zinsser, 2016), first published in 1976. Zinsser also pops up in Roy Peter Clark's excellent *Murder Your Darlings: And Other Gentle Writing Advice from Aristotle to Zinsser* (2020), which curates tips from a variety of authors.

If you need help with grammar, try *The Glamour of Grammar* (Clark, 2011), the classic *Eats, Shoots & Leaves: The Zero Tolerance Approach to Punctuation* (Truss, 2011), the grammar section of the Purdue Online Writing Lab (https://owl.purdue.edu/owl/general_writing/grammar/index.html), and the enjoyable Grammar Girl website (https://www.quickanddirtytips.com/grammar-girl).

Writing something—an article, a paper, a blog, or even a book chapter—can be daunting, especially if it's not something you learned in nursing school. Think back to when you learned a new skill, such as inserting a nasogastric tube. The first time, it was mentally tiring and probably more than a bit stressful: You had to consciously think about each step because you wanted to do it correctly. Each time thereafter, though, the procedure became easier and easier for you until you felt comfortable with it, and it came naturally. Here are ideas for boosting your confidence.

Call in an expert. Consider choosing an expert to accompany you on your first writing excursion. Having an experienced coauthor, coach, or mentor for your first article makes sense and fits with nurses' values. After all, you wouldn't insert a midline catheter for the first time without having someone verify you were doing it correctly. A note of caution: Choose your collaborator carefully, and if you choose to have one or more coauthors, follow the suggestions in the next section on collaborative writing.

> **Confidence Booster**
>
> We tell our patients to use positive self-talk to help them make lifestyle changes, and you can do the same to build your confidence with writing for publication. Tell yourself, "I can write!" and, "I can become a published author!" When potholes mar the road (e.g., you just had two staff nurses resign, leaving you short-staffed), think of them as temporary setbacks and plan how you'll get back on track.
>
> Reward yourself for small accomplishments. You wrote two paragraphs today? Enjoy a chapter or two in the latest fiction bestseller. Finished formatting your reference list? Go for a walk to take in a nice day. Of course, you'll need to match your rewards to what is meaningful for you. There's one reward you should avoid, however, and that's the reward of skipping your scheduled writing time (Silvia, 2019).

Write. The way to be more comfortable with writing is to just do it: to just write. Practice helps, which is why writing exercises are included in this book. And amazingly, the more you write, the easier it becomes.

Lack of Time

We're all busy these days, rushing to work, driving children to activities ranging from soccer to dance class, volunteering in our community, working out, and more. The trick is not to think of *finding* time to write, but instead think of *allotting* time to write (Silvia, 2019). After all, you don't find the time to attend a committee meeting—you just schedule it.

Here are a few ways to fracture the time barrier.

Think before you write. Don't waste time sitting in front of a blank computer screen waiting for inspiration. Mull over your topic while you are taking a shower or riding the subway to work. Watch for gifts of time: for example, when you are waiting in line at the grocery store or stuck in traffic. Think about the key points that you want to make and how you want to structure the article. You might map out an entire article on compassion fatigue during a pleasant bike ride.

Q *I always have great ideas, but when I don't write them down, I forget them. What are some techniques for capturing these thoughts?*

A The good news is that the solution is probably right at hand—your smartphone. Dictate your ideas into your phone for later access. Take advantage of apps, such as Evernote, Google Keep, Microsoft OneNote, and Apple Note, that let you organize your notes and, in most cases, sync them across platforms such as your smartphone, tablet, and computer so you can easily retrieve them. If you prefer a low-tech solution, start carrying a small blank book in your purse or pocket so it's ready to go for you to scribble in your ideas and observations. (Don't forget to keep a pen and pad of paper by the side of your bed.)

Schedule your writing. Schedule writing time on your calendar just as you would do for any meeting. Don't expect to be able to devote hours at a time to your writing efforts; that just sets you up for failure. Instead, try 60-, 30-, or even 15-minute blocks of time. What's most important is regularity, not the specific amount of time (Silvia, 2019). It's best to write at the same time, if possible. Some people prefer to write first thing in the morning, before the workday starts, while others turn to evening hours; find what works best for you. Be ready for people who don't respect your scheduled writing time (Silvia, 2019). If you need to put a sign on the door or near where you're working that says, "No interruptions!", do so. Keeping track of how many words you write may increase what you produce.

Negotiate. Talk to friends, family members, and significant others. Explain what you are trying to accomplish and ask for their help. We delegate at work, but too often fail to do so at home. After all, how clean does your house really need to be? Talk to your supervisor at work. Some organizations offer time to work on articles as part of staff retention efforts.

Manage the project. Treat your article as you would any other project you expect to accomplish, from developing a new policy and procedure to painting the house. Make a timeline of interim steps and set goals. Examples of goals for a writing session include: write at least 200 words, write the first two paragraphs of the discussion, review three articles and note how they fit into the article, or format references (Silvia, 2019).

Developing a Writing Timeline

If you don't create a timeline for your writing project, it's likely you will never have a final product. The level of detail for your timeline depends on how much direction you need. You might want to simply enter major milestones, like: choose topic, send query, research, write, revise, and submit. Or, you might want more detail, such as what is included here:

- Research possible ideas.
- Narrow and choose your topic. (See Chapter 2.)
- Decide if you will have coauthors; if so, confirm them and meet to establish the ground rules for the collaboration.
- Research possible publications.
- Decide on your target publication and read the author guidelines. (See Chapters 2 and 3.)
- Write a query letter to the appropriate person. (See Chapter 3.)

If your query is accepted:

- Conduct a literature search. (See Chapter 4.) (Even if you completed a literature search for the project you'll be writing about, you'll want to update it.)
- Review the results of the search and any other sources of information you may have found.
- Create an outline. (See Chapters 2 and 19.)
- Divide the outline into sections you will write—for example: introduction, literature review, methods, results, and discussion. List each section. Or, simply divide your time into a number of segments, such as five to ten, and be more open about what you will work on during those segments. For instance:

- Writing time #1
- Writing time # 2, etc.

- Write the manuscript, including text and graphics. (See Chapters 6 and 7.)
- Put the manuscript away for one to two weeks before you revise.
- Revise and edit the manuscript. You'll typically need two to three rounds. You may want to focus on a particular aspect with each round. For example, you might first focus on organization, then clarity, and then accuracy.
- Ask at least two people to review; be sure one is a member of your target reader group.
- Revise based on comments from the reviewers.
- Set the article aside for about three days.
- Read again for clarity and revise as needed.
- Proofread.
- Submit the manuscript.

Assign each task a corresponding deadline and treat those dates with the same respect you would other important work or personal projects.

Find a space. You can save time by dedicating one area of your home or office for your writing. That way, all your materials can stay in one place, ready to go. Take steps to avoid interruptions. If you have a door, close it. If you are in a cubicle, hang a "Do not disturb! Genius at work!" sign on the cubicle wall. If someone does interrupt, don't give into temptation to respond. Instead, say when you can get back to them. On the other hand, keep in mind that you can write anywhere you have a laptop or a paper and pen. Writers can work on planes, trains, and even boats. Writing is a mindset, not a location.

Be flexible. Don't feel that you have to start at the beginning, which is often the hardest part of the article to write. Instead of taking time fretting over that, just start writing. For example, say you're writing an article about your study on how your online education program increased knowledge of hypertension among Asian women. Instead of starting with the introduction, you might decide to start with the methods section, which is often the easiest section of a research article to write because you're simply describing what you did (Lang, 2017; Nicosia, 2023); another easier place to start for a research article is the results section, which tends to be straightforward (Nicosia, 2023). One professional medical writer sometimes alternates work on different sections (Nicosia, 2023). However, others feel that strategy slows down the process. The key is to find what works best for you.

Consider an accountability partner. Most of us have busy lives, so it can be difficult to hold ourselves accountable for meeting our publication goals. An accountability partnership can help you meet your goal and provides an opportunity for you to help someone else meet their goals (Saver, 2023). An accountability partner should be willing to push you and be honest when you're not meeting a goal (Capano, 2021; Mantel, 2023). Avoid picking a friend but do look for someone, such as a trusted colleague, who can gently point out when you're falling short (Capano, 2021). Your partner can be someone with a goal other than publishing (such as completing a quality improvement project) because the purpose is accountability, not critiquing your work. Establish a plan that includes how often you'll communicate and how (e.g., face-to-face vs. online).

Give yourself a break. Writing isn't easy (or everyone would do it, right?). Do not expect perfection; editors and peer reviewers can help you polish your manuscript. Be forgiving if your writing session doesn't go as planned. Although some deadlines must be met, there will be other times when the words just don't come. Understanding that this can happen and planning accordingly will keep you from getting discouraged.

Collaborative or Team Writing

Given today's emphasis on collaboration in all areas of healthcare, from quality improvement projects to research studies, it's likely that at some point you'll be writing with others as part of a writing team. In addition to writing with other nurses, you may be writing with other healthcare professionals, such as physicians, social workers, physical therapists, and respiratory therapists, as part of an interprofessional team. Serving on a writing team can be a wonderful experience, but it also can be more difficult than helpful if the project isn't well managed. If you're the one starting the team, follow these steps to ensure a positive experience.

Choose the Right Collaborators

If you don't choose the right people to work with, you may end up spending excessive time on your writing project—time you can ill afford to lose. In some cases, collaborators will be near at hand, such as those who worked on an evidence-based project with you. In other cases, such as clinical articles, you can look for those who have expertise in areas outside of your own. For instance, you may want to collaborate with a pharmacist when writing an article on lung cancer, so you have expert advice when it comes to discussing combination chemotherapy options. If you're new to writing, avoid choosing only other inexperienced writers (Jalongo, 2023). Instead, seek out at least one person with some publishing experience.

You also want those who mesh well with your work style: If you like to have everything done at least a day before a deadline, you're likely to be frustrated with someone who pushes it to the last minute.

Red flags that signal you don't have the right person include multiple cancellations of meetings you set up to discuss the project, which can be a sign of overcommitment; don't expect those commitments to lessen once the project starts. Also beware of someone who seems overly enthusiastic (Silvia, 2015). This person may be excited and happy to agree to the project, but then lose interest when it comes to the hard part of actually doing the writing. The ideal collaborator knows that writing is worth making a time commitment to and shares the team's goal for publishing.

Hold a Kickoff Meeting

You wouldn't launch a major quality improvement project without a planning meeting, and it's the same with a writing project. The kickoff meeting can be in person, by phone, or online, depending on the geographic location of the participants. If you opt for an online meeting, consider using video technology such as Zoom, Skype, or Webex to host the get-together. Being able to put a face to a name can foster "buy-in" and support the collaboration right from the start. Send out an agenda to participants ahead of time.

At the kickoff meeting, discuss the overall goals and direction of the project. You want to be sure everyone is clear about the manuscript's scope and purpose (Silvia, 2015). It's a good idea to have one person take notes or minutes to document the discussion and any decisions that are made at the meeting.

> ### Successful Interprofessional Writing
>
> Each person on an interprofessional writing team brings a different perspective to the topic, which can strengthen the effectiveness of the article and enrich the writing experience. But these teams aren't without their pitfalls. Cindy Munro, a nurse who shares the editor-in-chief role for the American Journal of Critical Care with physician Aluko Hope, notes that different disciplines may differ on expectations when it comes to the publishing process (personal communication, January 19, 2017). And, it can be hard to find a journal equally valued by all participants.
>
> You can take the following steps to foster collaboration (Knapp et al., 2015; Suttle et al., 2023; Vicens & Bourne, 2007; Vogel et al., 2019):
>
> - Respect your collaborators for their expertise and leverage their strengths.
> - Communicate consistently. Doing so will keep your project on track.
> - Learn the language of your collaboration partners. Every specialty in healthcare has its own jargon; understanding it promotes communication.
> - Know that different fields move at different speeds. For instance, the time from acceptance to publication of a manuscript may vary according to discipline. Understanding this will help you tamp down impatience.
>
> As is the case with any collaboration, it's important to talk early in the process about how to work together so you have the best possible synergy (Knapp et al., 2015; Suttle et al., 2023; Vogel et al., 2019). Respect each other's viewpoints, and keep in mind that once you establish a successful team, that team can collaborate on many future manuscripts.

This is also a good time to determine authorship, including lead author, corresponding author, and coauthors, along with the order of authorship.

The *lead author*, who isn't necessarily the same as the person who led the project or study—but who should be a major contributor to the article—will come first in the list of authors and shoulder the bulk of the work. The lead author agrees to take on multiple responsibilities, the most important of which are to help ensure the manuscript reads like it was written by one person instead of several and to keep the process moving. A good lead author facilitates group discussion; delegates tasks; and makes any difficult decisions about manuscript structure, content, and author contributions (Frassl et al., 2018). The lead author typically also coordinates manuscript review by the team members, checks that the manuscript meets the journal's submission guidelines, obtains final sign-off from all authors, and keeps the project files, although some of these tasks may be assumed by the corresponding author (see below).

Team members should speak up during the project if it seems that someone other than the lead author is doing most of the work. Sometimes a change is needed, but waiting until the end of the project to raise the issue can cause distress within the team.

The *corresponding author*—who is often, but not always, the same as the lead author—is responsible for ongoing communication with the journal. The corresponding author ensures that the submission meets the journal's requirements, such as authorship information; documentation of permissions granted and ethics committee approval (if applicable); and completion of disclosure forms, which stipulate financial and nonfinancial relationships and activities, including conflicts of interest, of the authors (International Committee of Medical Journal Editors, 2024). (See Chapter 11 for more information about disclosure forms.)

The *coauthors* are listed after the lead author. (See Chapter 11 for guidance as to who qualifies to be an author.) No hard or fast rules exist for the order of coauthors. The team should jointly decide the order and have a rationale for the decision. Tscharntke and colleagues (2007) offer some options:

- **Sequence Determines Credit (SDC):** The sequence of authors reflects the declining importance of their contribution.
- **Equal Contribution Norm (ECN):** Authors are listed alphabetically, and each person's contribution is considered equally.

- **First-Last-Author-Emphasis (FLAE):** The first and last authors are the major contributors, and everyone in the middle takes remaining credit; these names may be listed alphabetically.
- **Percent-Contribution-Indicated (PCI):** Each author specifies their contribution and the respective percent, which is included as a statement at the end of the article.

In general, the author listed first does the most work and holds the most prestige, but the importance of the remaining authors varies among disciplines and author teams (Phillippi et al., 2018; Thurston et al., 2023). For example, author teams writing about their research results often reserve the last position on the list for the team member who oversaw the project. In this case, being last is highly prestigious. However, the most common format is to list the person who contributed the most to the article in the first position, with the remaining authors listed in descending order of contribution (American Psychological Association, 2020; JAMA Network Editors, 2020).

If you have an interprofessional writing team, you may have plans for several manuscripts, with the lead author the representative of the discipline and journal that you target for submission. For example, you, as the nurse, would be the lead author for the manuscript to be sent to a nursing journal; a pharmacist might be the lead for an article for a pharmacy journal, and so on. Just remember that all of these articles need to be original and different from each other. You don't want to fall into the trap of "salami slicing" or duplicate publication. These ethical lapses are discussed in more detail in Chapter 11, which also contains information about determining who qualifies as an author.

Define each person's responsibilities for the manuscript. Match strengths to tasks. For example, the most detail-oriented team member might be the perfect person to take responsibility for verifying and finalizing the reference list. The clearer it is as to who is supposed to do what and by when, the more likely it is that you'll have an effective collaboration. An option is to use one of the author grids developed by Phillippi et al. (2018). The grids address key components of ethical authorship, link "work effort" with attribution, and guide any required future data sharing (e.g., to meet National Institutes of Health requirements for larger federal grants). Grids, which can be adapted to meet the writing team's needs, are available for quantitative studies, qualitative studies, and literature synthesis. While your team may not need quite the level of detail in the grids, having one will ensure you cover all the bases.

Another resource for writing research articles is the Contributor Roles Taxonomy (CRediT, n.d.), which provides 14 roles, such as conceptualization, methodology, and writing—original draft, that contributors typically play when engaged in research output. Identifying who will be fulfilling one or more of these roles can help avoid conflict later in the project. Many journals require you to identify how each author contributed to the submitted article, and CRediT can help with that as well.

Whatever format you use to identify responsibilities, you need to have a formal agreement for the writing team. Shellenbarger and Robb (2015) recommend the agreement include the order of the authors, expectations for each author, approach to writing, timeline, and guidelines for the group. The agreement promotes engagement in the writing process (Vogel et al., 2019).

Guidelines should detail what will happen if someone doesn't meet the team's expectations. For example, you might decide that if a person misses the deadline for comments by more than four days, their comments aren't considered; if this happens twice, the person is dropped from the team. It may seem harsh, but you don't want one person holding back the entire team and project. One strategy for managing deadlines is to take what Silvia (2015) calls an "opt-in" approach: If someone doesn't respond by the deadline, the manuscript continues to move forward without their input. The team also should decide now to resolve disputes that may arise (Herron, 2023). For example, you and your coauthors may agree to a neutral third-party person not directly involved in the work.

Set a timeline and schedule at least one interim meeting (more may be needed, depending on the nature of the project) and a final meeting before submission. Don't schedule too many meetings; you want to finish the manuscript, not spend your time talking about what you're going to do. Beware of trying to make too many decisions as a group (L. Nicoll, personal communication, October 6, 2013) or copying every team member on every email. The lead author can contact individual contributors as needed. You may also choose to use an app such as Asana (https://asana.com) or Trello (https://trello.com) to help you manage the tasks involved.

> **The Writing Team Kickoff Meeting**
>
> Use this checklist to ensure you have a productive meeting that sets up the team for a positive writing experience.
>
> ☐ Agree on the goals of the project.
>
> ☐ Define each person's responsibilities.
>
> ☐ Decide on the lead and corresponding authors.
>
> ☐ Determine the order in which all authors will be listed.
>
> ☐ Set a timeline and schedule an interim meeting and a final meeting.
>
> ☐ Establish ground rules up front, including expectations for meeting deadlines.
>
> ☐ Agree on a collaboration method.
>
> ☐ Decide which technology will be used for document review.
>
> ☐ Identify who will be working on the file at various points in the project (to avoid having multiple document versions).
>
> ☐ Put assignments and expectations in writing.

A resource for managing collaborative writing teams is the toolkit available from the University of Washington Center for Health Sciences Interprofessional Education, Research and Practice (Vogel et al., n.d.). It includes a project planning checklist and a sample author agreement form.

Decide on the Collaboration Method

There's no one best way to write collaboratively, but at the kickoff meeting, you'll need to decide what is best for the group. Silvia (2015) advocates having one person, or possibly two people, write the full first draft, so the manuscript has better flow. The coauthors can review the draft, adding their input and adding any small sections they may have been assigned. This works best when there is a solid understanding of the expected product among team members and can be an efficient way to complete a first draft (Lingard, 2021).

Other approaches for collaborative writing include parallel writing and hand-off (also called "each-in-sequence"). With *parallel writing*, each person completes an assigned section of the article (Lingard, 2021; Shellenbarger & Robb, 2015). This has the apparent advantage of moving the project along quickly but has two pitfalls: First, people write at different speeds, and second, the work can read like different people wrote it, which of course is the case. It's the lead author's responsibility to ensure the latter problem doesn't occur by editing sections to give them a consistent voice. Parallel writing works best when writers have distinct areas of expertise (Lingard, 2021; Shellenbarger & Robb, 2015). For example, a person with a strong background in statistics would be the ideal choice to write the data analysis section of a research paper. Or, the person who created the online brochure used in a quality improvement project to enhance communication with family members of patients in the emergency department (ED) at your hospital might be the best person to write the section on strategies as part of a larger article on family communication in the ED.

With the *hand-off method*, one person starts the manuscript, typically the person responsible for the introduction, then hands it off to the next author, who reviews what has been done and writes the next section (Lingard, 2021; Shellenbarger & Robb, 2015). This helps authors see the flow of the article but can cause bottlenecks if someone doesn't complete their section on time (Lingard, 2021).

Some writing teams choose to use more than one method. For example, one person writes the first draft, then others review the document sequentially (Lingard, 2021).

However you choose to collaborate, consider how technology can help facilitate the project (Yilmaz et al., 2022). A simple example is using a Doodle poll (https://doodle.com/en/product/polls/) to determine the best time for your kickoff meeting, rather than exchanging multiple emails. In addition, instead of emailing a document, which results in several sets of comments to manage, use document-sharing tools, such as Dropbox Paper, Google Docs, or OneDrive so everyone is working on the same version. You may want to use the Track Changes feature in Microsoft Word to allow everyone to see who made what changes when, or assign authors different font colors.

If you have several authors, you might want to consider tools specifically designed for collaborative writing, such as Manubot (https://manubot.org) and Overleaf (www.overleaf.com), which facilitate group editing and allow for easier reference management (Perkel, 2020).

Establish a system for labeling files to avoid confusion. For example, the person working on the file could name it with their initials and the date, so that the most current version would be the one with the most recent date. It's also often helpful to use a reference management system such as Mendeley or Zotero; you can learn more about these systems in Chapter 4.

Remember to build in time to have someone outside the group review the article to obtain a fresh perspective.

Celebrate Your Successes

Once you have your article published, don't forget to get the group together to celebrate—and plan your next project!

Publishing Process

Just like the nursing process (assessment, diagnosis, planning, implementation, and evaluation), the publishing process has defined steps: submission, peer review, revision, editing and layout, author review and approval, and publication. Upcoming chapters will provide more details, but here is an overview.

Submission

Submission occurs after you have made a final proof of your manuscript. (See Appendix B for a checklist to help you with this.) Once that's done, you'll need to email your manuscript to an editor or upload it via the publication's online editorial management system. (If you're blogging, you can create your article directly in a special web-based editing interface, inserting photos, illustrations, and hyperlinks as you go.)

When submitting to a journal, magazine, website, or book publisher, follow the publication's author guidelines (also called information for authors). Make sure that your article or chapter has all the required elements, including abstract and cover letter with complete contact information. Many journals will have additional guidelines if the article is being submitted for peer review. Carefully review author guidelines, too, for submitting illustrations or figures with your written work.

To give yourself the best possible chance for your work to be accepted, save time and energy by avoiding these common submission errors. (Don't worry—most authors have made one or more of these mistakes.):

- **Manuscript is not an appropriate fit for the publication.** The content may be good, but the topic isn't appropriate for the publication's audience, so the article is rejected.

- **Manuscript is too "rough" in its current state; in other words, it feels unfinished or incomplete.** The manuscript will take significant time to edit, so it might be rejected or sent back to the author for edits before it can be reviewed. Possible reasons for "roughness" include too broad a topic, overstating conclusions, or failing to make connections that would resonate with readers.

- **Manuscript doesn't have enough meaning for readers.** In the case of a study, it might be that the scope of the project was too small to have wider implications. Or, an article might not bring any new perspectives to the topic.

- **Manuscript does not meet or greatly exceeds suggested word count.** Don't send a textbook or a memo instead of a journal article. Publications use established word counts to ensure a consistency of coverage within their publication. Plus, they know how much they need to fill the pages, or in the case of online, to be sure an article isn't too long or short for the topic. You don't have to hit the requested number of words exactly, but be fairly close. For example, if 3,500 words are requested, it's acceptable to submit about 3,800, but don't submit 5,000. A good guideline is to be within 5% to 10%.

- **Manuscript uses fancy fonts and formatting styles.** This can make your submission difficult for the editor to read or accurately gauge its length. Stick to using basic fonts, such as Times New Roman or Calibri, and consult the publication's guidelines for specific requirements.

- **Author didn't follow directions for online submission.** In many cases, you'll submit your manuscript via an online portal. Online submission can be frustrating for authors unfamiliar with it. The good news is that these systems allow you to track the progress of your manuscript. And, you'll feel more comfortable with this type of submission the more you do it.

- **Manuscript isn't formatted according to the guidelines.** It's a small problem but a frustrating one, nonetheless. Check page sizes, margins, spacing, numbering, and other requirements. Use the reference style that the publication requires—and include all the information required for each reference. The publication might use the American Psychological Association (APA) style instead of the American Medical Association (also called "Vancouver") style, where references are cited in the text by number with a complete citation at the end. If your references are incomplete, your editor will likely return your manuscript to you. (See Chapter 4 for more information about references.)

- **Cover letter doesn't include title of manuscript and complete contact information.** Make sure to include the name, address, phone number, and email address for each author.

- **Cover letter doesn't indicate the corresponding author.** When submitting to a journal, the editors want to work with just one author so that the process is streamlined. This does not have to be the lead author.

- **Submission is incomplete.** Editors cannot begin work on a project until all elements—including photos, illustrations, tables, charts, and parts of the article or book—are submitted.

- **Author hasn't obtained necessary permissions for photos, illustrations, or text.** Most publications request that you submit letters of permission with your submission, say for a previously published figure.

Q *Is it ever acceptable to submit a manuscript for publication if I don't have all permissions in place?*

A If you will have to pay for a permission, it's usually acceptable to note the situation, indicating that you will obtain permission should the article be accepted for publication.

- **Artwork files are not prepared according to specifications.** Publications will include specific requirements in their guidelines for preparing images, including dots per inch (dpi) resolution, file sizes, and file formats. (See Chapter 7 for more information.)

- **Citations are weak.** Be sure citations are sufficient and support your work but are not excessive. Use the citation where the information originally appeared (primary source) rather than a publication that cites the article (secondary source).

- **Manuscript doesn't link content to practice.** Nursing is a practice-driven profession, whether clinical, education, or research. Be sure readers will be able to understand how the information applies to their practice, particularly when presenting study results.

- **Submission is late.** Just like you plan your schedule, editors plan a schedule, too, and they count on submissions arriving on time.

After you submit your work, the editor will review the manuscript and decide whether it should be sent for peer review. With most journals, your manuscript is not accepted for publication at this stage. It's just moving to the next step.

Peer Review

Nurses can't be experts in all areas of practice, and it's the same with editors. Editors use peer reviewers to tap into experts who can give them feedback on your submission. Reviewer feedback often includes a recommendation as to whether the work should be rejected, be published, or is acceptable for publication if certain revisions are made.

The peer-review process is common in scholarly or academic research journals (i.e., journals with a focus on research and evidence-based practice). Faculty members usually must publish in peer-reviewed journals as part of meeting tenure requirements. Although peer review is common for journals, many publishers will also use a similar process to assess the quality of your work for other outlets such as books and websites.

Q *How long does peer review take?*

A Peer review typically takes six to eight weeks, but this time frame varies considerably by publication. Peer reviewers, who receive either nothing or a small honorarium for their work, must fit the task around their already-busy schedules. If you haven't received peer-review feedback after 10 weeks, you can send the editor a quick email to check status.

The editor reviews the peer-reviewer comments, and authors see them as well. If it seems unfair that comments from outside reviewers hold so much weight, keep in mind that it's generally agreed that peer review improves the quality of the final product.

Revision

If the peer reviews are favorable, you will be asked to revise your manuscript. You'll base your revisions on comments from the peer reviewers and the publication's editorial staff. It can be stressful to see comments on the manuscript you put so much work into. Remember that it's highly unusual for any manuscript to be accepted without any revision. Editors say that too many times, authors become discouraged at this point and give up. Don't. If you complete the revisions satisfactorily, you have a good chance of being published.

Editing and Layout

After your manuscript has been accepted, publishing staff edit it and prepare it for layout, whether in print, online, or both. No matter what you have written and where it will be published, your work will be edited. Here are the most common types of editing:

- **Substantive or developmental editing (macroediting).** With this type of editing, the editor focuses on the big picture of your work, from the flow and organization to the tone and style of the text. The editor plays the role of an orthopedic surgeon faced with a complicated fracture, examining the article from all angles, deciding what works to deliver the content so the reader can grasp it, and what might need repair. The editor also makes sure that the style of your article fits the style of the journal or magazine—and in the case of a book, matches the outline of the work the publication expected to receive.

- **Line editing.** Some editors refer to the subset of substantive editing that focuses on paragraphs and sentences as *line editing*.

- **Copyediting (microediting).** Ever wonder about those miraculous editors who seem to catch every small grammar, spelling, and punctuation mistake? They are *copy editors*, and the process is similar to checking for bleeding before closing a surgical incision. The copy editor eases a weight from your shoulders. Unless you work in communications on a daily basis, no one can keep up on the latest rules of English. Copy editors also check for clarity and consistency in the tone of a manuscript.

Editing is followed by proofing to catch any mistakes that were missed. After your manuscript has been edited and proofed, it will be returned to you for your author review.

Author Review and Approval

When your edited article is returned to you for review, you will see questions—often called *queries*—included for you to answer. Queries often relate to one or more of the following areas (Saver & Cullen, 2021):

- **References.** Questions related to incomplete, incorrect, or missing information.

- **Terminology.** Authors sometimes use terminology that is familiar to them, but not necessarily to the publication's readers. Examples are terms for new concepts and terms used by nurses in one specialty writing for those in a different one.

- **Verification of editing changes.** The editor might want to verify that a change or addition they made didn't affect the meaning of the text.

- **Additional text.** An editor might suggest adding text to clarify points. For example, if the author writes that patients can use behavioral strategies to prevent diverging from dietary or physical activity goals, the editor might ask for examples of these strategies.

- **Clarification.** Although you might feel what you wrote is crystal clear, sometimes an editor will ask you to clarify a point to facilitate reader understanding.

> ### Confidence Booster
>
> Sometime in your writing experience, you're likely to have a manuscript rejected. While you might be tempted to cry or dump your beloved manuscript into your computer's trash can, don't give in to your emotions. Remember, your worth is not defined by any manuscript, whether or not it's published. In many cases you'll receive at least a summary of the peer-review comments that led to the rejection. View these comments as free advice from experts (Silvia, 2015). Revise your article and submit to another journal, following that journal's guidelines. If you are rejected again, consult with a trusted colleague as to whether you should try a third time or simply move on to another project.

> **Publication Timing**
>
> Several factors go into the decision of when to publish an article. One is the importance of the article to the reader. Some journals assign each article a priority number for publication; those with the highest priority are more likely to be published first. Other factors include how often the journal is published and the number of articles that a journal receives and accepts. Finally, unique innovation or cutting-edge research typically goes to the head of the publishing line and may be published on the journal's website before appearing in print. For example, during the COVID-19 pandemic, editors gave high priority to articles that could help clinicians better care for patients.

- **Inconsistencies.** An editor might pick up on contradictory information in your manuscript. For example, an author might use the term subspecialty palliative care in one section and secondary palliative care in another when referring to the same type of care.

You typically answer the queries within the manuscript. Sometimes an editorial change can inadvertently change the meaning of a sentence, so in addition to answering queries, review all edits carefully. This is not the time to reorganize your article or add substantial material, but rather the time to focus on accuracy, such as drug dosages and correct figure labels. Remember that you are responsible for the final accuracy of the article.

The time you have to review the edited manuscript varies considerably, depending on the type of publication. For a blog, you might have only a few hours. For a journal, you might have five to ten days. For a book or a chapter in a book, you might have two to four weeks. In some cases, you will review a Word document of the article; other times, you will review the article in its laid-out version as a PDF document or on a website that is not yet "live." You also might review the edited article in Word and then complete another review at the PDF stage.

Q *What if I have a change to my article after I've sent in my final submission?*

A Contact your editor immediately. Depending on the type of publication and stage your paper is in the process, you might have to hold on to your correction for an errata or addendum after publication. In this digital age, the good news is that corrections can be made quickly to articles online. But it's best to avoid the situation by making sure your final changes are truly your final changes.

You might also be asked to sign a form attesting that you have reviewed the article either with no changes or the minor changes noted on the form.

Publication

The best part of writing an article is seeing it in print or online! It can take anywhere from a few weeks to two years or longer for your final article to be published. Online publication is usually faster because websites don't have the same restrictions on number of pages per issue that journals and other print outlets do. Some journals publish some articles online and others in print, and others might publish an article online, then print it in a future issue. Still other journals publish only online.

After your handiwork is published, be sure to add your accomplishment to your professional portfolio, resume, and curriculum vitae.

Q *What I was taught as "good writing" in high school doesn't always match with what editors seem to prefer. What's going on?*

A English is a living, evolving language, and styles are different for different audiences. For example, many nurses were taught in high school that starting a sentence with a conjunction (and, or, or but) is an error. It is now acceptable to do so in more informal publications. Scholarly journals typically won't accept informal usages, though. The trick is to tailor your writing to the style required by the publication you're targeting. For instance, if contractions aren't used in your target journal, do not use them.

All About the Publishing Team

Publishing is a team sport. As with a multidisciplinary healthcare team, each person on the team has a specific role.

- **Author:** Supplies content expertise.

- **Peer reviewer:** Contributes knowledge expertise that helps authors strengthen their manuscript.

- **Editor:** Provides editorial expertise so that the article is editorially correct and is presented most effectively to readers. Editors understand what their readers prefer as far as topics and style of article. Editors plan the content of the publication; in most cases the planning is done months in advance. These professionals follow codes of editorial conduct such as those from the Committee on Publication Ethics (2022), the International Committee of Medical Journal Editors (2024), and the Council of Science Editors (Council of Science Editors Editorial Policy Committee, 2023). Within an editorial department, different editors have different responsibilities, but common roles include:

    - *Editor-in-chief*: Has primary responsibility for the overall content of the publication and strategic planning for the mission of the publication. In some cases, the editor is full time; in other situations, the editor might be part time and hold another job such as faculty member or dean at a college of nursing.

    - *Managing editor*: Oversees the general editorial operations of the publication, ensuring that articles undergo peer review and are edited, designed, and laid out.

    - *Acquisitions editor*: Consults with content experts who have expertise in specific areas relevant to the mission of the publication and asks them to submit a manuscript for potential publication, typically in a journal or as a book. The manuscript generally must still undergo peer review before it's accepted for publication.

    - *Developmental editor*: Assists the author to ensure that the manuscript meets the expectations of the publication and guides the author in focusing the manuscript to ensure quality of the content. The role may also be called the *clinical editor*, when the person has expertise in the clinical area of the publication (e.g., a nurse clinical editor for a nursing publication).

    - *Content editor*: Focuses on ensuring that the writing style of the manuscript is consistent with the publication guidelines. This editor may revise the organization of content and change the way it is written to ensure the content is understandable to the reader and follows the style guidelines of the publication. While changing the wording in some cases, this editor is careful not to change the meaning of the content.

    - *Project editor*: Responsible for tracking the manuscript through the editorial process, ensuring that it is sent for peer review, and ensuring that authors receive the feedback. This editor also works with other editors or copy editors as well as the art and production departments to ensure that the manuscript is complete and that all the content needed for final publication is included.

    - *Copy editor*: Performs copyediting and proofreading services for your manuscript.

- **Art director, designer, or graphics designer:** Creates the visual elements, such as illustrations, graphs, and tables. The editorial staff and the art director work closely together to ensure that your information is presented clearly.

- **Production assistant:** Lays out the publication on the page for printing or web design.

- **Editorial board member:** Provides strategic input into the direction of the publication and may serve as a peer reviewer or as a coordinator for a department or column.

Sometimes members of the publishing team forget and use jargon when communicating with authors. If you don't know what "crop marks," "folio," "marginalia," or other terms mean, refer to Appendix C.

Q *How can I best work with my editor?*

A Understand that, like you, editors are busy people with multiple deadlines. You will endear yourself to the editor (who, after all, can help make your article shine) by following the author guidelines (the most common complaint of editors is that authors don't do this); responding promptly to emails, texts, and phone calls; and meeting your deadlines. The good news is that most editors welcome the opportunity to nurture their relationship with you. That means they welcome your questions.

Collaboration within the publishing team is just as important as it is for a healthcare team. Respect each person's expertise and know that all of you have the same goal: an outstanding published product.

Get Ready to Write

You now have a solid overview of what it takes to write for publication, all based on something you already know—anatomy and physiology. You also know how to break down barriers to writing and how the publishing process works.

In upcoming chapters, you will learn much more about writing, submitting, and revising your work for publication. It's certainly true that writing can be hard work (Gennaro, 2020), but remember—if you passed anatomy and physiology, you can write!

Write Now!

1. List three benefits that you feel will come from writing an article. It might be personal satisfaction, a desire to learn more about a topic, or something else. The point is that it should be personal to you.
2. Now, write a few sentences about how you will carve out time in your schedule to write. Create action steps: for example, when you will set your first writing date in your calendar.

References

American Nurses Association. (2015). *Code of ethics for nurses with interpretive statements*. https://www.nursingworld.org/practice-policy/nursing-excellence/ethics/code-of-ethics-for-nurses/

American Psychological Association. (2020). *Publication manual of the American Psychological Association* (7th ed.). https://doi.org/10.1037/0000165-000

Capano, C. (2021, May 21). Accountability works if you do: Five tips for finding the right accountability partner. *Forbes*. https://www.forbes.com/sites/forbescoachescouncil/2021/05/21/accountability-works-if-you-do-five-tips-for-finding-the-right-accountability-partner/?sh=24e98d6b7d6f

Clark, R. P. (2011). *The glamour of grammar: A guide to the magic and mystery of practical English*. Little, Brown and Company.

Clark, R. P. (2020). *Murder your darlings: And other gentle writing advice from Aristotle to Zinsser*. Little, Brown Spark.

Committee on Publication Ethics. (2022). *Principles of transparency and best practice in scholarly publication*. https://doi.org/10.24318/cope.2019.1.12

Council of Science Editors Editorial Policy Committee. (2023). *CSE's recommendations for promoting integrity in scientific journal publications*. https://www.councilscienceeditors.org/recommendations-for-promoting-integrity-in-scientific-journal-publications

Crawford, C. L., Rondinelli, J., Zuniga, S., Valdez, R. M., Cullen, L., Hanrahan, K., & Titler, M. G. (2020). Testing of the nursing evidence-based practice survey. *Worldviews on Evidence-Based Nursing, 17*(2), 118–128. https://doi.org/10.1111/wvn.12432

CRediT. (n.d.). *Contributor Roles Taxonomy*. https://credit.niso.org/

Ellison, R. (1995). *Invisible man*. Vintage Classic.

Frassl, M. A., Hamilton, D. P., Denfeld B. A., deEyto, E., Hampton, S. E., Keller, P. S., Sharma, S., Lewis, A. S. L., Weyhanmeyer G. A., O'Reilly, C. M., Lofton, M. E., & Catalán, N. (2018). Ten simple rules for collaboratively writing a multi-authored paper. *PLOS Computational Biology, 14*(11), e1006508. https://doi.org/10.1371/journal.pcbi.1006508

Gastel, B. (2015). Editing and proofreading your own work. *AMWA Journal, 30*(4), 147–151.

Gastel, B., & Day, R. A. (2022). *How to write and publish a scientific paper* (9th ed.). Greenwood.

Gennaro, S. (2016a). Mistakes to avoid in scientific writing [Editorial]. *Journal of Nursing Scholarship, 48*(5), 435–436. https://doi.org/10.1111/jnu.12235

Gennaro, S. (2016b). Why write? [Editorial]. *Journal of Nursing Scholarship, 48*(2), 117. https://doi.org/10.1111/jnu.12200

Gennaro, S. (2020). Your scientific legacy [Editorial]. *Journal of Nursing Scholarship, 52*(2), 127. https://doi.org/10.1111/jnu.12543

Herron, C. R. (2023). Best practices to guide decisions of authorship and author order in a research manuscript. *AMWA Journal, 38*(4), 38–40.

Hill, M., Moreda, M., Navarro, J., & Mulkey, M. (2023). Assessing patients with altered level of consciousness. *Critical Care Nurse, 43*(4), 58–65. https://doi.org/10.4037/ccn2023449

International Committee of Medical Journal Editors. (2024). *Recommendations for the conduct, reporting, editing, and publication of scholarly work in medical journals*. http://www.icmje.org/recommendations

Jalongo, M. R. (2023). Writing together: Collaborative work. In M. R. Jalongo & O. N. Saracho (Eds.), *Scholarly writing: Publishing manuscripts that are read, downloaded, and cited* (pp. 301–321). Springer.

JAMA Network Editors. (2020). *AMA manual of style: A guide for authors and editors* (11th ed.). Oxford University Press.

King, S. (2010). *On writing: A memoir of the craft* (10th anniversary ed.). Scribner.

Knapp, B., Bardenet, R., Bernabeu, M. O., Bordas, R., Bruna, M., Calderhead, B., Cooper, J., Fletcher, A. G., Groen, D., Kuijper, B., Lewis, J., McInerny, G., Minssen, T., Osborne, J., Paulitschke, V., Pitt-Francis, J., Todoric, J., Yates, C. A., Gavaghan, D., & Deane, C. M. (2015). Ten simple rules for a successful cross-disciplinary collaboration. *PLoS Computational Biology, 11*(4), e1004214. https://doi.org/10.1371/journal.pcbi.1004214

Lang, T. A. (2017). Writing a better research article. *Journal of Public Health and Emergency, 1*(12), 88. http://dx.doi.org/10.21037/jphe.2017.11.06

Lee, C. J., Herrera, J., Miller, J., Moffit, C., & Wiczynski, H. (2023). The role of nurses in firearm safety. *American Nurse Journal, 18*(11), 12–15. https//doi.org/10.51256/ANJ112312

Lingard, L. (2021). Collaborative writing: Strategies and activities for writing productively together. *Perspectives on Medical Education, 10*(3), 163–166. https//doi.org/10.1007/S40037-021-00668-7

Mantel, B. (2023, May 10). Tips for finding and keeping accountability partners. *Association of Health Care Journalists.* https://healthjournalism.org/blog/2023/05/tips-for-finding-and-keepinga-accountability-partners

Morrison, T. (2006). *Beloved.* Everyman's Library.

Nguyen, S. C., Suba, S., Hu, X., & Pelter, M. M. (2020). Double trouble: Patients with both true and false arrhythmia alarms. *Critical Care Nurse, 40*(2), 14–23. https://doi.org/10.4037/ccn2020363

Nicosia, M. (2023). A medical writer's guide: Working on clinical research manuscripts for submission to peer-reviewed medical journals. *American Medical Writers Association Journal, 38*(2), 13–21. https://doi.org/10.55752/amwa.2023.249

Perkel, J. M. (2020, April 2). Collaborative writing: Beyond Google docs. *Nature, 580,* 154–155. https://media.nature.com/original/magazine-assets/d41586-020-00916-6/d41586-020-00916-6.pdf

Phillippi, J. C., Likis F. E., & Tilden, E. L. (2018). Authorship grids: Practical tools to facilitate ethical publication. *Research in Nursing & Health, 41*(2), 195–208. https://doi.org/10.1002/nur.21856

Pinker, S. (2015). *The sense of style: The thinking person's guide to writing in the 21st century.* Penguin Books.

Resnick, B., Boltz, M., Galik, E., Kuzmik, A., Drazich, B. F., McPherson, R., & Wells, C. L. (2023). Factors associated with function-focused care among hospitalized older adults with dementia. *American Journal of Critical Care, 32*(4), 264–273. https://doi.org/10.4037/ajcc2023440

Ruhland, J., Dähnert, E., Zilezinski, M., & Hauss, M. (2023). Pressure injury prevention in patients in prone position with acute respiratory distress syndrome and COVID-19. *Critical Care Nurse, 43*(2), 46–54. https://doi.org/10.4037/ccn2023559

Saver, C. (2023, July). Common questions about accountability partners. *American Nurse Journal.* https://www.myamericannurse.com/common-questions-about-writing-accountability-partners/

Saver, C., & Cullen, J. (2021). Two sides of editorial queries: Editors and authors. *Nurse Author & Editor, 31*(1), 5–9. https://doi.org/10.1111/nae2.14

Shellenbarger, T., & Chicca, J. (2020). More meaningful meetings. *American Nurse Journal, 15*(4), 22–24. https://www.myamericannurse.com/more-meaningful-meetings/

Shellenbarger, T., & Robb, M. (2015). Collaborative writing: Strategies to promote successful shared authorship. *Nurse Author & Editor, 25*(2), 1–8. http://naepub.com/student-authorship/2015-25-2-4/

Silvia, P. J. (2007). *How to write a lot: A practical guide to productive academic writing.* American Psychological Association.

Silvia, P. J. (2015). *Write it up: Practical strategies for writing and publishing journal articles.* American Psychological Association.

Silvia, P. J. (2019). *How to write a lot: A practical guide to productive academic writing* (2nd ed.). American Psychological Association.

Stephens, T. M. (2019). Building personal resilience. *American Nurse Journal, 14*(8), 10–15. https://www.myamericannurse.com/building-personal-resilience/

Suttle, R., Armstrong, G., Headrick, L., Miltner, R., Ogrinc, G. (2023). Key strategies to publishing your quality improvement work. *The Joint Commission Journal on Quality and Patients Safety, 29*(12), 706–711. https://doi.org/10.1016/j.jcjq.2023.08.002

Thurston, M. M., Moniri, N. H., Bown, J. P., Winkles, C. L., & Miller, S. W. (2023). Managing the "three Cs" of academic literature authorship: Contributions, credit, and conflict. *American Journal of Pharmaceutical Education, 87*(5). https://doi.org/10.1016/j.ajpe.2022.10.002

Truss, L. (2011). *Eats, shoots & leaves: The zero tolerance approach to punctuation.* Avery.

Tscharntke, T., Hochberg, M. E., Rand, T. A., Resh, V. H., & Krauss, J. (2007). Author sequence and credit for contributions in multiauthored publications. *PLoS Biology, 5*(1), e18. https://doi.org/10.1371/journal.pbio.0050018

Vicens, Q., & Bourne, P. E. (2007). Ten simple rules for a successful collaboration. *PLoS Computational Biology*, *3*(3), e44. https://doi.org/10.1371/journal.pcbi.0030044

Vogel, M. T., Blakeney, E. A-R., Willgerodt, M. A., Odegard, P. S., Johnson, E. L., Shrader, S., Liner, D., Dyer, C. A., Hall, L. W., & Zierler, B. (n.d.). *Interprofessional team writing toolkit*. University of Washington Center for Health Sciences Interprofessional Education, Research and Practice. https://collaborate.uw.edu/programs/team-science-initiative/interprofessional-team-writing-toolkit/

Vogel, M. T., Blakeney, E. A-R., Willgerodt, M. A., Odegard, P. S., Johnson, E. L., Shrader, S., Liner, D., Dyer, C. A., Hall, L. W., & Zierler, B. (2019). Interprofessional education and practice guide: Interprofessional team writing to promote dissemination of interprofessional education scholarship and products. *Journal of Interprofessional Care, 33*(5), 406–413. https://doi.org/10.1080/13561820.2018.1538111

Wu, K. J. (2021, May 18). The body's most embarrassing organ is an evolutionary marvel. *The Atlantic*. https://www.theatlantic.com/science/archive/2021/05/evolution-butts/618915/

Yilmaz, Y., Gottlieb, M., Haas, M. R. C., Thoma, B, & Chan, T. M. Remote collaborative writing: A guide to writing within a virtual community of practice. (2022). *Journal of Graduate Medical Education, 14*(3), 256–259. https://doi.org/10.4300/JGME-D-21-01108.1

Zinsser, W. (2016). *On writing well: The classic guide to writing nonfiction* (30th anniversary ed.). Harper Perennial.

Finding, Refining, and Defining a Topic

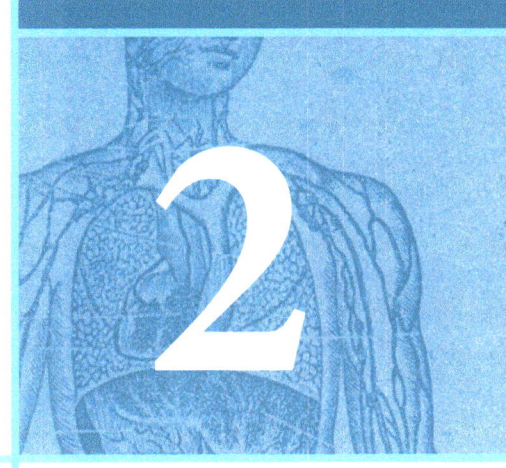

–Patricia Dwyer Schull, MSN, BS
–Cynthia Saver, MS, RN

WHAT YOU'LL LEARN IN THIS CHAPTER

- A three-step process can help you develop your topic.
- Mind maps and summary statements are useful for focusing and evaluating a topic.
- Use author guidelines to develop specifications for your article.

"Get a good idea, and stay with it.
Dog it, and work at it until it's done, and done right."
–Walt Disney

Every good article starts with a good idea. Finding the right topic, and then refining and defining it, makes writing easier. The right topic serves as the nervous system for your article; just as your brain, spinal column, and nerves keep you balanced, the right topic keeps you steady on your writing course and guides the entire creation of your article. This chapter describes a three-step process for developing a topic: finding your topic, refining your topic, and defining your topic.

Finding a Topic

A question first-time authors might ask is simply: What should I write about? Picking a topic requires thought and effort. If you plan to publish a study you just completed or you want to write about a recent important clinical experience on a topic you have expertise in, you have an easy answer. But what if you don't have a specific idea? The good news is that ideas are all around you: in your life, your practice, the literature you read—even your local news.

Think about how you would handle an emergency situation during your everyday practice. It's automatic, right? First, you assess the situation. The same applies to writing: Assess your motivation for writing an article. When you write down your thoughts and ideas in an organized and systematic fashion, it causes you to describe them more fully and coherently. Just as in nursing, practice makes perfect. The more times you work through the exercise of defining your idea, the easier it will become.

Use the questions shown in Figure 2.1 (these questions are described in detail in the following sections) to conduct your assessment. Write your responses to each question in the space provided.

Why Should I Write an Article?

As a practitioner or expert in your field, writing and sharing your ideas with professional colleagues can be a good way to increase your professional recognition, career opportunities, and advancement. You will also gain personal satisfaction and improve your confidence. We need to share our knowledge with our colleagues so we can learn from each other and build the best evidence to improve patient outcomes, further validating the nursing profession and what nurses do day to day. In essence, we have a duty to disseminate our knowledge.

Now that you are thinking about disseminating knowledge, consider what knowledge you have to share. What is your area of expertise? Is there a

Assessment

Why should I write an article? _____

Who will read my article? _____

What interests me? _____

What might interest others the most? _____

What can others learn from what I'm doing? _____

What is happening at work or in my specialty? _____

What writing style should I use for a topic? _____

What is the best timing for my article? _____

What publication is right for my article? _____

FIGURE 2.1 Writing assessment worksheet.

new procedure that your hospital is doing? Have you implemented a new hospital-to-home transition policy that is highly effective? Have you recently presented an in-service that you had to research and develop? What are common knowledge deficits that you have the expertise to correct? For example, perhaps you have noticed that many of your colleagues lack the knowledge to identify patients who harm themselves. You are passionate about helping these patients, so last year you honed your skills through research and by listening to webinars on the topic of self-harm or mutilation, which led to you identifying several colleagues who needed to learn more about this issue. Now you're ready to pass on your knowledge to others.

Who Will Read My Article?

Be clear about who the reader—the audience—is. Knowing who reads a journal, magazine, blog, or book will make it easier for you to write an article that the publication's audience will find useful. For example, is the reader a clinical staff nurse? A student? A critical care nurse? A nurse practitioner? A researcher? An educator? A manager? Don't make the mistake of writing before knowing the answer; otherwise, you'll have to rework your writing—or your article will be rejected. For example, an article on managing Stage 4 pressure injuries in patients with diabetes will be developed differently when intended for staff nurses, as opposed to nurse practitioners.

What Interests Me?

It's often best to write about topics you are most familiar with and enjoy working in, especially at the start of your efforts. What area(s) are you most knowledgeable and experienced in? Are you an expert? What do you have an interest in? Have you had an interesting patient experience recently? These questions are starting places for deciding what you could write about. Your experience, expertise, or interest in the topic will sustain you through planning, researching, writing, and revising. Editors often look for the voice of experience from an author. Keep in mind, however, that you don't have to be widely published to be an "expert." If you have cared for patients with chronic obstructive pulmonary disease (COPD) for 10 years, for example, you have developed expertise in areas such as oxygen therapy, nebulizer and inhaled medications, and smoking cessation. On the other hand, if you're interested in something that you don't have expertise in, it's best to work with a coauthor who is knowledgeable about the topic.

What Might Interest Others the Most?

Nurse editors and publishers spend a lot of time talking to nurses about what core topics interest them. For clinical journals, those topics usually include drugs, emergency situations, and care related to patients with common medical conditions. Clinical experiences or case studies on these topics are often sought after by editors. Also always of interest are any new breakthroughs or controversies related to diseases, treatments, and best practices. Keep up by reading articles currently published on your topic and searching general nursing journals, as well as journals specific to your topic area, and by following what is being presented at regional and national conferences. Note what specifics are included in these sources, especially any new information.

Q *I emailed an editor of a popular nursing journal suggesting what I thought was a high-interest topic idea. She sent me a reply saying they'd just published an article on the same topic. What should I do to avoid this in the future?*

A Subscribe to the journal (or other type of publication or website you are targeting) or access it online or at the library. Before you send an idea (a query) to an editor, make sure you know what that journal has published in the past six months or more. Better yet, do an online search to see whether the journal has published an article on a similar topic and what the approach was. Then, modify your focus to include how your article will differ and pitch your idea accordingly.

You might think that common topics aren't as interesting as uncommon ones, but that's not always true. Common topics involve the most prevalent disease states (e.g. COPD, diabetes, cardiovascular disease, and cancer) and their treatments. Healthcare professionals spend most of their time caring for patients with these diseases, so interest is high for these topics—both with readers and editors of general clinical nursing journals. And don't forget hot topics that relate to patient safety and urgent situations, such as an emergency event or the latest disease epidemic. For example, journals were highly interested in articles related to COVID-19 during the pandemic, and interest in articles related to the long-term impact of COVID-19 and implications for nursing care remains high.

> **From the Editor's Perspective**
>
> What makes a good idea? Thinking like an editor will help you choose a topic more likely to be accepted for publication. Here are some questions that an editor considers when evaluating your idea. Is your idea:
>
> - New?
> - Timely?
> - Relevant to the publication's readers?
> - Interesting?
> - Controversial?
> - Consistent with the publication's mission?

You might also consider a literature review or synthesis of material already published to help readers gain a broader understanding of a topic or to summarize evidence-based interventions. For example, you could summarize and analyze effective techniques for motivational interviewing, which encourages changes in behavior to improve health outcomes.

What Can Others Learn From What I'm Doing?

Nurses often seek ways to improve what they're already doing. Perhaps your specialty is diabetes, and you have developed a detailed protocol for helping patients with a new insulin pump, or you specialize in critically ill neonates and have expertise in caring for infants with neonatal abstinence syndrome. Or maybe you fine-tuned a proposal that addresses the management of community healthcare programs or conducted a survey with interesting results. You might assume that your new methods or fresh discoveries are of interest only to those in your immediate environment, but having your findings published can help others learn from you and build on your findings.

What Is Happening at Work or in My Specialty?

When you're looking for a journal topic, concentrate on the problems, issues, challenges, and trends that your colleagues speak of or write about most often. Access websites and social media posts focused on your specialty for topics of interest; look for repeated comments or questions on discussion forums. While there, read the featured topic presentations and overviews for recent or upcoming meetings, because these tend to present the most popular topics and latest developments in a field. Reading abstracts and overviews of the presentations will help you to narrow your focus by deciding what aspects of your topic to include. Many national associations post abstracts from previous meetings online. Because there is a lag time between a new innovation and its publication in a journal, this information might help you discover a topic not yet published. Take note of the presenters and consider one of them as a possible coauthor or mentor.

Don't ignore the general media when looking for trends and issues. *The Wall Street Journal* and *The New York Times* both frequently publish articles in print and online about new developments in healthcare. And the National Institute of Health website is a reliable and accurate source for current health information and, therefore, topic ideas.

Q *I have an idea, but what is the best way to research what others have written about it?*

A Many excellent sources of nursing publications and literature are available, including CINAHL (Cumulative Index to Nursing and Allied Health Literature), Ovid, Scopus, and PubMed (https://pubmed.ncbi.nlm.nih.gov). PubMed alone has more than 36 million citations from MEDLINE, life science journals, and online books. Citations can include links to full-text articles from PubMed Central (https://www.ncbi.nlm.nih.gov/pmc) and to publisher websites. Not all nursing publications are listed in this database, so look at other sources, such as the *Nurse Author & Editor* and International Academy of Nurse Editors' list of vetted nursing journals (https://nursingeditors.com/journals-directory). You also can use general search engines such as Google (www.google.com) and Google Scholar (http://scholar.google.com). Learn more about finding information in Chapter 4.

What Writing Style Should I Use for a Topic?

After you decide on a topic, you need to know whether your topic, expertise, and writing style are best suited for a scholarly or a clinical how-to journal, a soft piece (a human-interest story about a past experience), a case study, or a healthcare–related piece for consumers. If your expertise, for example, lends itself to a hands-on, practical article that focuses on useful information that helps readers deal with problems they face, then by all means plan to write a piece for the clinical or consumer markets. The specific tone of the article depends on the type of publication. For example, an article for *Nursing Research*, a scholarly journal, will be written in a different style than one for *American Nurse Journal*, which is clinically focused. Nursing journals often use *Publication Manual of the American Psychological Association* (APA, 2020) or the American Medical Association (AMA) style guide, *AMA Manual of Style: A Guide For Authors and Editors* (JAMA Network Editors, 2020). Keep in mind that the style and format of text and reference citations are essential for manuscript acceptance in scholarly journals.

What Is the Best Timing for My Article?

If you are writing a blog post or an article that will be quickly published online, you need to be timely. For example, if your organization developed a new protocol for assisting victims of a recent national disaster, you would want to write about it quickly. Timing considerations apply in print, too. If, for instance, your operating room is one of the few sites doing an innovative procedure, you would want to get the word out before it becomes more common in practice.

The bottom line: No one wants to read about a topic that is dated.

What Publication Is Right for My Article?

You need to know the publisher's mission, audience, types of articles published, manuscript format, and editorial process. Most journals have an editor who acts as the major decision-maker for what is considered acceptable. Keep in mind that some journal staffs spend considerable time editing, rewriting, and copyediting. In these cases, it's your clinical knowledge and expertise that interest the publisher, not necessarily your writing ability. But others don't—meaning that some journals require a fairly well-written initial submission and will provide only light copyediting and proofreading. In Chapter 3, you can read more about selecting the appropriate publisher for your work.

Q *Do journals and other publications publish lists of the topics that they are interested in?*

A Check the publication's author guidelines to see whether they specify desired types of topics. You should also search online for "call for manuscripts," "call for papers," or "call for topics" in journals— these alert you to what the editor needs for an upcoming issue with a special focus. Some journals also publish an annual editorial calendar that lists issue themes. If you see something of interest, a query letter to the editor is usually appreciated and sometimes required. Send your letter several months in advance of the issue you are interested in because editors plan ahead. (Learn more about query letters in Chapter 3.)

Refining a Topic

Now that you have answered the questions related to finding a topic, identify a topic that you want to explore further. Keep this topic in mind while you move to the next step—refining your topic.

With a working knowledge of your topic, you can begin your research by reviewing the literature for current and new information to start refining your idea. Reading articles related to the topic, especially those that are particularly interesting, factual, and well written, will help you better understand where your idea fits. While you're analyzing your topic area, check for the number of citations your search yields— a good indication of the depth of interest and coverage. Remember to review titles in the reference list for ideas on what specifics within the topic you might focus on.

When your research is completed, consider how the article you want to write can provide information that fills a void or offers a new perspective. Don't despair if your search turns up several articles within your expertise on what you thought was a unique topic. You might be able to take the topic and refocus it to a more specific discussion. For example, if you look for articles on neurological assessment, the sheer number might deter you from thinking that this would be a good topic. But differentiating or assessing a cerebrovascular accident versus a transient ischemic attack will narrow the scope of your article. Or, you might find that few articles on neurological assessment target a specific group of patients, such as children or those with dementia. Looking at popular topics from new angles provides you with the opportunity to revisit the topic of neurological assessment in a new light.

Focus Your Topic

Part of refining your topic is ensuring it is focused and not too broad. Writing about the patient with diabetes undergoing surgery could fill a book, but strategies for managing hypoglycemia in the outpatient surgical patient would be a topic that a standard journal article could accommodate. Although focusing usually involves narrowing a topic, that's not always the case. Sometimes you also have to turn the topic around a bit and focus on an aspect that is new, different, or unseen. For example, you could adjust the topic "the benefits/advantages of manual chest percussion for the patient with chronic obstructive pulmonary disease" to "the benefits of manual percussion versus mechanical percussors."

Mind mapping is an excellent tool to focus your topic. It helps you identify and understand the structure of a subject and how the main topics fit together. Further, it taps into how your brain works by allowing your thoughts to flow freely. First, you start with a central idea or a main topic in the middle of a large sheet of paper (Mind Tools, n.d.). Then you add branches and sub-branches to further represent subtopics and your ideas. You can then look at relationships to see possible linkages.

When you examine your topic, remember that it's brainstorming time. Don't critique your thoughts—just write down everything related to your topic, including ancillary ideas and research. This step should be the fun part; use colored pencils or markers to stimulate your creativity or to prioritize subtopics.

For example, start with the broad topic of Managing Heart Failure. The topic on its own is too large for most journals, but a mind map can be used to develop several subtopics, such as assessment, diagnostic tests, and differential diagnoses (see Figure 2.2). Based on

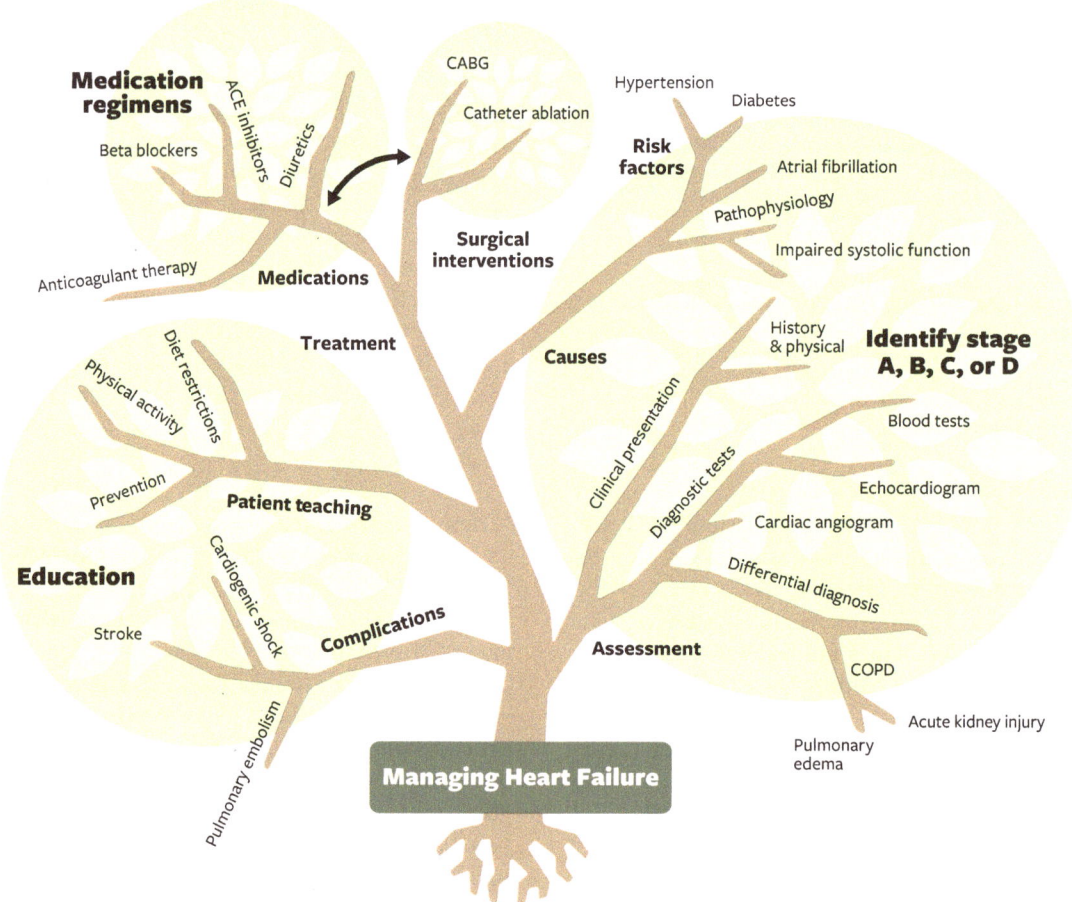

FIGURE 2.2 A mind map can help you visually analyze your topic and shed new light on how you might focus it.

this breakdown, options for possible articles include diagnosing heart failure, managing medication regimens, and nursing care related to surgical interventions. The final decision based on the results of a mind map will depend on what your earlier research revealed about your topic and the length of a typical article in your target publication.

You might also try other techniques for creating a successful mind map. Use single words or simple phrases and then draw lines to show linkages. On a separate sheet of paper, keep track of new concepts you think of while looking at these relationships and where they might fit. You might even find a new phrase or name for a concept that provides a solid foundation for your paper.

If you're technology-oriented, consider using a digital tool for your mind map, such as MindMeister, GitMind, Creately, and Coggle (Aston, 2023; Saigal, 2023). Many offer a free version with limited functionality, which may include the ability to download your map as a PDF so you can share it with others.

Most writers struggle with narrowing a topic, but it's also possible to choose a topic that is so narrow, it doesn't have wide enough applicability. For example, post-traumatic stress disorder in children who are in first grade is probably too narrow; post-traumatic stress disorder in elementary school–aged children would be better.

Scope of applicability is an essential part of evaluating any topic. Journal editors frequently report receiving articles about quality improvement projects that relate only to the author's organization and can't be replicated in other situations. (Learn more about writing articles about quality improvement projects that may qualify for publication in Chapter 16.)

Confidence Booster

Nurses are taught to write short, brief notes, so making the transition to writing an article can be challenging. The next time you're feeling discouraged, read the bios for some of the authors in the publication you're targeting. Chances are, you'll see many of them come from work settings similar to your own. They found a way to make the transition, and so can you!

Write and Test a Summary Statement

After you have your topic sufficiently focused or you think you might be on the right track, you can see whether it works on paper. Write one sentence that summarizes the article. Think of your sentence like a goal statement in a patient care plan. The statement should include the purpose and target audience for the article (be specific). For example, consider some sample original summary statements and notice how the revised statements are more specific than the original.

Original statement: This chapter covers how to pick a topic for an article.

Revised statement: This chapter explains how a nurse new to publishing should find, refine, and define a topic for publication.

Original statement: This article discusses the newest antihypertensive drugs.

Revised statement: This article provides staff nurses with an overview of three new antihypertensive drugs including pharmacokinetics, indications, dosage, adverse effects, contraindications, and patient education.

After you write your own summary statement, test its effectiveness by answering the question: Does it pass the "So what?" test? Although you might know what you want to accomplish, you must be sure that readers will be able to answer the question "So what?" with a response that has meaning to them in their professional or personal lives. Share your summary statement with those you want to read your article to see if it resonates with them or needs to be further revised (Saver, 2023).

Q *The peer reviewers for my manuscript for a general nursing journal said it wasn't relevant to clinical nurses. How can I refocus it?*

A It sounds like you didn't fully answer the "So what?" question before you wrote your article. Double back and ask it again. Check with your target audience to determine what is important to them and then see how your topic could be refined to better relate to their practice. You might try writing statements to answer the "So what?" question. Soon you will be back on track.

Defining a Topic

Now that you have focused your topic, you're ready to further define it with specifications and an outline.

Determine Specifications

By now, you have determined what kind of article you're writing—research, case study, or how-to, for example—and what sort of publication you're going to target—say, a general nursing magazine versus a specialty nursing journal. Now you need to check the publisher's author guidelines for the publication you are considering. (See Chapter 1 and Chapter 5 for more information about types of articles and Chapter 3 for more information on how to select a publication.)

Author guidelines detail what the publisher expects to see in a submission, including length of your piece (in words or both words and pages), and will usually offer suggestions as well as expectations for other main features of your submission, such as figures, tables, and illustration. Following the author guidelines will increase the likelihood your article will be suitable for the publication you are targeting, which, in turn, increases the likelihood it will be accepted for publication.

About Author Guidelines

Think of author guidelines as the policies and procedures for the publication. You'll want to read the author guidelines to ensure you write and submit your article correctly. As a nurse, if you switch from one organization to another, you refer to the new organization's policies and procedures to ensure your clinical practice is in alignment with them. That's why it's important to read the author guidelines for each publication you submit to. Don't assume that Journal A will have the same requirements as Journal B (Saver, 2020).

Here is a list of what is typically included in the author guidelines:

- Types of articles published and any regular departments. Regular departments, such as case studies and drug updates, are often an ideal entry point for a new author because they are usually shorter pieces, and the editor needs to have content for each issue.

- Whether the publication adheres to certain standards related to the type of manuscript you are submitting. For example, some journals require use of the Standards for QUality Improvement Reporting (SQUIRE) guidelines (Ogrinc et al., 2015) for quality improvement reports.

- Editorial standards the journal adheres to. For example, many nursing journals follow the International Committee of Medical Journal Editors (ICMJE) criteria for authorship (2024).

- Editorial style the publisher uses. Many academic journals follow the APA or the AMA style format, while your city magazine might use The Associated Press Stylebook (The Associated Press, 2022).

- How to prepare your manuscript, including format, length, sidebars, tables, figures, and references.

- How to submit your manuscript, including cover letter, contact information, author names, affiliations and credentials, and the publisher's submission process. Many of the major publishers use online editorial management systems such as ScholarOne or Editorial Manager to improve efficiencies of journal processes, including manuscript submission.

- What happens to your manuscript after submission, including confirmation of receipt, the peer-review process, and (if your article is accepted) the editing process.

Take time to read—and follow—the author guidelines to avoid delay (e.g., some journals will require you to fix references in the wrong format before sending your article for peer review) and possible rejection (a topic that doesn't fit with the publication's mission.)

You can locate author guidelines on the publisher's website. Look under "Submissions," "Author guidelines" (or "Information for authors"), or even "Contact us." Typically, author guidelines are available in a PDF or other downloadable file. If you can't find them on the website, try a broader Google search.

Most journal publishers will reject a manuscript if your submission doesn't conform to the basics:

- Importance, timeliness, and relevance of the topic
- Sufficient rationale for the topic and/or literature review
- Logical organization of ideas and thoroughness of presentation
- Congruence between the questions or issues investigated and implications/conclusions stated
- Clarity and consistency of writing
- Adherence to the publisher's editorial style guide

Having a clear focus on the specifics of your planned article will help you craft a more effective query letter and write a better article after your topic is approved for submission.

Draft an Outline

Your next step is to create an outline of your article. The outline may seem like a throwback to junior high English class, but in reality, it will guide you through the writing process. Just like a care pathway is a plan for a patient, an outline is a plan for an article. At this stage, forget about rules, such as every Roman numeral I must have at least a Roman numeral II beneath it. Instead, organize your thoughts into broad categories, expanding on what you came up with in the mind-mapping exercise.

To begin, put your summary statement at the top of the outline to serve as a touchstone while you write. Make a rough outline of your topic, writing down each major section with a topic sentence. After you have your major topics listed, you can organize them into an orderly flow of information by adding appropriate headings and subheads, helping the reader to understand each topic in a logical order. Include any tables, figures, or illustrations in each section as appropriate.

Figure 2.3 shows a short example of an outline that you would flesh out as you developed your article.

If you have difficulties with creating an outline, you may want to try an artificial intelligence (AI) program to help you organize your thoughts. When using these programs, you need to make your instructions, or "prompt," as specific as possible. For example, typing in the prompt "Please write a content outline for an article that tells critical care nurses how to identify a patient with pulmonary embolism" into an AI chatbot yields better results than "Please write a content outline about pulmonary embolism," which results in a less focused outline. One possible usefulness of AI for developing the content outline is that it may help identify content areas that you have overlooked.

At this stage of development, avoid using AI to write your article because of the many problems (e.g., inaccuracies, plagiarism, irrelevance, and bias) that can occur (Hosseini et al., 2023; ICJME, 2024; Kacena et al, 2024). If you do use AI in preparing an aspect of your work (e.g., data collection, data analysis, figure generation), you need to disclose that when you submit the article (Flanagin et al., 2024; Hosseini et al., 2023; ICJME, 2024; International Society for Medical Publication Professionals, 2024).

The Value of a Good Idea

It's important to take time in the beginning of your writing project to find a topic that you feel passionate about. Finding the right topic and approach will sustain you throughout the project. If you're working on a book proposal, your topic will guide you on the next steps of your journey. If you're preparing a journal article, it will help you choose a journal and prepare a query letter. And if you're submitting an idea to a magazine, an online-only publication, a blog, or a newsletter, you'll be ready to send a query letter to the editor.

Subsequent chapters provide detailed information about how to further organize your article, create good flow, and supplement or enhance your article with such tools as tables, graphs, and illustrations. Starting with a good idea, though, will give you the wings you need to launch you on a successful writing career.

Write Now!

1. Identify an idea for an article.
2. Use a mind map to narrow the focus of your idea.
3. Write a summary statement.
4. Create an outline.

Summary statement: This article tells nurses how to identify a patient with pulmonary embolism (PE) by assessing clinical presentation, diagnostic test results, and ruling out differential diagnoses.

I. **Introduction** (Importance of prompt diagnosis and presentation of a case situation)

II. **Clinical presentation** (How does the patient with PE present?)

    Relevant history (e.g., risk factors)

    Signs and symptoms
        Abrupt onset of pleuritic chest pain
        Shortness of breath
        Hypoxia
        Anxiety
        Possible atypical or no symptoms

    Physical examination (common findings)
        Tachypnea, tachycardia
        Fever
        Rales
        Heart sound abnormalities

III. **Diagnostic tests** (What results indicate PE?)

    Laboratory tests such as:
        D-dimer testing
        Arterial blood gases
        Serum troponin level

    Imaging studies, such as:
        Computed tomography angiography
        Pulmonary angiography
        Chest radiography
        Electrocardiogram
        MRI
        Echocardiography

IV. **Differential diagnoses** (What else could this be? Focus on more common ones)

    Myocardial infarction

    Acute pericarditis

    Fat embolism

    Atrial fibrillation

V. **Conclusion** (What two or three key points should nurses remember?)

    Hallmark signs and symptoms

    Importance of nursing role in prompt diagnosis

FIGURE 2.3 Sample outline.

References

American Psychological Association. (2020). *Publication manual of the American Psychological Association* (7th ed.). https://doi.org/10.1037/0000165-000

The Associated Press. (2022). *The Associated Press stylebook: 2022–2024* (56th ed.). Basic Books.

Aston, B. (2023, Jan. 1). 10 best mind mapping software to plan projects in 2023. *DPM.* https://thedigitalprojectmanager.com/tools/mind-mapping-software/

Flanagin, A., Pirrachio, R., Khera, R., Berkwits, M., Hswen, Y., & Bibbens-Domingo, K. (2024). Reporting use of AI in research and scholarly publication—JAMA Network guidance [Editorial]. *JAMA.* https://jamanetwork.com/journals/jama/fullarticle/2816213

Hosseini, M., Rasmussen, L. M., & Resnik, D. B. (2023). Using AI to write scholarly publications [Editorial]. *Accountability in Research.* https://doi.org/10.1080/08989621.2023.2168535

International Committee of Medical Journal Editors. (2024). *Recommendations for the conduct, reporting, editing, and publication of scholarly work in medical journals.* http://www.icmje.org/recommendations

International Society for Medical Publication Professionals. (2024, Jan. 3). International Society for Medical Publication Professionals (ISMPP) position statement and call to action on artificial intelligence. *Current Medical Research and Opinion.* https://doi.org/10.1080/03007995.2023.2273139

JAMA Network Editors. (2020). *AMA manual of style: A guide for authors and editors* (11th ed.). Oxford University Press.

Kacena, M. A., Plotkin, L. I., & Fehrenbacher, J. C. (2024). The use of artificial intelligence in writing scientific review articles. *Current Osteoporosis Reports.* https://doi.org/10.1007/s11914-023-00852-0

Mind Tools. (n.d.). *Mind Maps: A powerful approach to note-taking.* http://www.mindtools.com/pages/article/newISS_01.htm

Ogrinc, G., Davies, L., Goodman, D., Batalden, P., Davidoff, F., & Stevens, D. (2015). SQUIRE 2.0 (Standards for QUality Improvement Reporting Excellence): Revised publication guidelines from a detailed consensus process. *BMJ Quality & Safety, 25,* 986–992. https://doi.org/10.1136/bmjqs-2015-004411

Saigal, R. (2023, July 18). The 7 best free mind map tools (and how to best use them). *Make Use Of.* https://www.makeuseof.com/tag/8-free-mind-map-tools-best-use/

Saver, C. (2020, Feb. 24). Why author guidelines matter. *American Nurse Journal.* https://www.myamericannurse.com/why-author-guidelines-matter/

Saver, C. (2023, May 19). Summing up your article in one statement: A powerful writing tool. *American Nurse Journal.* https://www.myamericannurse.com/summing-up-your-article-in-one-statement-a-powerful-writing-tool/

How to Select and Query a Publication

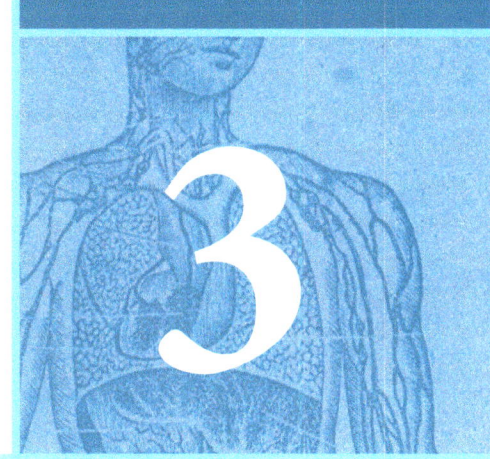

–Cynthia Saver, MS, RN

"A word after a word after a word is power."
—Margaret Atwood

WHAT YOU'LL LEARN IN THIS CHAPTER

- Use the five rights to choose a publication for your article idea.
- Be alert to the danger of predatory journals.
- A query should promote your idea and why you should be the one to write about it.
- Match the tone of the query to the tone of the publication.

When you choose a dressing for a wound, you carefully weigh the options to determine the best match for the patient. For example, you would never put a transparent film dressing on a wound with a lot of exudate—it just wouldn't do the job.

In the same way, you need to carefully select the publication, such as a journal, where you want your article to appear. After you decide that, you should see whether the publication editor accepts queries or reviews manuscripts only after they've been submitted. If the editor is open to a query, your next step is to prepare a *query letter* (ironically, sent via email) to see whether they are interested in the article. But first, take a look at what goes into selecting the best publication fit for your idea.

Q *Is the term "journal" limited to peer-reviewed, academic, scholarly, text-heavy publications?*

A Journals vary in appearance and tone. Some journals look more like magazines, even though they publish scholarly or evidence-based material. The term *journal* is a broad one, which means that more and more nursing information is accessible to more and more nurses. Although this chapter uses *journal* because most nurses are familiar with the term, the principles discussed also apply to other publications. For example, as you read, you'll see you can often substitute *publication*, *website*, or *newsletter* for the word *journal*. Consider many outlets for your writing. (You can learn more about these outlets in Chapter 21.)

Finding a Journal

The good news for authors is that there are more than 270 nursing journals in the Directory of Nursing Journals (https://nursingeditors.com/journals-directory), a vetted list from the International Academy of Nurse Editors (INANE) and the publication *Nurse Author & Editor*. While not an all-inclusive list, it shows that you have many opportunities for getting published. The easiest place to start is your own mailbox (physical or online) with the journals you currently receive and know the most about. You might also take a trip to a local nursing school's library—or, if you are fortunate to have one, your organization's medical library. In addition to the INANE site, you can visit these sites to see the wide range of available journals:

- **Directory of Open Access Journals** (https://www.doaj.org/about): Lists open-access journals from around the world; you can search by keyword such as "nursing." ("Open access" is discussed later in this chapter.) The Enago Open Access Journal Finder (https://www.enago.com/academy/journal-finder) uses this directory to enable authors to search for open-access journals by pasting their abstract into a search box.
- **Cumulative Index to Nursing and Allied Health Literature (CINAHL;** https://www.ebsco.com/products/research-databases/cinahl-database): One of the most helpful for nurses, CINAHL is accessed through EBSCO. You can download an Excel file or view in HTML a list of journals covered in CINAHL.
- **EBSCO** (https://www.ebsco.com/title-lists): As with CINAHL, you can download an Excel file or view in HTML a list of journals for a specific area.
- **PLOS** (http://www.plos.org): Publishes a suite of open-access journals, with *PLOS Medicine* the most applicable for nurses.
- **National Center for Biotechnology Information (NCBI;** https://www.ncbi.nlm.nih.gov/nlmcatalog/journals): Contains journals indexed in the NCBI databases, which includes PubMed; keep in mind that not all quality nursing journals are indexed here.
- **ScienceDirect** (https://www.sciencedirect.com/browse/journals-and-books): Includes more than 4,700 journals; you can search by keyword such as "nursing."
- **Scopus** (https://www.elsevier.com/products/scopus/content#4-titles-on-scopus): Includes a large number of journals.
- **Web of Science** (https://mjl.clarivate.com/home): Indexes a wide range of journals.

Many of these are more helpful for interprofessional topics than for nursing topics, but they provide more options beyond the INANE directory. Some require a subscription; in that case, you might be able to access through your organization's library. Keep in mind that it's not enough to simply find a journal; you want to be sure you choose the right journal for your topic.

Choosing the Right Journal

Choosing the right journal is just as important as choosing a partner for a project. Start by considering your goals. One goal of writing might be to reach the widest possible audience. Another might be to direct your information specifically at a narrow target audience of nurses. At the same time, you want to do everything possible to boost the likelihood an editor will be interested in your idea. That includes analyzing your possible journal selection with a critical eye.

Like the traditional "rights of medication administration" (right medication, right patient, right dose, right time, right route, and right documentation), these "rights of choosing a journal" should help you make the best decision.

When selecting the right journal for your idea, ask yourself whether each potential journal has the right:

- Audience
- Access
- Timing
- Review process
- Metrics

Completing this analysis will help you match your idea with the best journal. You can find most of the information you need on the journal's website in the "about" and author guidelines (also called information for authors) sections.

Right Audience

Who are you trying to reach with your article? If you want to reach clinicians, choose a journal that appeals to them directly (Wiley, 2019). Articles in clinical journals are typically shorter, include easy-to-read features—such as boxes and bullet points—and include a clear link of the information to clinical practice. If you want to reach researchers, scholarly journals (also called academic journals) might be more appropriate. *Scholarly journals* tend to have longer articles as well as a specific structure for research reports. They primarily reach nurses in academic and research settings. In some cases, non-scholarly journals also will publish research, but they tend to focus more on practice.

Know that these differences are a bit arbitrary. Clinicians read scholarly journals, for example, when they are working on evidence-based projects. And researchers read clinical journals to learn about the latest innovations and application. The terms are simply a way of locating your primary target audience.

Sometimes you might have more than one audience for your article. For instance, you recently completed a research study on a new suctioning technique for an intensive care unit (ICU) patient on mechanical ventilation. Those who would benefit from reading your study include critical care nurse researchers, critical care staff nurses, and critical care educators, among others. Immediately, you know that your article should appear in a critical care journal, but to target an editor, you need to narrow the options. If you want to reach critical care nurse researchers and staff nurses, a good choice might be *Critical Care Nurse* (*CCN*), a journal packed with research studies related to clinical practice. Another option might be *Dimensions in Critical Care Nursing*. One advantage of *CCN* is that it is from the American Association of Critical-Care Nurses, which gives you guaranteed access to members of the large specialty association.

What if your article relates to suctioning of ICU patients with heart failure? In that case, you might choose *Heart & Lung: The Journal of Cardiopulmonary and Acute Care*, the official publication of the American Association of Heart Failure Nurses. Although the audience for the latter journal is decidedly smaller, you are directly targeting the nurses who need your information the most.

Right Access

Publishing is partly a numbers game. For example, you narrow your possible journals to three, all of which seem to fit well with your manuscript. Checking each journal's circulation number, typically found in the "about" section on the journal's website or in marketing materials, gives you more information to help you make your decision.

Consider that *Journal A* is published every month and has a circulation of 15,000 nurses—that's 180,000 possible readers in a year. *Journal B* is published every month and has a circulation of 10,000 nurses—that means 120,000 annual possible readers. *Journal C* is published quarterly, with a circulation of 15,000, making the total possible hits 60,000. In this case, *Journal A* would give you the best opportunity for reaching the most nurses with your information and would be the best pick of the three journals that fit with your topic. Generally, journals and magazines that are published more frequently provide greater opportunities for publication.

Numbers are affected by more than subscribers—*access* is a key factor determining how far your message will go and how many people it will reach. According to the *HowOpenIsIt? Open Access Guide* (developed by the Scholarly Publishing and Academic Resources Coalition [SPARC], Public Library of Science, and Open Access Scholarly Publishers Association), access can be viewed as a spectrum, with open access (OA) on one end and closed access on the other (SPARC et al., 2014). *Open access* means an article is available at no charge; *closed access* means the article is available only to subscribers, those who can access a copy through a subscription database (which an organization typically pays for), or those who are willing to pay for a copy.

Factors such as reuse rights, copyrights, author posting rights, and automatic posting can vary along that spectrum. For instance, one journal might give readers access to articles when they are published, but another might restrict free access to articles to after a set time, such as six months or one year (referred to as an *embargo*). Another variation is the ability for the author to post the article on a website or a repository. Depending on the publisher, an author may be able to post the article upon acceptance, upon publication, after a specified time frame has elapsed, or not at all. The version the author will be allowed to post varies by journal and publisher. Most publishers don't allow authors to repost a PDF of the final published version of record unless it's on a university repository or personal website.

OA options continue to grow in publishing. A significant advantage of OA is that giving wider access to information can, ideally, speed implementation of changes that ultimately improve patient care. For example, nurses in settings without access to full-text articles, because their organizations can't afford a subscription to a database, would be able to read your

What Is a Preprint?

Authors may choose to submit their article to a preprint server (an online site) either before submitting it to a journal or at the same time as submission. Preprint servers, which are typically free to authors, facilitate rapid dissemination of information by making articles available for anyone to read and comment on, which provides authors feedback (American Medical Writers Association, European Medical Writers Association & International Society for Medical Publication Professionals [AMWA–EMWA–ISMPP], 2021; Gastel & Day, 2022). Authors can revise the preprint and repost the article.

However, preprints have not undergone peer review, so are not meant to be relied on to guide clinical practice (medRxiv, n.d.). Although most preprint servers have authors complete a screening checklist, authors of one study (Malički et al., 2020) found they "have little explicit guidance on issues that are important for transparency in reporting and research integrity." Factors such as these have made the role of preprints somewhat controversial. Information that turns out to be incorrect or misleading can be widely spread through social and traditional media with little follow-up to correct the original dissemination. Other issues include authors failing to make revisions and the fact that only about a third to a half of articles are ever fully published (AMWA–EMWA–ISMPP, 2021).

Check the author guidelines (sometimes called information for authors) of the journal you're targeting before posting to see if there are any instructions related to preprints. In most cases, the preprint won't affect your chances of being published, but journals might not welcome preprints or have caveats (Gastel & Day, 2022). For example, the author guidelines for *Nursing Research* state:

> We do not consider these unrefereed manuscripts [preprints] posted by an author on a preprint server to be a prior publication, provided that the following conditions are met: (a) during submission, authors must acknowledge to have placed a version of the manuscript on a preprint server deposition and provide any associated accession numbers or DOIs (Digital Object Identifier); (b) versions of a manuscript that have been altered as a result of the peer review process may not be deposited; (c) the preprint version itself cannot have been indexed in MEDLINE or PubMed; (d) upon publication, authors are responsible for updating the archived preprint with a DOI and link to the published version of the article. (*Nursing Research*, n.d.)

Preprint servers offer different licensing terms, which can affect a publisher's decision. On the other hand, many preprint servers are either run by or partially owned by traditional publishers or well-respected institutions (Schonfeld & Rieger, 2020), so journals are becoming more accepting of the practice. For example, medRxiv, which has a nursing section (https://www.medrxiv.org/collection/nursing), was founded by Cold Spring Harbor Laboratory (CSHL), Yale University, and BM. Authorea is a Wiley preprint service, and Springer Nature owns Research Square. Some preprint servers will automatically submit preprints to select journals they have partnered with.

Once an article is posted, it is considered to be published and receives a DOI number, which makes it easier for people to find. Note that not all bibliographic databases include preprints (AMWA–EMWA–ISMPP, 2021), although as part of pilot project, as of January 30, 2023, the National Library of Medicine includes preprints that acknowledge direct support from the National Institutes of Health (NIH) or have an NIH-affiliated author (and that are posted in an eligible preprint server) in PubMed (National Library of Medicine, 2023).

A link should be added to any article that is subsequently published in a traditional journal. In some cases, the preprint service will do this, but it's the author's responsibility to ensure the link is added.

work. But OA also has its detractors. Many articles on the blog "The Scholarly Kitchen" explain potential issues with OA. Watson (2019) notes that although OA has been seen as a way around what some perceived as "excessive" profits by large publishers, some OA organizations charge large amounts of money for article editing, processing, and publication.

OA articles may have great freedom from copyright restrictions. For instance, the Open Access Scholarly Publishers Association (n.d.) recommends publishers use the Creative Commons-BY license, which allows for unrestricted reuse of content, although the source work must be appropriately attributed. However, Creative Commons also has more restrictive license options, and publishers may have other copyright restrictions.

OA journals have different business models, with some including an article processing charge (APC). The fee is paid through a variety of sources, including the author's employer or affiliated institution (either through dedicated funds or through the institution's [often via the institution's library] membership arrangement with the publisher), the author's personal funds, or research funders (Borrego, 2023). A survey of more than 1,000 Springer Nature authors found that nearly half combined two or more sources to fund the APC (Monaghan et al., 2020).

Research funders, especially those supporting publicly funded research, often require that study results must be published as OA, so researchers can sometimes build publication costs into their budget. Many institutions have signed the Compact for Open-Access Publishing Equity (http://www.oacompact.org), which states that universities and funding agencies can support authors by paying fees in the same way they pay for subscriptions to journals. SHERPA Services (https://beta.sherpa.ac.uk) provides tools to help authors learn about a journal's OA policies and whether a journal complies with requirements from major funders such as Wellcome Trust, but the number of nursing journals included is limited.

Plan S, an open access initiative launched in 2018 by cOAlition S, a consortium of international funders, is designed to fast-track the OA movement (Plan S, 2023a; Singh, 2022). It originally called on its funders to mandate that all scholarly publications funded by public grants should be OA upon publication under the Creative Commons-BY license. In October 2023, cOAlition S released a proposal stating that all articles and associated peer-review reports should be OA upon publication, without authors having to pay any fees, and that authors (not publishers) should decide when and where to publish their articles (Liverpool, 2023; Plan S, 2023b).

Plan S has had more impact in Europe, but the United States government also is promoting OA. Starting in 2026, articles related to taxpayer-supported research must be freely available upon publication (Office of Science and Technology Policy, 2022).

Another factor related to access is how active the journal is in using other platforms to get the word out about what has been published. Ask:

- How often are articles in the journal mentioned in other publications or even the general media?
- How active is the journal on social media?
- Does the journal offer graphical (also call visual) abstracts, infographics, or plain-language summaries? These can be distributed via social media to extend the reach of your article, but you may need to pay development costs. (See Chapters 5, 7, and 12 for more information about graphical abstracts.)
- Does the journal offer the ability to post videos of you discussing your article (referred to as a video abstract)?
- Is the journal indexed in commonly used databases? Those in schools and healthcare organizations search these databases for information, increasing the likelihood your article will be found and shared, although many students and clinicians are now choosing instead to use major search engines such as Google Scholar.

Of course, numbers aren't everything. You should balance "who" with "how many." For example, you've completed a study on the financial impact of a program to retain new graduates and want to see it implemented in other hospitals. A good journal choice might be *Nursing Economic$*, read by nurse leaders who have the ability to green light such a program in their own organization, as opposed to *Nursing*, which probably has more subscribers, but is read by a broader audience.

Finally, be aware of *predatory* (also called fraudulent) journals. There is no universal agreement on a definition of a predatory journal, but a group of 43 participants from 10 countries and representing a wide range of stakeholders (including researchers, funders,

> ### A Primer on Publishing Business Models
>
> Understanding publishing business models can help you decide where to publish your article (Baffy et al., 2020; Linacre, 2022; Penn Libraries, 2023; SPARC et al., n.d.; Suber, 2015):
>
> - **Traditional:** Publishers earn money through subscription fees, advertising (in some cases), and by charging nonsubscribers and libraries to access articles.
>
> - **Green:** This OA model allows posting of the final edited article in a digital or an institutional repository, or, in some cases, by authors themselves through blogs or websites. (You can search for OA repositories at the website for the Directory of Open Access Repositories: www.opendoar.org.) There is no charge for the author or reader. Many universities now require faculty to deposit their research in the university repository, but the article may be embargoed until the publisher's version is printed. Preprint servers operate under this model.
>
> - **Gold:** In this open-access (OA) model, the journal makes the article freely available on publication and allows the author to retain copyright. To fund this model, many journals charge a fee (referred to as an "article processing charge" or "article publication charge" [APC] that is paid after an article is accepted for publication). Sometimes the fee is paid by the author, but it's more typically paid by the author's employer or a funder (i.e., the entity that funded the research study the article is reporting on).
>
> - **Platinum or Diamond:** The journal receives funding from grants, institutions, professional associations, and/or foundations, so the authors don't pay a fee and articles are free to read.
>
> - **Hybrid:** A journal charges a subscription fee, but authors may also choose to pay to make their article OA.
>
> Most nursing journals currently operate under the traditional or hybrid model; however, be prepared to navigate many more OA options if you choose to publish in a field other than nursing, which may be the case depending on your area of interest and the backgrounds of the other members of your writing team.
>
> One more publishing model you should know is transformative (also call transformational) agreements (TAs), which several major publishers are using as a means to transition from the traditional subscription model to OA. In a TA, a consortium (e.g., group of universities) forms a partnership with a publisher. The agreement typically allows researchers who are members of the consortium unlimited access to the publisher's journals and funding or discounts for APCs (Seymour, 2022). These agreements also can be with a single library or national organization (although that arrangement is less common), and most require the author retain copyright (Eugene McDermott Library, 2023). Terms of the agreement can vary. For example, not all of the publisher's journals may be available, and the consortium's payment of APCs may apply to a limited number of articles (Eugene McDermott Library, 2023). It's a good idea to check if your university has a TA because information about the agreement is sometimes not widely shared.

librarians, policymakers, and patients) created this definition that sums up the key elements (Grudniewicz et al., 2019, p. 211):

> Predatory journals and publishers are entities that prioritize self-interest at the expense of scholarship and are characterized by false or misleading information, deviation from best editorial and publication practices, a lack of transparency, and/or the use of aggressive and indiscriminate solicitation practices.

Linacre (2022, p. 11) offers this more succinct definition.

> Predatory journals are deceptive and often fake, giving the appearance of legitimate peer-reviewed journals and impact academic stakeholders by exploiting the open access model while using misleading tactics to solicit article submissions.

Predatory for-profit journals prey on unsuspecting authors, luring them with promises of quick publication (e.g., within a week or even 48 hours) in exchange for a fee. Unfortunately, unlike legitimate APCs, these fees don't support the editorial process, making these journals low quality. Predatory journals might not disclose the fees on their websites and may even claim "no submission fee." However, after manuscript submission, the author learns that a fee is required to pay for services such as peer review and editing, which either aren't done or are of low quality (Committee on Publication Ethics [COPE], 2019). When the author refuses to pay, the journal may ignore the request or even demand a withdrawal fee.

To mislead authors, journals may claim to be indexed in reputable databases when they are not (although unfortunately, some have made their way in), create fake impact factor scores, hijack a reputable journal by using its name and website (but with a slightly different URL), or attempt to mirror legitimate journals in name or website design to mislead authors (COPE, 2019; Solomon, 2023; Umlauf, 2016).

A predatory journal is often low quality, but not all low-quality journals are predatory. A 2022 report from the InterAcademy Partnership (IAP) includes a spectrum of predatory behaviors for journals, with fraudulent journals on one end and low-quality journals on the other (see Figure 3.1). The spectrum approach recognizes that some of the poor practices associated with predatory journals also can occur in journals not considered "predatory."

It can be tempting to succumb to promises of quick publication, particularly if you are under pressure to publish from your employer. But publication in a predatory journal damages your reputation and usually precludes you from republishing the article in a legitimate journal (AMWA–EMWA–ISMPP, 2019; COPE, 2019), although Linacre (2022) notes that an author could write an entirely new article for a

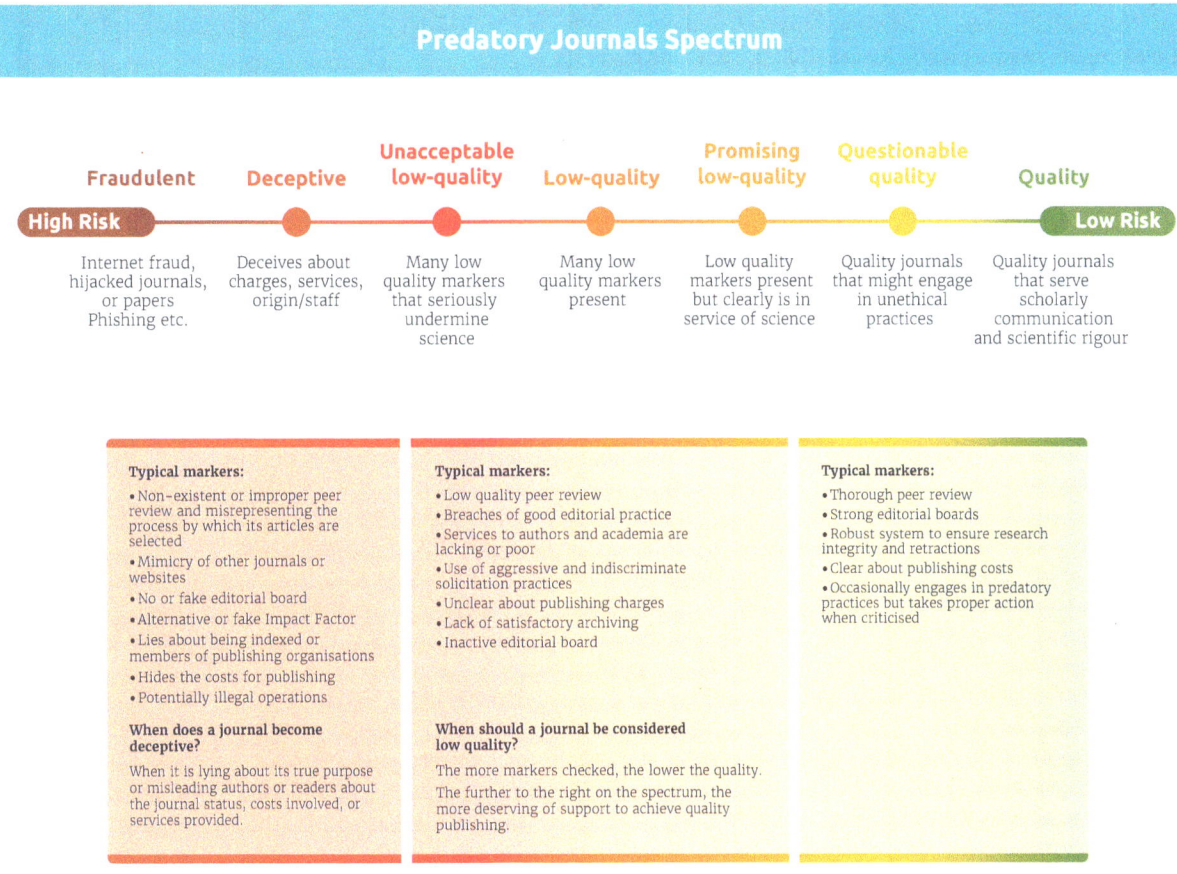

FIGURE 3.1 Spectrum of predatory journals (InterAcademy Partnership, 2022).

legitimate journal. (The author would need to disclose to the editors the experience with the predatory journal.) Publishing in a predatory journal also can result in disqualification for tenure or return of research funding (IAP, 2022). In addition, long-term archiving often doesn't exist, so your article might vanish when the journal ceases publication (Nicoll & Chinn, 2015).

From a global perspective, predatory journals often permit low-quality information to land in legitimate databases, where they are retrieved and cited by other authors ("citation pollution" or "citation contamination"), perpetuating the dissemination of misinformation (Anderson, 2019; Hinchliffe & Clarke, 2019; Linacre, 2022). Ultimately, this can undermine people's trust in science and even cause harm if patients make treatment decisions based on poor study results they find online (Bucceri et al., 2019; Linacre, 2022). Another issue is the loss of funding resources when fees are paid to predatory journals (Linacre, 2022).

The problem of predatory journals is a serious one. As of May 2022, Cabells *Predatory Reports* listed over 16,000 predatory journals (Linacre, 2022). In a study of 358 articles (most of which were research reports) published in predatory nursing journals, 96.3% were rated poor or average, based on a tool the researchers developed (Oermann et al., 2018). Another study found that articles in predatory nursing journals have been cited in nonpredatory nursing journals (Oermann et al., 2019).

Q *How can I avoid falling into the predatory journal trap?*

A To avoid becoming a victim, check to see if the journal is listed in one of the directories mentioned at the start of this chapter. If your organization has a subscription, you can also turn to Cabells' *Journalytics Academic & Predatory Reports* or *Journalytics Medicine & Predatory Reports* (https://cabells.com/). Unfortunately, some predatory journals have penetrated directories, and Cabells and the Directory of Open Access Journals have disagreed on whether a journal is predatory (Grudniewicz et al., 2019). However, publication in the directory is certainly a good sign of legitimacy, as is membership in the Committee on Publication Ethics. You also can check for hijacked journals (journals that mimic legitimate journals by adopting their titles and other metadata) by using the Retraction Watch Hijacked Journals Checker at https://docs.google.com/spreadsheets/d/1ak985WGOgGbJRJbZFanoktAN_UFeExpE/edit#gid=5255084 (Retraction Watch, 2022).

Use resources for evaluating journals, including checklists (one for journals and another for books and book chapters) found on the website Think. Check. Submit. (http://thinkchecksubmit.org), part of a campaign to help researchers identify trusted journals. A short video on the home page explains the think, check, submit process.

Another resource is the journal evaluation guidelines from the International Academy of Nurse Editors (INANE "Predatory Publishing Practices" Collaborative, 2014). Factors to check for include the following (AMWA–EMWA–ISMPP, 2019; Amsen, 2024; IAP, 2022; INANE "Predatory Publishing Practices" Collaborative, 2014; Shamseer et al., 2017; Think. Check. Submit., 2023):

- The editor and editorial board members have a good reputation within the specialty.
- Information for contacting the editor is easily accessible.
- Any impact factor mentioned is valid. (In a study by Shamseer et al. [2017], 33% of predatory journals promoted a bogus impact factor.)
- The journal is produced by a reputable publisher (is an established publishing firm or is publishing on behalf of a trusted association).
- The journal is transparent about the publication process, including fees and the peer-review process; it doesn't promise unrealistic review times.
- The journal provides examples of how it adheres to ethical standards. Examples include being a member of the Committee of Publication Ethics (COPE) or Open Access Scholarly Publishers Association, and policies related to author conflict-of-interest disclosure.
- The website is professional, and both it and the journal are free from multiple spelling and grammatical errors.

Beware of the flattering email that asks you to submit an article to a journal you have never heard of or wants you to recruit colleagues to prepare a special issue (Umlauf, 2016). Evaluate what the journal is publishing: Do the articles meet your own standards for excellence? Discuss your choice with trusted colleagues and healthcare librarians (Linacre, 2022); if they haven't heard of the journal, is it something you would want to be published in?

Right Timing

Timing might vary, depending on the type of publication, but editors generally plan their issues 6 months to 18 months ahead. For a magazine and for some journals, editors establish a general outline of topics they would like to include in an issue. Others, including more formal research journals, compile an issue based on the papers submitted, peer reviewed, and edited. Still others have a "call for manuscripts" or "call for submissions," which alerts readers to an upcoming special issue. For instance, *Orthopedic Nursing* might plan a special issue on pediatric fracture, or the *Journal of Radiology Nursing* might want to do a special issue on radiologic interventions for stroke. Sending a query in response to a call for manuscripts increases your opportunity for being heard above the background noise of a busy editor's day.

Q *Where can I find calls for manuscripts?*

A Calls for manuscripts are usually listed in the journal or on its website. Another source is the nursing writing resource by the University of Connecticut School of Nursing (http://nursingwriting.wordpress.com). You can also search for "call for manuscript" or "call for submissions" and "nursing" in search engines.

Keep in mind that many journals or magazines publish monthly, but others publish quarterly. If you have two journals that are roughly equal as good options for your article, you would likely want to give preference to the journal published monthly.

Certain diseases or conditions can be seasonal. If you have a manuscript on the care of heat stroke, most editors will want to publish it in the summer. As a rule, start sending queries related to seasonal conditions to editors about a year before you would like to see it published.

Timing of events can also affect your topic. When a major national disaster occurs, it often prompts interest in articles related to disaster response or prevention topics. Other events that receive widespread media coverage can also be a factor. For example, the COVID-19 pandemic brought a sharper focus on the role of social distancing as a public health measure.

Don't forget about online publications. They often have much shorter lead times than traditional print publications, and they can be a great venue for your work. Many editors publish topics that they find of interest, and often your article can be published within a matter of weeks or days—not months.

Finally, if the clock is ticking for you to publish as part of your tenure track, check the time between acceptance and publication for several articles in the journals you are considering. That information isn't always available, but if it is, it can give you a good idea of how long it might take for your article to be published.

Right Review Process

Most scholarly journals use a formal peer-review process (described more fully in Chapter 9). After your manuscript is fully finished and submitted, a panel of experts in your area will review it and offer comments or suggestions. Peer reviewers offer a journal a way to validate what you have written. If you're a faculty member required to publish for tenure, or even a graduate student looking for a prestigious outlet for your research, you will probably want a journal that uses peer review. Journals clearly state in the author guidelines whether the article will be peer reviewed or *refereed* (another term for the same process).

Right Metrics

Metrics are tools used to determine the impact of a journal or article. Metrics can affect how your work is disseminated (Smith & Watson, 2016). They can be divided into four categories: author metrics, traditional journal metrics, and journal- and article-level altmetrics (SPARC, 2023; Suelzer & Jackson, 2022). Here's a closer look at each.

Author metrics measure the impact of an author over time. The most common is the h-index. Author metrics usually do not factor into journal choice, although publishing in journals that are commonly cited can help increase your scores, which, in turn, can help you increase the reach of your work. (Learn more about promoting your work in Chapter 12.)

Traditional journal metrics aim to measure the impact of a journal. Examples include impact factor (IF), SCImago Journal Rank (SJR), CiteScore, and Eigenfactor metrics.

IF, the best known of these metrics, is based on the *Journal of Citation Reports* (*JCR*) published by Clarivate Analytics. The IF is based on a two-year period and is calculated by dividing the number of citations by the total number of articles published during those two years (University of Illinois at Chicago, 2023). There also is a five-year IF version. A significant drawback of IF is that citation data are limited to journals indexed in the Web of Science.

You cannot access the list of IFs without being a subscriber to *JCR*; however, a medical librarian might be able to answer your questions. You can also check whether a specific journal is included in Web of Science by doing a search at their website (https://mjl.clarivate.com/home).

SJR uses citation data from the Elsevier database Scopus but is managed by SCImago, a research group from the Consejo Superior de Investigaciones Científicas (CSIC), University of Granada, Extremadura, Carlos III (Madrid) and Alcalá de Henares. You can access various indicators on a publicly available portal, where journals can be compared or analyzed separately; some data can also be displayed visually (SCImago Journal & Country Rank, n.d.).

CiteScore is based on citations made in a given year to documents published in the past four years and includes all types of documents, not just articles and reviews. A journal's score is updated monthly, instead of annually as is the case with the *JCR* IF, but the ranking only uses journals in the Scopus database, owned by Elsevier, and has been criticized for its results (Bergstrom & West, 2016; Davis, 2016; University of Illinois at Chicago, 2023).

Eigenfactor metrics, including the Eigenfactor Score (EF) and Article Influence Score (AI), use information from the entire citation network to measure the importance of each journal. It includes journals in the *JCR* since 1996. You can search for a journal's scores at Eigenfactor.org, although this journal-level metric is not used as much as the others.

Many publishers and editors consider journal-level metrics a measure of how heavily their journal is used. Librarians and university researchers may consider these metrics when choosing which journals to subscribe to, although demand, cost, and access are typically more important. Journal-level metrics can play a role in promotion and tenure decisions for a faculty member or funding decisions for a researcher.

But recent years have brought increasing criticism that these citation-based metrics are relied on too much for making those decisions even though they have limitations. For instance, Larivière et al. (2016) report that IF is heavily influenced by a small number of articles that are highly cited. Other limitations of metrics include:

- Each database has its own criteria as to what types of articles are included when calculating journal metrics. For example, one may include editorials or letters to the editor, while another may not, which will affect citation count (Sugimoto & Larivière, 2018).
- A score owned by a publishing company may only include journals indexed in its particular database, which might favor its own journals when calculating metrics.
- Impact factors typically look at only two to three years of citation data, but articles may start to be cited or be more highly cited after that time has passed.
- Citations only paint part of a picture. For example, an article may have had a significant impact on a national policy change but not have been frequently cited.
- Studies show that impact factor is not a proxy for quality (Triggle et al., 2022).

Just because a journal doesn't have an IF or some other metric doesn't mean you should automatically strike it from your list as a possible publishing outlet; it may still produce excellent content. Some journals are simply too new to have received a full assessment to be listed in a database; others might focus on material, such as case studies, that are less likely to contribute to a favorable journal-level metric (Wiley, 2019). In addition, nursing journals have been traditionally underrepresented in some databases, such as Web of Science. Fortunately, thanks to the efforts of librarians and nurse editors, that is changing, but much more work needs to be done.

The bottom line is that journal-level metrics should be only one factor in deciding where to publish, and in most cases, not at the top of your list—that spot should be reserved for your target reader. If you are in academia, it may be an important consideration because it often affects tenure. Publishing in journals with high IF can also help you win grants to fund your research. However, you also want to reach a wide audience with your work. So if you're a researcher, publish in research-based journals, but don't forget to also publish in clinical practice journals to reach a wider audience with an article that has a different focus.

The San Francisco Declaration on Research Assessment (DORA), signed by more than 24,000 individuals and organizations in more than 160 countries, calls for eliminating IFs as a way of measuring the quality of research articles. DORA (Declaration of Research Assessment, n.d.) encourages the use of other measures, such as article-level metrics (altmetrics).

Altmetrics are a way to determine the impact of an article sooner than a citation-based metric allows. Altmetrics incorporate traditional, scholarly data sources, such as number of citations, with nontraditional data sources, such as tweets or blog posts, to determine the impact of an article (SPARC, 2023). Altmetrics also may take into account the number of times an article is exported to a citation management system such as Mendeley or Zotero. (Learn more about these systems in Chapter 4.) Altmetrics focus on articles, but by looking at results for several articles, they also help in assessing the impact of a journal.

Many publishers and databases are now providing altmetrics publicly, including Public Library of Science (PLoS), Scopus, and BioMed Central. (Some only share them with authors.) The data are usually provided by a company such as Altmetric, Impactstory, and Plum Analytics (Suelzer & Jackson, 2022; Sugimoto & Larivière, 2018), and the information is posted near the article on the journal's website. Because you can track your impact, choosing a journal that provides altmetrics can be helpful, especially if you're a career researcher.

Key Steps to Making a Choice

In the classic 2009 article, "Avoid Rejection: Write for the Audience and the Journal," Charon Pierson distills making the choice into three key steps:

1. Read several articles from the journal you plan to target.
2. Look at the table of contents for the issues from the past two years.
3. Read the journal's mission statement.

Unfortunately, as Pierson says, "Regardless of how widely publicized this advice is, it is the exception rather than the rule that authors follow one or more of the suggestions" (Pierson, 2009, p. 2).

Bond (2023) suggests creating a comparison chart for your top three options. The chart can include the elements discussed in this chapter, such as frequency of publication, timing, and metrics.

Q *Isn't there a faster way to pick a journal than going through all the steps discussed?*

A It's important to thoughtfully select your journal, and that takes time. However, you can also turn to journal selection tools that act as a matchmaker for your topic. These tools ask you to enter information such as the keywords of your topic or the title/abstract of an article; they then generate a list of journals where your article might fit. An advantage is that the results of the search are presented in a consistent format, making it easier to compare journals. Here are a few examples of free journal selection tools:

- **Clarivate Manuscript Matcher** (https://mjl.clarivate.com/home): Only includes journals listed in Web of Science and requires free subscription
- **Genamics JournalSeek** (http://journalseek.net): Supported by OCLC, a global library organization
- **Jane: Journal/Author Name Estimator** (http://jane.biosemantics.org): Only includes journals in MEDLINE; provides impact factor and link to sample articles
- **JournalGuide** (https://www.journalguide.com): Maintained by Research Square, an independent company

Examples of publishers' tools include:

- **Elsevier Journal Finder** (http://journalfinder.elsevier.com)
- **Sage Journal Recommender** (https://journal-recommender.sagepub.com)
- **Wiley Journal Finder** (https://journalfinder.wiley.com

Unfortunately, these tools have significant limitations. Some include few or no nursing journals, those developed by publishers may contain only their own journals, and too many of the results are not a good fit for the article. Consider them as a supplement, not a substitute for researching your options (Bond, 2023).

Whichever journal you choose, tailor your manuscript to that journal. For example, if you plan to write about how to assess pain in cognitively impaired older adults for a clinically focused journal, focus on the step-by-step process of assessing pain in clinical practice. However, if the journal is more scholarly, you might want to write a review of current pain assessment tools for older adults and include recommendations for practice.

After you have chosen a journal, the next step is to see if the editor is interested in your idea.

Framing a Good Query

After you select your target journal, send a query letter to the editor to determine interest in the topic. A query letter, which is typically sent by email, includes an overview of your article and the reasons why an editor should publish it.

The query is usually placed in the body of the email. Some authors send a letter as an attachment; however, an email with an attachment sent to someone you have not previously corresponded with could end up in the person's spam folder. That's why it's probably best to keep your query to the body of the email.

You want to query before you start writing because (Saver, 2016):

- You won't waste time writing if the editor isn't interested in your topic.
- The editor can give you feedback on your idea, helping you to tweak it to make it the most effective possible for the journal's target audience.
- If the editor gives you a positive response, you can then tailor your manuscript to that particular journal, enhancing the likelihood of acceptance for publication. An important note of caution, however: Editor interest in an idea does *not* ensure publication.

A query letter is your opportunity to sell your idea to the editor. We nurses don't typically think of ourselves as salespeople, but consider what you do when you teach patients—you have to sell them on why it's important to follow the prescribed treatment plan. What's more difficult can be the self-promotion needed to convince the editor that you should be the one to write the article.

Q *Do all editors accept queries?*

A Some editors of journals don't see the value of queries. They may receive too many or have seen too many that were poorly written. If a journal has a narrow focus and publishes traditional research articles, which tend to have a standard format no matter what the journal, the editor may view query letters as unnecessary (Saver, 2016). However, many editors do welcome queries. The author guidelines, available on the journal's website, usually state whether queries are accepted. If not, a simple note to the editor asking whether they accept queries will get you the answer you need.

A query consists of several elements—addressing the right person/right journal, promoting your topic, promoting yourself, and wrapping up. To begin, consider one nurse's letter (Example 3.1, adapted from an actual email). As you read the next section, think about how you would make over Terry's query to convert it from one that doesn't work to one that sells the editor on her article.

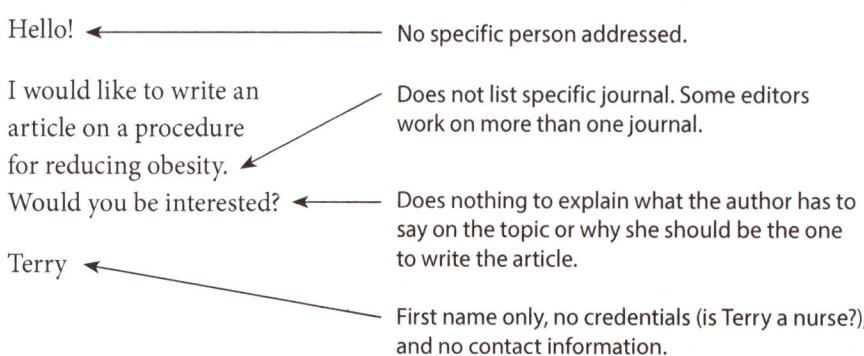

EXAMPLE 3.1 Poorly written query letter.

Addressing the Right Person/Right Journal

Be sure to address the correct contact person, which is typically the editor or editor-in-chief. This person's name will be in the author guidelines, which are usually posted on the journal's website. You can also check the journal's *masthead*, the section in the front of the journal that lists the names of staff members, editorial board members, and contact information. Always spell the person's name correctly and use the appropriate title. For example, if the person has a doctorate degree, use "Dear Dr. Jones" instead of "Dear Mary." If the editor is also a dean, opt for "Dear Dean White." Err on the side of formality at first. Also be sure to get the name of the journal right. Unfortunately, this is a common mistake (Gennaro, 2016). It's frustrating for an editor to receive a query addressed to the wrong journal or with the wrong publication in the text. It also doesn't give the editor confidence that you will provide an accurate article.

Q *Can I use the same query for several publications?*

A You can use parts of it, but your query is too generic if you don't have to make a few changes to appeal to one publication or another. Although it might seem many publications are similar, their editors and readers know the subtle differences. And no matter what, make sure you match the correct editor and title to your letter.

The subject line of an email should clearly state that you are inquiring about publishing an article. For example, which subject line do you think would generate more editor interest?

> *Staffing article idea for* Journal of Nursing Administration

> or

> *Journal of Nursing Administration*: Query for article on new technique for staffing off-shifts that reduced costs

You probably chose the second subject line. The word "new" will catch an editor's eye (just be sure what you are writing about is truly new), and the topic is not only clearly stated but is also obviously something of interest to the journal's readers.

Unfortunately (and all too often), editors receive queries for topics that are not suited for their journals. An editor of a practice-focused journal received a query to publish a research article related to cellular changes in heart failure, clearly not something of interest to the publication's typical reader. On the other hand, the editor might have been interested in the topic of assessing a patient with heart failure, something that the query author could likely write about given their implicit knowledge of the physiologic effects of the condition.

Q *Can I submit my idea to two or more different journals at the same time?*

A Some editors believe that sending multiple queries simultaneously to multiple journals is acceptable; others do not. If you do decide to send simultaneous queries, send each email individually, rather than sending a group email (Saver, 2016). (You should *not* submit your manuscript to more than one journal at a time.)

Promoting Your Topic

Most editors don't sit around waiting for writers to contact them. They work their networks to get ideas and articles from readers, editorial board members, conference speakers, local and national media, social media (e.g., X, LinkedIn, and Facebook), and more. Then they choose the topics that best fit the journal's mission and will interest the reader.

Make your topic stand out from the others first by clearly stating what your take on the topic will be. Again, which of the following statements will more likely get the editor's attention?

> I would like to submit an article that would describe the results of a research study on how to reduce hospital readmissions.

> I would like to submit an article that would describe the results of a research study showing how regular telemedicine follow-ups from a nurse practitioner for patients with heart failure reduced hospital readmissions by one-third.

The first statement certainly states the topic, but notice how the second tells the editor what the study found as well as the results that would make them want to read it. Next, explain why the topic is important to the journal's readers. If your article is about "hands only" CPR in people in the community, for example, you might write something like the following:

> Cardiac disease remains the leading cause of death in the US, with many patients dying from acute myocardial infarction (MI) even before they reach the hospital. "Hands only" CPR provides a way to improve survival. The readers of *Home Healthcare Nurse* may encounter patients in cardiac arrest in the home, where state-of-the-art equipment is lacking, and all nurses have to rely on is themselves.

Include statistics on how many people experience cardiac arrest in the home to strengthen your case.

Here is another example of how you might pitch an article—this one on childhood diabetes:

> The manuscript describes a new program for managing children with diabetes in an outpatient clinic. We conducted a survey of children and parents to determine unmet needs of the child, designed the program to address those needs, and then conducted a follow-up survey six months later. The needs we identified included management of diet in school and at parties, participating in sports, talking with friends about diabetes, and monitoring blood glucose.
>
> We found that our program, designed by a multidisciplinary team, increased overall satisfaction with care by 50%.

Note that the potential author provided a *hook* by telling the editor the program's effectiveness.

Depending on the publication, you can have a bit of fun with the opening of your query letter. Think about this when you skim through a magazine or journal. The first few lines can prove to be an important factor in whether you read the article. It's no different for the query letter. Here is a possible opening:

> Amid the nursing shortage, nurses struggle to deliver care with fewer numbers. What if they could count on an extra nurse on two of their three shifts? Better yet, what if the nurse didn't have to be paid?
>
> That's the situation at Anytown Medical Center, where we have a volunteer program for retired registered nurses. After an orientation, the nurses work mornings and afternoons, helping out with morning or afternoon physical care, vital signs, and limited physical assessments. We now have more than 60 volunteers in our program.
>
> An article on this program would be of interest to the readers of *American Nurse Journal* because they would have the information they need to replicate the program in their own institutions and reap the benefits.

It's hard to imagine an editor turning down this request. However, the same idea pitched to a more scholarly journal would require a much different letter. Match the formality of your query to the tone of the publication.

Describing the Article

Give the editor a short description of what the article will include so that they know what to expect. This also gives the editor the opportunity to guide the direction of the manuscript.

Here is an example of a query letter, adapted from one received by the editor of a nursing journal, that illustrates how to promote your topic (second paragraph) and the type of information about content that you should include (third paragraph):

> I am writing to inquire about your interest in publishing a case study of a young adult who acquired Lyme carditis through a tick bite.
>
> The prevalence of Lyme disease has steadily increased in recent years and can lead to neurological and cardiovascular complications that can significantly impair patients' quality of life. Education on prevention strategies and recognition of early signs and symptoms are key to mitigating this disease and preventing complications.
>
> The case study would describe a common scenario in which a person can experience a tick bite and subsequently develop Lyme disease,

leading to Lyme carditis. I would then outline the clinical manifestations, diagnosis, and management of the disease and the role of the nurse in providing education.

I am a clinical nurse specialist with more than 10 years of clinical experience. Over the years I have cared for a variety of patients with acute and complex cardiovascular problems

This query resulted in a published article.

Selling Yourself as an Author

Your query letter is not the time to be shy. Tell the editor why you should be the one to write the article (see the last paragraph of the sample query letter in the previous section). For example, if you want to write an article on transcatheter aortic valve replacement, you might write:

I have more than 15 years of experience in critical care, including 5 years in the surgical ICU, where I have been caring for patients undergoing this procedure. [If the volume of patients is high, it would be good to include the average number per month or year.] I also presented a program on this topic at our local chapter of the American Association of Critical-Care Nurses.

Include any past writing experience. For example, "I have had three articles published in nursing journals, including *Critical Care Nurse*." If the topics were cardiovascular related, say so. It's best not to note that you wrote the paper as a class assignment and would now like to publish it. A class assignment differs from a published article. (See Chapter 18 to learn how you can turn an assignment into an article.) Opinions differ as to whether to mention that the topic is based on a dissertation or capstone project. Some feel the idea should stand on its own, and others feel that mentioning the source can even be detrimental because of the frequent failure of authors to adapt the work for a journal. On the other hand, the disclosure can support your claim that you have expertise in the topic. If you decide to include the origins of the topic, state that you will be adapting the information to be suitable for a journal article (Saver, 2016, 2019).

Q *What if I have never been published? Is it more likely my idea will be rejected?*

A Don't despair if you have not been published. Every writer had to start with one article. You might consider listing nonpublished writing experience. For example, perhaps you write your hospital's or clinic's newsletter. Even though the style of the article is likely to be different, it at least shows that you have an interest in writing. Another option is to choose a coauthor who has been published.

Closing Your Query Letter

Let the editor know when you could have the manuscript done: "I could have the manuscript ready by September 30."

If you have any flexibility with the date, change the sentence to read, "I could have the manuscript ready by September 30, or sooner if that better meets your needs."

Be honest when it comes to deadlines. Editors expect manuscripts to arrive on time. They might have even tentatively scheduled the article for a particular issue, pending peer review, so a late article disrupts the schedule.

If you can't write the article before September 30, don't say that you can. There is no faster way to take the gloss off the relationship between editor and writer than to miss your deadline. You can still see your article published (unless you miss the deadline repeatedly), but the editor will be more cautious about accepting ideas from you in the future. Communicate if you know you will miss your deadline.

To finish your letter, give your complete contact information, including full name, email and mailing addresses, and phone numbers, including which number is best for reaching you.

Q *How long before I receive a response to a query letter?*

A Many editors respond to query emails within a week, often sooner, but others do not. If you haven't heard back after one week, you can resend the email, saying you want to verify it was received. If you still don't receive a response a few days later, move on to another journal (Saver, 2019).

What If You're Going to Miss Your Deadline?

Life happens, and editors understand that you might have to miss a deadline because of illness or a family emergency. Here is how to handle this situation professionally.

- **Notify the editor as soon as you know you will be late.** This sounds like common sense, but many authors fail to do this under the mistaken impression that they will somehow be able to salvage the project or because they simply don't want to admit defeat.

- **Give an estimate for a new deadline.** The editor may be able to simply reschedule your article for a later issue. If you are unable to commit to a new deadline, say so. That way, the editor can decide whether to pursue another author.

- **If possible, find a replacement author.** Ask your editor whether they wish for you to find a new author if you can commit to doing so. Depending on your topic, you might be able to find a colleague who is willing to pinch-hit for you. This will make you an instant hero with your editor. However, most editors understand that your circumstances will likely preclude you from finding a replacement.

You do not need to state why you will miss the deadline. The bottom line: Try to honor your commitment, but your health, family, and friends must come first.

Finally, be sure to spell-check and grammar-check your query. This is your only chance to make a good first impression on the editor. A query riddled with typos could cause the editor to wonder whether you will submit a quality manuscript.

Keep in mind that you want to keep the letter short so the editor is more likely to read it.

Example 3.2, which follows, is a "makeover" of the query letter from earlier in the chapter. The letter pitches the fictitious procedure adipose supra-ablation (used in this letter for illustration purposes only) to a fictitious journal. A query letter such as this one will hopefully result in the editor responding that they are interested in the article. Even if they decide to decline the idea, you should thank them for their time (Bond, 2023).

Choose Wisely

Choosing the right target publication journal requires careful thought and analysis. After you select your publication, write your query letter in an appropriate style, and email it to the appropriate person. Writing an effective query will boost the likelihood the editor will respond positively, and you will be ready to start writing. Keep in mind that your manuscript will still need to be reviewed before it is accepted for publication.

Write Now!

1. Make a list of journals that would fit your idea for an article. Then narrow the list to three and rank them in order of best fit.

2. Write a query letter, including the topic, a brief description of the article, why you should write the article, and your contact information.

Note: This is the text of an email sent on April 8, 2024, to Carter Smith, PhD, CNOR, Editor-in-Chief, *Perioperative Services Journal*.

Dear Dr. Smith, ⟵——————————— Correct name of editor.

I would like to submit a manuscript to *Perioperative* ⟵——— Correct name of journal.
Services Journal. The manuscript describes a new surgical
procedure for reducing obesity: adipose supra-ablation. ⟵——— Proposed topic.

Obesity is a leading cause of death in the United States, with more than 25% of Americans classified as obese. Techniques such as bariatric surgery have been used to treat patients who are obese; these surgeries are associated with serious complications and can be used in only a select patient population. Adipose supra-ablation, a less extensive surgical option for those who are obese, is associated ⟵——— Explains why the article is important to readers.
with only minor complications and can be performed in children and adults. My article would include indications ⟵——— Briefly states what the article will include.
for adipose supra-ablation, a description of the procedure, risks and benefits, and the perioperative nurse's role.

I have more than 10 years' experience in the perioperative setting. For the past three years, I have been the nurse ⟵——— Briefly explains why she should write the article. If Terry has published any articles previously, she should mention her writing experience here.
leader of our perioperative team for adipose supra-ablation. Our surgeons perform an average of 10 adipose supra-ablations each month, twice the national average.

I could have the manuscript ready by June 7, 2024. ⟵——— States when the article will be ready. If Terry has some flexibility with the date, she should add that.
Please call me at (555) 888-0000 or email me at
t.lee@nowhere.com if you have any questions. ⟵——— Provides several ways to contact.

Thank you for your consideration.

Sincerely,
Terry Lee, RN, MS, CNOR ⟵——— Author's full name and credentials.

Adapted from Saver, 2006. Reprinted with permission.

EXAMPLE 3.2 A well-written, effective query letter.

References

American Medical Writers Association, European Medical Writers Association & International Society for Medical Publication Professionals. (2019). AMWA–EMWA–ISMPP joint position statement on predatory publishing. *Current Medical Research and Opinion, 35*(9), 1657–1658. https://doi.org/10.1080/03007995.2019.1646535

American Medical Writers Association, European Medical Writers Association & International Society for Medical Publication Professionals. (2021). AMWA–EMWA–ISMPP joint position statement on medical publications, preprints, and peer review. *Current Medical Research and Opinion, 37*(5), 861–866. https://doi.org/10.1080/03007995.2021.1900365

Amsen, E. (2024). How to avoid being duped by predatory journals. *BMJ, 384*(q452). https://doi.org/10.1136/bmj.q452

Anderson, R. (2019, Oct. 28). Citation contamination: References to predatory journals in the legitimate scientific literature. *The Scholarly Kitchen.* https://scholarlykitchen.sspnet.org/2019/10/28/citation-contamination-references-to-predatory-journals-in-the-legitimate-scientific-literature/

Baffy, G., Burns, M. M., Hoffmann, B., Ramani, S., Sabharwal, S., Borus J. F., Pories, S. Quan, S. F., & Ingelfinger, J. R. (2020). Scientific authors in a changing world of scholarly communication: What does the future hold? *The American Journal of Medicine, 133*(1), 26–31. https://doi.org/10.1016/j.amjmed.2019.07.028

Bergstrom, C. T., & West, J. (2016, Dec. 8). Comparing impact factor and Scopus CiteScore. *Eigenfactor.org.* http://eigenfactor.org/projects/posts/citescore.php

Bond, J. (2023). *The little guide to getting your journal article published.* Rowman & Littlefield.

Borrego, A. (2023). Article processing charges for open access journal publishing: A review. *Learned Publishing, 36*(3), 331–488. https://doi.org/10.1002/leap.1558

Bucceri, A., Hornung, P., & Schindler, M. (2019). Predatory publishing—What medical communicators need to know. *Medical Writing, 28*(3), 28–33. https://journal.emwa.org/trends-in-medical-writing/predatory-publishing-what-medical-communicators-need-to-know/

Committee on Publication Ethics. (2019). *COPE discussion document: Predatory publishing.* https://doi.org/10.24318/cope.2019.3.6

Davis, P. (2016, Dec. 12). CiteScore—Flawed but still a game changer. *The Scholarly Kitchen.* https://scholarlykitchen.sspnet.org/2016/12/12/citescore-flawed-but-still-a-game-changer

Declaration of Research Assessment. (n.d.). *San Francisco Declaration of Research Assessment.* https://sfdora.org/read/

Eigenfactor.org. (n.d.). *About the Eigenfactor® project.* http://www.eigenfactor.org/about.php

Eugene McDermott Library (2023, Oct. 20). *Transformative agreements in publishing.* https://libguides.utdallas.edu/transformative-agreements-in-publishing/introduction

Gastel, B., & Day, R. A. (2022). *How to write and publish a scientific paper* (9th ed.). Greenwood.

Gennaro, S. (2016). Mistakes to avoid in scientific writing [Editorial]. *Journal of Nursing Scholarship, 48*(5), 435–436. https://doi.org/10.1111/jnu.12235

Grudniewicz, A., Moher, D., Cobey, K. D., Bryson, G. L., Cukier, S., Allen, K., Ardern, C., Balcom, L., Barros, T., Berger, M., Buitrago Ciro, J., Cugusi, L. Donaldson, M. R., Egger, M., Graham, I. D., Hodgkinson, M., Khan, K. M., Mabizela, M., Manca, A., Milzow, K., Mouton, J., Muchenje, M., Olijhoek, T., Ommaya, A., Patwardhan, B., Poff, D., Proulx, L., Rodger, M., Severin, A., Strinzel, M., Sylos-Labini, M., Tamblyn, R., van Niekerk, M., Wicherts, J. M., & Lalu, M. M. (2019). Predatory journals: No definition, no defence. *Nature, 576,* 210–212. https://doi.org/10.1038/d41586-019-03759-y

Hinchliffe, L. J., & Clarke, M. (2019, Sept. 25). Citation pollution—The challenge of detecting fraudulent journals in works cited. *The Scholarly Kitchen.* https://scholarlykitchen.sspnet.org/2019/09/25/fighting-citation-pollution/

INANE & *Nurse Author & Editor.* (2023, Sept. 9). Directory of nursing journals. *Nurse Author & Editor.* https://nursingeditors.com/journals-directory/

INANE "Predatory Publishing Practices" Collaborative. (2014). Predatory publishing: What editors need to know. *Nurse Author & Editor, 24*(3), 2. https://doi.org/10.1111/j.1750-4910.2014.tb00183.x

InterAcademy Partnership. (2022). *Combatting predatory academic journals and conferences. Summary report.* https://palast.ps/sites/default/files/inline-files/2.%20Summary%20report%20-%20English.pdf

Larivière, V., Kiermer, V., MacCallum, C. J., McNutt, M., Patterson, M., Pulverer, B., Swaminathan, S., Taylor, S., & Curry, S. (2016). A simple proposal for the publication of journal citation distributions. *bioRxiv.* https://doi.org/10.1101/062109

Linacre, S. (2022). *The predator effect: Understanding the past, present and future of deceptive academic journals.* ATG LCC.

Liverpool, L. (2023). Open-access reformers launch next bold publishing plan. *Nature, 623,* 238–240. https://doi.org/10.1038/d41586-023-03342-6

Maličk, M., Jerončić,, A., & ter Riet, G, Bouter, L. M., Loannidis, J. P. A., Goodman, S. N., & Aalbersberg, I. J. (2020). Preprint servers' policies, submission requirements, and transparency in reporting and research integrity recommendations. *JAMA, 324*(18), 1901–1903. https://doi.org/10.1001/jama.2020.17195

medRxiv. (n.d.). *About medRxiv.* https://www.medrxiv.org/content/about-medrxiv

Monaghan, J., Lucraft, M., Allin, K., van der Graf, M., & Clarke, T. (2020, June 4). 'APCs in the wild': Could increased monitoring and consolidation of funding accelerate the transition to open access? *Springer Nature.* https://figshare.com/articles/_APCs_in_the_Wild_Could_Increased_Monitoring_and_Consolidation_of_Funding_Accelerate_the_Transition_to_Open_Access_/11988123/4

National Library of Medicine. (2023, April 5). *NIH preprint pilot.* https://www.ncbi.nlm.nih.gov/pmc/about/nihpreprints/

Nicoll, L. H., & Chinn, P. L. (2015). Caught in the trap: The allure of deceptive publishers. *Nurse Author & Editor, 25*(4), 1–11. https://doi.org/10.1111/j.1750-4910.2015.tb00568.x

Nursing Research. (n.d.). Preprints policy. https://journals.lww.com/nursingresearchonline/Pages/informationforauthors.aspx#overlap_with_other_manuscripts

Oermann, M. H., Nicoll, L. H., Carter-Templeton, H., Woodward, A., Kidayi P. L., Neal, L. B., Edie, A. H., Ashton, K. S., Chinn, P. L., & Amarasekara, S. (2019). Citations of articles in predatory journals. *Nursing Outlook, 67*(6), 664–667. https://doi.org/10.1016/j.outlook.2019.05.001

Oermann, M. H., Nicoll, L. H., Chinn, P. L., Ashton, K. S., Conklin, J. L., Edie, A. H., Amarasekara, S., & Williams, B. L. (2018). Quality of articles published in predatory nursing journals. *Nursing Outlook, 66*(1), 4–10. https://doi.org/10.1016/j.outlook.2017.05.005

Office of Science and Technology Policy. (2022, Aug. 25). *OSTP issues guidance to make federally funded research freely available without delay* [Press release]. https://www.whitehouse.gov/ostp/news-updates/2022/08/25/ostp-issues-guidance-to-make-federally-funded-research-freely-available-without-delay/

Open Access Scholarly Publishers Association. (n.d.). *Licensing FAQ.* http://oaspa.org/information-resources/frequently-asked-questions/

Penn Libraries. (2023). *Services for authors at the Penn Libraries: Open access publishing.* https://guides.library.upenn.edu/Authors/open_access

Pierson, C. (2009). Avoid rejection: Write for the audience and the journal. *Nurse Author & Editor, 19*(2), 1. http://naepub.com/writing-basics/2009-19-2-1/

Plan S. (2023a). *FAQ.* https://www.coalition-s.org/faq/

Plan S. (2023b). *Towards responsible publishing: A proposal from cOAlition S.* https://doi.org/10.5281/zenodo.8398480

Retraction Watch (2022, May 29). Want to know whether that journal is scanning you? Introducing the Retraction Watch Journal Checker. *Retraction Watch.* https://retractionwatch.com/2022/05/29/want-to-know-whether-that-journal-is-scamming-you-introducing-the-retraction-watch-hijacked-journal-checker/

Saver, C. (2006). Choosing a journal and submitting your manuscript. *AORN Journal, 84*(1), 27–30. https://doi.org/10.1016/S0001-2092(06)60095-1

Saver, C. (2016). Effective queries can save authors time and effort. *Nurse Author & Editor, 26*(3), 4. https://doi.org/10.1111/j.1750-4910.2016.tb00225.x

Saver, C. (2019, March 9). Ask before you write: Crafting the query. *American Nurse Journal: The writing mind.* https://www.myamericannurse.com/ask-before-your-write-crafting-the-query/

Scholarly Publishing and Academic Resources Coalition. (2023). *Article-level metrics?* https://sparcopen.org/our-work/article-level-metrics/

Scholarly Publishing and Academic Resources Coalition, Public Library of Science, & Open Access Scholarly Publishers Association. (2014). *HowOpenIsIt? Version 2.0.* https://sparcopen.org/wp-content/uploads/2015/12/hoii-guide_V2_FINAL-1.pdf

Schonfeld, R. C., & Rieger, O. Y. (2020, May 27). Publishers invest in preprints. *The Scholarly Kitchen.* https://scholarlykitchen.sspnet.org/2020/05/27/publishers-invest-in-preprints/?informz=1

SCImago Journal & Country Rank. (n.d.). *About us.* http://www.scimagojr.com/aboutus.php

Seymour, H. (2022, May 19). *Transformational agreements: An introduction for editors, 2022 update.* The Wiley Network. https://www.wiley.com/en-us/network/publishing/research-publishing/editors/transformational-agreements-an-introduction-for-editors-2022-update

Shamseer, L., Moher, D., Maduekwe, O., Turner, L., Barbour, V., Burch, R., Clark, J., Galipeau, J., Roberts, J., & Shea, B. J. (2017). Potential predatory and legitimate biomedical journals: Can you tell the difference? A cross-sectional comparison. *BMC Medicine, 15*(1), 28. https://doi.org/10.1186/s12916-017-0785-9

Singh, S. (2022, June 3). Plan S: An update on what's happening and what's in store. *Editage Insights.* https://www.editage.com/insights/plan-s-an-update-on-whats-happening-and-whats-in-store

Smith, D. R., & Watson, R. (2016). Career development tips for today's nursing academic: Bibliometrics, altmetrics and social media. *Journal of Advanced Nursing, 72*(11), 2654–2661. https://doi.org/10.1111/jan.13067

Solomon, R. V. (2023). Breaking free from academic scams: Five key reflections on the cloned journal conundrum. *Learned Publishing, 37*(1), 44–48. https://doi.org/10.1002/leap.1590

Suber, P. (2015). *Open access overview.* http://legacy.earlham.edu/~peters/fos/overview.htm

Suelzer, E. M., & Jackson, J. L. (2022). Measures of impact for journals, articles, and authors. *Journal of General Internal Medicine, 37*(7), 1593–1597. https://doi.org/10.1007/s11606-022-07475-8

Sugimoto, C. R., & Larivière, V. (2018). *Measuring research: What everyone needs to know.* Oxford University Press.

Think. Check. Submit. (2023). *Journals.* https://thinkchecksubmit.org/journals/

Triggle, C. R., MacDonald, R., Triggle, D. J., & Grierson, D. (2022). Requiem for impact factors and high publication charges. *Accountability in Research, 29*(3), 133–164. https://doi.org/10.1080/08989621.2021.1909481

Umlauf, M. G. (2016). Predatory open access journals: Avoiding profiteers, wasted effort and fraud. *International Journal of Nursing Practice, 22*(S1), 3–4. https://doi.org/10.1111/ijn.12433

University of Illinois at Chicago. (2023). *Measuring your impact: Impact factor, citation analysis, and other metrics: Journal impact factor (IF).* https://researchguides.uic.edu/if/impact

Watson, R. (2019). Evolving trends in open access. *Compliance Elliance Journal, 5*(1), 91–98. https://ul.qucosa.de/api/qucosa%3A33909/attachment/ATT-0/

Wiley. (2019). *Writing for publication: An easy-to-follow guide for any nurse thinking of publishing their work.* Wiley. https://www.wiley.com/en-us/network/publishing/research-publishing/writing-and-conducting-research/writing-for-publication-for-nurses-english-edition

Finding and Documenting Sources

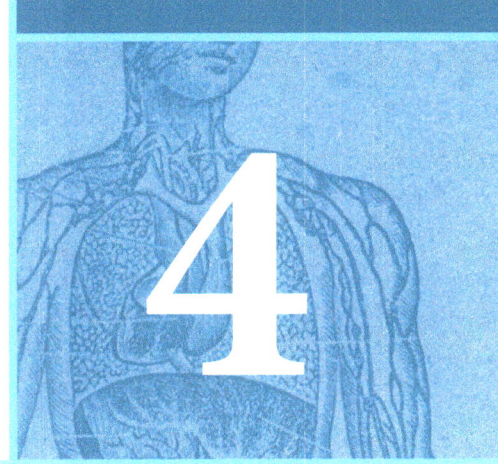

4

–Leslie H. Nicoll, PhD, MBA, RN, FAAN

*"The most important thing is to begin. Once you start,
you can always correct, revise, and improve later."*
–Jodi Picoult

WHAT YOU'LL LEARN IN THIS CHAPTER

- Authors need to find sources, and cite and organize them correctly, to meet publishing standards.

- It's important to know the different types of sources and when each is appropriate to use in a manuscript.

- You can use several strategies to help keep your reference library organized.

Whether you're writing a journal article, a book chapter, or an online education program, accurately documenting what you write is the gold standard of professional publication. Good sources help you develop and support the arguments and opinions you present in your article. In this chapter, you'll learn why references are important as well as how to find them, cite them, and keep them organized. Citations presented in the proper format will be one of the first things that an editor looks for in your submission—and one of the elements that is most often wrong or incomplete in a published paper. After all the hard work you've put into writing your article, paying attention to your references helps ensure that it isn't rejected for publication because of careless errors.

Why Citations Are Necessary

In scientific writing, citations serve two important purposes. First, they document where you obtained the information you are reporting. Second, they provide the information that a reader needs to be able to find the original source material.

> **Q** *I'm writing an article on my evidence-based practice project for a journal. My colleagues tell me that I won't need to worry about formatting my references because the publisher will do it. Is that correct?*
>
> **A** In general, publishers do not format references, although some offer manuscript formatting services that include formatting references. However, the fees for these services are pricey. Even if you choose to go this route, furnishing a complete and properly styled reference list remains *your* responsibility. A manuscript may be rejected because the reference list is incomplete or inaccurate. The reference list is integral to the manuscript and is as important as the abstract and data that are reported, so it's best to handle this task yourself.

By documenting where you obtained your information, you protect yourself against plagiarism and give credit to the original researchers for their work. *Plagiarism* is the practice of presenting another person's thoughts or ideas as your own. By providing a citation to the primary source material, you recognize the originators of the material and protect yourself.

Providing a reference to the source material is also important so that a reader can check the original report. A reader might want to verify that you interpreted the original source material correctly, or a researcher might also use your article and its associated reference list as a starting point for further exploration or study.

Finally, the references you cite provide a foundational basis for your conclusions. References show your peers, colleagues, and others interested in your topic the path you followed as you synthesized the literature.

Q *Does the use of references vary by type of article?*

A References cited within the text, and then listed in detail at the end of the article, are essential in academic writing, including articles for scholarly journals, school papers, and textbook chapters. Although formal references are not typically part of opinion pieces, or certain online writing such as blog posts, you should still cite sources that support your points. Rather than use the citation method for academic work, you can simply work the source into the text or, in the case of an online reference, insert a link to the relevant information. Magazine articles incorporate references in more subtle ways, which may include statistics from well-respected organizations, such as the American Heart Association or commentary by experts. For example, "Lori Stein, a nurse practitioner whose research on women and heart disease has been published in leading academic journals, says women often experience a heart attack differently than men."

If you fail to reference your material sufficiently, your professional reputation could suffer. Those with an interest in your subject area keep a close eye on what is published and may choose to send a letter to the editor if they see something not properly credited.

Omission is a serious mistake, but falsifying references is worse and can set you up for professional failure. Falsified references can be the basis for retraction of a published article. If an editor is forced to retract something you have written, you will be banned from publishing in the journal. The journal world is a small one, so it is highly likely that you would find a cold reception at other journals as well. Depending on the circumstance, plagiarism, falsifying references, and retractions may prompt an editor to contact your employer to report the issue, which could have negative repercussions for your work situation as well. Prevent all these problems by being thorough, careful, and accurate when referencing your paper. "I didn't know," is not a sufficient defense. If you are going to write and publish in the professional literature, you need to understand these issues. (You can learn more about legal and ethical issues related to publishing in Chapter 11.)

Primary, Secondary, and Tertiary Sources

The three kinds of sources are primary, secondary, and tertiary. A *primary source* document is the original written report, such as a research report published in a journal like *Nursing Research*. Primary sources can also include letters, diary entries, data from patient records or surveys, and so on—essentially anything that serves as an original source for information.

Secondary sources are those citations that quote the primary source document—for example, textbooks or literature review articles.

Tertiary sources are distillations of information from primary and secondary sources, such as almanacs, fact books, dictionaries, and encyclopedias. Tertiary sources can be handy to obtain a quick overview of a topic, but you should not cite them in your paper as an authoritative source.

You should try to rely on and quote primary documents, from research articles to firsthand interviews. Sometimes, admittedly, this is impossible. For example, not many of us have access to Florence Nightingale's original letters—but you may read a letter in a secondary source. In this case, acknowledge both the letter and the secondary source in which it is cited. However, if you want to quote a study cited in a textbook, do the legwork to obtain the primary source document.

Q *Can I use Wikipedia as a source?*

A Wikipedia is a tertiary source that describes itself as an encyclopedia—it should generally not be used as a source in an article or paper. Even Wikipedia acknowledges this on the page "Researching with Wikipedia" (n.d.), which states that Wikipedia should not be used for primary research unless you are writing a paper about Wikipedia.

References for Student Writing

Another key reason to provide citations illustrates the fundamental difference between a student paper and a paper for publication in a professional journal. A student paper is, essentially, a document that conveys to your faculty what you have learned. A paper in a professional journal conveys new information to readers, whether that information is a synthesis of the literature or a primary research report.

If you are a student, the references that you cite provide evidence to the faculty that you collected information on a topic, read the associated articles, synthesized the data, and can provide a comprehensive analysis of what you have studied. This analysis should go beyond just a simple regurgitation of the articles that you read. The ability to analyze ideas and synthesize new ones is the core of critical thinking (Shellenbarger, 2016).

A student paper may contain information that would be appropriate for publication in a professional journal, but the paper, as written, most likely will not be suitable. You need to do the work to edit the paper to journal style and, at the same time, transform the content in such a way that it provides new information to the audience of readers. (You can learn more about how to do this in Chapter 18.)

The Essence of Documentation

How many sources should you document? That's an excellent question, and one that novice authors struggle with. Certainly, you want to be comprehensive and appropriately cite the sources that you have used. However, you want to find a balance and not over-cite references in an article for publication. Take a look at these examples to help you find your own middle ground:

- Many different organizations, such as the American Cancer Society and the National Cancer Institute, collect statistics on the incidence of breast cancer. If you quote a statistic, you do not need to include two, three, or four organizational references to support it. One authoritative and up-to-date reference should be sufficient—and you should cite the actual source you used. Although this sounds obvious, different organizations report statistics in different ways, so you want to make sure the citation you use matches the data you report.

- As another example, the SF-36 is a measure of health outcomes and quality of life that has been widely used and has well-established psychometric properties. A quick search using the MEDLINE online database reveals it's been cited more than 25,000 times in articles since 1989. If you were using this instrument in a research study, would you cite all these articles? Of course not. You should include only the most salient, recent, and relevant citations that are illustrative of how and why the instrument is appropriate for your study.

Q *What about common knowledge? Do I need to cite every statement?*

A If something is common knowledge, it does not need to be cited. But what is considered "common knowledge"? It depends on your audience. If you are writing for clinicians, you can assume that they will know and accept certain things as facts, such as, "Nursing is an art and a science," and, "A diagnosis of breast cancer is a devastating moment in a woman's life." On the other hand, even though it's widely stated and accepted as truth, the statement, "One in eight women will be diagnosed with breast cancer during her lifetime," should be supported with a citation.

Editors of journals are beginning to react to overcitation, and some editors have taken steps to limit the number of references in an article. When you encounter this limitation, the number is firm. If the publication's author guidelines list a maximum of 50 references, that means 50—not 51 or 52. Even though you believe that every reference is absolutely essential, you need to delete some if you go over the limit. How do you do that? Remember the earlier example: It is not necessary to provide multiple citations to document a single statement. Read with a critical eye—you will see where references can be pared.

Also, consider how often you cite a single source. For example, say you have a five-sentence paragraph, and all the ideas in that paragraph come from the same source. Write the paragraph to make the source of the information clear, and then include the citation at the end of the paragraph instead of at the end of every sentence. However, if several sources contribute to the content of the paragraph make sure to add citations appropriately so the reader will be able to follow your line of thinking and documentation.

Q *How far back do I need to go in my literature search and citation of references?*

A While you certainly want to read thoroughly and deeply to master the topic area you're researching, how far back you go depends on your project. If you are writing a literature review, you need to seek out articles from a wider time range, going back a number of years, in addition to more recent works. If you are writing an article on a quality improvement project or a clinical condition, the general rule is to use sources no older than three to five years.

No matter how many articles you've read, you need to synthesize the literature and cite only those sources that are key to your presentation. So even if you have read dozens of articles dating back 20, 30, or 50 years, be selective in what you cite. Some editors ask you to only include references written in the last five years, unless it is a classic source that requires citation. This is particularly true for clinical articles, where treatment and interventions change based on research findings. You want to make sure you have the most up-to-date information on the topic you are presenting.

Style Manuals

A *style manual* or *stylebook* provides a set of guidelines and standards for written documents. *Style* is an inclusive term that can encompasses everything from punctuation and capitalization to citation formatting specifics. Style manuals include much more than directions on how to reference citations. They also provide guidance on structure, writing style, preferred abbreviations, and how to report statistics, as well as ethical issues related to publication. The idea is to standardize formatting issues for authors, editors, publishers, reviewers, and anyone else involved in the process of disseminating information through publication. Most newspapers (and some magazines) use *The Associated Press Stylebook* (2022). Another heavily used style guide—especially in mainstream book publishing—is *The Chicago Manual of Style* (2017), published by the University of Chicago Press. Both of these guides have websites with subscription fees. The *Associated Press Stylebook* website is updated as changes are made.

The two manuals that are most widely used in nursing and other healthcare publications are the *Publication Manual of the American Psychological Association* (7th ed.), published by the American Psychological Association (APA, 2020), and the *AMA Manual of Style* (11th ed.), produced by the American Medical Association (JAMA Network Editors, 2020). These also have websites with subscription fees. The websites are updated between print editions as changes are made, so they are a valuable resource. Do not use older editions of style guides, which may contain outdated information.

Some journals use a selected style manual for certain aspects of their articles, such as citing references, but differ in other areas of guidance. Thus, remember to carefully read the information for authors or author guidelines to understand what exceptions (if any) are made, and then format your paper accordingly.

The most important issue, no matter which style manual you use, is to be complete and accurate in your citations. Check and double-check that you have authors' names spelled correctly; the correct year of publication; and complete citation information, including title of the article (or book), the journal where it was published, and volume, issue, and page numbers. The AMA and APA style manuals handle citations differently, and most editors are adamant that the guidelines be followed.

Confidence Booster

When you have a working knowledge of more than one style, you won't feel restricted to selecting only journals that use the one you know. This gives you many more options, increasing your chances for publication success, because you will have strategically chosen the best journal for your article.

Anatomy of a Reference

When gathering citations, carefully document all the information related to the reference. When you compose the actual citation, some information may not be required, but it's easier to edit out information rather than search for missing information at the last minute.

You can organize your references in a bibliography database manager (BDM, discussed later in this chapter), an Excel spreadsheet, a table in Word, or another system that you develop. If you can import citation information from an online source, or cut-and-paste into your library or spreadsheet, do so. Errors caused by retyping are common and a major source of inaccurate citations. Keep a copy of the article as a PDF (or as a paper copy) and organize the articles by topic or author so you can easily locate what you need.

Whatever method you choose, make sure your notes are complete. Essential elements include:

- **Author(s') names:** Include complete information for all authors: first and last names and middle initials. Even though the style might only require last name and first initial, you should have complete data in your notes. Double-check that you have spelled names correctly and have included any accents or other diacritical marks (signs that are added to letters).

- **Title of article:** Include the complete title.

- **Title of journal:** Be sure you have the complete title of the journal. If the journal title is abbreviated, make sure you find the correct, full name. For citations in MEDLINE, you can click on the link of the journal abbreviation to obtain the full name. Even if you need to abbreviate the title (according to style guidelines) when you create the reference list, in your database you should have the complete title.

- **Date of publication:** This is when the article was either published in print or posted online. An article may have been "published ahead of print" and posted on the journal website before being assigned to an issue. In this case, the date of publication may change, so it is important to double-check and make updates as needed.

- **Volume:** In general, the volume number changes each year; for example, the first year a journal is published is volume 1, year five would be volume 5. An article that is "published ahead of print" may not have a volume or issue number, or assigned pages. Again, keep checking to see if this information is added to the citation and to ensure that your data are current.

- **Issue number:** The issue number changes each time an issue is published within a volume; for example, the first issue of the year is issue 1, the second is issue 2, and so on. As a rule, if the publication is monthly, the issues match the months (e.g., issue 5 is May, issue 12 is December).

- **Page numbers:** Include all page numbers even if an article "jumps" to a nonconsecutive page.

- **URL or Uniform Resource Locator:** For online sources, you will need the complete URL. Some style manuals require the specific date you retrieved a source, such as May 15, 2024.

- **DOI, or Digital Object Identifier:** The DOI (discussed later in the chapter) is a unique code assigned to an article upon publication that enables a person to retrieve the article using the DOI in a search. The newest editions of the APA and AMA manuals include the DOI as part of the citation, so it is important to capture this information when you first retrieve the article.

Reference Formatting

When it comes to references, one major difference between AMA and APA is how they are cited in the text. AMA uses superscripted numbers that are consecutively numbered and listed in numerical order in the reference list. APA uses author and date citations within the text, followed by an alphabetical reference list.

The following examples illustrate what you might see in the text for each style.

AMA: Four studies reported that the treatment was effective.[1-4]

APA: Four studies reported that the treatment was effective (Allen et al., 2021; Grant & Jones, 2020; Peterson et al., 2019; Smith, 2023). [Citations are fictitious. Note that authors are listed in alphabetical order.]

Here are examples of a journal-article reference in each style:

AMA: Halm MA. Skin pigmentation and accuracy of pulse oximetry values. *Am J Crit Care*. 2023; 32(6): 459-462. doi: 10.4037/ajcc2023292

APA: Halm, M. A. (2023). Skin pigmentation and accuracy of pulse oximetry values. *American Journal of Critical Care*, *32*(6), 459–462. https://doi.org/10.4037/ajcc2023292

Here are examples of a book reference in each style:

AMA: Nicoll LH, Chinn PL. *The Editor's Handbook*. 3rd ed. Philadelphia, PA: Wolters Kluwer Health; 2019

APA: Nicoll, L. H., & Chinn, P. L. (2019). *The editor's handbook* (3rd ed). Wolters Kluwer Health.

Keep in mind is that reference lists in AMA are numbered in consecutive order of references appearing in the text; therefore, if you add a reference to the text, unless it's the last reference in the document, all the existing references need to be renumbered—another reason to use a bibliography database manager (BDM) to write your paper, as this digital tool will keep track of citations in the text and number them correctly on the reference list.

If you are using Microsoft Word as your word processing program, an alternative to a BDM is to use the software's auto-numbering feature to help with formatting. However, most journals won't accept manuscripts using the Word EndNote feature, so you'll need to convert these citations to plain text before submission. To do this, select all the text in the document using the following shortcut commands—for Mac: Cmd+A—for Windows: Ctrl+A. If you are using Microsoft Word, you can then remove the codes with these shortcuts—for Mac: Cmd+6—Windows: Ctrl+6. Make sure to save a copy of the document before removing the formatting codes.

Q *I read the* American Journal of Critical Care *on my iPad. How do I cite something I've read electronically, but not online?*

A When an article is published both in print and online, you should use the citation information associated with the print version, which will include volume, issue, and page numbers. A PDF of the issue on your iPad should have this information. If an article is available only online, you should cite that version, with complete citation information.

Remember, you provide citation information so a reader can go back to the same source you used for verification or further reading, so it is important to be complete and accurate. As noted previously, the AMA and APA manuals include DOI numbers as part of the citation. Journals using these manuals have followed suit, which means you need to include them. Having this number allows a reader to quickly find the article online.

The Scoop on Digital Object Identifiers

The DOI has been established as the standard to act as a permanent locator to retrieve an article online (Nicoll & Chinn, 2015). The standard was finalized in 2010, so any article published after that date will likely have an assigned DOI. Include this information in your citation database so it will be available when you create your reference list.

Many publishers are working backward to assign DOIs to previously published articles, so you should check to see if a DOI has been assigned to an older reference. Here are three options to do so:

- Use the *single citation matcher* in PubMed, shown in Figure 4.1 (https://www.ncbi.nlm.nih.gov/pubmed/citmatch). Type in some of the information about your article—you don't need to fill in every box, just enough to uniquely identify it—and press search. When you find your citation, you can see if there is a DOI assigned.
- Use CrossRef (https://www.crossref.org/guestquery). As shown in Figure 4.2, the screen is similar to the single citation matcher in PubMed. Type in the citation information, and if there is a DOI, it will be returned to you when the search is complete.
- Go to the original source of the article on the journal's website. Even if the DOI hasn't made it to PubMed or CrossRef, it may show up on the citation for the article where it's posted on the journal's website.

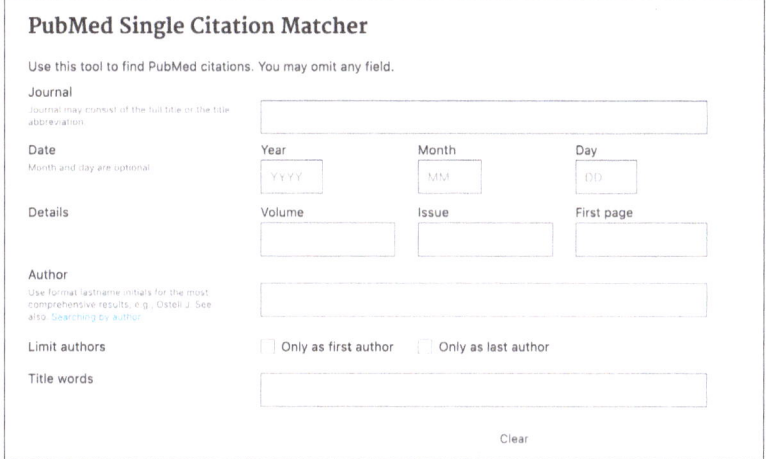

FIGURE 4.1 The PubMed single citation matcher search screen.

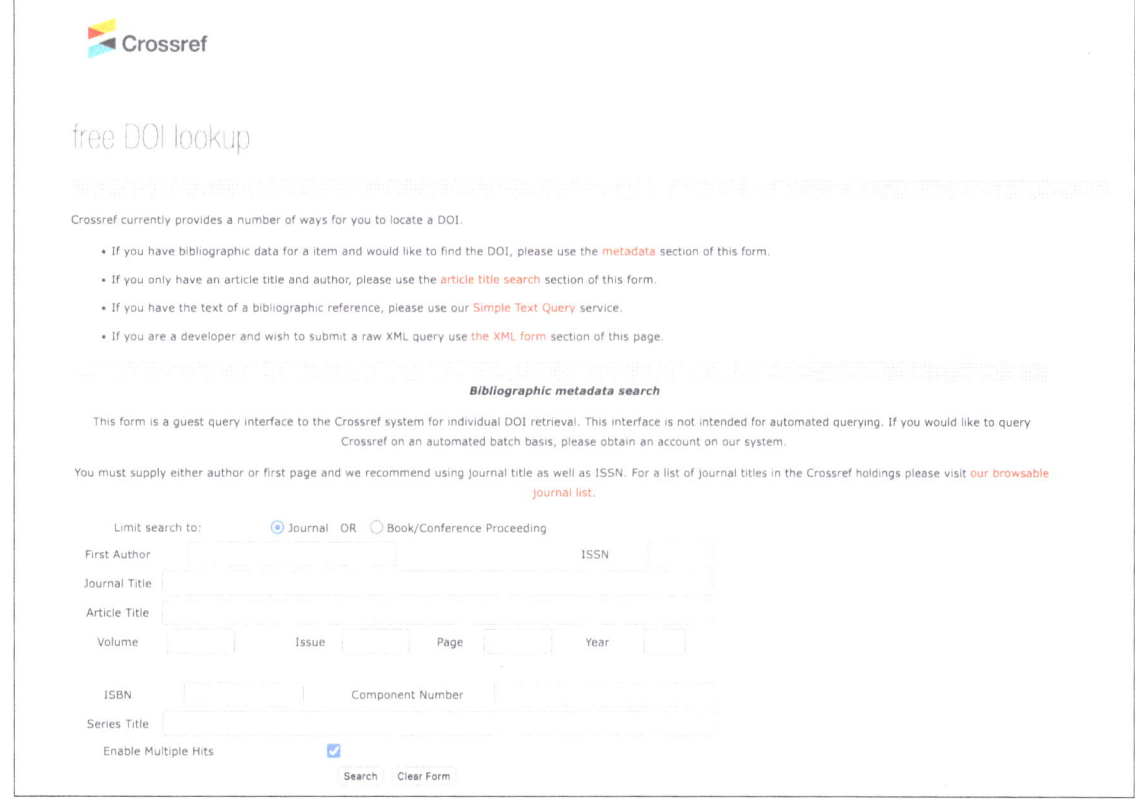

FIGURE 4.2 The CrossRef query search screen.

If you don't come up with a DOI after trying these three steps, you can safely assume that one has not been assigned to your citation.

Always use the DOI if one is available, even if you retrieved the article by using a database at your college or organization library. You might be tempted to use the URL associated with your search; however, because you had to log in to your library database, the URL is useless to someone who doesn't have that same access. Those who don't have access will get a 404 Error (page not found) or similar message. Remember, you want to provide information to readers so that they can find the sources you cite—at this time, the DOI is the standard for permanent retrieval of a citation. As an aside, you should check all URLs included in a manuscript to ensure that they direct you to the correct location. You should also check DOIs for accuracy.

> **Q** *Can I cite fugitive literature in my paper?*
>
> **A** *Fugitive literature*, also called *ephemeral literature* or *grey literature*, consists of documents that exist outside of traditional, peer-reviewed publications. A common example is an abstract (or paper) published as part of a conference program and distributed only to conference attendees.
>
> If you want to cite an abstract from a conference, first check whether the presentation has been published. A published article is preferable over citing the proceedings, as the latter would be hard for people who didn't attend the conference to access. If there is no published article, is something available online? If not, cite the materials you have in hand. Keep in mind, however, that as your source becomes more difficult to access, it becomes less valuable to your reader. Obscure references aren't necessarily better or more scholarly (although some people labor under that impression).

Databases as a Source of References

How do you go about finding references? Your first step is to learn what resources are available to you. If you are a student or if you work in a setting with a library, start there. Health sciences libraries have access to online databases that include citations and, often, full text. Students and employees can typically use these resources at no charge. In addition, the librarians will be able to assist, so that resources can be used most effectively. The top databases, except for MEDLINE, are licensed to institutions rather than individuals. If you have access through your institution, it's wise to take advantage of this resource.

MEDLINE and More

The National Library of Medicine (NLM) provides three important options for authors seeking information (NLM, 2023b):

MEDLINE is the most useful online database for health literature. It contains more than 30 million citations. The citations include complete reference information, abstract (when available), and Medical Subject Headings—or MeSH—the vocabulary of the NLM. (You'll learn about using MeSH for a more effective search later in this chapter.)

PubMed is the user interface for MEDLINE. In addition to the MEDLINE references, it includes citations for other materials, such as articles that have not yet been published in a journal, author manuscripts that have been submitted to comply with funding requirements related to making articles openly available, and preprints from eligible preprint servers. (Preprints facilitate rapid dissemination of information but have not undergone peer review. Learn more about preprints in Chapter 3.)

PubMed Central (PMC) contains free, full-text articles. These articles are provided by publishers or by authors to comply with any funding requirements.

You'll want to use PubMed (https://pubmed.ncbi.nlm.nih.gov) for your searching needs since the results will include MEDLINE and PMC articles. A number of tutorials can help you get started with searching PubMed (https://learn.nlm.nih.gov/rest/training-packets/T0042010P.html). One tutorial that focuses on using PubMed to answer clinical questions related to evidence-based practice includes scenarios and application exercises. You can access it at https://www.nlm.nih.gov/oet/ed/pubmed/pubmed_in_ebp/index.html. One note of caution: Not all peer-reviewed nursing journals are indexed by the National Library of Medicine.

Google Scholar

A resource that is not limited to the health science literature is Google Scholar (https://scholar.google.com):

Google Scholar provides a simple way to broadly search for scholarly literature. From one place, you can search across many disciplines and sources: articles, theses, books, abstracts and court opinions, from academic publishers, professional societies, online repositories, universities and other websites. Google Scholar helps you find relevant work across the world of scholarly research. (Google Scholar, n.d., para. 1)

As with PubMed, Google Scholar has tutorials and various levels of help to assist you with a literature search. An advantage of Google Scholar is that it searches a wider range of journals than PubMed; a disadvantage is that it is not a curated list, so it may include citations from predatory journals. (See Chapter 3 for more information on predatory journals.) Just as you want to carefully select a journal for publication, you also want to be careful with the citations you use as sources in your manuscript (Oermann et al., 2020).

Other Database Options

Other useful databases include the Cumulative Index to Nursing and Allied Health Literature (CINAHL), available through EBSCOhost; Scopus; Embase; Cochrane Library; and ProQuest Nursing & Allied Health Database. Remember, however, that you need to access these resources through an institution such as a medical library. You can find open-access journals by searching BioMed Central (https://www.biomedcentral.com) or the Directory of Open Access Journals (https://www.doaj.org). (Learn more about open-access journals in Chapter 3.) Table 4.1 provides a comparison of some of the major databases generally accessed when searching for nursing-relevant literature.

Search With Search Engines

Both PubMed and Google Scholar use similar search engines. You can search using any number of variables, including author name, words in the title, year of publication, keywords, volume, issue, and more. You can use Boolean operators, such as AND (narrow your search) or OR (expand your search). For example, let's say you want to write an article related to diabetes in children. Searching for "children AND diabetes" would result in articles that are about children with diabetes, excluding articles that don't have both words in them. This search makes it more likely you will find articles related specifically to your topic.

Putting quotes around a phrase, such as "myocardial infarction," cues the search engine to look for that exact phrase.

TABLE 4.1 Relevant Databases for Accessing Nursing Literature

Database	Scope	Citations	Journals	Time Frame	Access
MEDLINE	Journal articles in the life sciences with a concentration on biomedicine	31+ million, updated daily	5,200 journals in 40 languages	1966–present (1946–1966 Old MEDLINE)	Via PubMed, available at no cost to anyone with internet access
CINAHL	Nursing and allied health literature, including journals and publications from the National League for Nursing and the American Nurses Association. Literature covers a wide range of topics including nursing, biomedicine, health sciences librarianship, alternative/complementary medicine, consumer health, and several allied health disciplines.	6 million	Searchable cited references for more than 1,300 journals	1981–present	Via EBSCOhost, requires an institutional subscription

continues

TABLE 4.1 Relevant Databases for Accessing Nursing Literature (*continued*)

Database	Scope	Citations	Journals	Time Frame	Access
Scopus	Abstract and citation database published by Elsevier; established in 2004. Covers life sciences, physical sciences, health sciences, and social sciences. Sources covered: book series, journals, and trade journals.	93+ million	28,000+ titles; 327,000+ books	1970–present	Via Scopus, requires an institutional subscription
PsycInfo	Behavioral and social sciences, with a focus on psychology	5.4+ million, updated twice weekly	2,400 journals	1887–present	Individuals can subscribe to PsycInfo at a variety of price points (also available through institutional subscription)
Ovid Nursing Database	Nursing and allied health portal for practice, education, research, and administration	Based on the nursing and allied health sub-set of Ovid MEDLINE	800+ journals		Via Ovid through an institutional subscription
ProQuest Central	Comprehensive multidisciplinary database	Nursing & Allied Health premium includes scholarly literature, dissertations, systematic reviews, and more	Includes journals, magazines, trade publication, and news items		Via ProQuest through an institutional subscription

Some universities have their own open-access resource, such as the Digital Access to Scholarship at Harvard (https://dash.harvard.edu). And professional organizations often have repositories like the Sigma Repository, from Sigma Theta Tau International, which shares nursing research and evidence-based practice materials (www.nursinglibrary.org).

No matter what sources you use, beware of articles generated by artificial intelligence (AI), which often have fabricated or inaccurate references. One study found that among 115 references in 30 ChatGPT-generated medical articles, 47% were fabricated, 46% were authentic but inaccurate, and only 7% were authentic and accurate (Bhattacharyya et al., 2023). You should be wary of AI-generated content and not cite these articles in your manuscript.

Finding What You're Looking For

By now you have probably narrowed your topic and started your search for articles and data. Many people begin a search in a rather haphazard fashion, which is fine because it provides an idea of just how much information is out there on a given topic. For example, typing "breast cancer" in PubMed retrieves more than 506,600 citations—clearly more than you would ever need for a paper or could even read and synthesize.

The next step, then, is to begin to focus and refine your search. You might have specific aspects of your topic that you'd like to study, or you might want to use the suggestions many databases provide for you. Are you interested in breast cancer risk, or metastasis, or pain? You can narrow your results by year or discipline (e.g., nursing). As you begin to get a handle on your search, the results will become more focused—and more manageable.

Track your keywords, which will help give you additional avenues for searching. You may also want to review the reference lists of the articles you retrieve—a helpful trick that can make your search even more comprehensive. Are there certain authors or articles that keep showing up? This might be a pointer to a *classic reference*—one that is essential in the literature and that you should be familiar with. Your goal through this process is to achieve a level of saturation where you feel you have found all the relevant articles that exist on a topic.

Q *Is it acceptable to just cite the abstract of a full-text article so I don't have to pay for the article?*

A The abstract can help you determine how relevant the article is to your research topic. However, when citing a source, it is expected that you have read the entire article—not just the abstract—as a matter of good scholarship.

Using MeSH Terms to Maximize Your Search

MeSH is the controlled vocabulary thesaurus used by the NLM to index articles for MEDLINE. Learning this vocabulary will help you search more effectively. According to the NLM, MeSH is a "controlled vocabulary ... used for indexing, cataloging, and searching for biomedical and health-related information and documents" (NLM, 2023a, para. 1). The vocabulary refers to subject descriptors that are arranged both alphabetically and hierarchically.

MeSH terms help users find content with different terminology but the same concept. Assigning MeSH terms to an article is both a science and an art—there are specialists at the NLM whose sole task is to do just this. You needn't be an expert, but you should have a working familiarity with the MeSH vocabulary to get the most out of your literature search. Keep in mind that when you use MeSH terms with PubMed searches, you will only see MEDLINE citations in your results.

The simplest way to become acquainted with MeSH terms is to study those that are assigned to citations you retrieve through PubMed. When you find

Clinical Competence

The capability to perform acceptably those duties directly related to patient care.
Year introduced: 1975

PubMed search builder options
Subheadings:

- [ ] economics
- [ ] standards
- [ ] legislation and jurisprudence

- [ ] Restrict to MeSH Major Topic.
- [ ] Do not include MeSH terms found below this term in the MeSH hierarchy.

Tree Number(s): I02.399.630.210, N04.761.210, N05.715.175
MeSH Unique ID: D002983
Entry Terms:

- Competency, Clinical
- Competence, Clinical
- Clinical Competency
- Clinical Competencies
- Competencies, Clinical
- Clinical Skill
- Skill, Clinical
- Skills, Clinical
- Clinical Skills

Previous Indexing:

- Educational Measurement (1966-1974)

See Also:

- Culturally Competent Care

All MeSH Categories
Anthropology, Education, Sociology and Social Phenomena Category
Education

FIGURE 4.3 Definition and hierarchy of the MeSH term "clinical competence."

a citation, scroll down past the abstract to see the headline "MeSH Terms." You can go a step further and click on a term, which allows you to search either MEDLINE or MeSH for that specific term. If you choose the latter, you will retrieve a screen, such as shown in Figure 4.3, which provides the definition, history, and hierarchy of the MeSH term. This can be a helpful tactic for learning the proper indexing terms in your area of interest.

Another handy feature for learning more about MeSH terms is the MeSH browser (https://www.nlm.nih.gov/mesh/MBrowser.html). Here, you can type a term into the search field to find out if it is the correct MeSH term or, if not, what the correct term is. For example, a search for the term "breast cancer" will reveal the proper MeSH term—"Breast Neoplasms"—which is hierarchically arranged under Neoplasms, and then "Neoplasms by site." Many publishers ask you to include three to five keywords, using MeSH language, when you submit your manuscript. If you have used the MeSH browser, you would know that "breast neoplasms" is a more appropriate keyword than "breast cancer" and will enhance the likelihood that your article will appear in another person's search results.

One final, useful feature is MeSH on Demand (https://www.nlm.nih.gov/mesh/MeSHonDemand.html). In this case, you can type in text, up to 10,000 characters. Select "Find MeSH Terms" and the site will give you a list of suggested MeSH terms based on the content of the text you submitted. How would you use this? You could paste in the text of your abstract when you finish your article and find possible keywords using MeSH headings to submit with your manuscript. As with everything related to searching and citations, don't just blindly tick off the words from the list. You need to consider if they are the best descriptors for your topic—but MeSH on Demand can give you a starting point for identifying keywords, something that can be very challenging for novice and experienced authors alike.

Q *How can I be more efficient with my searching?*

A Keep track of what search terms you use and the order in which you used them so that you don't repeat terms unnecessarily. Also keep track of how many results you found and how you then narrowed your search—what inclusion and exclusion criteria did you use to keep or discard references? For example, you may choose to only include articles published in peer-reviewed journals and discard articles in newspapers or magazines. Document all this information in your notes or reference library.

One thing to keep in mind as you move toward saturation: Narrowing your focus is easier than trying to read hundreds or thousands of articles on a given topic. It is better to be comprehensive within a narrow range rather than superficial and arbitrary, such as selecting random cutoff years, or places where articles are published.

As you search, you will be retrieving as many as three things:

- Information for a complete article citation
- Abstract (i.e., the short summary of the article, presentation, or document)
- Full text

Q *How can I find out whether an article will be useful to me before I pay to access it online?*

A Databases like MEDLINE, online libraries, and others give free access to abstracts (often provided by the journal publisher) with links to the full-text versions of articles online. Although some articles may be available at no cost, many publishers charge a fee. Even if you're on a budget, all is not lost. Your university, community college, or hospital library might maintain an institutional subscription to the journal for which you need access.

If you are working in a setting that does not provide access to a health sciences library, check with your alma mater to see if library access is available to you as an alumni benefit. In this case, you may be able to access and search online through the university library portal, obtain the full-text version of articles, and even request articles through interlibrary loan.

If you belong to a professional organization (like Sigma Theta Tau International), you might receive a journal subscription as part of your member benefits. You might also receive substantial discounts on other journals you'd like to receive. Your membership may give you free access to full-text published articles online. Similarly, if you subscribe to a journal, part of your subscription may include online access to full text of the articles at no charge.

Another possible source is your local public library. It may have access to medical journals or be able to help you obtain an article through the local library loan at no charge or for a small fee.

Another time-honored tradition is to write the first author and request a copy of the article. Most authors receive a PDF at the time an article is published and will send you a copy upon request. Be polite, address the author by name with an appropriate salutation (e.g., Dear Dr. Smith), and briefly explain why you are asking for the article. Most authors are flattered to be asked and will send you the PDF file.

The bottom line: Do a little sleuthing before pulling out your credit card to pay for access to an online full-text article.

Information for a complete citation has been discussed previously—see the box on "Anatomy of a Reference" earlier in this chapter. *Abstracts* are the summaries of full-text articles written by the authors and made available at no cost. They will help you determine whether it would be useful to retrieve the full text of the research paper, chapter, presentation, or other source. Databases like MEDLINE include an abstract if it was published with the article. Certain types of journal articles—such as letters to the editor, editorials, and columns—do not include abstracts. You also won't often find abstracts for magazine articles, profiles, personal interviews, and so on.

Full text is just what the name implies: the full text of an article. Just about everything published in scholarly journals is available online, but the ability to access the full text of a given work varies depending on the publisher, the topic of the article, and the database in which it is maintained. Some articles are available at no charge; however, many require a fee (often called "pay per view") or a subscription to the journal.

Bibliography Database Managers

A study found that researchers spend a median of 14 hours formatting their manuscript before publication, including references, tables, and figures (LeBlanc et al., 2019). You can help avoid much formatting time by being accurate and organized with your references.

Before computers, authors used use *bib cards* (short for *bibliography cards*) to organize their references. These were hand-written index cards with the complete citation, where it was obtained, notes, and even portions of the abstract. Bib cards are an anachronism, but the concept is not. Paper cards have just been replaced by software. Many writers create their own systems, spreadsheets, or databases for references, but a more common option is to use a commercially available bibliography database manager (BDM), such as EndNote (a product of Clarivate Analytics), Mendeley (a product of Elsevier), or Paperpile. There are other similar programs available—some free for public use, others for purchase. These programs may help improve accuracy of citations (Nicoll et al., 2022).

A detailed description of all available BDM programs is beyond the scope of this chapter. However, Wikipedia (2023) has a helpful comparison chart of many of the programs that currently exist, the associated costs (many are free), and whether the resource resides on your computer as software or is housed "in the cloud." You can access the information at https://en.wikipedia.org/wiki/Comparison_of_reference_management_software.

Q *Earlier you said not to quote Wikipedia, but you just did. What's up with that?*

A Good catch. Wikipedia is a tertiary source, and thus a compilation of facts and information from multiple sources. It should not be used as a primary source for scholarly writing. However, this particular table is a good synthesis of reference management software and can easily be verified by going to each named company's website. Because information on Wikipedia is updated regularly, this source will be accurate beyond the date this book is published. As a tertiary source that summarizes information on BDMs, Wikipedia, in this case, gives you a starting point to learn more.

What Does a BDM Do?

A BDM provides a database to maintain your references by creating a *library*, or internal reference database, on your own computer or in the cloud, creating an electronic substitute for bib cards. You can attach notes and keywords to each reference so that you can easily sort and access information. You can also attach PDFs of the article, and the pictures, figures, and annotations therein. How much or how little you include depends on your need and the extent of the writing. Nothing is required—although a citation without the minimum, basic information, as discussed earlier, is not going to be very useful.

BDM programs work in conjunction with your word processor, helping you format your references and making sure that they are presented correctly in your paper. Other functionalities vary depending on the software, but a good BDM also makes it easy to change between required styles, such as APA or AMA. For example, if you write a paper for Journal A that uses APA style and the paper is not accepted, you can easily revise the references in the paper to AMA style, which might be required for Journal B. Your BDM also helps keep your references numbered properly, if that is the citation style, no matter how many references you move around while editing and revising your manuscript.

After you get comfortable with the program, whichever one you decide to use, you'll be able to work with online search engines such as PubMed and Google Scholar, which have the capability to import references into a BDM. This can save you time because you don't have to retype the citation; more importantly, it increases accuracy by minimizing room for error when typing an author's name or the year of publication, for instance. By using this feature, you can also have a more complete citation in your library. For example, by default, PubMed includes abstracts, keywords, and MeSH terms. Citations from MEDLINE also include the DOI for an article as well as the PubMed ID (PMID). Many BDMs enable you to search online databases from within the program and import citations directly into the program.

Another feature of many BDMs is the capability to share and sync libraries among users. This makes collaboration among coauthors easier.

Q *I am writing a short article with maybe 10 or 12 references. But I have never heard of any of these programs. Should I take the time to learn how to use one in this case?*

A Yes, it would be a good idea to do so. As noted in the beginning of this chapter, citing references accurately is the gold standard for authors, and it's your responsibility to do this. Because of the wide variety of types of citations that exist, ranging from journal articles and chapters in books, to online white papers and blogs, it's difficult to learn all the "ins and outs" and style references by rote. A BDM makes this task much easier, and a short article with just a few references is a great way to learn how to use a BDM program. That way, you'll already be familiar with the program when writing a longer, more complex article in the future. If you access the Wikipedia comparison table, referenced earlier, you can find programs that are free or have free trial periods.

> **Confidence Booster**
>
> To feel confident that your information is as current as possible, keep a list of your search terms and run them monthly to retrieve anything new that has been published on your topic. Import the citations into your BDM. In doing so, you will always be up to date on the relevant literature.

BDMs have some drawbacks, too—but there are resources to help you overcome the following obstacles:

- **Learning curve:** For many people, BDMs are not naturally intuitive or easy to use. They do require time to learn; for some users, the learning curve is so steep that they think using one is not worth the effort, but don't give up—the payoff is big. If you find a BDM challenging, ask a colleague for help. The program you use may also have a tutorial to get you started, an FAQ database, or an online forum where you can connect with other users. All these resources are designed to help you become a "power user" in no time.

- **Time:** Maintaining a library and using it effectively requires a time investment up front, although ultimately, you'll save formatting time later. Keeping citations up to date allows you to make the most of what a BDM has to offer. Fortunately, there are an increasing number of online tools to help you do this. Figure 4.4 shows an online citation to a recent article published in the *Journal of Nursing Scholarship*. As you can see, you can download and save the citation in six different formats: plain text, RIS (format for ProCite, Reference Manager, and Paperpile), EndNote, BibTex, Medlars, and RefWorks. The site also provides tips on downloading, as shown on the right.

- **Sloppy data entry:** If you put references into the BDM incorrectly, the resulting citation will be inaccurate. Take time to edit as you go, correcting capitalization and punctuation and ensuring that journal titles are correctly entered. Even when you download citations directly from the internet, double-check to ensure each element of the citation is accurate and in the appropriate field (e.g., the author's name is complete, and the year of publication is in the date box).

If you are embarking on a project, particularly one that is expected to encompass years of work (such as a dissertation), or you know that you will work in a specialty area for a significant amount of time, a BDM is the best way to maintain and organize your reference data.

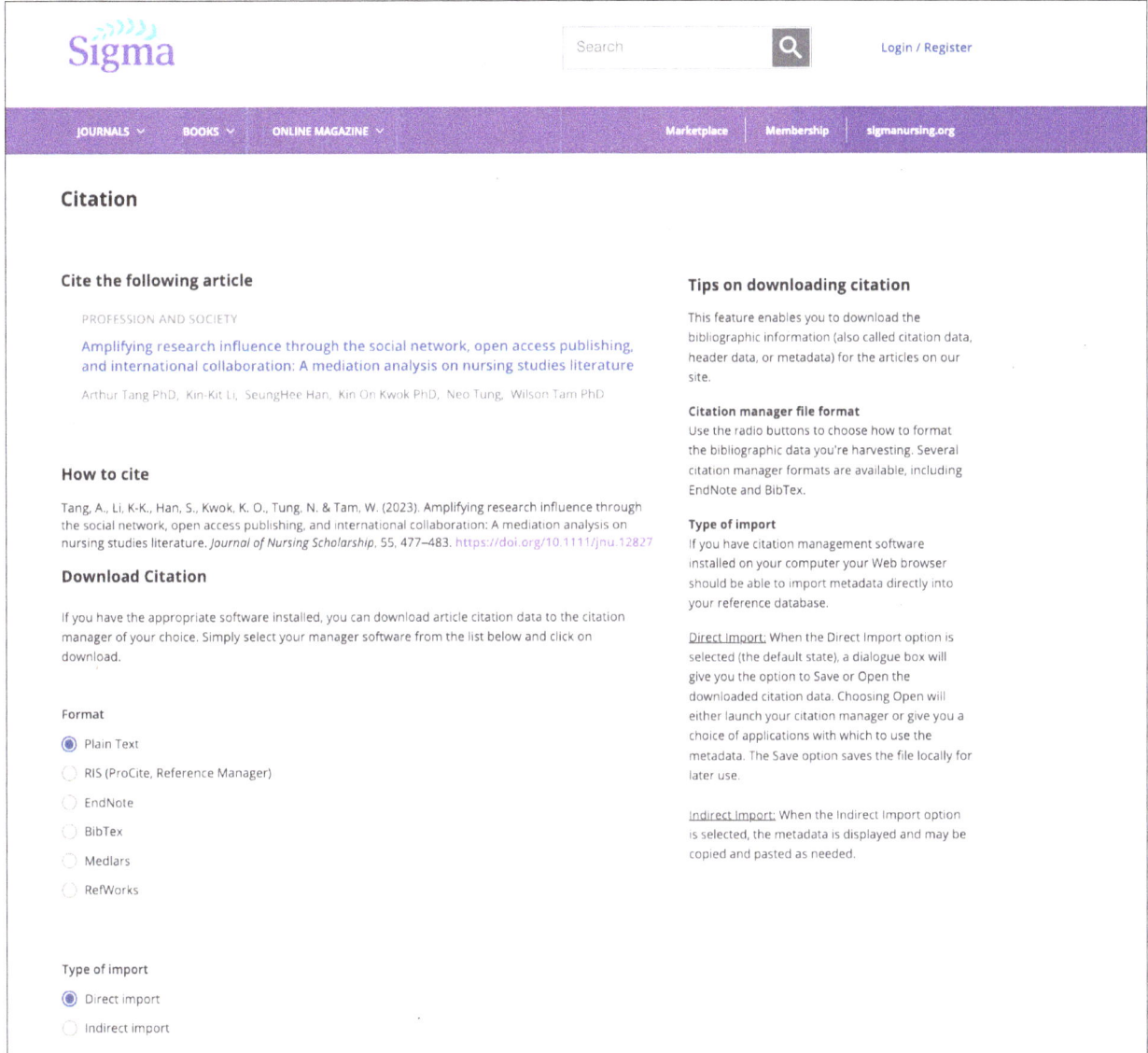

FIGURE 4.4 Citation tools for the *Journal of Nursing Scholarship*.

Q *I've used a BDM to format my references for my article, but the author guidelines say not to include citations from an automatic reference system. Now what do I do?*

A You need to remove the citation codes before you submit your manuscript. This should be your very last step, after you have ensured that all your final edits have been made. First save a copy of the document with a new file name (you might include "no codes" in the file name as a reminder which version this is). Then, select all the text in the document using the following shortcut commands—for Mac: Cmd+A—for Windows: Ctrl+A. If you are using Microsoft Word, you can then remove the codes with these shortcuts—for Mac: Cmd+6—for Windows: Ctrl+6. If you are using Google Docs, the shortcut Ctrl+\ will clear the formatting, as will selecting "Clear Formatting" from the Format dropdown menu.

Solid Researching

Now you know the usefulness of style guides, and how to find sources, organize them, and cite them appropriately. Just like writing, searching and managing your sources take practice. Your payoff is a high-quality article useful to readers—and isn't that your ultimate goal?

Write Now!

1. Conduct a search in PubMed and Google Scholar, and compare your results.

2. Access a free BDM, or one that has a free trial. Import some citations from the search you did in #1 into your library. Change the output style to APA, then AMA. Compare how the citations look.

3. Select three journals and look at some articles to identify the style of reference citation that each uses. Then look at the Information for Authors for the journals. Do the guidelines specify which style manual to use for citations? Did you pick the right ones?

References

American Psychological Association. (2020). *Publication manual of the American Psychological Association* (7th ed.). https://doi.org/10.1037/0000165-000

The Associated Press. (2022). *The Associated Press stylebook: 2022–2024* (56th ed.). Basic Books.

Bhattacharyya, M., Miller, V. M., Bhattacharyya, D, & Miller, L. E. (2023). High rates of fabricated and inaccurate references in ChatGPT-generated medical content. *Cureus, 15*(5), e39238. https://doi.org/10.7759/cureus.39238

Google Scholar. (n.d.). www.google.com/intl/en/scholar/about.html

JAMA Network Editors. (2020). *AMA manual of style: A guide for authors and editors* (11th ed.). Oxford University Press. https://doi.org/10.1093/jama/9780190246556.001.0001

LeBlanc, A. G., Barnes, J. D., Saunders, T. J., Tremblay, M. S., & Chaput, J.-P. (2019). Scientific sinkhole: The pernicious price of formatting. *PLoS One, 14*(9), e0223116. https://doi.org/10.1371/journal.pone.0223116

National Library of Medicine. (2023a). *Medical subject headings: Preface.* https://www.nlm.nih.gov/mesh/intro_preface.html#pref_rem

National Library of Medicine. (2023b). *MEDLINE, PubMed, and PMC (PubMed Central): How are they different?* https://www.nlm.nih.gov/bsd/difference.html

Nicoll, L. H., & Chinn, P. L. (2015). *Writing in the digital age: Savvy publishing for healthcare professionals.* Wolters Kluwer Health.

Nicoll, L. H., Oermann, M. H., Carter-Templeton, H., Wrigley, J., & Owens, J. K. (2022). Exploring the accuracy of cited references in a selected data set of nursing journal articles. *Advances in Nursing Science, 45*(3), 209–217. https://doi.org/10.1097/ANS.0000000000000408

Oermann, M. H., Nicoll, L. H., Ashton, K. S., Edie, A. H., Amarasekara, S., Chinn, P. L., Carter-Templeton, H., & Ledbetter, L. S. (2020). Analysis of citation patterns and impact of predatory sources in the nursing literature. *Journal of Nursing Scholarship, 52*(3), 311–319. https://doi.org/10.1111/jnu.12557

Shellenbarger, T. (2016). Simplifying synthesis. *Nurse Author & Editor, 26*(3), 1–10. https://doi.org/10.1111/j.1750-4910.2016.tb00224.x

University of Chicago Press Editorial Staff (Eds.). (2017). *The Chicago manual of style* (17th ed.). University of Chicago Press.

Wikipedia. (n.d.). *Wikipedia: Researching with Wikipedia.* https://en.wikipedia.org/wiki/Wikipedia:Researching_with_Wikipedia

Wikipedia. (2023). *Comparison of reference management software.* http://en.wikipedia.org/wiki/Comparison_of_reference_management_software

Organizing the Article

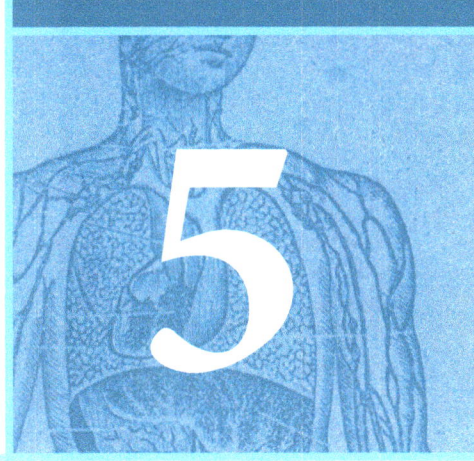

–Kayla Little, MSN, APRN, AGCNS-BC, PCCN
–Mary Alexander, MA, RN, CRNI, CAE, FAAN

"Writing is a skill, not a gift."
–Paul J. Silvia

WHAT YOU'LL LEARN IN THIS CHAPTER

- The type of article that you write will depend on the data you have and the key messages that you want to convey to readers.
- Using a standard template to organize your content makes it easier for readers to follow your article.
- Each type of article has a different template.

You gathered all your data from your research project. You implemented a novel idea to improve patient care. Or maybe you reviewed several articles on a single topic. What now? You need to disseminate this wealth of knowledge by writing an article for publication.

As you look to contribute to the body of nursing literature by publishing your research or sharing relevant clinical experiences, the articles that you write should be presented in a coherent and logical manner with evidence to support your conclusions. Organizing your content in a predictable manner allows the reader to follow your line of reasoning and makes understanding your message easier. Different types of articles lend themselves to different types of organization.

Although there is some flexibility in writing, following a structured format—or rather, a *template*—will help you include all the necessary components, thereby minimizing the chance of omitting an essential part of the article. Some authors believe that using templates can stifle a writer's creativity, but Graff and Birkenstein (2014, p. 11) state that "templates do not dictate the content of what you say, which can be as original as you want it, but only suggest a way of formatting how you say it."

When the content of an article flows in an organized way, your reader can easily follow your train of thought and better understand your message. This chapter explains types of articles and describes the typical format that each one should follow.

Basic Format of the Article

Your article should have a title, a beginning, a middle, and an end. Headings are also usually helpful, and, depending on where the article is published, you might need an abstract. When you follow this format, you enable the reader to understand and follow the logic of the information presented. Writing an organized piece also keeps the reader engaged and more apt to read the entire article.

Title

The style of your title might vary depending on whether you're writing an article for a nursing magazine or submitting to a scholarly journal. Either way, your title tells the reader about the information presented in the article by simply summarizing the main idea.

For less formal publications, you can be clever and create a title that draws readers' attention. For a scholarly work, such as a research report, your title should summarize the main idea of the article while still engaging the reader (American Psychological Association [APA], 2020; Watson, 2021). Consider placing the main idea towards the front of the title, or left-hand side, so it is read first (Watson, 2021). Titles for scholarly articles are typically longer and more descriptive than less formal articles; however, in both situations, it's important to include keywords that will prompt the article to appear in the results box when someone searches the literature for a particular topic.

Avoid using unnecessary words and phrases that needlessly increase title length, such as "a study of" and "method," and avoid abbreviations to ensure accurate and complete indexing of an article in reference databases (Ali, 2021; APA, 2020). If you're reporting your research, include the study population (JAMA Network Editors, 2020)—for example, "Prediction of Smoking Abstinence in Women Living With Human Immunodeficiency Virus Infection" (Kim et al., 2020).

Keep titles specific, but don't provide excessive details (JAMA Network Editors, 2020). For example, the following original title goes into too much detail for a general nursing journal focused on clinical practice. The revised title is more concise.

Original title: Management of the Patient With Phlebitis and the Nursing Interventions Needed to Treat the Problem After Assessing Needs: Utilizing the INS Phlebitis Scale

Revised title: Effective Management of the Patient With Phlebitis

It's usually best to keep titles of scholarly articles to 10 to 12 words so that the title is easier to read, but no hard and fast rules exist (APA, 2020; Bahadoran et al., 2019). Some journals specify a maximum length for titles. For example, the *Journal of Clinical Nursing* limits title length to 20 words (*Journal of Clinical Nursing*, 2023), and *JAMA* limits title length to 100 characters (including spaces) for research reports and 60 characters for shorter articles such as opinion pieces and letters (*JAMA*, n.d.). Any information about title restrictions will be in the author guidelines (sometimes called information for authors). A study by Heßler and Ziegler (2023) found that the nature of titles varies substantially across five major medical journals, so be sure to study the titles of articles in the publication you are targeting.

Consider writing the title last because it represents the entire article. Bahadoran and colleagues (2019) suggest the following five-step process:

1. Describe the content of the article in two to three sentences, using essential keywords and phrases.

2. Summarize the sentences by removing unnecessary and nonspecific words (such as "the" and "a") when possible and compacting necessary words, using category terms and adjectives rather than nouns (such as "reduced" instead of "reduction in").

3. Write an initial tentative title. Put the most important concept at or near the start to catch the reader's attention.

4. Review and refine the title.

5. Check that the title is clear, concise, specific, engaging, and informative.

The title gives the reader an initial impression of the article (Ali, 2021). Determine what makes your article unique and emphasize it in your title so that it stands out from other literature in the field (Cals & Kotz, 2013).

Examples of effective titles include:

> "Risk Factors Associated with Pressure Injury in Critically Ill Children with Congenital Heart Disease" (Shields & Lin, 2023)—describes what is in the article

> "The Effect of Immediate Versus Delayed Port Access on 30-Day Infection Rate" (Tancredi et al., 2020)—implies that there will be results from a study or quality improvement project

> "The Influence of Stigma on Suicide Bereavement: A Systematic Review" (Evans & Abrahamson, 2020)—phrases such as "meta-analysis" and "systematic review" are attractive for those seeking summary of information to apply in practice

> "Stroke Impact Symptoms Are Associated With Sleep-Related Impairment" (Byun et al., 2020)—states the conclusion of the study

> "Tables, Figures, and Graphs—Oh My: How to Best Display Data" (Siedlecki, 2023b)—catchier title more appropriate for practice-based journal; still conveys what the article will cover

Although you'll want to do your best to give your article the right title, don't be concerned if an editor changes your title; this happens frequently to best fit the publication's style.

Headings

Think of headings as "mini-titles" that can be used to organize the flow of the article or highlight important items within a section. Headings are like signposts along the road—they guide the reader from one topic to the next by providing a transition (APA, 2020; JAMA Network Editors, 2020). Headings also break up the text, making it more attractive and easier to read (JAMA Network Editors, 2020). There is no required number of headings for an article; however, since they divide a section into parts, there should be a minimum of two. If at least two headings are not needed, then they should not be added (JAMA Network Editors, 2020). For some types of articles, the format follows predetermined headings. For example, a research paper often uses the IMRAD format and uses the following headings: **I**ntroduction, **M**ethods, **R**esults, and **D**iscussion.

Beginning

Whether it's a paragraph, a section, or just a good opening line, the *introduction* sets the tone of the article. It tells readers what the article is about and entices them—formally or informally—to continue reading. Ultimately, the introductory statement should stimulate interest in the subject so that the reader will want to read the entire article.

There are a number of techniques for writing a *lede*—writer parlance for that strong opening line or paragraph—but some examples you might use in an introduction include providing relevant background information, giving pertinent statistics, or asking a provocative question (Troyka & Hesse, 2016). Your introduction should reflect the style of the publication, journal, or online resource. For example, in an article published in *Clinical Nurse Specialist*, Fischer-Cartlidge and Hoffman (2023) introduce the challenges of clinical nurse specialist practice that will be explained further in the article:

> The clinical nurse specialist (CNS) is the oldest advanced practice nursing role, discussed in the literature in 1949, with a defined role and educational programs established in 1969. Even with this established history, it can be difficult to articulate the value of the CNS within an organization. Clinical nurse specialist practice is shaped by the nature of the specialty population, organizational priorities, and external influences such as state-level regulations. Because of this variability, CNSs are often underutilized, leaving the CNS vulnerable to staffing and budgeting decisions within the organization. (p. 78)

In an introduction of an article on a mindfulness intervention that was published in *Critical Care Nurse*, the authors (Vandenbogaart et al., 2023) use statistics to reinforce the prevalence of anxiety in patients awaiting heart transplant. Note that only a few, well-chosen numbers are used; you don't want to overwhelm your reader with too many:

> The patient journey to heart transplant is arduous. These clinically tenuous patients have a mortality risk of 10% to 15% on the transplant waiting list given the limited donor heart availability. Coping with the uncertain timing of a donor match, threat to survival, and extensive time in critical care environments with little

control or independence intensifies an inherently stressful period. Separation from family, home, and social network contributes to patients' feelings of isolation. This constant exposure to unavoidable stressors coupled with social isolation frequently increases anxiety and depression. In patients with advanced heart failure (HF) awaiting transplant, the estimated incidence of anxiety is 20% to 36%; of depression, 18% to 50%. (p. 16)

Middle

The *middle* is the main portion of the article. To maintain the flow of the article, paragraphs and subtopics should address the points in your article outline. Each paragraph will have a "topic" sentence, which is the main point of the paragraph, with subsequent sentences supporting the main idea. Each separate, distinct paragraph aids the reader, signaling a new step in the development of the subject (Strunk & De A'Morelli, 2018). The body of the paragraph might include examples, reasons, facts, and details directly related to the topic (Troyka & Hesse, 2016).

A paragraph can be as short as one sentence—for example, when you want to emphasize a point or make a dramatic change—but tends to be no more than four to six sentences long. The main point to keep in mind is that each sentence should relate to the topic sentence. (Learn more about paragraphs and other writing tips in Chapter 6.)

End

All articles have a conclusion, which contains key message(s) you want your readers to glean from the article. The conclusion brings the article to an end and should flow logically while simultaneously reinforcing your message. Some options for endings include a summary of key points, a call to action, or suggested future directions for research.

You want to avoid introducing new ideas or facts in your ending that belong in the body of the article. In addition, your conclusion should not be only a reiteration of your introduction (Troyka & Hesse, 2016).

The following conclusion of "Artificial Intelligence, Digital Health Research and the Clinical Nurse Specialist" effectively summarizes the key points of the article:

> The clinical nurse specialist should be an active participant in the development and refinement of digital interventions, digital content, and

---

Consider this: Writing from the Middle

Authors typically approach writing a manuscript by starting with the introduction followed by the methods, results, and discussion, and ending with the abstract and graphics. But readers usually start with the abstract and graphics and then proceed to the body of the article. It's important the abstract and graphics are enticing and tell enough of the story to invite the reader to dig deeper into the article. Additionally, graphics are often the easiest to share when discussing the work. Because of this, Gerstein and colleagues (2022) recommend creating graphics as the first step in writing a manuscript, which they refer to as starting in the middle, then working outward.

Consider this process when writing from the middle:

1. **Create graphics.** Think about the main points and key outcomes you want the reader to understand.

2. **Write the results section.** Reference the graphics and provide a narrative.

3. **Write the methods section.** The graphics and results section will guide writing the methods. Simply describe what was done to achieve the outcomes.

4. **Write the discussion.** Share rationales for the findings, next steps, strengths and limitations, and conclusion.

5. **Write the introduction.** This section foreshadows information conveyed in other parts of the manuscript.

6. **Write the abstract.** Provide a summary sentence, or two, of each section.

Starting with the graphics may be challenging and different from your usual technique, but this approach creates a strong foundation that facilitates the writing process.

the use of sensor technology. Their clinical expertise and knowledge of nursing workflow are an invaluable asset. Thus, it will become more and more important for the clinical nurse specialist to stay abreast of new developments in digital health and the use of digital technology in the years to come and to offer their guidance to safeguard patients. Artificial intelligence has the potential to improve lives and health, but it is not without hazards. Advances in digital health through artificial intelligence are complex and evolving at a very rapid pace. Knowledge of artificial intelligence is essential to prepare the clinical nurse specialist to advocate for the rational and ethical use of digital technology in clinical practice and research. (Siedlecki, 2023a, p. 217)

Abstract

Although not a formal part of the body of your article, for many publications, you will need to prepare an abstract. An *abstract* is a brief, comprehensive summary of the contents of an article, allowing the reader to survey the article contents quickly. The abstract creates an important first impression for editors, who will decide whether your article should proceed to the peer-review stage; for reviewers, who will form an initial impression of your article based on it; and, most importantly, for readers, who frequently decide based on the abstract whether to read the entire article (Alspach, 2017; Watson, 2021). A poor abstract can lead to indexing errors or omissions, which can make the article harder to find for researchers and others interested in your topic (Alspach, 2017). To make the best first impression and improve the life span of your article, the abstract should be accurate, concise, coherent, and compelling.

Abstracts may be structured or unstructured in format. The headings for a *structured* abstract are typically: Objective, Design, Setting, Participants, Interventions, Outcomes, Results, and Conclusions (JAMA Network Editors, 2020). Be sure to adhere to the word count for the abstract. Word count for an abstract varies from journal to journal, ranging from 150 to 350 words (APA, 2020; JAMA Network Editors, 2020; Gerstein et al., 2022). Refer to Chapter 14 for an example of a structured abstract.

An *unstructured* abstract does not use headings, is written in paragraph form, and has a word count that typically does not exceed 200 words (JAMA Network Editors, 2020). An unstructured abstract may be used for columns, case studies, brief reports, and education articles (Curry, 2019).

No matter which type of abstract you are writing, be sure to write it after you write the article so that it is consistent with the content (Curry, 2019; Gerstein et al., 2022), and follow these tips (Alspach, 2017):

- Include key information (e.g., sample, research instrument), but do not exceed the specified word limit.
- Do not include information that isn't in the article.
- Do not overstate the results.
- Carefully check grammar, spelling, and punctuation.
- Spell out abbreviations.
- Emphasize the most important points. For instance, the results section of an abstract for a research study should constitute the largest percentage of the total length.
- Tailor your abstract to the type of article—an abstract for a case study will differ from an abstract for a quality improvement report. Reporting guidelines, discussed later in this chapter, can help you with this.

You may need to add keywords at the end of your abstract—a short list of 3 to 10 words or phrases that represent the key topics in the article (JAMA Network Editors, 2020). Keywords supplied by the author are not used by PubMed or other indexing databases. Editors may use your keywords to help choose a peer reviewer or to ensure appropriate tagging for the journal's website so that the article can be easily found (JAMA Network Editors, 2020). (Chapter 14 has more information about writing abstracts.)

An Additional Option: Graphical Abstracts

The goal of an abstract is to capture the attention of readers and invite them to read the article in its entirety. In today's fast-paced environment, we need to quickly connect with readers. Graphical abstracts (GA; also called visual abstracts) provide an avenue for that quick connection. Similar to an infographic, GAs use design elements and visual-spatial reorganization of content to share key findings of an article on social media (Oska et al., 2020; Trivedi et al., 2021). Figure 5.1 reflects some typical elements of a GA: methods, treatment, and outcomes (results).

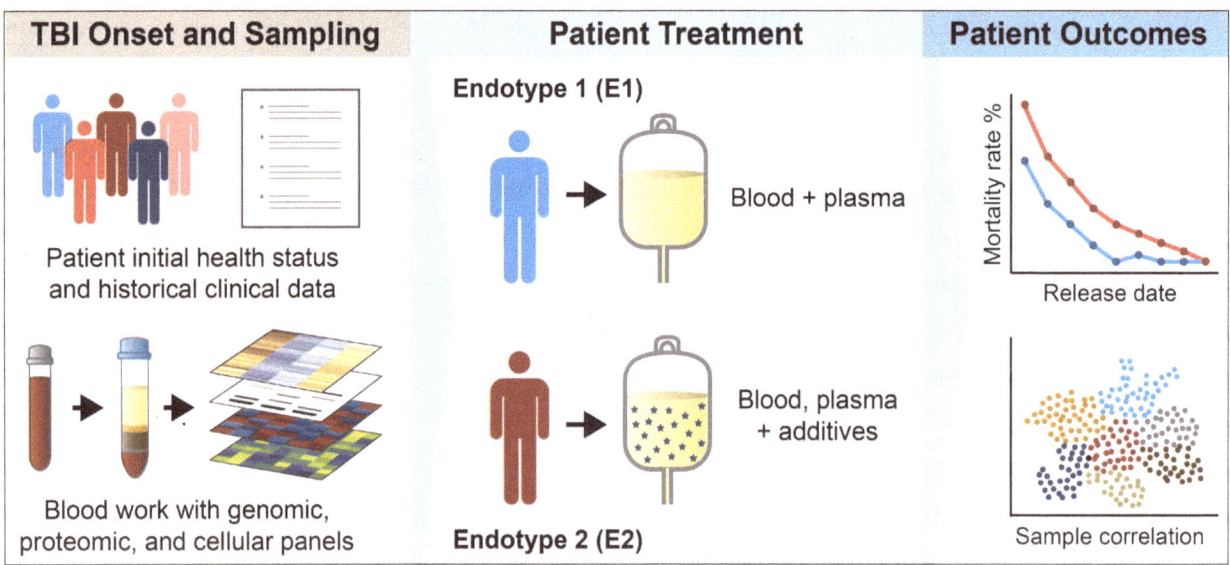

FIGURE 5.1 Elements of a graphical abstract (Simplified Science Publishing, 2024).

The premise behind GAs is that people recall information better when it's presented visually than as text (Martin, 2020; Trivedi et al., 2021). Readers are more likely to ignore long text because it takes approximately six seconds to read 20 words whereas it takes a quarter of a second to establish the meaning of a visual symbol (Oska et al., 2020). The goal of a GA is to "provide a single, concise, pictorial summary of the main findings" (Martin, 2020, p. 29) to a broad audience, including those who feel they don't have time to read the article in its entirety (Lee & Yoo, 2023). A strong GA can prompt readers to invest time in reading the full article.

Originally designed for visual representation of studies in slide presentations, GAs have been adapted to promote research reports (and other types of articles) on social media (Oska et al., 2020). Journals share GAs via social media to promote your work and will typically allow you to share them as well, which can vastly extend the reach of your article. Oska et al. (2020) found that GAs had five times the engagement of citation-only tweets. Another study found that in the case of randomized clinical trial articles published in JAMA Network journals, using GAs, rather than a figure from the article, as part of a social media post that included a summary of the conclusions and a link to the article increased the number of clicks (Trueger et al., 2023). The display of GAs attracts readers because vision accounts for 87% of the five human senses, and color accounts for more than 60% of vision (Lee & Yoo, 2023). This time-efficient and visually appealing tool promotes knowledge transfer and retention, and decreases cognitive workload (Trivedi et al., 2021).

Check the journal's guidelines to see if it accepts GAs, which will undergo the same scrutiny as your manuscript, although they will not necessarily undergo peer review. You can design these abstracts in Microsoft PowerPoint, although online design tools can be helpful, such as Mind the Graph (https://mindthegraph.com) and Canva (https://www.canva.com). You also can access free courses in design principles from Stanford (https://dschool.stanford.edu/resources/get-started-with-design). Explore design ideas used outside the medical field. Find and save layouts and visual strategies you find attractive to use as a reference when creating your own GA. You'll also want to collaborate with a team to gain different perspectives (Trivedi et al., 2021).

The format of a GA varies depending on the message of the article and the target audience (Lee & Yoo, 2023). The following are common types:

- **Conceptual diagram:** Best for complex information, such as mathematics or scientific concepts. Uses illustrations and diagrams.

- **Flowchart:** Best for delineating methods or procedures. Information is conveyed using arrows.
- **Infographic:** Best for summarizing an extensive amount of data in a compact method. Illustrations, text, and other design elements are used.
- **Iconographic:** The simplest visual abstract; best for targeting a broader audience. Icons are used to represent key findings and present data so it's easy to understand.

Keep these principles in mind when creating a GA (Ibrahim, 2018; Lee & Yoo, 2023; Martin, 2020; Saver, 2023):

- Identify the main message. For a research article, that includes summarizing the research question and key outcomes.
- Provide a visual display of outcomes using simple icons. This includes stating the outcome with directionality and providing a numeric value with clear labeling of the units.
- Keep the design simple. Use color and design elements to capture attention but avoid too much text and too many colors.
- Be sure text is readable online.
- Identify author of article and visual abstract.

Ibrahim (2018), Trivedi et al. (2021), and Lee and Yoo (2023) give detailed instructions for creating a GA, including finding images, and provide examples of completed abstracts. Several free GA templates are available through Simplified Science Publishing (www.simplifiedsciencepublishing.com), and you can search online for "free graphical abstract templates."

More journals are beginning to require GAs as the first step of submission. Check the author guidelines because there is no universal standard for GAs (Lee & Yoo, 2023). Mastering the art of creating enticing GAs will optimize dissemination of your hard work.

Types of Flow

For the reader to understand and follow your train of thought, you must consider the flow of the article. In Chapter 1, you learned about these types of flow: how-to, case studies, IMRAD, disease process, and chronology. Take a closer look at a few of these. Remember that you can use a single approach or a combination of methods to get your point across.

How-To

Quality improvement projects and clinical tips can be best described in *how-to* articles. Using the nursing process, you can organize your article by writing about your assessment of the problem, plan of action, implementation, and evaluation of the process/procedure/practice. For example, you might write about how you implemented an in-service education program to address the problem of occluded central lines. Be sure to include "lessons learned" so that readers know what to avoid. (You can learn more about clinical how-to articles in Chapter 13.)

Case Studies

Case studies provide information on nursing practice and how that information can be applied to a specific patient problem. You may organize the entire article around the case study, or the case study may be part of a manuscript. The flow of this type of article typically includes a patient history, assessment, diagnosis, treatment, nursing interventions, and outcomes with implications for clinical practice. (Case studies are described in more detail in Chapter 13.)

IMRAD

Just as you learn the scientific method for research and experiments, you'll use IMRAD if you're writing a research article. IMRAD is the standard flow for a research article, especially those that report on quantitative studies. (IMRAD is discussed later in this chapter and in Chapter 14.)

Disease Process

You may choose to organize your article according to the traditional topics for discussing a disease, including incidence, signs and symptoms, diagnosis, medical treatment, and nursing care. This format can be particularly helpful when you are writing an educational program about a specific disease.

Chronological

Time can serve as an organizing tool for an article, either as a timeline (what happened when) or as a process (e.g., preoperative, perioperative, and postoperative).

> **Confidence Booster**
>
> Keep writing. Keep submitting your work. Some of the most well-known works of literature were initially rejected—multiple times. Among manuscripts originally rejected are *Harry Potter and the Sorcerer's Stone* by J. K. Rowling (rejected by 12 publishers), *Dubliners* by James Joyce (22 rejections), and *Gone with the Wind* by Margaret Mitchell (rejected by an amazing 38 publishers). Thankfully, these authors kept writing—and offering their work for publication.

Types of Articles

The kind of article that you write depends upon the topic you have selected and the message you want to convey. (The following sections provide an overview of these types. You'll learn more about each type in more detail in subsequent chapters.) The most common types of articles are:

- Research articles
- Quantitative and qualitative articles
- Evidence-based practice articles
- Quality improvement articles
- Clinical articles
- Literature reviews
- Case studies
- Nursing narratives and exemplars

When matching the style of article, you also need to consider the type of publication that you're targeting. Not all journals accept nursing narratives and exemplars, and an evidence-based practice article, for example, wouldn't necessarily fit in some research journals. If you completed a study evaluating the effectiveness of saline versus heparin solutions to flush central IV catheters in multiple hospitals, you would write a research article that describes the statistical analysis and significance of your results. If the rate of occluded central IV catheters increased on your unit because of improper flushing techniques, a description of how you resolved this issue would be appropriate in a quality improvement article. Each category has a general format, or template, that is useful in developing a concise, organized article that will generate interest for the reader.

Q *There are so many types of articles. How can I pick the one that best fits my message?*

A Some factors that you can consider are your specific message, who you want to read that message, how much information you have, and your general purpose. Realize that there isn't always one answer. For example, say that you just saw a patient with an unusual disease in your emergency department. You might choose to present this as a case study, or perhaps provide a broader picture by writing about the disease itself and using the patient as an example.

Research Articles

Research articles are reports of original data, findings, and results. They summarize a study, its purpose, methods, and findings. The typical format for a research article is the IMRAD format—introduction, methods, results, and discussion. This format follows the stages of the research process, enabling the author to easily organize the article.

Introduction. The *introduction* should present the problem and gaps noted in the research. A *literature review*, or presentation of the existing research on the topic, can be part of the introduction or written as a separate section following the introduction. Stating the problem early in the introduction explains why particular concepts or theories were used to direct the research. A statement of the problem should be clear to readers in the beginning of the introduction.

Methods. The section describing your research methods should be written in subsections, which generally follow a specific order: study design, subjects, measures, procedures, and data analysis. The reader can easily follow the research methodology.

Results. The *results* section describes the findings of the study and should both address the purpose of the study and answer the research questions. Typically, you present the main findings first, followed by any secondary findings. Keep in mind that the data results belong in the "Results" section, and the *implications* of those results belong in the "Discussion" section.

Q *Some of my results run counter to what I expected to find. Can I omit those results?*

A No. All findings, even those that run counter to expectations, are to be reported. Uncomfortable results or those that do not support your hypothesis should not be omitted (APA, 2020). Reasons for those results can be explained in the "Discussion" section.

Discussion. In this section, the author interprets the results of the study and explains the findings in relation to the original hypotheses. Begin this section with a clear statement of support or nonsupport for your original hypotheses. Discuss whether this research is consistent with previous research. Acknowledge any limitations of your research, such as a small sample size. Describe the implications of the research for clinical practice. Remember that your statements and conclusions need to be supported by your data. Suggestions for future research can be included in this section. End this section with a clear, direct statement on the importance of your findings. (For more on writing research articles, see Chapter 14.)

Quantitative and Qualitative Articles

Research articles can be reported as quantitative or qualitative. *Quantitative* research studies are used to test a theory or to build on one. They focus on measurement and statistical analysis of data to test a hypothesis with a goal of discovering relationships or cause and effect between variables. Quantitative research papers typically follow the IMRAD format (Luby & Southern, 2022). When presenting results of quantitative studies, the findings and related discussion are organized according to the purposes, questions, or hypotheses. The data analysis is numerical. Quantitative research methods include surveys and experimental manipulation of variables. These studies can include interventions between two or more groups, with one group acting as a control group (Saver, 2006).

In comparison, a *qualitative* study attempts to better understand a phenomenon, such as a clinical problem, rather than focus on cause and effect. A qualitative study, which can help identify key concepts, focuses on the individual's relationship with their surroundings and their interactions with others (Chicca, 2020). Research methods include interviews, observation, and analysis documents such as journals.

In a qualitative study, the format depends on the purpose of the research, the methods used, and the data obtained from the research. There is no one style for presenting qualitative research; you may use one of the following formats:

- **IMRAD:** Introduction, Methods, Results, and Discussion
- **Time:** Findings are organized as they happen, or what was learned at different points in time.
- **Prevalence:** The most frequently occurring themes are presented first.
- **Concept:** Describe or test a theory noted in the study.

A valuable resource are the Standards for Reporting QUalitative Research (SRQR) guidelines, which can help you organize and prepare your manuscript (O'Brien et al., 2014).

Evidence-Based Practice (EBP) Articles

Evidence comes from a variety of sources, including published and unpublished reports, internal quality improvement project summaries, and expert opinion (Dang et al., 2022; Hagle & Senk, 2010). An *evidence-based practice* (EBP) article, or evidence report, includes knowledge synthesis, review, and documentation of how evidence-based practices are used in a clinical area. It can also include a discussion of the clinical relevance to a proposed change in practice (Benefield, 2002). The format for an EBP article is similar to the IMRAD format and should include the following information (Benefield, 2002; Hagle & Senk, 2010):

- **Summary statement:** Succinctly describe the clinical question that is being addressed and what the evidence reports.
- **Analysis of the scientific data:** Describe the review of the published and unpublished reports, target populations who were studied, type of clinical interventions that were investigated, and strength of the individual or collective study results.
- **Critical appraisal of the evidence:** Summarize the scientific reports, including the rank and strength of the evidence.

- **Practice recommendations:** Based on the cumulative information from the analyzed evidence, state the practice recommendations suggested for integration into clinical practice. Should a recommendation be suggested for implementation into practice, the benefits versus risks to the patient are discussed in this section.

To ensure you include what's needed in your manuscript, turn to resources such as the Evidence-Based Practice Process Quality Assessment: EPQA Guidelines (Lee et al., 2013) and the Evidence-Based Practice Dissemination Guide (Dean & Gallagher-Ford, 2021). Another resource is a template for publishing an EBP project that you can find in the book by Dang and colleagues (2021) listed in the references. (For more on writing about EBP, see Chapter 16.)

Quality Improvement (QI) Articles

Quality improvement (QI) articles describe how to improve care or solve a problem. Like a research article, data are used to support the information presented in a QI article. However, some differences exist between a QI and a research or an EBP article. For example, a research article must put the study in context with prior research by including a comprehensive literature review. Research methodology tries to control the variables in the study, but there is less control over variability in a QI project. Also, the statistical analysis required for a research study is typically more extensive than that used for a QI study.

Because QI projects tend to be narrow in scope, focusing on a single unit or organization, it can be more challenging to find a publication outlet. Check the journal's author guidelines and past issues to determine if QI articles are welcome; if they are, the guidelines may specify that you follow SQUIRE 2.0 guidelines. Examples of nursing journals that accept QI submissions are *American Nurse Journal*, *American Journal of Nursing*, *Critical Care Nurse*, *Journal of Pediatric Nursing*, and the *Journal of Nursing Care Quality*. QI projects may also be suitable as short articles for journals with departments that focus on tips or lessons learned. (For more on writing about QI projects, see Chapter 16.)

All About Reporting Guidelines

Reporting guidelines, typically developed with input from an expert panel, exist to improve the consistency and usefulness of published information. For example, many journals require authors follow the Standards for QUality Improvement Reporting Excellence—the SQUIRE 2.0 guidelines—when writing quality improvement articles (Ogrinc et al., 2016).

Reporting guidelines such as SQUIRE 2.0 and the ones below are excellent resources to help you organize your article.

- **CARE (CAse REport).** These guidelines for case studies are discussed later in this chapter (Gagnier et al., 2013; Riley et al., 2017).

- **CONSORT (Consolidated Standards of Reporting Trials) and CONSORT-Outcomes 2022 Extension.** For reporting on clinical trials, these guidelines detail information that should be included in a research report (Butcher et al., 2022).

- **EPQA (Evidence-Based Practice Process Quality Assessment).** These guidelines consist of a 34-item checklist (Lee et al., 2013).

- **PRISMA (Preferred Reporting Items for Systematic reviews and Meta-Analyses).** These guidelines consist of a 27-item checklist and flow diagram (Page et al., 2021).

- **SAGER (Sex and Gender Equity in Research).** These guidelines are used for reporting of sex and gender information in study design, data analyses, results, and interpretation of findings (Heidari et al., 2016).

Your choice of guidelines depends on the journal's requirements and the type of article (Buccheri & Sharifi, 2017). For example, the PRISMA guidelines work well for a systematic review, and the CONSORT guidelines are a good fit for a randomized controlled trial (Butcher et al., 2022; Page et al., 2021).

You can learn more about reporting guidelines through the Enhancing the QUAlity and Transparency Of health Research (EQUATOR) network (EQUATOR Network, n.d.) and by accessing a summary of guidelines in Appendix D. The EQUATOR website offers a flowchart to help you choose the right guidelines for your article.

Clinical Articles

Clinical articles address topics that are relevant to clinical practice. They might present new skills or knowledge related to patient care, provide an empirically or clinically based review of a disease state or procedure, or analyze current literature related to a topic. Research findings, if available, or other evidence should be included to support the rationale for recommended interventions.

The format for writing clinical articles varies among journals. Unlike research articles, there is no specific format; however, some general guidelines are helpful as you develop your manuscript.

Begin the article with an *introduction*, which may be a brief presentation of a patient or situation that a nurse might experience. Describe the purpose of your article, an overview of the topics, the relevance of the content for clinical practice, and the value of the article to the reader. Here, you tell the readers that the article will present useful information that can be applied to clinical practice.

In the *body* of the article, tell readers the key points. For example, if you are writing about a specific procedure, you might include a review of the disease or condition associated with the procedure, its incidence and pathophysiology, information about the procedure, and a care plan—and then conclude with a summary of information. If you are presenting a new procedure, discuss the steps in the order in which they occur. Organize the content from simple to complex and from known to unknown. To help the reader understand your decision to recommend a particular intervention, provide sufficient background information and data. Describe the evidence and research that support the changes in practice. And remember the purpose of the article—nursing management of a patient's problem, not medical management—to ensure your content reflects your nursing interventions.

Each clinical article ends with a *conclusion* that summarizes the information presented. Although your conclusion might suggest areas of further study, do not add new information at this point. The conclusion for these types of articles should show the value to the nurse in clinical practice when a new intervention is implemented or a change in nursing practice is endorsed. (For more on clinical articles, see Chapter 13.)

Literature Reviews

One type of literature review is part of the research process, but a formal, written *literature review* is another type of article that you can submit for publication. This literature review is a summary and synthesis of current knowledge about a topic that has already been published. By evaluating previously published literature, authors of literature reviews inform readers of the state of research in a particular area (APA, 2020). Clinicians often use review articles as guides for clinical decisions (JAMA Network Editors, 2020), so be sure your reviews are systematic, include relevant data, and aren't influenced by your own opinions and biases.

Here is a handy format for writing a literature review:

Beginning. Begin with an introductory statement about the literature that you will present and its importance to the problem or purpose of the manuscript. This statement should not be too broad; keep it specific enough so the reader knows what literature will be discussed. A more-specific statement gives the reader a better idea of the content of the article. Compare these examples of too-broad and more-specific introductory statements:

> **Not specific enough:** The authors conducted a literature review of studies published on glycemic control in adults with type 2 diabetes.
>
> **Good overview:** A systematic literature review of studies published between 2012 and 2022 was conducted to evaluate the impact of isolated telephone interventions on glycemic control in adults with type 2 diabetes.

Middle. In the body of the literature review, summarize previous publications to inform the reader of the state of the research. Highlight important studies and describe their significance to the research. Note classic studies and how they have contributed to the research. If you can't locate relevant literature about a topic, note the dearth of literature in your review as well as any relationships, contradictions, gaps, and inconsistencies that you identify in the literature.

End. In your conclusion, describe how the review closes a gap in the literature and extends existing research. Address how this work will contribute knowledge to the profession.

(For more on writing literature review articles, see Chapter 15.)

Case Studies

Case studies, or *case reports*, provide new information on nursing practice or patient care problems. Case studies can appear in more formal journals, but also in less formal venues like magazines. They can be used to describe patient care; illustrate how concepts, theories, and research are used in practice; present issues in a patient's care and strategies for resolving them; or apply information to a real or hypothetical case. Case studies illustrate a problem, indicate a means for solving a problem, or shed light on needed research, clinical applications, or theoretical matters.

The case study article begins with why the case was selected and its importance to nursing practice. Then the article continues with a description of the patient and related care given. Case studies are used to promote clinical judgment, decision-making, and critical-thinking skills. As previously noted, when providing illustrative material, be sure not to disclose information that would identify a specific patient (APA, 2020).

The CARE (CAse REport) guidelines contain a checklist for items that should be part of a case study (Gagnier et al., 2013; Riley et al., 2017). You can use the following elements from the checklist as a guide when writing your article:

- **Title:** Gives the primary diagnosis or intervention of focus followed by "case report"
- **Keywords:** Lists two to five words that identify the diagnosis or intervention of focus
- **Abstract:** Includes contributions of the case study to literature, important clinical findings, and one take-away lesson
- **Introduction:** Provides a summary of the case and why it's important
- **Patient information:** Includes demographic information; main signs and symptoms; and medical, family, and psychosocial history
- **Clinical findings:** Presents the relevant results of the physical examination
- **Timeline:** Includes key time frames
- **Diagnostic assessment:** Provides information about diagnostic methods and reasoning
- **Therapeutic intervention:** Describes medical, surgical, and nursing interventions, including modifications made as needed
- **Follow-up and outcomes:** Tells what happened to the patient and what kinds of follow-up testing or visiting were done
- **Discussion:** Summarizes the strengths and limitations of what was done and should include relevant literature and main "lessons learned" from the case

If possible, it's also helpful to share the patient's perspective.

The CARE guidelines recommend obtaining informed consent from the patient even when they are not named. If the patient is unable to provide consent, the alternative is to contact a relative. If neither the patient nor a relative is available, the guidelines recommend obtaining consent from an ethics committee or institutional review board. The step of obtaining patient consent for a case study is an unusual requirement for nursing publications, particularly because authors are typically asked to make adjustments to

Preserving Patient Privacy

When writing a case study about a real person, it's important to preserve patient privacy by not publishing identifying patient information, such as names, initials, or hospital numbers, unless the information is essential for the article's purpose. In that case, patients should provide written informed consent (International Committee of Medical Journal Editors, 2024). Avoid any details that might make it possible to identify someone, such as writing about a patient with blunt chest trauma as a result of wrecking his car during a high-speed car chase through a rural town. The events are likely to have been published online and in print. You should simply state the patient was someone involved in a high-speed auto accident. Another option is to change the gender of the patient if it isn't germane to the case study. To protect yourself, it's best to obtain the patient's consent before writing an article, although that's not always practical. (Learn more about privacy rights in Chapter 11.)

> Case examples can teach nurses new to the emergency department to have a heightened index of suspicion for signs and symptoms that appear to be one thing but are actually another. ← Introduction
>
> A 78-year-old man was brought to the emergency department by his family because his behavior had suddenly changed, and his family was frightened by the way he was acting. Upon awakening from a nap, he became very agitated and told his family that he wanted "those strangers who are talking to me out of my bedroom." Despite his family's reassurances that there were no strangers in the room, he was insistent that there was an entire family in the bedroom, and they were all talking to him. ← Description of the patient
>
> A comprehensive assessment of the patient's physical condition and consideration of potential side effects from a recently prescribed antidepressant medication were evaluated. Within two days after the antidepressant was discontinued, the agitation and hallucinations were gone, and the patient was "back to normal." ← Nursing care
>
> A thorough medical history and the appropriate laboratory tests can reveal that an apparent psychiatric patient is really a medical patient with psychiatric symptoms. ← Conclusion
>
> *Source: Pestka et al., 2002*

EXAMPLE 5.1 Shorter case study illustrating key points.

protect patient privacy. However, it will be interesting to see if adoption of the CARE guidelines by journals affects future practice.

Keep in mind that in addition to being the entire article, shorter case studies can be used to illustrate key points in other types of articles, as shown in Example 5.1.

Nursing Narratives or Exemplars

If you are a novice author, a way to gain experience and confidence in your writing skills is to write a *nursing narrative* or *exemplar*, which is a personal account that describes outstanding examples of the actions of individuals in clinical settings that have enhanced patient care. A discussion of difficult interpersonal, ethical, or clinical judgments is the basis for these articles (Saver, 2006). (Learn more about this type of article in Chapter 20.)

Q *I was recently invited to contribute to a regular department for a journal. What format should I use?*

A Many publications include regular columns or departments. Departments make a good target for your ideas because they are published frequently and feature shorter articles.

You can usually identify the format by studying two or three past articles for the specific department. Stick to the same length, style, and tone—and if in doubt, ask the editor to verify that you're on the right track.

Organize for Success

As an author contributing to the body of nursing literature, you must write in a logical and coherent manner. Articles fall into many different categories, from detailed research articles written in a formal style to an opinion piece not longer than one page. The type of article that you write will depend upon factors such as data you have and key messages you want to convey to readers. Templates can help you organize your information more easily. When your article is written in a predictable pattern, the reader can more easily follow your line of reasoning. General characteristics of articles with corresponding formats exist, making it easier for the author to organize the information. Keeping in mind the elements of organizing your article will foster your success as an author.

Write Now!

1. Choose a journal in your specialty. Read two to three articles and identify the types of articles you've read.
2. Identify three types of articles that you would like to write. For each one, create an overview of what you would include.

References

Ali, M. (2021). The "title" of a manuscript: Guidelines for its construction. *Seminars in Ophthalmology, 36*(7), 459–460. https://doi.org/10.1080/08820538.2021.1966725

Alspach, J. G. (2017). Writing for publication 101: Why the abstract is so important [Editorial]. *Critical Care Nurse, 37*(4), 12–15. https://doi.org/10.4037/ccn2017466

American Psychological Association. (2020). *Publication manual of the American Psychological Association* (7th ed.). https://doi.org/10.1037/0000165-000

Bahadoran, Z., Mirmiran, P., Kashfi, K., & Ghasemi, A. (2019). The principles of biomedical scientific writing: Title. *International Journal of Endocrinology and Metabolism, 17*(4), e98326. https://doi.org/10.5812/ijem.98326

Benefield, L. E. (2002). Evidence-based practice: Basic strategies for success. *Home Healthcare Nurse, 20*(12), 803–807. https://doi.org/10.1097/00004045-200212000-00011

Buccheri, R. K., & Sharifi, C. (2017). Critical appraisal tools and reporting guidelines for evidence-based practice. *Worldviews on Evidence-Based Nursing, 14*(6), 463–472. https://doi.org/10.1111/wvn.12258

Butcher, N. J., Monsour, A., Mew, E. J., Chan, A., Moher, D., Mayo-Wilson, E., Terwee, C. B., Chee-A-Tow, A., Baba, A., Gavin, F., Grimshaw, J. M., Kelly, L. E., Saeed, L., Thabane, L., Askie, L., Smith, M., Farid-Kapadia, M., Williamson, P. R., Szatmari, P., Tugwell, P., Golub, R. M., Monga, S., Vohra, S., Marlin, S., Ungar, W. J., & Offringa, M. (2022). Guidelines for reporting outcomes in trial reports: The CONSORT-Outcomes 2022 extension. *The Journal of the American Medical Association, 328*(22), 2252–2264. https://doi.org/10.1001/jama.2022.21022

Byun, E., Kohen, R., Becker, K. J., Kirkness, C. J., Khot, S., & Mitchell, P. H. (2020). Stroke impact symptoms are associated with sleep-related impairment. *Heart & Lung, 49*(2), 117–122. https://doi.org/10.1016/j.hrtlng.2019.10.010

Cals, J. W. L., & Kotz, D. (2013). Effective writing and publishing scientific papers, part II: Title and abstract. *Journal of Clinical Epidemiology, 66*(6), 585. https://doi.org/10.1016/j.jclinepi.2013.01.005

Chicca, J. (2020). Introduction to qualitative nursing research. *American Nurse Journal, 15*(6), 28–32. https://www.myamericannurse.com/introduction-to-qualitative-nursing-research

Curry, K. (2019). Crafting a compelling abstract [Editorial]. *Journal of the American Association of Nurse Practitioners, 31*(5), 279. https://doi.org/10.1097/JXX.0000000000000233

Dang, D., Dearholt, S. L., Bissett, K., Ascenzi, J., & Whalen, M. (2022). *Johns Hopkins evidence-based practice for nurses and healthcare professionals: Model & guidelines* (4th ed.). Sigma Theta Tau International.

Dean, J., & Gallagher-Ford, L. (2021). Evidence-based practice: A new dissemination guide [Editorial]. *Worldviews on Evidence-Based Nursing, 18*(1), 4–7. https://doi.org/10.1111/wvn.12489

EQUATOR Network. (n.d.). *Enhancing the QUAlity and Transparency Of health Research.* http://www.equator-network.org

Evans, A., & Abrahamson, K. (2020). The influence of stigma on suicide bereavement: A systematic review. *Journal of Psychosocial Nursing and Mental Health Services, 58*(4), 21–27. https://doi.org/10.3928/02793695-20200127-02

Fischer-Cartlidge, E., & Hoffman, M. (2023). Demonstrating the value of the clinical nurse specialist: A how-to guide. *Clinical Nurse Specialist, 37*(2), 78–82. https://doi.org/10.1097/NUR.0000000000000732

Gagnier, J. J., Kienle, G., Altman, D. G., Moher, D., Sox, H., & Riley, D. (2013). The CARE guidelines: Consensus-based clinical case reporting guideline development. *Global Advances in Health and Medicine, 2*(5), 38–43. https://doi.org/10.7453/gahmj.2013.008

Gerstein, H. C., Sherifali, D., & Satia, I. (2022). Writing your paper from the middle. *American Medical Writers Association Journal, 37*(2), 19–20. https://doi.org/10.55752/amwa.2022.159

Graff, G., & Birkenstein, C. (2014). *They say/I say: The moves that matter in academic writing* (3rd ed.). Gildan Media.

Hagle, M., & Senk, P. (2010). Evidence-based practice. In M. Alexander, A. Corrigan, L. Gorski, J. Hankins, & R. Perucca (Eds.). *Infusion nursing: An evidence-based approach* (3rd ed.; pp. 10–21). Saunders/Elsevier.

Heidari, S., Barbor, T. F., De Castro, P., Tort, S., & Curno, M. (2016). Sex and gender equity in research: Rationale for the SAGER guidelines and recommended use. *Research Integrity and Peer Review, 1*(2). https://doi.org/10.1186/s41073-016-0007-6

Heßler, N., & Ziegler, A. (2023). Content and form of original research articles in general major medical journals. *PLoS One, 18*(6), e0287677. https://doi.org/10.1371/journal.pone.0287677

Ibrahim, A. M. (Ed) (2018). *Use of a visual abstract to disseminate scientific research* (Version 4). https://static1.squarespace.com/static/5854aaa044024321a353bb0d/t/5a527aa89140b76bbfb2028a/1515354827682/VisualAbstract_Primer_v4_1.pdf

International Committee of Medical Journal Editors. (2024). *Recommendations for the conduct, reporting, editing, and publication of scholarly work in medical journals.* http://www.icmje.org/recommendations

JAMA. (n.d.). *Instructions for authors: Title page.* https://jamanetwork.com/journals/jama/pages/instructions-for-authors

JAMA Network Editors. (2020). *AMA manual of style: A guide for authors and editors* (11th ed.). Oxford University Press.

Journal of Clinical Nursing. (2023) *Author guidelines.* https://onlinelibrary.wiley.com/page/journal/13652702/homepage/forauthors.html

Kim, S., Cooley, M. E., Lee, S. A., & DeMarco, R. F. (2020). Prediction of smoking abstinence in women living with human immunodeficiency virus infection. *Nursing Research, 69*(3), 167–175. https://doi.org/10.1097/NNR.0000000000000421

Lee, J., & Yoo, J.-J. (2023). The current state of graphical abstracts and how to create good graphical abstracts. *Science Editing, 10*(1), 19–26. https://doi.org/10.6087/kcse.293

Lee, M. C., Johnson, K. L., Newhouse, R. P., & Warren, J. I. (2013). Evidence-based practice process quality assessment: EPQA guidelines. *Worldviews on Evidence-Based Nursing, 10*(3), 140–149. https://doi.org/10.1111/j.1741-6787.2012.00264.x

Luby, S., & Southern, D. (2022). *The pathway to publishing: A guide to quantitative writing in the health sciences.* Springer, Cham.

Martin, K. (2020). A picture is worth a thousand words. *Medical Writing, 29*(1), 28–34.

O'Brien, B. C., Harris, I. B., Beckman, T. J., Reed, D. A., & Cook, D. A. (2014). Standards for reporting qualitative research: A synthesis of recommendations. *Academic Medicine, 89*(9), 1245–1251. https://doi.org/10.1097/ACM.0000000000000388

Ogrinc, G., Davies, L., Goodman, D., Batalden, P., Davidoff, F., & Stevens, D. (2016). SQUIRE 2.0 (Standards for QUality Improvement Reporting Excellence): Revised publication guidelines from a detailed consensus process. *BMJ Quality & Safety, 25*, 986–992. https://doi.org/10.1136/bmjqs-2015-004411

Oska, S., Lerma, E., & Topf, J. (2020). A picture is worth a thousand views: A triple crossover trial of visual abstracts to examine their impact on research dissemination. *Journal of Medical Internet Research, 22*(12),1-7. https://www.jmir.org/2020/12/e22327

Page, M. J., McKenzie, J., Bossuyt, P. M., Boutron, I., Hoffmann, T. C, Mulrow, C. D., Shamseer, L., Tetzlaff, J. M., Akl, E. A., Brennan S. E., Chou, R., Glanville, J., Grimshaw, J. M., Hróbjartsson, A., Lalu, M. M., Li, T., Loder, E. W., Mayo-Wilson, E., McDonald, S., McGuinness, L. A., Stewart, L. A., Thomas, J., Tricco, A. C., Welch, V. A., Whiting, P., & Moher, D. (2021). The PRISMA 2020 statement: An updated guideline for reporting systematic reviews. *The British Medical Journal, 372*, n71. https://doi.org/10.1136/bmj.n71

Pestka, E. L., Billman, R. R., Alexander, J. M., & Rosenblad, M. K. (2002). Acute medical crises masquerading as psychiatric illness. *Journal of Emergency Nursing, 28*(6), 531–535. https://doi.org/10.1067/men.2002.128438

Riley, D. S., Barber, M. S., Kienle, G. S., Aronson, J. K., von Schoen-Angerer, T., Tugwell, P., Kiene, H., Helfand, M., Altman, D. G., Sox, H., Werthmann, P. G., Moher, D., Rison, R. A., Shamseer, L., Koch, C. A., Sun, G. H., Hanaway, P., Sudak, N. L., Kaszkin-Bettag, M., Carpenter, J. E., & Gagnier, J. J. (2017). CARE guidelines for case reports: Explanation and elaboration document. *Journal of Clinical Epidemiology, 89*, 218–235. https://doi.org/10.1016/j.jclinepi.2017.04.026

Saver, C. (2006). Determining what type of article to write. *AORN Journal, 84*(5), 751–757. https://doi.org/10.1016/s0001-2092(06)63962-8

Saver, C. (2023, March 23). Grab readers' attention with graphical abstracts. *American Nurse Journal.* https://www.myamericannurse.com/grab-readers-attention-with-graphical-abstracts/

Shields, A., & Lin, J.-H. (2023). Risk factors associated with pressure injury in critically ill children with congenital heart disease. *American Journal of Critical Care, 32*(3), 216–7220. https://doi.org/10.4037/ajcc2023811

Siedlecki, S. L. (2023a). Artificial intelligence, digital health research, and the clinical nurse specialist. *Clinical Nurse Specialist, 37*(5), 214–217. https://doi.org/10.1097/NUR.0000000000000763

Siedlecki, S. L. (2023b). Tables, figures, and graphs—Oh my: How to best display data. *Clinical Nurse Specialist, 37*(4), 160–163. https://doi.org/10.1097/NUR.0000000000000751

Silvia, P. J. (2019). *How to write a lot: A practical guide to productive academic writing* (2nd ed.). American Psychological Association.

Simplified Science Publishing. (2024). *Best graphical abstract examples with free templates*. https://www.simplifiedsciencepublishing.com/resources/best-graphical-abstract-examples-with-free-templates

Strunk, W., Jr., & De A'Morelli, R. (2018). *The elements of style*. Spectrum Ink.

Tancredi, T. S., Kissane, J. L., Lynch, F. C., Li, M., Kong, L., & Waybill, P. N. (2020). The effect of immediate versus delayed port access on 30-day infection rate. *Journal of Infusion Nursing, 43*(3), 167–171. https://doi.org/10.1097/NAN.0000000000000370

Trivedi, S., Chin, A., Ibrahim, A., & Ou, A. (2021). Infographics and visual abstracts. *Journal of Graduate Medical Education, 13*(4), 581–582. https://doi.org/10.4300/JGME-D-21-00590

Troyka, L. Q., & Hesse, D. (2016). *Simon & Schuster handbook for writers* (11th ed.). Pearson.

Trueger, N. S., Aly. E. Haneuse, S., Haung, E., & Berkwits, M. (2023, Sept. 29). Randomized clinical trial visual abstract and social media-driven website traffic [Letter]. *JAMA*. https://doi.org/10.1001/jama.2023.16839

Vandenbogaart, E., Gawlinski, A., Grimley, K. A., Lewis, M. A., & Pavlish, C. (2023). App-based mindfulness intervention to improve psychological outcomes in pretransplant patients with heart failure. *Critical Care Nurse, 43*(2), 15–25. https://doi.org/10.4037/ccn2023411

von Elm, E., Altman, D. G., Egger, M., Pocock, S. J., Gøtzsche, P. C., & Vandenbroucke, J. P. (2007). The Strengthening the Reporting of Observational Studies in Epidemiology (STROBE) statement: Guidelines for reporting observational studies. *Annals of Internal Medicine, 147*(8), 573–577. https://doi.org/10.7326/0003-4819-147-8-200710160-00010

Watson, R. (2021). Writing for publication: The journal article. In K. Holland & R. Watson (Eds.), *Writing for publication in nursing and healthcare* (pp. 62–97) Wiley-Blackwell.

Writing Skills Lab

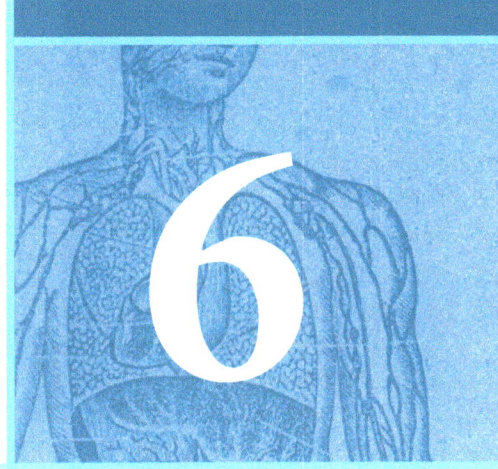

–Cynthia Saver, MS, RN

WHAT YOU'LL LEARN IN THIS CHAPTER

- The four Cs of writing can guide you in producing an effective manuscript.
- Self-editing is challenging, but it will improve your work.
- Proofreading is an essential step to achieve optimal quality.

"Written words can also sing."
–Ngũgĩ wa Thiong'o

As mentioned in Chapter 1, writing is a skill, something you can learn. In your nursing studies, you applied your classroom education in the skills lab, becoming proficient in the procedures you would later use to care for patients. This chapter discusses basic writing techniques that will help you produce a worthwhile manuscript. As when you were a student, you'll need to practice these skills to become a better writer.

Developing writing skills relies on the ability to effectively use the tools of written communication. In nursing school, you learned that proteins are made up of chains of amino acids joined end to end. In writing, amino acids = words, chains of amino acids = sentences, joined chains = paragraphs, and protein = the finished product, whether it is a book, an article, or even a letter to the editor (Saver, 2019). Words, sentences, and paragraphs are the essential amino acids (tools) you can use to create a powerful impression on the reader through writing that is clear, concise, correct, and compelling—the four Cs.

Clear

You can use several techniques to ensure your writing is clear, including limiting passive voice, choosing effective words, providing signposts for the reader, and using parallel structure.

Limit Passive Voice

Active voice promotes reader engagement. A sentence written in the active voice has a structure of subject/verb/object. Passive voice changes that order to object/verb/subject, flipping the positions of the subject (the "actor") and object (what is being acted upon), so that the subject comes after the object. Here is a simple example:

Passive voice: "A neurological assessment was performed by the nurse every 2 hours." The order is: object = assessment, verb = was, subject = nurse.

Active voice: "The nurse performed a neurologic assessment every 2 hours." Now the order is subject = nurse, verb = performed, object = assessment.

Passive voice can create ambiguity. Consider this case of the missing physician:

Passive voice: The catheter is advanced through the artery until it reaches the blockage. (Who advanced the catheter?)

Active voice: The cardiologist advances the catheter through the artery until it reaches the blockage. (Through active voice, the cardiologist appears.)

One way to detect passive voice is to watch for what are referred to as "be" verbs, such as was, are, is, could be, and will be. These often, but not always, indicate passive voice. Another warning sign of passive voice is "by the…" Note that the earlier example had two of these signposts: A neurological assessment *was* performed *by the* nurse every two hours.

To convert a passive sentence into an active one, ask, "Who does what to whom?" (Redish, 2012). The person or thing doing the action (subject) goes before the verb. A simple illustration is:

Passive voice: Several steps can be taken by nurse educators to improve nurses' expertise in pain management.

Active voice: Nurse educators can take several steps to improve nurses' expertise in pain management.

Writing Terminology

Each healthcare specialty has its associated terminology—for example, "antenatal care" for nurses in maternal/child health and "cognitive dissonance" for nurses in psychiatric specialties. Similarly, writing has its own terminology, some of which might be familiar to you from high school. Understanding this terminology helps you be a better writer (Fogarty, 2018; Purdue Online Writing Lab, n.d.-b):

- **Noun:** A noun is a person, place, thing, or concept. Nouns answer the questions who and what. For example, in the sentence "The nurse changed the dressing," nurse and dressing are nouns. In "Honesty is an important attribute of the nurse-patient relationship," honesty is a noun that represents a concept.

- **Pronoun:** A pronoun takes the place of a noun. For example, in "She changed the dressing," she is a pronoun.

- **Verb:** A verb shows action or a state of being. For example, in "The nurse changed the dressing," changed is a verb.

- **Adjective:** An adjective modifies (describes) a noun or pronoun. For example, in "The dialysis nurse changed the dressing," dialysis is an adjective.

- **Adverb:** An adverb modifies a verb or an adjective. They usually, but not always, end in ly. For example, in "The nurse carefully changed the dressing," carefully is an adverb.

- **Conjunction:** A conjunction joins items and can create transitions. For example, in "The nurse administered pain medication and changed the dressing," and is a conjunction joining two actions.

The basic sentence structure is subject, verb, object, as in: Nurses care for patients. In this case, "Nurses" is the subject, "care" is the verb, and "patients" is the object. The subject is the "actor" (the person or thing doing something), and the object is what is being acted on. This structure is usually the strongest way to convey your thoughts.

Adjectives and adverbs can round out a sentence, such as "Critical care (adjective) nurses care for seriously (adverb) ill patients," but they need to be used thoughtfully. Adverbs in particular are prone to overuse. Think of them as a strong spice to be used sparingly.

Notice that the nurse educator is the "who" doing the action ("take several steps") directed at nurses. Here is another example.

> **Passive voice:** Phenomenological evidence of suffering and limitations caused by pancreatic cancer that has been found in qualitative study results has resulted in an increased knowledge of living with pancreatic cancer.
>
> **Active voice:** Results of qualitative studies have increased our knowledge of living with pancreatic cancer by providing phenomenological evidence of the suffering and limitations caused by the disease.

This example illustrates that "who" (subject) isn't always a person; in this case, it's "qualitative studies" that "increased our knowledge."

Not all sentences need to be active—that would be as off-putting as having all passive sentences. For example, passive voice is useful if the subject performing an action is obvious, unimportant, or unknown (Lang, 2017; Purdue Online Writing Lab, n.d.-a). One example is the methods section of a research report. For instance, in the sentence, "An adapted PICO (population-intervention-comparison-outcome) structure was used to determine the eligibility of the studies," the important point is the tool that was used (PICO), not who used it. In this case, "We used an adapted PICO..." puts the emphasis in the wrong place. Remember that the advice is to *limit*, not *eliminate*, passive voice.

Choose Effective Words

Mark Twain said, "The difference between the right word and the almost right word is the difference between lightning and a lightning bug." Choose your words with care, particularly when it comes to verbs, which usually do the heavy lifting in a sentence. Avoid turning strong verbs into weak nouns or adjectives that can't do a verb's job. (The technical term for this is *nominalization*.) For example, "Inhibition of HIV replication is induced by antiretroviral therapy" is cumbersome, but "Antiretroviral therapy inhibits HIV replication," which converts "inhibition" to "inhibits," is easier to comprehend (Every, 2017). Consider also the words "increase" and "decrease": Instead of "An increase in patients' scores was observed," consider "The patients' scores increased"

(Every, 2017). In addition, avoid "ize" words such as "utilize"; "use" is stronger.

Effective words are specific. Instead of a "small" wound, give the dimensions or compare it to something readers would know, such as a quarter. Replace "many" and "some" with numbers, if possible; what is the age range for "older" patients? "Show" what you mean rather than simply "tell" something to the reader. For instance, give the formula for calculating the infusion rate, then provide an example. Below is another example of providing specifics.

> **Before:** Make sure the graft is intact.
>
> **After:** Inject 20 mL of saline into the graft and watch for leaking in the sutured areas.

Stick to words that your readers will understand instead of trying to impress them with your vocabulary. Your goal is to communicate clearly (Gould, 2019).

Be careful of vague jargon, such as, "Shared governance structures provide continuous bidirectional feedback." What exactly is meant by "continuous bidirectional feedback"? It would be better to state who provides the feedback and how often, for example, "Leaders and staff give and receive feedback during weekly shared governance committee meetings."

The bottom line: Make every word in your manuscript pull its weight.

Provide Signposts

Use transitions between sentences and paragraphs as signposts to guide readers on their reading journey; think of transitions as a literary GPS. For example:

> Hemostasis comprises three steps. *First*, vascular spasm occurs; *second*, the platelet plug forms; and *third*, coagulation begins. (This is an example of sequencing to promote easy understanding.)
>
> The project's primary goal was to reduce waiting time in the clinic. Secondary goals included improving the physical environment and improving communication with the family. (*Primary* and *secondary* lead the reader through the goals.)

Transitions

Here are examples of words and phrases that help with transitions between sentences and from one paragraph to another.

Type of transition	Sample words or phrases
Addition	Furthermore, moreover, in addition
Cause and effect	As a result, because, consequently, therefore
Contrast	Alternatively, despite, however, in contrast, on the other hand, yet
Compare	By comparison, compared to, compared with
Example	For example, for instance, particularly, specifically, such as
Sequence	First, second, third
Similarity	Similarly, likewise
Time	Then, after, later, subsequently

Conjunctions (if, and, but, yet, so) also provide transitions by connecting words, phrases (which do not have a subject and verb), and sentences (which have a subject and verb). For example, "Leaders completed simulation training, and they conducted at least two simulations under the guidance of an experienced instructor."

Transitions are particularly important when explaining complicated concepts. Whereat and Leventhal (2017) refer to transitions as "linking words" that show the relationship between one idea and another and guide the reader.

Another way to create signposts is to craft effective paragraphs. Each paragraph should have a topic sentence, which conveys the main point of the paragraph (Whereat & Leventhal, 2017). The topic sentence usually (but not always) comes first, followed by sentences with supporting information such as data or examples, then a final sentence that bridges to the next paragraph (or ends the article).

You can build paragraphs based on the outline you created for your article. For example, if you are writing an article about identifying a patient with pulmonary embolism, one of your outline entries is likely to be diagnostic tests. You might start your paragraph with: "Common imaging tests for pulmonary embolism are computed tomography angiography and pulmonary angiography." You could then go to explain how each is used and typical findings. Depending on the level of detail you need to include, you might end up writing a paragraph for each test.

Use Parallel Structure

Parallelism, or *parallel structure*, refers to keeping words and phrases within a sentence or a bulleted or numbered list consistent; doing creates a pattern that makes it easier for readers to follow the information (Saver, 2020; Whereat & Leventhal, 2017).

> **Not parallel:** The parts of the nursing process are *assessing*, *to plan*, *implement*, and *evaluating*.
>
> **Parallel:** The parts of the nursing process are to *assess*, *plan*, *implement*, and *evaluate*.

Note that in the first example, the words in italics don't have the same structure. For example: *implement* and *evaluating* don't match. But in the parallel version, all the italicized words match, including *assess* and *evaluate*.

Here is another example:

> **Not parallel:** The patients *warmed up*, *were asked* to walk 2 miles, and a notebook *was used* to record the activity.
>
> **Parallel:** The patients *warmed up*, *walked* 2 miles, and *recorded* their activity.

Notice that in the parallel version, the verbs are still in the past tense (as they were in the nonparallel version), but because the format for each is the same ("ed" at the end), the sentence is easier to read. The parallel version has the additional advantage of clarifying who recorded the activity. It also only has 11 words versus 19, another plus.

Parallel structure makes it easier for a reader to understand what you are saying. In both examples above, the nonparallel example is harder to follow, so the reader has to work harder to comprehend what's written. Here is an example of how to apply parallelism to a list of bullet points.

Not parallel

Research supports providing staff with a specific oral care protocol for patients to reduce the incidence of hospital-acquired pneumonia:

- Use a soft-bristle toothbrush or an electric suction toothbrush if patients can't brush their own teeth.
- The toothpaste should contain sodium bicarbonate.
- It's important to examine the oral cavity, including the teeth and gingiva, thoroughly; for patients receiving antibiotics, watch for oropharyngeal candidiasis.
- Ensure that patients' dentures are cleaned after each meal and before bedtime.
- A mouthwash without alcohol is preferred to complete oral care.

Parallel

Research supports providing staff with a specific oral care protocol for patients to reduce the incidence of hospital-acquired pneumonia. Nurses should:

- *Use* a soft-bristle toothbrush or an electric suction toothbrush if patients can't brush their own teeth.
- *Use* toothpaste that contains sodium bicarbonate.
- *Examine* the oral cavity, including the teeth and gingiva, thoroughly; for patients receiving antibiotics, watch for oropharyngeal candidiasis.
- *Ensure* that patients' dentures are cleaned after each meal and before bedtime.
- *Use* a mouthwash without alcohol to complete oral care.

In the parallel case, each bullet point starts with a verb (in italics; Meehan & McKenna, 2020). Also note that every bulleted item is a sentence and thus should end with a period.

Parallelism also is useful for two related ideas joined by a conjunction. For example, "Staff satisfaction improved by 50%, but physician satisfaction didn't increase as much—it only rose 10%," can be improved by writing, "Staff satisfaction increased by 50%, but physician satisfaction increased by only 10%." (Data are fictitious.)

Parallel structure is a simple tool that is easy to learn.

Concise

One of the hardest lessons for writers to learn, whether new or experienced, is to focus on what the reader *needs* to know as opposed to what is *nice* to know. Readers want information they can use, and they want to access it in the most efficient way possible. Being concise will help readers absorb what you have written. Here are some suggestions.

Think Shorter (Usually)

The length of your sentences and paragraphs can affect comprehension. It's best to avoid long, convoluted sentences and paragraphs, although there are no hard and fast rules about how many words make a sentence or paragraph too long. Lang (2017) points out that length is only one factor in comprehension—nominalization also plays a role.

A useful strategy is to evaluate how easy it is for a reader to follow what you have written. Consider breaking long sentences into two shorter ones, or use punctuation to provide mental pauses.

Keep in mind, however that shorter isn't always better, as illustrated in this example:

The new shorter, smaller catheter is superior to the one used now.

The new catheter is shorter and smaller, which makes it easier to insert into the hepatic vein of older adult patients.

> ### Punctuation Basics
>
> A period is usually the best way to end a sentence (reserve those exclamation points for social media), but what about punctuation within the sentence? You can use commas, colons, dashes, parentheses, and semicolons to link parts of a sentence, emphasize key elements, and make a longer sentence easier to understand (Saver, 2019).
>
> - **Commas** can be used to separate items in a list, connect two short sentences, or mark the end of an introductory phrase, as in "Although patients identified their objectives before the support group started, many refined their goals midway through the intervention." Note that most publications use what is called the Oxford comma in a list of items. The Oxford comma is placed after the next-to-the-last item on the list. For example, in the sentence "Symptoms of a myocardial infarction include chest pain, nausea, fatigue, and shortness of breath," the Oxford comma is after fatigue. Some publications would not use a comma in this situation.
>
> - **Parentheses** give readers additional information (words, phrases, or sentences) that is helpful but of less importance than the main sentence. Removing what is in parentheses should not change the meaning of a sentence, as in: "We determined glycemia (based on A1C) before enrolling the patients into the study."
>
> - **Semicolons** can be used connect two independent clauses (a clause consists of a noun and verb) that could stand alone as two sentences but have a close connection. Be careful not to overuse them. Semicolons also are used when items in a list already contain commas, such as: "created a detailed, two-page algorithm; provided education sessions; and followed up to determine effectiveness."
>
> - **Colons** tell the reader, "Pay attention to what comes next." A colon may introduce the reader to a bulleted list, or, more often, expand on the thought just expressed. For example: "Mindfulness practice mainly acts in 3 systems: emotional regulation, self-awareness, and attentional control" (Tripathi & Mulkey, 2023).
>
> - **Dashes** can be effective if used sparingly. Like colons, dashes call attention to themselves; for example, in the sentence "Helping patients establish their own goals—preferably ones that are measurable—will improve the likelihood of success," the dashes help emphasize the importance of having goals that can be measured.

The first sentence stacked too many adjectives (new, shorter, smaller) before the noun (catheter). The second sentence is longer, but easier to read, and more importantly, it provides a rationale for the change.

Another example of when shorter might not be better is the use of abbreviations and acronyms (*acronyms* are abbreviations that form a word that can be pronounced, e.g., HIPAA for the Health Insurance Portability and Accountability Act of 1996). Lang (2019) notes that abbreviations can shorten text, but they can also potentially confuse readers. For example, he found more than 50 meanings for the randomly chosen abbreviation "TD." Even if an abbreviation is defined the first time it appears, if it is used sparingly in a long document, the reader may forget the meaning and spend valuable time searching for the definition. Abbreviations also can be ambiguous. One example is CRF, which can refer to case report form, chronic renal failure, chronic respiratory failure, or corticotropin-releasing factor.

Overuse of abbreviations can be distracting to the reader, as in "If the patient with COPD is SOB, take his BP and call his MD." Most readers would know what the abbreviations mean but would need to take mental time to decode them. Another problem is that some abbreviations, such as LVPWT (left ventricular posterior wall thickness, an echocardiographic measure of cardiac structure), can't be easily read as words or letters (Lang, 2019). Lang offers suggestions to guide use of abbreviations, including:

- Use abbreviations sparingly.

- Use only common abbreviations whose meanings are readily available in standard references.

- Use abbreviations only when they appear often enough to be helpful. For example, if "emergency department" only appears twice in a 2,000-word document, use both words instead of ED.
- Don't use abbreviations in titles and headings unless they are well known.

Another consideration is your target audience. For example, nurses new to oncology are less likely to be familiar with abbreviations common to the specialty, so limit their use.

Cut the Clutter

Be aggressive in cutting the clutter in your sentence by removing extraneous words. For example:

Before: It is important to remember that bystanders may confuse a seizure with behavioral problems or the inappropriate use of drugs.

After: Bystanders and first responders may confuse seizures with behavior problems or illicit drug use.

"It is important to remember" is probably not necessary; if it weren't important, you wouldn't have included it, although alternatively, you could write, "Remember that…" Here are other some examples of how to be more concise:

- "By" instead of "by the way of"
- "Most" instead of "a majority of"
- "Many" instead "of a large number of"
- "To" instead of "in order to"
- "Because" instead of "due to the fact that"
- "All" instead of "all four of"
- "Few" instead of "a small number of"
- "May" instead of "could potentially"

Qualifiers such as "very," "quite," "rather," "actually," "basically," "extremely," "generally," "largely," "mostly," "slightly," and "somewhat" can almost always be cut or replaced with a stronger adjective (Every, 2017). For example, replace "very hard" with "difficult." Another word that often simply takes up space is "that." For example, "Most (55%) of the nurses reported that they experienced moral distress in the past 30 days" would work better as, "Most (55%) nurses reported they experienced moral distress in the past 30 days."

Be alert to phrases such as "There are," There is," and "There were," which not only add words, but also weaken the opening of your sentence (Every, 2017) and are often followed by nominalized verbs (Lang, 2017). Most of the time the sentence can be recast; for instance, instead of, "The data confirm that there is an association between job satisfaction and shared governance," try, "The data confirm an association between job satisfaction and shared governance," which also makes the sentence more active in structure.

Another example of unnecessary words are what Nicoll (2015) calls "pizza pies," which are modifiers that become unnecessary after the first mention. For example, if your study participants were "junior level pre-licensure baccalaureate nursing students," you can simply call them "the students" or "the participants" once you have established who they are and why they were in the sample. There is no need to repeat the six-word description throughout the text.

Q *Does the order of the words in a sentence matter?*

A The strongest parts of the sentence are the beginning and the end, so avoid burying the most important information in the middle (Saver, 2019). Consider this sentence: "Peripheral vascular access device complications, including tissue injury, infection, emboli, and extravasations, can lead to increased morbidity and mortality." The actual complications are certainly important, but in this case, the most important point is that those complications cause illness and death.

Finally, consider replacing lengthy text with figures, tables, and other graphics. Graphics can often deliver background or complicated information more effectively. (See Chapter 7 for more information about graphics.)

> **Confidence Booster**
>
> You may feel intimidated by words and phrases such as "nominalization" and "passive voice." Remember that you have already learned complicated information. You can learn this too.

Correct

Accuracy matters. If peer reviewers find small errors such as the numbers in a pie chart not adding up to 100% without any explanation why, they may question your attention to other details. Check numbers, citations and their corresponding references, grammar, and spelling. Errors in references are common. While these may seem minor, such errors can make it more difficult for others to find the article cited.

A good time to check accuracy is when you edit your work (see Appendix A). Using a proofreading checklist, such as that in Appendix B, before you submit your manuscript will also promote accuracy.

Editing yourself is a key step in creating an effective manuscript, but it can be difficult given the time and effort you invested into your writing. Try to put your ego aside. Your goal is to ensure the reader has correct, useful information; every word, every sentence, and every paragraph must serve that goal. Editing a printed copy instead of viewing the document on a screen may give you a new perspective (Gastel, 2015). You may also want to change the typeface or font size and widen the margins so you can more easily make comments. Reading aloud can help you identify rough patches that need smoothed.

Proofreading is the final step before you submit the article. It's best to wait a day or so after you complete your manuscript so you can approach it with a fresh outlook. Before you start to proofread, find an environment that limits distractions (Zaman, 2018). Most people will need quiet, but others prefer to have at least some background noise, such as music. You can proofread either on your computer screen or on paper—experiment to see what works best for you.

Focus on details such as typographical errors, grammatical errors, and reference format. Run a spell- and grammar-check, but remember that because of features such as autocorrect and an author's momentary lapse in concentration, it will not detect all errors—for example, "pubic" vs. "public" or "lumber puncture" instead of "lumbar puncture" (Gastel, 2015; Gastel & Day, 2022). Take frequent breaks to keep your focus sharp. Another strategy is to start first with the overall title and headings, then focus on each section in detail. You may find it helpful to proof twice (with some time in between), first starting at the beginning of the manuscript and reading forward, and the second time starting at the end of the manuscript and reading each section in reverse order.

Q *What are resources to help me improve my editing and writing?*

A If you are seeking grammar advice, turn to the Grammar Girl website (www.quickanddirtytips.com/grammar-girl). Grammarly (https://app.grammarly.com) offers a free version of its software that you might find helpful. Many writing centers at top colleges offer free writing advice online, such as Purdue's Online Writing Lab (https://owl.purdue.edu/owl/purdue_owl.html). Two excellent books are Stephen King's *On Writing: A Memoir of the Craft* (2010) and William Zinsser's *On Writing Well* (30th anniversary edition, 2016), both classic resources for fiction and nonfiction authors alike. Finally, *Nurse Author & Editor* (http://naepub.com) is a free website with valuable articles on writing and editing that are written specifically for nurses.

Compelling

The idea of "compelling" writing may seem intimidating, but it is achievable by using techniques such as taking ownership, being positive, and being considerate.

Take Ownership

Effective writing requires you to use words that show you own your ideas. If you developed the curriculum for the education program you are writing about, say so; your writing will be the better for it, especially because your sentence will be active rather than passive (Saver, 2019). For example, instead of, "A new curriculum consisting of five modules was developed," write, "We developed a new curriculum of five modules." The latter sentence makes it clear that the authors created the modules, as opposed to someone else, and eliminates a few unnecessary words.

One caveat: Look at articles published in the journal you are considering for your manuscript. If you do not see any first-person pronouns in the articles, then you probably don't want to include them in your manuscript. In this case, it's more important to follow the journal's style. This information may also be in the author guidelines.

Ownership in research studies typically comes in the discussion and conclusion sections (rather than methods), as authors conclude what they have learned from the results of the study. However, the results section is another area where you should be wary of diluting your statements. Sometimes, "tend to" and "generally" are appropriate, depending on the strength of the results. However, if you had a major finding, say so. Consider this example from the results section of a study on the safety of temporary staff: "Temporary staffing was associated with significant increases in the hazard of death, particularly at higher levels" (Dall'Ora et al., 2020, p. 213).

Ownership means not being afraid to take a stand. Avoid words and phrases such as "apparently," "it appears," or "to a degree." State what you believe and back it up as needed.

> **Before:** It would appear that nurses are worried about their safety at work.
>
> **After:** "Based on our results, nurses are increasingly concerned about their safety at work." Or, to avoid the "our" (because of journal style): "Based on these results…"

Be Positive

In addition to taking up space, negatives can be misinterpreted. Try to recast the sentence or substitute a different word (Saver, 2019). For example, instead of, "Nurses did not believe the intervention was harmful," try, "Nurses believed the intervention was helpful." When a negative is called for, be precise and concise. For example, consider changing "did not remember" to "forgot."

> The intervention was found not to be harmful.
>
> The intervention was safe.

Notice that the second option also uses fewer words. Another example:

> The students did not want to complete the assignment incorrectly.
>
> The students wanted to complete the assignment correctly.

Be Considerate

Good writers are considerate of the reader's time and needs. For example, they don't waste readers' time with vague or obvious statements such as, "Nurses face ethical dilemmas." Instead, they provide more substance such as, "In a recent survey, 76% of labor and delivery nurses reported they encounter ethical dilemmas at least weekly." (Data are fictitious.)

It also is helpful to anticipate what questions readers might have about the information you are presenting. Consider sharing a draft with one or two people within the target group for the article and ask what questions they have.

Above all, tailor the article to the reader. For instance, if you're writing an article on acuity-based staffing for chief nurse executives, you do not need to define basic financial terms. In addition, keep in mind that writing for online publications is slightly different than writing for print.

Being considerate extends to those not reading the article, such as patients. Your writing should be inclusive and free from bias. For example, guidelines from the American Association of Diabetes Educators and the American Diabetes Association recommend that language, whether spoken or written, should foster collaboration between patients and providers and be (Dickinson et al., 2017):

- Neutral, nonjudgmental
- Based on facts, actions, or physiology/biology
- Free from stigma
- Strength-based, respectful, inclusive, and hopeful
- Person-centered

These guidelines do not only apply to patient education material. Authors have a responsibility to be inclusive no matter who is the target audience. In fact, the *Publication Manual of the American Psychological Association* (APA, 2020), a commonly used style guide, devotes an entire chapter to bias-free language. The chapter notes two important principles for reducing bias: describe at the appropriate level of specificity and be sensitive to labels.

It is the author's responsibility to avoid irrelevant or judgmental language when referring to those being written about. Sensitive areas include age, ability and disability, religion, race and ethnicity, sex and gender, sexual orientation, socioeconomic status, and immigration status (APA, 2020; Likis, 2021). The nursing profession provides a simple example: Most nurses are women, but using only "she" or "her" in your writing excludes men in the profession.

> **Online Writing**
>
> *Leslie H. Nicoll, PhD, MBA, RN, FAAN*
>
> The basic principles of good writing apply to both print and online. However, it's worth focusing on some unique principles of writing content that will primarily appear online.
>
> People tend to "read" differently online. Online text needs to be easily searched and cataloged, which also changes how people write. You need to adapt your writing so that it best meets the needs of online readers.
>
> A few hints: Break up your text into chunks to make it easier for readers to follow the material. Use lists and short paragraphs rather than multiple unbroken lines of text. A sentence should not contain more than 20 words, and a paragraph should not contain more than six sentences, according to Research-Based Web Design and Usability Guidelines from the US Department of Health and Human Services (2013).
>
> Graphics and multimedia features (e.g., audio and video) are excellent tools for illustrating your points, but they should be used appropriately to provide useful information instead of distracting the reader. The main image should be given dominance, with the others available through links within the text.
>
> For more success, try the following tips for writing for online publications (US Department of Health and Human Services, 2013):
>
> - Avoid jargon and use abbreviations sparingly.
> - Define any acronyms and abbreviations used.
> - Use conventional capitalization of sentences.
> - Keep sentences and paragraphs short.
> - Use active voice.
> - Make the first sentence in a paragraph descriptive because readers tend to skim these when scanning text.
> - Don't overdo graphics. Some writers have the mistaken impression that online readers only look for visuals. In fact, they will read text if it is of interest to them.
>
> Note that many of these tips, such as defining acronyms, are important when writing for print, too.

You can avoid bias by omitting unnecessary "labels" such as "nonadherent" or "failed to follow the treatment plan." For example, instead of "seniors" use "older adults," or better yet, "adults 65 years or older." Instead of "diabetics" use "persons with diabetes," which is an example of "person first" language. Person first examples related to socioeconomic status include "people with low income" rather than "needy" or "disadvantaged," and "people who are homeless" ("houseless" or "unhoused" are becoming more common) rather than "the homeless." Focus on what people have instead of what they don't have; for example, "people with some high school education" instead of "high school dropouts."

Be guided by respect for other people. For instance, when speaking about ability and disability, "uses a wheelchair" shows more respect than "wheelchair-bound." You'll also want to avoid terminology that can seem pejorative, such as "addiction"; choose more neutral words, such as "substance misuse."

Guidance for reporting factors such as race and ethnicity is available. For example, editors for the JAMA Network (Flanagin et al., 2021) write that if race and ethnicity categories were collected for a study, the reason for doing so should be noted. In addition, the term "minorities" should be avoided in writing; "underserved groups" is an example of a substitute. Others have suggested using "minoritized" rather than "minority." For example, the authors of a RAND report on addressing the impact of racism on patient safety (Schulson et al., 2022) used the term minoritized rather than minority "to acknowledge societal power structures that have conferred minority status on certain populations and to emphasize that race and ethnicity are social constructs rather than biological" (p. iv).

Be sure to use the terms "sex "and "gender" appropriately: Sex is a biological construct (based on anatomy, physiology, genetics, and hormones), while gender is a social and cultural construct (based on identity, roles, relationships, and expectations; National Institutes of Health [NIH], n.d.). Avoid gender and sex bias by using plurals, such as "they," instead of "she." In the past, "he or she" or "his or her" was used to be inclusive, but now these also should be avoided whenever possible because gender is not considered to be a binary state. In addition, it is now becoming acceptable to use "they" and "their" in the singular form to avoid bias, as well as awkward sentence structure (APA, 2020; JAMA Network Editors, 2020). For example, "Each patient turned in their survey," instead of, "Each patient turned in his or her survey."

Language has always evolved and will continue to do so; therefore, be aware of developments in this area. Some journals include information about bias-free writing in their author guidelines. General resources include the APA Bias-Free Language website (https://apastyle.apa.org/style-grammar-guidelines/bias-free-language), Conscious Style Guide (https://consciousstyleguide.com), and The Diversity Style Guide (www.diversitystyleguide.com).

Promoting Readership

Why do people read what they read? In attempting to answer that question, Wilbur Schramm, a communications expert, concluded that two factors influence what people read: expectation of rewards and effort required (Royse, 2021). In other words, how much value they expect to receive from the information and how much effort it takes to obtain it (Saver, 2021). For example, if I (the reader) think I'm going to learn what I need to know about a procedure I'm not familiar with, I'm predisposed to read the article. But if once I start reading, I encounter too many polysyllabic words or confusing sentences, or if I don't get the practical information I'm expecting, I'm unlikely to finish the article. Therefore, authors need to consider the two aspects of Schramm's formula: how to increase the rewards of the content in what you write and how you can make the content easier to read and absorb.

Increasing rewards includes being clear about the purpose of what you are writing and creating a title and introduction that indicates the benefits to come (Saver, 2021). Many of the tips in this chapter (such as using active voice) will help reduce effort. Combining higher rewards with lower efforts encourages wider dissemination of your work.

Q *Can I use artificial intelligence (AI) tools when I write?*

A AI technology like large language model tools and chatbots have the potential to assist authors with their writing endeavors. For example, they may be helpful in creating an outline and in developing certain sections of the manuscript, such as the methods section in a research report. AI technology also may be helpful for improving the title, abstract, and conclusion of your article; for identifying key points you may have missed; and for stimulating a new perspective (Buriak et al., 2023). AI tools with grammatical or structural editing capabilities may help streamline the writing process, and other tools can help with literature reviews (Golan et al., 2023). However, AI writing tools raise many concerns. Too often the information is incorrect, and it can stifle critical thinking.

If you use an AI writing tool, check all information carefully and don't use the text verbatim, which can lead to plagiarism (Buriak et al., 2023). Check the publication's guidelines related to use of AI. You'll need to disclose what tool you used and how you used it (International Committee of Medical Journal Editors [ICMJE], 2024; NIH, 2023; World Association of Medical Editors, 2023). Disclosure applies to more than just text. For example, *BMJ*'s policy states, "[This policy] applies to all formats, including, without limitation, all text, audio, video and audio-visual material, abstracts, databases, tables, data, diagrams, photographs and other images or illustrative materials" (BMJ Author Hub, n.d.).

Most importantly, AI tools are not considered authors because they can't be responsible for the accuracy, integrity, and originality of the work (ICMJE, 2024; International Society for Medical Publication Professionals, 2023; Jackson et al., 2023).

Write Now!

1. Pick an article from your favorite journal and identify active and passive sentences.
2. Compare research articles and clinical journals. Note how they differ in style.

References

American Psychological Association. (2020). *Publication manual of the American Psychological Association* (7th ed.). https://doi.org/10.1037/0000165-000

BMJ Author Hub. (n.d.). *AI use.* https://authors.bmj.com/policies/ai-use/

Buriak, J. M., Akinwande, D., Artiz, N., Brinker, C. J., Burrows, C. Chan, W. C. W., Chen, C., Chen, X., Chhowalla, M., Chi, L. Chueh, W., Crudden, C. M., Di Carlo, D., Glotzer, S. C., Hersam, M. C., Ho, D., Hu, T. Y., Huang, J., Javey, A. Kamat, P. V., Kim, I.-D., Kotov, N. A., Lee, T. R., Lee, Y. H., Li, Y., Liz-Marzan, L. M., Mulaney, P., Narang, P., Nordlander, P., Oklu, R., Parak, W. J., Rogach, A. L., Salanne, M., Samori, P., Schaak, R. E., Schanze, K. S., Sekitani, T., Skrabalak, S., Sood, A. K., Voets, I. K., Wang, S., Wang, S., Wee, A. T. S., & Ye, J. (2023). Best practices for using AI when writing scientific manuscripts [Editorial]. *CAN Nano, 17*, 4091-4093. https://doi.org/10.1021/acsnano.3c01544

Dall'Ora, C., Maruotti, A., & Griffiths, P. (2020). Temporary staffing and patient death in acute care hospitals: A retrospective longitudinal study. *Journal of Nursing Scholarship, 52*(2), 210–216. https://doi.org/10.1111/jnu.12537

Dickinson, J. K., Guzman, S. J., Maryniuk, M. D., O'Brian, C. A., Kadohiro, J. K., Jackson, R. A., D'Hondt, N., Montgomery, B., Close, K. L., & Funnell, M. M. (2017). The use of language in diabetes care and education. *Diabetes Care, 40*(12), 1790–1799. https://doi.org/10.2337/dci17-0041

Every, B. (2017). Writing economically in medicine and science: Tips for tackling wordiness. *Medical Writing, 26*(1), 17–20.

Flanagin, A., Frey, T., Christiansen, S. L., & Bauchner, H. The reporting of race and ethnicity in medical and science journals [Editorial]. (2021). *JAMA, 325*(11), 1049–1052. https://doi.org/10.1001/jama.2021.2104

Fogarty, M. (2018, March 22). Parts of speech. *Grammar Girl.* https://www.quickanddirtytips.com/education/grammar/parts-of-speech

Gastel, B. (2015). Editing and proofreading your own work. *AMWA Journal, 30*(4), 147–151.

Gastel, B., & Day, R. A. (2022). *How to write and publish a scientific paper* (9th ed.). Greenwood.

Golan, R., Reddy, R., Muthigi, A., & Ramasamy, R. (2023). Artificial intelligence in academic writing: A paradigm-shifting technological advance [Comment]. *Nature Reviews Urology, 20*(6), 327–328. https://doi.org/10.1038/s41585-023-00746-x

Gould, K. A. (2019). Writing for publication: Expanding professional practice [Editorial]. *Dimensions of Critical Care Nursing, 38*(5), 233–235. https://doi.org/10.1097/DCC.0000000000000376

International Committee of Medical Journal Editors. (2024). *Recommendations for the conduct, reporting, editing, and publication of scholarly work in medical journals.* http://www.icmje.org/recommendations

International Society for Medical Publication Professionals. (2024, Jan. 3). International Society for Medical Publication Professionals (ISMPP) position statement and call to action on artificial intelligence. *Current Medical Research and Opinion.* https://doi.org/10.1080/03007995.2023.2273139

Jackson, J., Landis, G., Baskin, P. K., Hadsell, K. A., English, M., CSE Editorial Policy Committee. (2023). CSE guidance on machine learning and artificial intelligence tools. *Science Editor, 46*, 72. https://doi.org/10.36591/SE-D-4602-07

JAMA Network Editors. (2020). *AMA manual of style: A guide for authors and editors* (11th ed.). Oxford University Press.

King, S. (2010). *On writing: A memoir of the craft* (10th anniversary ed.). Scribner.

Lang, T. (2017). How to shorten a text by up to 30% and improve clarity without losing information. *Medical Writing, 26*(1), 21–25.

Lang, T. (2019). Abbreviations: Expectations, permutations, revelations, reservations, and applications of shortened words and phrases. *AMWA Journal, 34*(4), 152–157, 160.

Likis, F. E. (2021). Inclusive language promotes equity: The power of words [Editorial]. *Journal of Midwifery & Women's Health, 66*(1), 7–9. https://doi.org/10.1111/jmwh.13225

Meehan, C. D., & McKenna, C. (2020). Preventing hospital-acquired pneumonia. *American Nurse Journal, 15*(2), 16–21. https://www.myamericannurse.com/preventing-hospital-acquired-pneumonia/

National Institutes of Health. (n.d.). *What are sex & gender?* https://orwh.od.nih.gov/sex-gender

National Institutes of Health Office of the Director. (2023). *Conduct of research in the intramural research program at NIH* (8th ed.). National Institutes of Health. https://oir.nih.gov/system/files/media/file/2023-08/guidelines-conduct_research.pdf

Nicoll, L. H. (2015). Becoming a ruthless editor. *Nurse Author & Editor, 25*(2), 2. http://naepub.com/writing-basics/2015-25-2-2/

Purdue Online Writing Lab. (n.d.-a). *Choosing passive voice.* https://owl.purdue.edu/owl/general_writing/academic_writing/active_and_passive_voice/choosing_passive_voice.html

Purdue Online Writing Lab. (n.d.-b). *Parts of speech overview.* https://owl.purdue.edu/owl/general_writing/mechanics/parts_of_speech_overview.html

Redish, J. (2012). *Letting go of the words: Writing web content that matters* (2nd ed.). Morgan Kaufmann.

Royse, M. (2021, March 9). How to get your readers to actually read your articles. *The Writing Cooperative.* writingcooperative.com/how-to-get-your-readers-to-actually-read-your-articles-7a313b377291

Saver, C. (2019). The humble sentence. *Nurse Author & Editor, 29*(4), 5. http://naepub.com/writing-basics/2019-29-4-5/

Saver, C. (2020, March 16). The power of parallelism. *American Nurse Journal.* https://www.myamericannurse.com/the-power-of-parallelism/

Saver, C. (2021, April). A formula for writing success. *American Nurse Journal.* https://www.myamericannurse.com/community-the-writing-mind-a-formula-for-writing-success/

Schulson, L. B., Thomas, A. D., Tsuei, J., & Etchegaray, J. M. (2022). *Identifying and understanding ways to address the impact of racism on patient safety in health care settings.* RAND Corporation. https://www.rand.org/pubs/research_reports/RRA1945-1.html

Tripathi, S. K., & Mulkey, D. C. (2023). Implementing brief mindfulness-based interventions to reduce compassion fatigue. *Critical Care Nurse, 43*(5), 32–40. https://doi.org/10.4037/ccn2023745

US Department of Health and Human Services. (2013). Research-based web design and usability guidelines. https://www.usability.gov/sites/default/files/documents/guidelines_book.pdf

Whereat, A., & Leventhal, P. S. (2017). Structuring paragraphs. *Medical Writing, 26*(1), 38–42.

World Association of Medical Editors. (2023). *Chatbots, generative AI, and scholarly manuscripts.* https://wame.org/page3.php?id=106

Zaman, N. (2018). Honing your proofreading skills. *Medical Writing, 27*(3), 6–9. https://journal.emwa.org/editing/honing-your-proofreading-skills/

Zinsser, W. (2016). *On writing well: The classic guide to writing nonfiction* (30th anniversary ed.). Harper Perennial.

All About Graphics

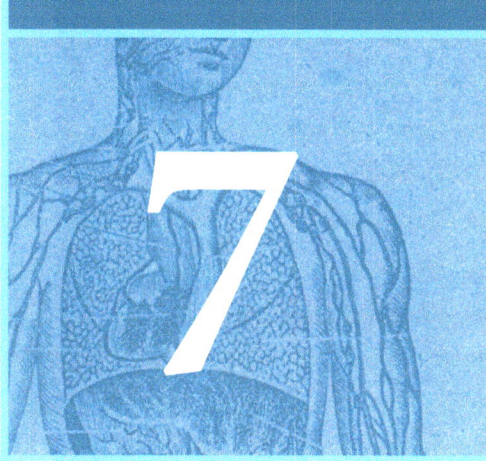

–Susanne J. Pavlovich-Danis, MSN, RN, APRN-C, CDCES

"Good design is a lot like clear thinking made visual."
–Edward R. Tufte

WHAT YOU'LL LEARN IN THIS CHAPTER

- Eye-catching graphics call attention to key points in your manuscript.
- Graphics should be labeled using standard conventions.
- Style the graphics in your manuscript to match those of the publication you are submitting to.
- To hold readers' attention, balance text with graphics.

You envision that every word in your manuscript will captivate readers. The truth is that many readers will skim an article or book chapter, concentrating on the introduction, graphics, and summary to focus on the key points. If you omit graphics or insert ones that don't emphasize your take-home points, you decrease your chances of making a lasting impression.

This chapter provides guidance for authors who want to include graphics in their manuscripts. *Graphics* is an inclusive term for tables, figures, graphs, illustrations, and photographs. When carefully selected, graphics provide visual enhancement, clarification, and an opportunity to stress significant points in your manuscript. Visual learners require them, and most readers appreciate how graphics break up text and allow for better content comprehension. Combining words and images improves your manuscript and can enhance greater retention of your key points.

Language of Graphics

Using graphics requires more effort than simply using an "Insert Table," "Insert Picture," or "Copy/Paste" command in a word processing program. Here are some key points authors must consider, including the purpose, number, and style of graphics:

- Graphics should captivate readers' attention and solidify key points.
- Use graphics to supplement—not completely replace, duplicate, or overshadow—your text.
- Use eye-catching graphics to draw in readers.
- Limit graphics to no more than one-third of your manuscript.

- Position graphics to provide readers with a visual break from reading text. Even in scholarly journals, readers expect to find graphics.
- Do your homework. Carefully study the format of the publication you are preparing your manuscript for and design your graphics in a similar fashion.
- Avoid biased wording when describing your graphics. For example, "This graph clearly identifies the superior skin care product."

You also should consider the needs and preferences of the publication's intended audience when you select graphics. Information must be tailored for that audience and presented in a clear, simple way. This is true for lay audiences who are unfamiliar with the concepts and for busy clinicians who don't always have time to decipher a complicated visual (Hafner et al., 2022). Consider that clinicians and patients have different levels of understanding, and interpret graphs differently. Patients prefer simpler graphs than do clinicians (Stonbraker et al., 2020) particularly when they have limited health literacy. If you were writing a manuscript on diabetes risk factors for a publication targeting advanced practice nurses, you might include graphics with detailed information and research findings, but if the publication targeted educators, you might include graphics that could be used for patient education instead.

If the publication targets patients or caregivers and the voice or tone of the magazine is less formal, you may even consider incorporating *emojis* (small images, symbols, or icons that communicate a message playfully without using words) to emphasize teaching points. A good example of this would be describing different levels of emotions with face emojis ranging from smiling to extreme sadness. Your editor will guide you if you have questions.

Q *Are graphics really necessary?*

A In general, yes. Graphics can provide valuable support to your article, making it easier for readers to absorb and retain information. However, not all publications use graphics, and some limit the number that can be submitted. Check the author guidelines and review past issues to gain a sense of the number and types of graphics used.

Q *I want to include graphics, but I notice the publication rarely includes them. What should I do?*

A Review the publication's specifications and contact the editor in advance if possible. Specify in your cover letter or early communications with editors that you can provide graphics and then follow their cue.

You must learn the language that editors use for graphics. Editors generally identify graphics by using standard conventions and numbering them consecutively: for example, Table 1, Table 2, and so on; Figure 1, Figure 2, and so on. Use this standard naming convention to identify the files that correspond to your graphics: for example, table1.pdf, figure1.jpg, figure2.tiff. Note that each graphic in this example tells the editor the kind of file by its *file extension*: those three or four letters after the file's name (.pdf, and .jpg, for example). An accurate file name, complete with its extension, helps you and the editor keep track of all graphics. For created graphics—such as in Photoshop or Illustrator—the file extension also tells an editor the host program.

Graphics also may be the product of generative artificial intelligence (AI), a technological advance used by tools such as ChatGPT and Midjourney. These tools use algorithms to analyze existing content to synthesize new content—in this case, creating new images and videos that may include data and descriptions based on the content from existing images and data. Images may be difficult to distinguish from original images, yet they may depict untrue, biased, or unfavorable characteristics (deep fakes), and accompanying data or graphic descriptions may be biased or out of context. Currently, measures to detect AI-generated content are insufficient, making fact-checking and proper source citation of images used to create an AI-generated image nearly impossible.

The use of AI-generated imagery in medical and nursing publication raises questions around integrity, consent, privacy, and intellectual-property protection (Alenichev et al., 2023; Otterbacher, 2023; Švab, 2023). AI images with unverifiable sources are likely to be rejected. For example, *Nature* does not allow the use of AI in images and videos. From an editorial perspective, AI-generated photography, video, or illustrations do not have transparent and verifiable sources and do not conform to current expectations for source citation, potentially violating copyright, privacy, and consent (Why *Nature* will not allow the use of generative AI in images and video, 2023).

Bottom line: Check the author guidelines for what file types are accepted; if none are listed, contact the editor. If you used AI in generating an image, disclose this use in the manuscript (International Committee of Medical Journal Editors, 2024).

Q *Can I submit my manuscript first and describe graphics I will create if my work is accepted?*

A This isn't a good idea unless you already have a working relationship with a publication and your editor has approved your plan. It's best to submit a manuscript for consideration in its entirety, with all graphics provided for review. It's hard for an editor or a peer reviewer to complete the review without seeing the graphics that accompany the text.

Before you submit your paper, article, or book chapter, consult the publication's guidelines. Most will ask you to go one step further and include a placement identifier for the book or article or even chapter. For example, in this book, Figure 2 for Chapter 7 is named Fig 7.2. Your editor will guide you if you have any questions.

You also want to maintain consistency when referring to graphics in your manuscript. Will you refer to the graphic in text as shown in the following example?

> The studies supporting the effectiveness of nursing telehealth visits are summarized in Table 1.

Or will you note it in parenthesis after the statement it supports?

> Many studies support the use of nursing telehealth visits (Table 1).

In some cases, you can use both approaches, but be sure to follow the publication's instructions and author guidelines.

If you're working on a book, larger publishers with in-house graphic design departments might be (but are not always) able to assist in creating images to accompany your manuscript. Be prepared to provide guidance or an example of what you want to depict.

Q *If I don't include graphics in my manuscript, can the editor add them later?*

A This varies by publication. Some publications offer graphics services (with or without a fee), but most do not. Keep in mind that if a publication has to use resources to locate graphics that authors should have provided, the likelihood of the manuscript being accepted and published may decline.

After you decide that you will use graphics, the next step is to decide which types. Graphics vary in effectiveness when it comes to communicating relationships, promoting nonbiased presentation of information, disseminating research results, and affecting reader task performance (Kiran et al., 2017; Rappaz, 2022). For example, a brightly colored infographic of the heart showing key statistics related to cardiac disease may better resonate with the reader than a graphic that simply presents the same information as numerical data in a chart. An *infographic* is a visually striking image that combines words and images to convey information in a simple, health-literacy friendly manner (Devraj et al., 2022). Size also matters, and often more is not better. Research indicates that large tables are dry and cumbersome to read and assimilate (Mignini et al., 2016), so keep your graphics clear.

Explore some of the unique graphic options available to enhance your manuscripts.

Q *I was so excited to write my first book chapter, but it was sent back as, "not accepted as submitted." I had copied my figures and pasted them into my Microsoft Word document, but my editor called these "embedded figures" and said they are a no-no. Shouldn't the editor be able to handle a common usage of Word?*

A It's not quite that simple. Your manuscript files will most likely be styled in a sophisticated template with all kinds of codes the publication uses for everything from layout programs to ebooks. Figures inserted in text don't necessarily convert—or *compute*, if you will—to publishing layout programs. Most editors will want you to submit all graphics separately so they can be assessed and redrawn if needed. Make sure to follow their instructions, or your submission might be sent back.

Tables

Tables, which are often used to compare data, are composed of rows and columns. Tables are also useful for emphasizing numbers rather than trends. Use tables when you want to show relationships or convey detailed information or complex relationships within specific data. Tables enable you to present raw data or statistical analysis of complex data that would otherwise require a lengthy narrative explanation (Hayes-Larson et al., 2019).

Word-processing programs make table creation easy. Take a minute to review the table shown in Figure 7.1, which illustrates the key parts of a table, including the title, column headings, row headings, body or data fields, and footnotes.

Keep these tips in mind for creating a table that works well for the reader:

- Avoid long table and row heading titles.
- Align and justify column content.
- Insert adequate spacing between columns for easy reading.

Two common types of tables are text and tabular tables:

- *Text tables* showcase information only in words.
- *Tabular tables* showcase figures or a combination of words and figures.

Text Tables

A text table can feature information that summarizes key points, which can help reduce the word count of the main body of the manuscript. You can also display comparisons, descriptions, and instructions. For example, a text table can list definitions of methodologies used to study metabolic syndrome (see the table shown in Figure 7.2). Note that this table has a title, column headings, data fields, and a footnote, providing any necessary explanations the reader will need to understand the table more clearly.

Tabular Tables

The tabular format features data sorted and compared by specific characteristics. The table shown in Figure 7.3 reports the estimated number of adults 18 years or older with diagnosed diabetes, undiagnosed diabetes, and total diabetes in the United States for 2018. Note that this tabular table also features a title, column headings, data fields, and a footnote.

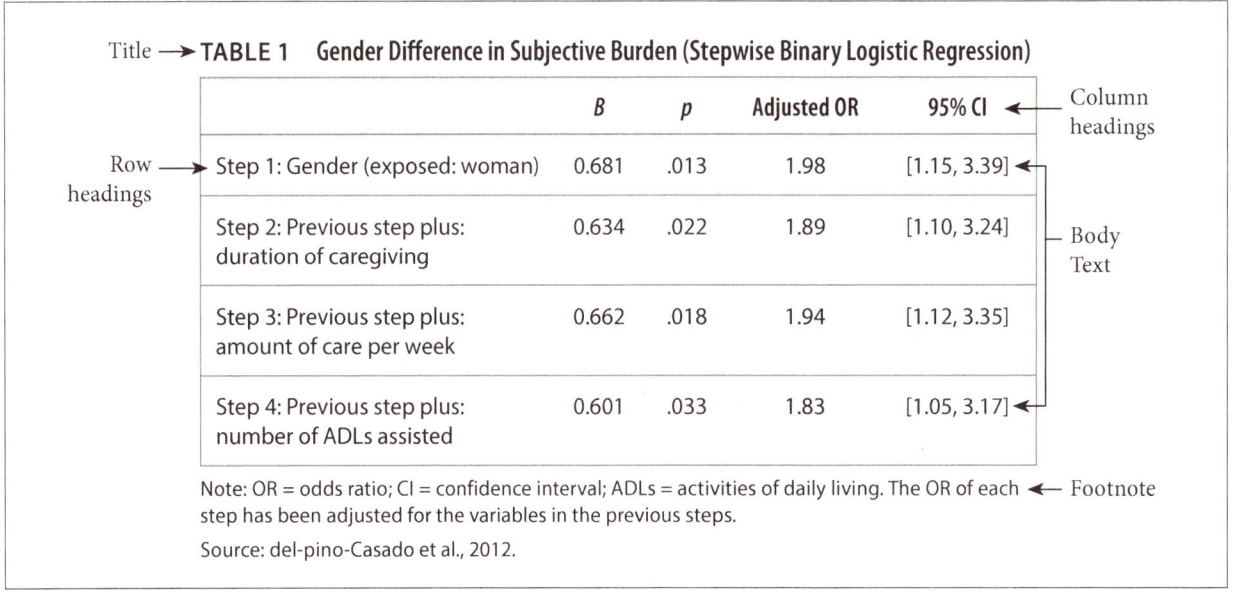

FIGURE 7.1 Sample table, including its key parts.

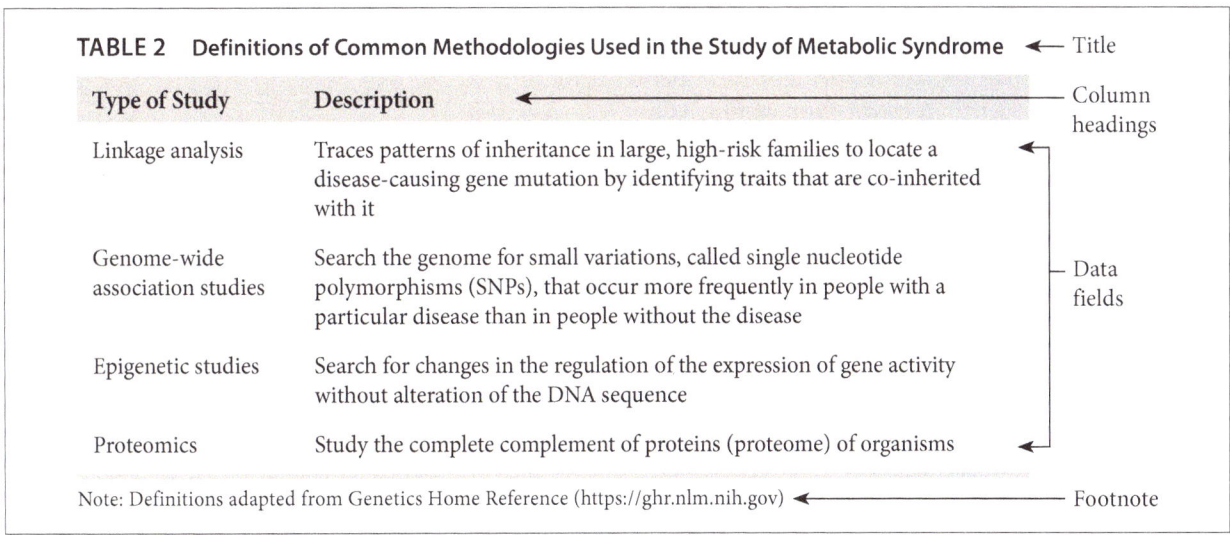

TABLE 2 Definitions of Common Methodologies Used in the Study of Metabolic Syndrome ← Title

Type of Study	Description
Linkage analysis	Traces patterns of inheritance in large, high-risk families to locate a disease-causing gene mutation by identifying traits that are co-inherited with it
Genome-wide association studies	Search the genome for small variations, called single nucleotide polymorphisms (SNPs), that occur more frequently in people with a particular disease than in people without the disease
Epigenetic studies	Search for changes in the regulation of the expression of gene activity without alteration of the DNA sequence
Proteomics	Study the complete complement of proteins (proteome) of organisms

Note: Definitions adapted from Genetics Home Reference (https://ghr.nlm.nih.gov) ← Footnote

FIGURE 7.2 Sample text table, including its key parts.

Table 1a. Estimated crude prevalence of diagnosed diabetes, undiagnosed diabetes, and total diabetes among adults aged 18 years or older, United States, 2017–2020

Characteristic	Diagnosed diabetes Percentage (95% CI)	Undiagnosed diabetes Percentage (95% CI)	Total diabetes Percentage (95% CI)
Total	11.3 (10.3–12.5)	3.4 (2.7–4.2)	14.7 (13.2–16.4)
Age in years			
18–44	3.0 (2.4–3.7)	1.9 (1.3–2.7))	4.8 (4.0–5.9)
45–64	14.5 (12.2–17.0)	4.5 (3.3–6.0)	18.9 (16.1–22.1)
≥65	24.4 (22.1–27.0)	4.7 (3.0–7.4)	29.2 (26.4–32.1)
Sex			
Men	12.6 (11.1–14.3)	2.8 (2.0–3.9)	15.4 (13.5–17.5)
Women	10.2 (8.8–11.7)	3.9 (2.7–5.5)	14.1 (11.8–16.7)
Race-Ethnicity			
White, non-Hispanic	11.0 (9.4–12.8)	2.7 (1.7–4.2)	13.6 (11.4–16.2)
Black, non-Hispanic	12.7 (10.7–15.0)	4.7 (3.3–6.5)	17.4 (15.2–19.8)
Asian, non-Hispanic	11.3 (9.7–13.1)	5.4 (3.5–8.3)	16.7 (14.0–19.8)
Hispanic	11.1 (9.5–13.0)	4.4 (3.3–5.8)	15.5 (13.8–17.3)

Notes: CI = confidence interval. Time period 2017–2020 covers January 2017 through March 2020 only. Diagnosed diabetes was based on self-report. Undiagnosed diabetes was based on fasting plasma glucose and A1C levels among people self-reporting no diabetes. Numbers for subgroups may not add up to the total because of rounding.
Data source: 2017–March 2020 National Health and Nutrition Examination Survey.

FIGURE 7.3 Sample tabular table, including its key parts. Centers for Disease Control and Prevention (CDC), 2022.

Figures

Figures is a collective term that includes all other graphic images—other than tables—you can include in your manuscripts. Figures can be graphs; charts; diagrams; illustrations; graphical abstracts; photographs; and diagnostic images, such as X-ray and ultrasound images. Here are some tips for using figures:

- Unlike tables, titles for figures are placed under the image.
- Don't describe visual images; describe the data. For example, do not say that the lines or the bars went up. Instead, explain what the line or bar changes represent.
- When describing graphics, use full sentences. Avoid using shorthand—or *chart speak*—which refers to abbreviated nursing language often used in health record documentation.

Choosing a Graph Type

You must select the appropriate graph type for the key point you want to highlight.

For example, look at the same information presented in two different formats: first as a table (see the table shown in Figure 7.4) and then as a line graph (Figure 7.5). Each quarter, a different staffing pattern was implemented on three intensive care units. Note the table focus is on detailed data and scores. The line graph emphasizes trends in patient satisfaction over time.

However, the line graph does not enable the reader to appreciate the actual quarterly percentage scores for each of the units. Therefore, in the main text of your article, you need to briefly describe the graph and summarize what it depicts. For example, Figure 7.5 reveals the highest satisfaction scores during the fourth quarter with a patient-to-nurse ratio of 1.75:1, which is not mentioned on the graph, but is what the data describes. All units experienced increases in satisfaction scores as nurse: patient ratios decreased. Do not describe the entire graph; just highlight the main or most significant points, allowing readers to explore the graph and arrive at their own conclusions.

TABLE 4 *2023 Patient Satisfaction Percentages Reported by Care Unit*

UNIT	1ST QUARTER 2.5:1 RATIO	2ND QUARTER 2.25:1 RATIO	3RD QUARTER 2:1 RATIO	4TH QUARTER 1.75:1 RATIO
Surgical ICU	48.2	54.2	62.1	88.4
Medical ICU	73.7	81.9	74.3	92.8
Trauma ICU	71.4	85.5	83.7	93.3
Average	**64.4**	**73.9**	**73.4**	**91.5**

Possible scores range from 0–100. (Note: Data are fictional.)

FIGURE 7.4 Data shown in a table.

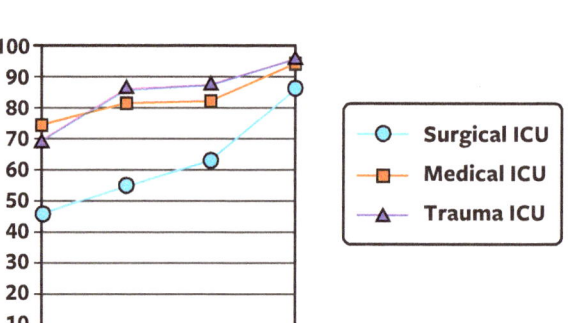

FIGURE 7.5 Sample line graph showing hypothetical comparison between three patient care units during four quarters. The vertical axis represents the level of satisfaction reported, and the horizontal axis represents the independent variable of the staffing pattern. (Note: Data are fictitious.)

Here is a closer look at some of the most common types of figures used.

Graphs

Graphs quickly draw the reader's attention, providing the visual impact that tables usually lack. They provide information about the relationship or frequency of specific variables. Use graphs to demonstrate how two or more sets of data are related. Select a graph that illustrates the point you are trying to make. For example, if you want to show how patient satisfaction levels fluctuate during the year on three different patient-care units, a line graph works well. However, if you want to compare the percentages of actual patient satisfaction levels on each of the individual units, using a table might be best. Keep reading to see the different types of graphs you can incorporate into your manuscript.

Line Graphs

Use *line graphs* to show the effect that an *independent variable* (the variable manipulated in the study) has upon a *dependent variable* (the variable being evaluated in response to the independent variable). For example, you can use a line graph to evaluate the effect of medications or placebo on pain levels or to show how staffing patterns affect patient satisfaction.

Independent variables are plotted on the horizontal (x) axis, and dependent variables are plotted on the vertical (y) axis. Data points are plotted along the corresponding x and y axes. Use a legend to describe what the data points represent. Figure 7.6 depicts the key features of a line graph.

Line graphs are created by entering data into a corresponding table, which displays data as points on the line graph along the corresponding x and y axes. Connecting data points allows the reader to see upward or downward trends, or the absence thereof. Line graphs clearly show trends in data and can allow the viewer to speculate on future trends.

Most publications have both print and online versions of an article (or are published entirely online), so capturing your audience's attention by incorporating interactivity is a desirable feature. *Interactive graphics* can allow the reader to control what is displayed when a large amount of information is presented—focusing only on information of interest to them while skipping over information they may not find useful. For example, a patient viewing an educational article that covers diabetes management may scroll over the blood glucose monitoring image in an interactive graphic to display content and learn about blood glucose meters but may opt not to scroll over the insulin image because they are not prescribed insulin.

This format for conveying information is especially good for learners who are better able to retain information when it incorporates physical activity. You don't need to be a statistician or programmer to incorporate interactivity for graphs in your manuscripts—one website (http://statistika.mfub.bg.ac.rs/interactive-linegraph) can help you create interactive line graphs in a few simple steps (Weissgerber et al., 2016). Multiple examples of interactive graphics can also be explored on the Centers for Disease Control and Prevention websites, such as https://www.cdc.gov/gis/interactive-applications.htm or https://www.cdc.gov/flu/weekly/fluviewinteractive.htm, which shows interactive graphics about the flu.

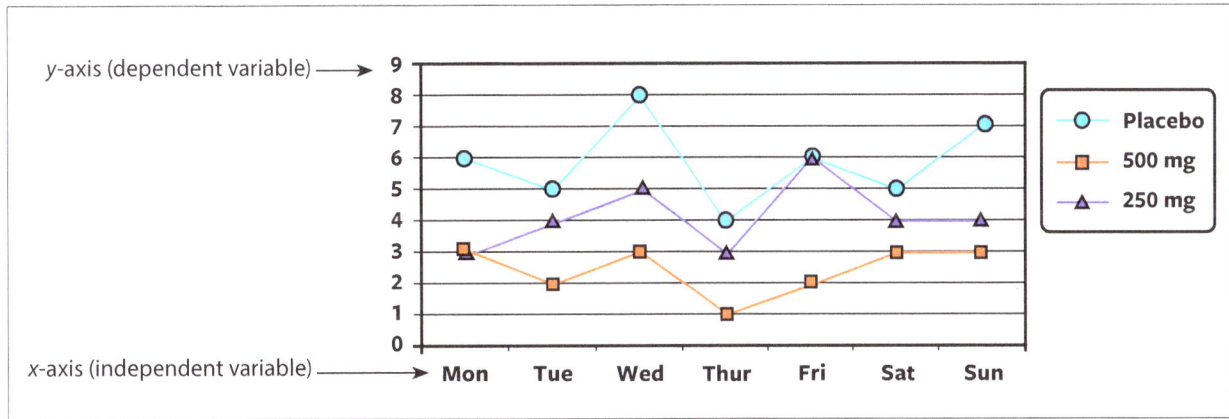

FIGURE 7.6 Pain level sorted by medication administered. (Note: Data are fictitious.)

Pie Graphs

Pie graphs, also known as *pie charts*, are circles divided into segments (see Figure 7.7). You'll find this type of graphic useful for displaying percentages of a whole. Pie charts must be clearly labeled, and those with many segments requiring excessive labeling may also need a corresponding legend. Use them only when you have a few slices to show; a pie chart with more than five to six slices becomes difficult to read.

Pie charts can misrepresent information when all components are not provided. For example, if a value is omitted, the values of remaining parts can be altered inappropriately. Figure 7.7 would inaccurately represent data if five vacancies in oncology and three vacancies in pediatrics were not reported in the pie chart.

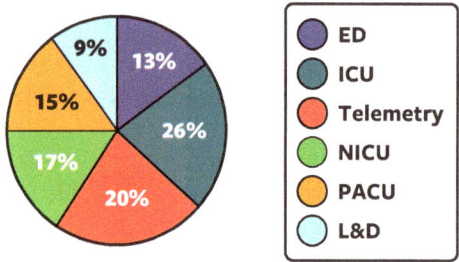

FIGURE 7.7 Sample pie graph showing hypothetical vacancies on nursing units at a hospital. (Note: Data are fictitious.)

Bar Graphs

Use *bar graphs* to compare individual groups of data that are discontinuous or categorical or classifying in nature, for example, to compare the number of cases of measles reported in the United States for different years. Bar charts are divided into columns that provide a visual comparison between two or more variables (see Figure 7.8). They can be displayed in horizontal or vertical orientation. This bar chart also provides an example of how preliminary data that may be subject to change would be identified.

Scatter Plots

You can use a *scatter plot*, also known as a *scatter gram* (see Figure 7.9), to show the relationship between two variables. This relationship is described as a *correlation*. These images are similar to line graphs in that they allow comparison along vertical and horizontal axes to determine a relationship (*positive* correlation), an opposite relationship (*negative* correlation), or no relationship. The x axis represents the independent variable, and the y axis represents the dependent variable. A perfect positive correlation on a scatter plot is from the origin to high values on the x and y axes (bottom left to top right). A perfect negative correlation on a scatter plot is from a high value on the y axis to a high value on the x axis (top left to bottom right).

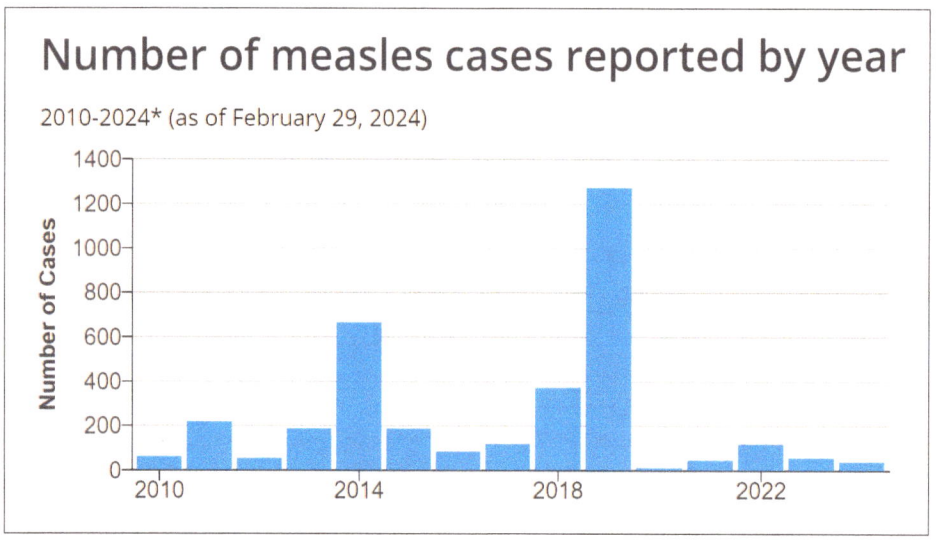

FIGURE 7.8 Sample bar graph comparing the number of measles cases reported by year from 2010 to February 2024 as reported by the CDC (2024).

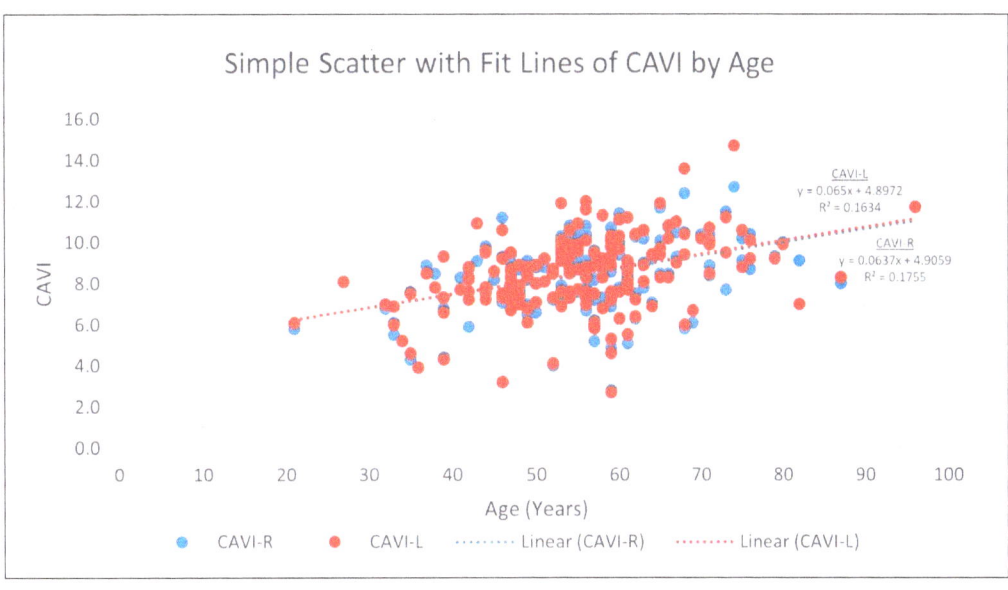

FIGURE 7.9 Sample of a scatter plot (Alghamdi et al., 2021).

How close the points on a scatter plot come to these ideal imaginary directions depicts correlation strength. For example, in Figure 7.9, the data points that represent cardio-ankle vascular index (CAVI) scores, a measure of arterial stiffness, are clustered more closely together along the line representing increasing age and increasing HbA1c. This tighter clustering results in a stronger correlation for older individuals with increasingly worse glucose control having arterial stiffness.

Illustrations

Several types of illustrations exist, including flowcharts and diagrams, graphical abstracts, photos, and created art or images. Videos/audio are also discussed in this section.

Flowcharts and Diagrams

Flowcharts and diagrams are useful ways to visually capture complex information, highlight relationships, describe a specific course of action, or provide instructions (see Figure 7.10). Flowcharts that include decision points are also called algorithms.

Use illustrations when you want to depict an image for which a photograph might not be suitable or space won't accommodate—for example, if you want to review the anatomical structure of the heart or visually depict the necessary steps to gather a blood sample.

Photographs

Photographs offer an additional dimension that tables, charts, and graphs don't provide. For example, say you want to compare melanoma lesions found among samples of adults in different areas of the country. A chart or table can feature size and stage data, but photographs can show discoloration, margins, and surrounding skin tone. Visuals can also provide information about variables that weren't included in an original study or observation but would be of note to suggest for future studies. Use photo captions to highlight what you want to emphasize. If measurement is important, include a ruler with the illustration.

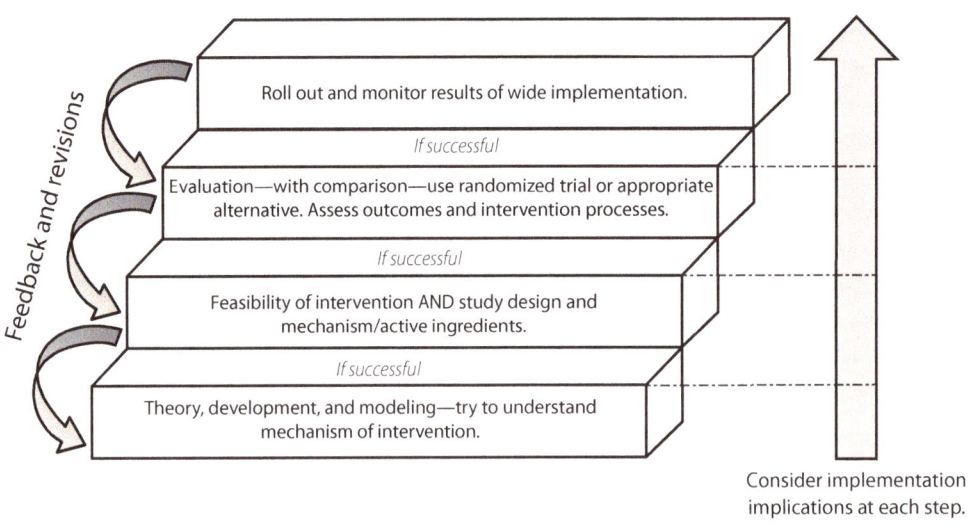

Key steps in developing and evaluating EoLC interventions. Although it is possible to begin at any step in the ladder, it is important to progress development with successful interventions. EoCL = end of life care.

FIGURE 7.10 Example of a flowchart (Higginson et al., 2013).

Here are some tips for photographs that you should keep in mind:

- Pictures should not reveal the patient's identity.

- Even if the person cannot be identified, you must comply with federal privacy laws (the Health Insurance Portability and Accountability Act [HIPAA]) and institutional policies—don't assume you have the right to take and use images in any clinical setting; doing so puts you and your employer at risk of a HIPAA violation.

- Obtain consent from all subjects in your photographs. You will need to use a special photo consent form provided by the editor. (For more information about consent, refer to Chapter 11.)

- Obtain permission to use any photographs you didn't personally take. Ask early and plan an alternative in case your request is denied.

- Most publications prefer high-resolution digital images for printing; online-only publications can use images of lower resolution, but it's best to send high resolution.

- If hard copy photographs are accepted (many publications do not accept them), they must be of high quality.

- If you scan a photograph, follow the software and author guidelines to ensure your file is of high enough quality for printing.

Created Art or Images

Graphics can be created in a variety of programs including Adobe Illustrator, Adobe Photoshop, CorelDraw, Microsoft PowerPoint, and Microsoft Excel. Before choosing graphic creation software, check to see if it will be acceptable to the publication by reviewing the author guidelines. Whatever program you decide to use, most editors will want you to send graphics in the original file format of that program, or as a Portable Document Format (PDF) file. To save PDF documents to your computer, you will need to install a PDF software program (usually Adobe Acrobat) first.

Infographics

Sometimes, you can combine text with different types of graphics to stress two points in the same space, referred to as an infographic. For example, you can use an image as a background for a text table that provides the impact of a behavior or practice on outcomes. Figure 7.11 combines the data from a table depicting the incidence of bathroom-associated microbial contamination via mobile phones even after handwashing.

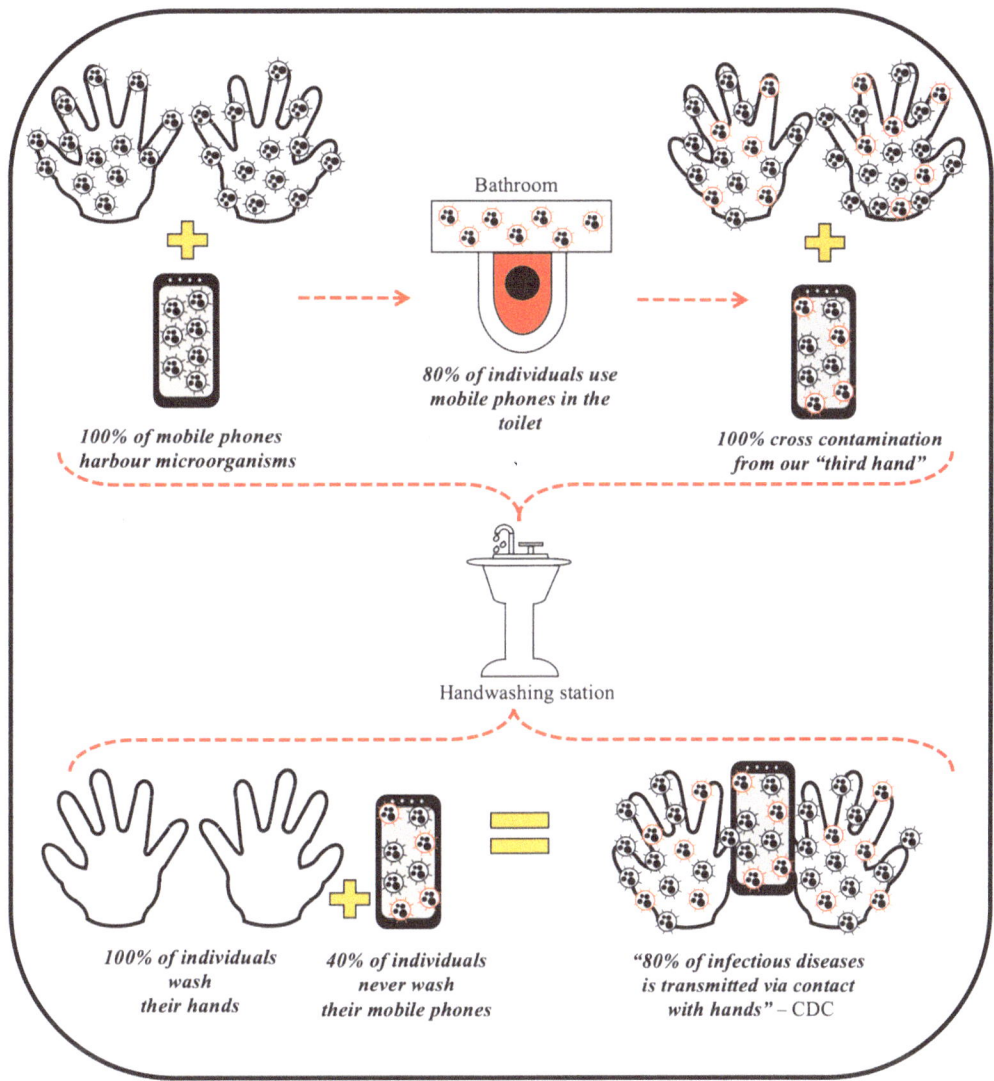

FIGURE 7.11 Sample infographic combining the data from a chart with images of contaminated hands and mobile phones (Olsen et al., 2021).

Infographics, which can be used in the form of graphical abstracts and in articles, should have a compelling title; emphasize key messages; and balance images, charts, and text (Murray et al., 2017). *Graphical abstracts*, also referred to as visual abstracts, are graphical summaries of the key points of an article, including key findings in the case of a study. These summaries help readers quickly gain an overview of the article's content.

When developing an infographic, consider the target audience and summarize the key message in one sentence (Spicer & Coleman, 2022). Think about what information needs to be included to support that message, then sketch out the infographic, choosing the best options, such as tables, charts, timelines, graphs, and icons, to illustrate your points.

Tools such as Canva or Inkscape can help you create your vision. It's best to keep to no more than three to five colors; use a neutral color for 60% of the space, a secondary color for 30%, and an accent color for 10% (Spicer & Coleman, 2022). Be sure to seek feedback from a few people in your target audience.

Learn more about creating infographics by reviewing the information on graphical abstracts in Chapter 5.

Digital Image Quality

Image quality is crucial. Your photos should be well lit, tightly cropped, in focus, and only include the important objects being discussed in the manuscript (Saver, 2007). Images taken with cellphones historically had low resolution and weren't acceptable. However, as smartphone camera quality and automated features evolved, it is hard now to tell the difference between a photo taken with a smartphone and one of the same image captured with a full-frame camera (DXOMARK, 2020). However, if your cellphone camera only produces low-quality images, you may need to invest in (or borrow) a digital camera.

High-resolution digital cameras often yield a large file size but the best-quality images. Cellphone photos also may result in larger image files, which often pose a problem when submitting them as an email attachment. Most publications require authors to upload files at the same time the manuscript is submitted through a designated website.

Dots per inch (dpi) defines how sharp the resolution of an image is. Images with low resolution will appear distorted or pixelated (have a box-like appearance with jagged edges for text or color transitions instead of smooth lines). Photographs must have at least 300 dpi resolution for the final layout. If images are enlarged, their resolution changes. You can calculate minimum image requirements by multiplying vertical and horizontal size in inches by 300. For example, if an image is to appear in a 3 x 4-inch space, it must have a resolution of at least 900 x 1200 pixels. If you have a 2 x 2-inch space for a photo, it must have a resolution of 600 x 600 pixels. (Resolution requirements for online use of photographs are not as strict.)

Common formats include Tagged Image File Format (TIFF), Joint Photographic Experts Group (JPG/JPEG), and Photoshop Document (PSD). Portable Network Graphics (PNG) and Bitmap (BMP) files are sometimes used in place of JPG/JPEG and TIFF images. Identify the publication's preferred format(s) before sending image files and send the highest resolution possible. TIFF is the most commonly used standard format for biomedical journals; however, these images taken with a high-quality digital camera can often be too large to handle. While images saved in the JPEG format can be a good alternative with minimal loss of quality, some journals do not accept JPEG images because these images lose quality as compression increases. (University of Michigan Library, 2021).

Video/Audio

If you're writing for an online publication that incorporates videos or animations, you should consult with the editor for any specific submission requirements for media footage or clips you wish to include with your manuscript. If you're creating or providing additional information to use on a website where your publication is posted, make sure that you clear the source and permissions for videos you use. Remember that the same rules that apply to photographs also apply to media clips: You must have permission to use them, and you must have releases from individuals who appear in the media clips.

Tips for Using Images

Whether it's a pie chart you found online or an algorithm you created, consider these tips for using images:

- Publication requirements differ significantly. Check online for author guidelines and review graphic requirements *before* you create or identify images you want to use.

- Study the publication to identify whether certain colors or color schemes are customary—and then design your graphics to conform.

- Avoid "chartjunk," which refers to elements in a graphic that don't add anything but instead distract from, rather than illuminate, your ideas (Tufte, 2001). Examples include unnecessary use of the three-dimensional effect for bar graphs and labels that are too long.

- For publications printed in black and white or in grayscale, design your graphics to emphasize differences with various shading or fill options. Again, study the publication first to detect any preferences.

- Images may be used in alternative venues. For example, you may want to include color images of a wound in a journal article, but you discover that it is published in black and white. An online version, however, includes color images. You might be asked to submit the images for the online version. You could alert the reader to additional online content with a callout, such as, "To view an online version of this article and all images in color, go to http://www.*sitenamehere*.com."

- Images abound on the internet, but beware that the vast majority of them are not considered to be public domain (i.e., freely available for use). For publication, you must find the owner and obtain permission to use any online image within your work, even if you properly cite the source. Some images can be purchased for a fee, but you must pay attention to what permissions are granted. For example, you might purchase an image to use in your manuscript and later find out that you are granted only personal use that does not allow for publication or commercial reproduction in an article or a book.

- Become familiar with sources for free images, including the Public Health Image Library (PHIL; https://phil.cdc.gov/default.aspx), the National Institutes of Health (NIH) photo galleries (https://www.flickr.com/photos/nihgov), US Department of Health and Human Services Image Galleries (https://www.hhs.gov/web/services-and-resources/image-galleries/index.html), and Wikimedia Commons (https://commons.wikimedia.org/wiki/Main_Page). Although the images are free, you should still credit the source. Be sure to check resolution of the image, particularly if it will be for a print publication.

- You may need to request permission for a graphic via a *clearinghouse*, a company that handles copyright permission requests for a specific journal, publisher, or organization; the most common is Copyright Clearance Center. (For more information about copyright and permissions, refer to Chapter 11.) In other cases, you may need to contact the publication directly. Keep a sample request template on hand to quickly customize a request (see Figure 7.12).

- Learn how images should be credited and whether permission to use a graphic also allows any manipulation or changes. For example, some images must be displayed with specific verbiage under them and must not be cropped or enhanced in any way, whereas others may be displayed as the author chooses. The restrictions depend upon what the owner of the image will allow.

Q *I want to include a graphic but have not yet received permission to use it in my manuscript. Should I include it and let the editor know that I'm seeking permission?*

A Yes, you should let the editor know you have not yet obtained permission. The editor might also be able to suggest a replacement graphic from a stock photo source that the publisher subscribes to, or one created by the publication's staff, although this latter option occurs rarely because of resource limitations.

- Don't embed text or insert lines–*callouts*—on your photos. Use a computer program, such as Illustrator or Photoshop, to create an additional layer that contains your descriptions or labels, or simply describe to the editor what you need. Send the unlabeled image along with the labeled image in case adjustments are needed.

- Lastly, you may be asked to provide an image of yourself. Carefully review the style of the publication to determine what type of photograph should be submitted. Most publications prefer a head-and-shoulders image with a solid background and professional attire. Others may accept less formal images that depict the author in a familiar setting or in surroundings fitting to the article's subject content. For example, if your article is about nursing on medical missions, an image taken in a field clinic may be a perfect choice.

Q *What if the publisher or clearinghouse granting permission for the figure or table I want to use in my manuscript charges a fee? Who pays?*

A Most publications expect the author to pay the permission fee, which in some cases can be costly. If there is a fee, you often can wait until you see that the article is accepted before making the purchase. Check the author guidelines or seek the editor's advice. Not all permissions come with a fee attached. Publishers who are members of STM (a trade association for academic and professional publishers) and have signed onto the STM Permissions Guidelines do not charge for certain items (e.g., three figures, tables, or images) if the new work will be reproduced in the journal or book of another publisher that also is part of STM (STM, 2022). Learn more about this in Chapter 11.

Dear Permissions Editor:

RE: Figure 4.1 appearing in Smith, R.: *Journal of Nursing History*

I am preparing an article titled "Dissemination of Lessons From Florence Nightingale" ("the Article") shortly to be published in the *Journal of Nursing Scholarship*, published by Sigma Theta Tau.

I request your permission to reproduce or, if it is necessary, to redraw or modify the material listed below within the article. Permission is requested in any form or medium, in all languages, for distribution throughout the world. Full credit will be given to the original source.

Material requested*:

> **Author:** Smith, R.
> **Journal or Book Title:** *Journal of Nursing History*
> **Volume No.:** 24
> **Article Title:** The Birth of Modern Nursing
> **Details of the illustration or other material required:** Image of Florence Nightingale caring for soldiers
> **Page No.:** 214
> **Publisher and Year of Copyright:** Sage Publications, 2024

Please provide any preferred credit line.

Sincerely,

Susanne Pavlovich-Danis, APRN
sauthor@internet.com

*Citation is fictitious.

FIGURE 7.12 Sample permission request.

Choosing and Submitting Graphics

You have learned about many different types of graphics, so at this stage, you may be wondering how to choose the most effective ones for your article. To make the right choices, match the graphic to the purpose. For example, if you want to compare data, a table or bar chart would be better than two pie charts. Table 7.1 can help you select the right graphic based on the purpose you want it to serve. The algorithm in Figure 7.13 is helpful for determining the most effective way to present data. These two tools will ensure your graphics support the goals of your article.

TABLE 7.1 Selecting the Right Graphic Based on Purpose

	Compare data	Provide detailed information	Emphasize numbers	Emphasize trends	Show relationships	Display percentage of a whole	Summarize key points	Provide descriptions	Provide steps or instructions
Table	✓	✓	✓		✓		✓	✓	✓
Line graph				✓	✓				
Pie graph						✓			
Bar graph	✓								
Scatter plot					✓				
Flow chart		✓			✓		✓	✓	✓
Diagram		✓						✓	✓
Photo or video								✓	✓

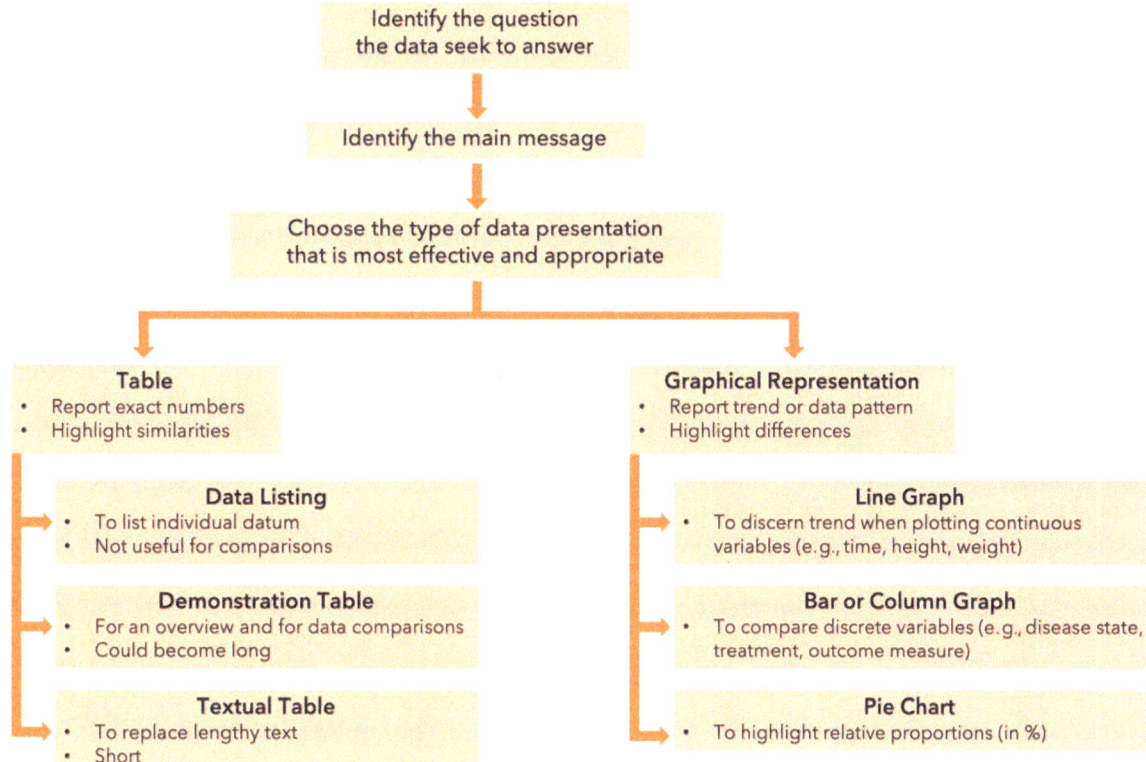

FIGURE 7.13 Algorithm for choosing how to present data (Rappaz, 2022). Reprinted with permission from *AMWA Journal*.

Saving and Submitting Images

Here are some tips to keep in mind when saving and submitting images:

- **Format.** When possible, save your graphics in a format that can be adjusted if necessary for color, shading, size, and font to accommodate style and space limitations. If your graphics can't be edited, your images might not be included or might display with reduced quality.
- **B&W.** Save images containing lines—such as tables, charts, graphs, and drawings—in black-and-white format, not grayscale.
- **Grayscale.** Save images or photographs that contain shading as grayscale format, not black and white.
- **Creation program information.** The more information you provide to a publication about your graphics, the better. Specify what software you used to create the graphic, including the operating system (PC or Mac) and its version, as well as the program name and version. You can often locate this information by clicking the top navigation bar of most programs and selecting "Help" and then "About."
- **Online source quality.** If you plan to use graphics from online sources, contact the publisher or the author of the online source for high-resolution, editable files. Images displayed online are typically inadequate for press-quality publication.
- **High resolution.** It's typically best to make your graphics large and of the highest resolution. Your graphics will be scaled to fit during the journal production process. Enlarging smaller graphics can result in a loss of image quality.
- **Publication guidelines.** Review the publication's graphic file size limits (usually found in the author guidelines) and don't exceed them.
- **Online storage and data transfer.** If you routinely send large files or graphics, consider subscribing to a virtual or cloud data storage service (e.g., Google Drive, Dropbox, or iCloud) that allows you to upload and share large data. As a last resort, store large images on a portable media device (burning to a CD or DVD, or saving on a data card or flash drive).

Q *Can I embed my graphics in the Word file of my manuscript?*

A Don't embed graphics within the word processing file of your manuscript. This can reduce image quality, make the file size too big, and eliminate editing options. As discussed earlier in this chapter, remember to use standard naming conventions and save each graphic as a separate file.

Once you have written the article, selected the graphics, and created and saved images, use this checklist as a final review to be sure figures and tables are properly prepared before submitting your manuscript.

- ☐ Are all figures and tables mentioned in the text?
- ☐ Are all figures and tables numbered in the order they are mentioned?
- ☐ Are all figures and tables numbered with Arabic numerals (1, 2, 3, and so on)?
- ☐ Do all tables and figures have titles?
- ☐ Does every table column have a heading?
- ☐ Are all tables and figures labeled using standard conventions?
- ☐ Is the font size acceptable for the publication (typically no smaller than 8 points and no larger than 14 points)?
- ☐ Are all data abbreviations spelled out in a descriptive legend (explanation key)?
- ☐ Are all figure elements large enough to remain legible if reduced to the width of the journal column or page?
- ☐ Is the figure resolution quality consistent with the publication guidelines?
- ☐ Have the figures and tables been saved in a format consistent with the publication guidelines?

Making the Most of Graphics

By including relevant, eye-catching graphics in your manuscript, you'll enhance your work and give readers a break from excessive reading. Tables, figures, graphs, illustrations, and photographs enhance communication with fewer words. As with every step of the writing process, it pays to be prepared.

Write Now!

1. Choose a research article and analyze the effectiveness of its graphics.
2. Choose a clinical article and note how the graphics differ. Are they effective?

References

Alenichev, A., Kingori, P., & Grietens, K. P. (2023). Reflections before the storm: The AI reproduction of biased imagery in global health visuals. *The Lancet. Global health*, S2214-109X(23)00329-7. Advance online publication. https://doi.org/10.1016/S2214-109X(23)00329-7

Alghamdi, Y. A., Al-Shahrani, F. S., Alanazi, S. S., Alshammari, F. A., Alkhudair, A. M., & Jatoi, N. A. (2021). The association of blood glucose levels and arterial stiffness (cardio-ankle vascular index) in patients with type 2 diabetes mellitus. *Cureus, 13*(12), e20408. https://www.ncbi.nlm.nih.gov/pmc/articles/PMC8671052/

Centers for Disease Control and Prevention. (2022). *National diabetes statistics report.* https://www.cdc.gov/diabetes/data/statistics-report/index.html

Centers for Disease Control and Prevention. (2024). *Measles cases and outbreaks.* https://www.cdc.gov/measles/cases-outbreaks.html

del-pino-Casado, R., Frias-Osuna, A., Palomino-Moral, P. A., & Martinez-Riera, J. R. (2012). Gender differences regarding informal caregivers of older people. *Journal of Nursing Scholarship, 44*(4), 349–357 (table on p. 354). doi: 10.1111/j.1547-5069.2012.01477.x

Devraj, R., Wilhelm, M., & Deshpande, M. (2022). Consumer perceptions of a shingles infograph intervention and vaccination plans in community pharmacy settings. *Innovations in Pharmacy, 13*(3). https://doi.org/10.24926/iip.v13i3.4918

DXOMARK. (2020). Smartphones vs cameras: Closing the gap on image quality. https://www.dxomark.com/smartphones-vs-cameras-closing-the-gap-on-image-quality/

Hafner, C., Schneider, J., Schindler, M., & Braillard, O. (2022). Visual aids in ambulatory clinical practice: Experiences, perceptions and needs of patients and healthcare professionals. *PloS One, 17*(2), e0263041. https://doi.org/10.1371/journal.pone.0263041

Hayes-Larson, E., Kezios, K. L., Mooney, S. J., & Lovasi, G. (2019). Who is in this study, anyway? Guidelines for a useful Table 1. *Journal of Clinical Epidemiology, 114*, 125–132. https://doi.org/10.1016/j.jclinepi.2019.06.011

Higginson, I. J., Evans, C. J., Grande, G., Preston, N., Morgan, Myfanwy, McCrone, P., Lewis, P., Fayers, P., Harding, R., Hotopf, M., Murray, S. A., Benalia, H., Gysels, M., Farquhar, M., & Todd, C. (2013). Evaluating complex interventions in end of life care: The MORECare statement on good practice generated by a synthesis of transparent expert consultations and systematic reviews. *BMC Medicine, 11*, 111. https://doi.org/10.1186/1741-7015-11-111

International Committee of Medical Journal Editors. (2024). *Recommendations for the conduct, reporting, editing, and publication of scholarly work in medical journals.* http://www.icmje.org/recommendations

Kiran, A., Craspillo, A. P., & Rahimi, K. (2017). Graphics and statistics for cardiology: Data visualization for meta-analysis. *Heart, 103*(1), 19–23. https://doi.org/10.1136/heartjnl-2016-309685

Mignini, L., Champaneria, R., Miskanina, E., Kahn, K. S., & EBM_CONNECT Collaboration. (2016). Graphical displays for effective reporting of evidence quality tables in research syntheses. *Reproductive Health, 13*, 21. https://doi.org/10.1186/s12978-016-0130-3

Murray, I. R., Murray A. D., Wordie, S. J., Oliver, C. W., Murray, A. W., & Simpson, A. H. R. W. (2017). Maximizing the impact of your work using infographics [Editorial]. *Bone & Joint Research, 6*(11), 619–620. https://doi.org/10.1302/2046-3758.611.BJR-2017-0313

Olsen, M., Nassar, R., Senok, A., Albastaki, A., Leggett, J., Lohning, A., Campos, M., Jones, P., McKirdy, S., Tajouri, L., & Alghafri, R. (2021). A pilot metagenomic study reveals that community derived mobile phones are reservoirs of viable pathogenic microbes. *Scientific Reports, 11*(1), 14102. https://doi.org/10.1038/s41598-021-93622-w

Otterbacher, J. (2023). Why technical solutions for detecting AI-generated content in research and education are insufficient. *Patterns (N Y), 4*(7), 100796. https://www.ncbi.nlm.nih.gov/pmc/articles/PMC10382978/

Rappaz, S. (2022). The importance of data presentation. *American Medical Writers Association Journal, 37*(2), 17–18. https://doi.org/10.55752/amwa.2022.99

Saver, C. (2007). More strategies for enhancing your message. *AORN Journal, 85*(1), 131–134. https://doi.org/10.1016/S0001-2092(07)60018-0

Spicer, J. O., & Coleman, C. G. (2022). Creating effective infographics and visual abstracts to disseminate research and facilitate medical education on social media. *Clinical Infectious Diseases, 74*(S3), e14–22. https://doi.org/10.1093/cid/ciac058

STM. (2022). STM permissions guidelines. https://www.stm-assoc.org/2022_01_27_STM_Permission_Guidelines_2022.pdf

Stonbraker, S., Porras, T., & Schnall, R. (2020). Patient preferences for visualization of longitudinal patient-reported outcomes data. *Journal of the American Medical Informatics Association*, *27*(2), 212–224. https://doi.org/10.1093/jamia/ocz189

Švab, I., Klemenc-Ketiš, Z., Zupanič, S. (2023). New challenges in scientific publications: Referencing, artificial intelligence and ChatGPT. *Zdr Varst*. *62*(3), 109–112. https://www.ncbi.nlm.nih.gov/pmc/articles/PMC10263368/

Tufte, E. R. (2001). *The visual display of quantitative information* (2nd ed.). Graphics Press.

University of Michigan Library. (2021). *All about images: Image file formats*. https://guides.lib.umich.edu/c.php?g=282942&p=1885348.

Weissgerber, T. L., Garovic, V. D., Savic, M. D., Winham, S. J., & Milic, N. M. (2016). From static to interactive: Transforming data visualization to improve transparency. *PLoS Biology*, *14*(8), e1002484. https://doi.org/10.1371/journal.pbio.1002484

Why *Nature* will not allow the use of generative AI in images and video [Editorial]. (2023). *Nature*, *618*(7964), 214. https://doi.org/10.1038/d41586-023-01546-4

Submissions and Revisions

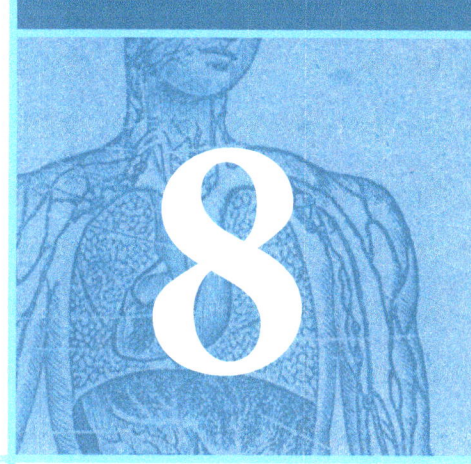

–Patricia Gonce Morton, PhD, RN, ACNP-BC, FAAN
–Tina M. Marrelli, MSN, MA, RN, FAAN

"A piece of writing must be viewed as a constantly evolving organism."
–William Zinsser

WHAT YOU'LL LEARN IN THIS CHAPTER

- Follow the journal's author guidelines when you submit your manuscript.
- An editor(s) and, usually, peer reviewers will review your manuscript.
- Most articles require some revision before final acceptance for publication.
- Follow a systematic approach when making requested revisions.
- Responding to editors' queries is an essential step in the revision process.

Having worked hard on crafting your manuscript and choosing a journal, you smile with satisfaction as you click the save button. Your article is done; your blood, sweat, and tears have been poured into this manuscript submission. Now you're ready to submit the manuscript to the journal editor whom perhaps you met at a conference last year. Or to the colleague who asked you to write a chapter for an upcoming book. Or to the journal that you've carefully researched and chosen. What can you do at the submission stage to be successful?

Or maybe you're at the point where you have already submitted to a nursing journal and just received the peer-reviewer comments about your manuscript with a request from the editor for a revision. After taking a deep breath, you wonder how you're going to revise the article to boost your chances of final acceptance—the point at which a submission or manuscript becomes an accepted article.

This chapter describes how to successfully navigate these scenarios and explains how the submission and revisions process works. Even though the process covered here is typical for peer-reviewed journals, the overall submission and revision process is similar for most magazines and books. Be aware that if you are writing about a project completed in the organization you work for, you should notify your supervisor of your plans before you submit. In some cases, the organization may have a nurse scientist or other experts review the manuscript before submission; they typically check for items such as obtaining proper permission for forms and noting institutional review board approval, as needed.

First Impressions Count

At this point, you may already have corresponded with the editor of your target publication, who was receptive to your topic. This acknowledgement is not a guarantee of acceptance, however. You'll need to create an effective submission to enhance the likelihood that your manuscript will be well received by the editor and any peer reviewers.

A good first step is to review the author guidelines (also called information for authors) for the journal before you submit. Strictly adhering to the rules within this document is the best way to make your submission stand out and shine. Editors want to help prospective authors get published. But one easy way to get rejected is to send a manuscript that shows you didn't take the time to read the guidelines you can easily find online (Mikhail, 2021). Using the spell-check option for your document is essential, but you also must carefully proofread the entire manuscript one last time before submitting. Think of a submission like a job interview: First impressions count.

Author guidelines vary from publication to publication, but each has a few common elements you should look for, including word count, keywords, editorial style (including requirements for references), and submission requirements for figures and tables. You'll also want to add a cover letter before submitting (Seals, 2023).

Word Count

Double-check the publication's word or page count limit requirements—minimum and maximum—for the article and, if required, abstract. Take the example of *Journal A*'s guidelines, which specify that your article be no more than 3,500 words. If your submission is 6,000 words, the editor is faced with either asking you to trim your manuscript to fit the requirements, or, since it so greatly exceeds the specified word count, not reading it and sending you a rejection decision. Remember, more is not better when it comes to publishing a journal article. Such a large departure from the stated author guidelines conveys to the editor that you either didn't read the guidelines—or read them but didn't respect them. If you believe that you must have (a few!) more words, first discuss this with the journal editor. Remember, the editor is the expert on the journal and its content, vision, and mission.

Alternatively, don't shortchange your chances for acceptance by turning in a manuscript far less than the desired word or page count. The peer reviewers will likely find your article lacking in substance, depth, and development.

Keywords

Many journals will ask you to provide three to five keywords (words or phrases), which are used to index your article in databases and search engines (Saver, 2023). Keywords help others find your article more easily. Some journals specify that keywords should be drawn from Medical Subject Headings (MeSH). In this case, you might want to try the MeSH on Demand tool (https://www.nlm.nih.gov/pubs/techbull/mj14/mj14_mesh_on_demand.html) to identify terms relevant for your article. (You can learn more about MeSH in Chapter 4.)

When choosing keywords, think about words and phrases that you used in your research. Then test your words (Saver, 2023). Run them in a search engine to see if the articles you find align with the topic of your article. You also might want to check how your keywords score on Google Trends (https://trends.google.com/trends).

Editorial Style

All journals have a preferred editorial style, with the most common styles being the American Psychological Association (APA, 2020) and American Medical Association ([AMA], JAMA Network Editors, 2020). Don't expect the editor to format the text and reference list for you into the correct style. You can research style rules simply by searching online by the name of the style. Be sure to use the most recent version of the style guide.

Using the correct style is particularly important for references. Make sure you use the preferred style that was specified in the journal's guidelines, and check that each reference has the elements required by the journal's reference style: typically, author name(s), title of article, journal title, year published, volume, issue number, and page numbers. You'll also likely need the Digital Object Identifier (DOI) number for the reference, which is a series of numbers, letters, and symbols used to identify electronically a journal article and to provide it with a permanent web address (URL). One of the most common mistakes is not including page numbers when citing a chapter within a book. Another common mistake is not including quotation marks on direct quotes within the text of the manuscript. (Learn more about references in Chapter 4.)

Submission Checklist

Here are key questions to answer before submitting your manuscript to an editor:

Title/Headings
- ☐ Is the title succinct, and does the title support the content in the manuscript?
- ☐ Are there headers to divide specific information and content areas logically?

Content
- ☐ Have I stayed within 5% to 10% of the requested word or page count per author guidelines?
- ☐ Did I proofread and spell-check the final submission? (See Appendix B for a proofing checklist.)
- ☐ Did I read the article through for clarity?
- ☐ Did I check for consistency in each section of the manuscript and the manuscript overall? (Iwaz, 2022)
- ☐ Is my math correct (for any calculations included)?
- ☐ Does the manuscript support my purpose in writing it?
- ☐ Is the organization logical?
- ☐ Is the tone and level appropriate for the readers of the journal?
- ☐ Did I correct simple grammar mistakes?
- ☐ If this is a nursing continuing professional development (NCPD, previously referred to as continuing nursing education [CNE]) submission, does the content have the depth and specific information needed?
- ☐ Did I give the manuscript to a trusted colleague to read with "new eyes"? Did I then make changes in the areas identified as needing improvement or have a rationale for not making a change?
- ☐ If the manuscript was written by more than one author, did one author edit the entire manuscript for a consistent writing style and to remove any redundancies?
- ☐ Did I run the manuscript through a plagiarism checker to be sure I didn't accidentally engage in plagiarism?

References
- ☐ Are statements cited in the text as needed?
- ☐ Did I use the correct citation style within the text and for listing the references at the end of the text?
- ☐ Does each reference entry have complete information per the style specifications?
- ☐ Is each listed reference also mentioned in the text, and does the citation in the text match with what is in the reference list?
- ☐ Are author and journal names spelled correctly?

Tables and Figures
- ☐ Are my figures in the correct electronic format for submission?
- ☐ Do the numbers for tables and figures match what is called out in the manuscript and are they numbered consecutively?
- ☐ Are the figures complete, including captions?

Format
- ☐ Did I write an abstract or summary according to the journal's format (if requested in the author guidelines)?
- ☐ Did I include a cover letter or cover email to the editor? Did I proof it?
- ☐ Have I included a title page with author names and contact information, but omitted names or other identifying information on the actual manuscript?
- ☐ Have I double-checked the correct spellings, credentials, and affiliations for all my coauthors?
- ☐ Is the manuscript formatted properly according to the author guidelines? (This includes such items as being double-spaced and having running heads and page numbers.)

Avoid citation errors and ensure that each reference is correct. Common citation errors include factual errors such as an incorrect interpretation of information from the source, use of secondary rather than primary citations, or failure to cite a source. Errors in the reference list often involve inaccurate author names, journal names, dates, and page numbers of the cited work (Agarwal et al., 2023).

Tables and Figures

Tables, figures, and other data are handled in various ways from publication to publication. A book publisher might want you to submit these elements as separate graphics or as attachments, with placeholders in the text indicating where they should be inserted. Online publications might want figures embedded. Many journals require authors to put tables at the end of the manuscript, with one table on each page. Figures and tables are often created in Microsoft Word, Excel, or PowerPoint. (See Chapter 7 for more information about figures, tables, and other types of graphics.) The publication's preferences will be in the author guidelines.

Be sure that figures and tables are "called out" in the body of the manuscript submission in numerical order—for instance, "A participatory leadership style increased nurse retention by 20% (Table 2)," or "Figure 3 shows the internal workings of the cardiovascular system." Simply put, "called out" means there is a place in the text of the manuscript that clearly refers the reader to the table, figure, tool, or other data that is a part of the manuscript.

Cover Letter

A cover letter is another opportunity to create a good first impression of you and your manuscript. Address the letter to the right person (usually the editor) and include key points, such as manuscript title, authors (and order of authorship), corresponding author (with contact information), any conflicts of interest, and a note about approval related to treatment of human subjects, if applicable (APA, 2020). In the latter case, this approval might be noted as, "The study received approval from the University of Smith institutional review board." Note if your article has been posted on a preprint server or in a repository before submission (International Committee of Medical Journal Editors [ICMJE], 2024). This type of early dissemination doesn't usually disqualify the article from being considered for publication. For more information about preprints, see Chapter 3.

Some journals require "boilerplate" statements. For example, you may be asked to include a written assurance that the manuscript is not under consideration by any other journal. Additionally, you may be asked to state that the manuscript will not be submitted to another journal until the present review process is completed. Check the author guidelines carefully for any such cover letter requirements (Author Services, n.d.; Seals, 2023).

The cover letter also provides an opportunity to highlight the value of your manuscript. Example 8.1 shows an effective cover letter, which should be kept to no more than one page. Although called a "letter," you will upload it into a submissions portal or email it to the editor.

After you prepare your submission, spell-check and proofread your work one last time for accuracy before you submit. In addition, consider having a trusted colleague review your submission for items such as clarity and typos.

Formal Submission

The norm for most publishers is that manuscripts are submitted electronically either via an online portal or by email. The author guidelines will give you the specifics. If the journal is published with a large publishing company, you'll find yourself using a standardized electronic system that enables authors, reviewers, and editors to work with manuscripts online from all over the world (Seals, 2023).

After creating an account in the editorial management system, you upload the required documents and files. Because many of these items need to be uploaded separately, some authors find online submission a little daunting at first, but if you work through the process step by step, it begins to make sense. If you get stuck, chances are that the journal has a staff person who can help. The greatest advantage of these automated systems is that you, as an author, can track the progress of your manuscript submission throughout the entire review and publication process.

Most book publishers, magazine publishers, and online publications, as well as some journals, want the text and related files, such as tables and signed copyright agreement, submitted by email to the editor or managing editor.

Ann Miller, DNP, RN, FNP-C
1234 Universal Rd.
Salt Lake City, Utah 84108

April 14, 2024

Terry Norton, PhD, RN, FAAN ← Correct spelling and name of editor (not "to whom it may concern").
Editor-in-Chief
Families Together Journal
Mobile, Alabama 36609

Dear Dr. Norton,

I am pleased to submit the manuscript "Strategies for Helping Families Meet Vaccination Requirements" for publication in *Families Together Journal*.

— Name of manuscript and correct title of journal.

This manuscript summarizes the national guidelines for vaccinations for children and adults and strategies to help families comply with the guidelines. This quality improvement project resulted in a 20% increase in compliance with vaccinations at a clinic serving a rural population.

— Succinctly explains what was done and the main outcome.

With recent pandemics and infectious disease outbreaks, compliance with recommended vaccinations has become even more important in maintaining the health of populations. My manuscript offers readers effective strategies to achieve this goal.

— States why the journal's readers would be interested.

The manuscript I am submitting is an original work; it has not been published elsewhere and is not under consideration by another journal. The authors listed in the byline have agreed on the author order and on the submission of the manuscript. I am the corresponding author. Neither I nor my coauthors have any conflicts of interest.

— Assures editor that the work is original and has not been submitted for publication elsewhere.

— Notes that authors have agreed on order and manuscript submission, and who will be the corresponding author (the editor's contact).

— Most journals have a separate conflict of interest form you'll need to sign, but it's good to note this point here as well. (Of course, you should also disclose any conflicts.)

Thank you for considering our manuscript. I look forward to hearing from you.

— A thank-you is always appreciated.

Sincerely,
Ann Miller, DNP, RN, FNP-BC
(555) 888-0000
amiller@email.com

— Full name and credentials.
— Provides two contact options.

EXAMPLE 8.1 An effective cover letter.

Whether submitting by email or by an online editorial management system, know that most publications require you to submit the following items in addition to your manuscript:

- Title page, including the name of the manuscript, author names and affiliations, and contact information for the corresponding author
- Abstract (if not included at the top of the manuscript)
- Keywords
- Signed transfer of copyright agreement
- Digital files of artwork
- Evidence of permission for you to use or adapt any copyright materials that you have included in your manuscript. Some publishers allow you to wait and submit these forms with the revised version of the manuscript.
- Completed author profile form (so that the editor has the correct information for your byline and biographical statement at the end of the article). Authors who have an Open Researcher and Contributor ID (ORCID) should include it with their submission. Some journals require authors to have an ORCID, which is a unique identification number that helps ensure researchers obtain credit for their contributions and share information with other researchers (ORCID, n.d.) Non-researchers also can benefit from having an ORCID number.
- Signed conflict of interest form (Learn more about conflict of interest in Chapter 11.)

Some scholarly publications require completion of a form that outlines the areas of responsibility for each author. A resource that might be helpful for this part is the Contributor Roles Taxonomy (CRediT, n.d.), which provides 14 roles contributors play when working on an article. (Some journals specify use of this taxonomy in their submission guidelines.)

Most journals state that all authors must meet certain requirements, usually based on guidelines from the International Committee of Medical Journal Editors (ICMJE, 2024). Publications often include an acknowledgement section, where you can recognize those who provided assistance (e.g., data analysis or writing assistance) but do not meet the author criteria established by the journal. Many of these use the ICMJE guidelines (2024, p. 2) to determine authorship versus acknowledgement, with acknowledgement reserved for those who do not meet all four criteria for authorship:

- "Substantial contributions to the conception or design of the work; or the acquisition, analysis, or interpretation of data for the work; AND
- Drafting the work or reviewing it critically for important intellectual content; AND
- Final approval of the version to be published; AND
- Agreement to be accountable for all aspects of the work in ensuring that questions related to the accuracy or integrity of any part of the work are appropriately investigated and resolved."

Journals may ask for authors to provide evidence that the person being acknowledged agreed with the plan. The reason for this requirement is that acknowledgment may imply endorsement of a study's data and conclusions (ICMJE, 2024).

Many journals ask authors to disclose if artificial intelligence (AI) technology was used in producing the manuscript (e.g., data collection or analysis, helping to draft the methodology section), based on editorial guidance from well-respected organizations (ICMJE, 2024; International Society for Medical Publication Professionals, 2023; National Institutes of Health Office of the Director, 2023; World Association of Medical Editors, 2023). Even if you are not specifically asked to do so, it's best to be transparent about the use of AI and specify how it was used.

AI technologies should not be listed as authors because they can't be responsible for the accuracy, integrity, and originality of the work (Council of Science Editors Editorial Policy Committee, 2023; ICMJE, 2024).

Q *I just uploaded my manuscript to the editorial management system, but I see a passage that I need to revise. Should I resubmit or just wait until I receive the manuscript back?*

A Check with your editor. It's best to avoid this situation. Submitting multiple manuscripts—or even revised passages, piecemeal—can cause confusion. Keep track of any correction you need to make in a file. Then, when you begin the revisions process, all changes can be made at one time.

Editorial Review

Editorial workflows vary from publication to publication and from editor to editor. Some editors like to thoroughly read all submissions right away, and others read quickly to determine if the article is suitable for the next step, then wait until after peer review for a more detailed reading. Editors may reject your manuscript at this stage and not send it out for peer review. Rejection at this stage is referred to as *desk rejection* or *editorial rejection* (Fisher et al., 2017; Seals, 2023; Shah, 2015). At some point before sending for peer review, your manuscript will likely be run through a plagiarism detector.

Common reasons for rejection either at this stage or after peer review (Balch et al., 2018; Fisher et al., 2017; Morton, 2020) and follow-up actions are listed in Table 8.1.

If you submitted your work to a book, magazine, or newsletter, it may not be peer reviewed; the editor to whom you submitted your manuscript will tell you about the next step. The editor will most likely read through your work, edit it, and then send you notes, along with the text, to revise. Your editor will also provide you with a deadline, and a publication date (if known) when your piece might be likely to publish, run, or appear.

Peer Review

When you're submitting a manuscript to a journal that uses peer review, the process is more formal. After an initial positive evaluation, the editor will usually send your manuscript out for peer review. During the peer-review process, "peer" experts thoughtfully review and evaluate your manuscript against specific criteria such as logic, content, accuracy, and consistency with the journal's purpose (Chicca & Shellenbarger, 2023).

Peer reviewers provide an invaluable volunteer service to journals, editors, publishers, authors, and readers. A good reviewer clarifies information, identifies missing content, catches problematic references, suggests revisions when needed, adds headers for clarification, helps connect the dots for readers, and generally improves the quality of the manuscript. The primary role for reviewers is to focus on content, which is another reason why manuscripts should be carefully proofread before submission. Reviewers should not have to copyedit or wordsmith your work. You want them focused on the information and content and not distracted by typos, sentence fragments, poor sentence structure, punctuation errors, and so on. Finding such items as grammar errors and typos doesn't generally support a positive peer-review process (Sempokuya et al., 2022).

TABLE 8.1 Responses to Common Reasons for Rejection

Reason for Rejection	Action to Take
The topic is not appropriate for the journal.	Consult the journal directory on the website of *Nurse Author & Editor* (http://naepub.com/journals-directory) and select a more appropriate journal.
The manuscript offers no new information and does not answer the "Who cares?" or "So what?" question.	Revise the manuscript to offer readers new information or new solutions to an old problem.
The manuscript is poorly written or contains multiple writing styles.	Hire an editor or ask an experienced author to help.
The data have been published previously.	Data can only be published once. Aim to publish another aspect of the study, such as challenges in recruiting a pediatric sample.
An article too similar to yours has recently been published or will soon be published by the targeted journal.	Submit your manuscript to a different journal.
There is evidence of plagiarism.	Rewrite the manuscript in your own words and cite sources for the ideas.

In essence, reviewers are another source of help on your way to being published:

- Peer reviewers are chosen for their expertise in the content area.

- Usually the review is anonymized. In most cases, the review will be double-anonymous (preferred over the older term of double-blind), that is, neither author nor reviewer is identified to each other. Although rare in nursing publishing, some scientific journals use open peer review, where authors and reviewers know each other's identities; reviews also may be published with the final article (Author Services, n.d.).

- Peer reviewers for journals are usually volunteers; reviewers for books and book chapters may be paid a small stipend.

- Peer review typically takes about six to eight weeks, depending on the journal and the reviewers.

- Journals usually have two to four peer professionals reviewing any one manuscript.

Most peer-reviewed manuscripts need some amount of revision. You can learn more about peer review in Chapter 9, but here are some common questions reviewers are asked to answer; consider what their answers might be when it comes to your manuscript:

- Does the manuscript align with the purpose of the journal and have relevance to the journal's intended readers?

- Is the topic timely? Does it have a new or unique slant?

- Is the organization clear and logical?

- Does the information flow logically?

- Are references used when needed? Are they current? Are they accurate?

- Is the manuscript developed in adequate depth?

- Are illustrations, figures, or tables appropriate? (And do they support the information in the manuscript?)

- Was the manuscript interesting to read?

- Is the manuscript innovative, or does it provide a better presentation of what is already in the literature?

- Is the title relevant, and does it explain the topic?

- What are the manuscript's positive points?

- What are areas for improvement?

- Why is this topic important from a practice, research, or education perspective?

The Editor's Decision

After peer review, the editor examines the reviewers' comments, reads the manuscript and makes comments, and then places your manuscript into one of three categories:

- **Accept:** The editor might ask for minor corrections or revisions, but the manuscript is generally ready to publish. It is rare that any manuscript is completely accepted at this stage.

- **Revise:** The editor is sending you a message that your manuscript is worthwhile but will take some work to make it better. When they return your manuscript, some editors will use the term "minor revisions" or "major revisions" to signal the amount of work that will be required. You have a high likelihood of having your manuscript accepted if you make the requested revisions.

- **Reject:** Rejection after peer review doesn't mean failure. Perhaps your manuscript was rejected because reviewers had difficulty understanding the point of the manuscript or too many questions were raised but not answered. Manuscripts also are rejected if your study violates the principles of research methods or statistics. Note that not all journals share peer-review comments when a manuscript is rejected.

Your editor might use slightly different terms and reasons than these, but the intent is the same. Sorting manuscripts by category helps keep them flowing back to authors while the editor can compile a journal issue based on quality content that is available and ready to publish.

Be glad if the editor asks you to revise your manuscript. It's an exciting day when the peer reviews are back, and the editor indicates your manuscript is worth revising. Some authors get overwhelmed when they receive a large number of comments from the peer reviewers and the editor. Take a deep breath, tackle the comments one at a time, and remember, the editor wants to help you produce a publishable manuscript. If your revisions are satisfactory, you are on your way to being published.

> **The Emotional Side of Reviews**
>
> Reviewer comments are intended to improve manuscripts. Reviewers do this by identifying positive aspects of the submitted article and by listing recommendations that would improve it in the revision stage.
>
> That does not mean it's always easy to read the reviewers' comments. The positive ones make your heart soar; negative ones make it plummet to your toes. It can be an emotional roller coaster. And, unfortunately, not all reviewers are as tactful as they should be.
>
> First-time (and even experienced) authors can get discouraged and never make the suggested revisions. That's too bad because being asked to revise—instead of receiving a rejection—is a good sign that the editor is interested in publishing your article.
>
> After you read through the reviews, put them away for a day if you feel frustrated. Then look at them with fresh eyes. The good news is that because you have not read the article for a while, you, too, might see areas for improvement. Put aside your ego and remember that the article is not about you—it's about delivering great information or interesting content to readers. Think of yourself as part of a team that includes you; the editor; and the peer reviewers, who are experts in the subject matter of the article. Each of you brings a unique perspective, and your article can be improved when you consider these various points of view (Chicca & Shellenbarger, 2020;; Su'a et al., 2017).

In the case of minor revisions, you will likely be asked to make them after the article is edited or when the article is laid out and ready for publication (sometimes referred to as "page proofs"). If you're making page proof edits, you'll be asked to make your corrections electronically, using a PDF markup program. Don't worry about this part of the process, though; your editor or journal staff will give you instructions for accessing your pages, making your corrections, and returning them. Not all journals send page proofs to authors; in that case your final review will be when you see the edited copy.

When more detailed revisions are required, which is much more common, the editor will send you copies of the review forms or a summary of the comments for you to use in making revisions. If you're working in a journal's online editorial management system, you'll receive an email notification that your manuscript is ready for you to log in and "pick up" for revision. Comments might also be embedded into the actual manuscript pages.

Q *My manuscript went through the peer-review process and was rejected. I am devastated. Now what do I do?*

A Yes, you may be feeling a variety of emotions such as anger, disappointment, and frustration. Read the comments carefully and then perhaps put them aside for a day or two. Remember, the reviewers did not provide a negative critique of you as a person. Instead, they provided valuable feedback to help you learn. If you believe the reviewers' comments are totally off base and unfair, you can politely contact the editor to discuss. Avoid any urges to write a hostile email telling the editor the reviewers are wrong. You can send your paper to another journal; however, if you ignore the reviewers' comments and make no changes, it's likely that your manuscript will be rejected by the next journal. Instead, use the comments to improve the quality of your manuscript and boost the chances of acceptance by another journal. You also may want to consider whether you simply chose the wrong journal in the first place. (For more about selecting a journal, see Chapter 3.)

The Revision Process

Now that you have received the editor's and reviewers' feedback, it is time to get busy. Pierson (2016) suggests using the four R's of revising a manuscript: *read, reflect, revise/rewrite,* and *respond.*

Read: Carefully *read* the editor's and reviewers' comments. Keep in mind that the volunteer reviewers gave their precious time to provide comments intended to help you improve your manuscript. Each comment is meant to be helpful advice to make your manuscript better.

Reflect: Take time to *reflect* on the feedback and be sure you have a clear understanding of what you have been asked to do. If needed, seek the guidance of a mentor or an experienced author, or contact the editor if you are confused. At this stage, some authors feel overwhelmed and discouraged. They refuse to spend any more time on the manuscript and never make the requested revisions (Morton, 2022). Don't let this happen to you. You have put too much time and effort into the manuscript to quit now. Plan a timeline for revisions and stick to it.

Revise and rewrite: Now start to *revise and rewrite*, addressing each comment one by one. Start with the easy fixes such as reference inaccuracies, then move to the more complex revisions. If you choose not to make some of the requested revisions because you feel they aren't appropriate, you must provide excellent justification by clearly explaining your rationale when resubmitting the manuscript (Author Services, n.d.; Conn, 2022).

Making your revisions can include rewriting, reorganizing, adding content, or deleting content (Morton, 2013; Saver, 2006). Reviewers will comment, ask questions, and sometimes suggest alternative wording. Here are a few examples of the types of comments you might receive:

- Correct or update references (this is particularly common if references for a clinical topic are more than five years old).
- Remove redundant information.
- Clarify information and be sure to distinguish fact from your opinion.
- Provide more background on the topic. Add more in the literature review so it is clear to readers what is known about the topic, what is not known, and how your work fills a gap.
- Check information (that the reviewer thinks might be inaccurate).
- Explain more the model you are using as a framework.
- Define terms.
- Add a patient case scenario (particularly for clinical journals) or other illustrative examples.
- Strengthen by adding tables, figures, tools (e.g., assessment tips), or more examples.
- Include a section at the end on implications for nursing practice for clinical journals or implications for nursing education for education-focused journals.
- Explain in more detail the statistical test used to analyze the data.

As noted in this list, reviewers may request clarification of information or definition of terms you wrote. Remember, readers may not be as familiar with the topic as you are, so clarification can only be helpful (Saver & Cullen, 2021). Reviewers also may point out how the article could be better organized or spot gaps in information (e.g., no patient education tips in a clinical article on a surgical procedure).

Unfortunately, sometimes feedback is conflicting. For example, one reviewer may recommend additional tables while another claims you have too many. If the editor has not already addressed this conflict when returning the materials, contact them for guidance. If you contact the editor for this or another point of clarification, do not fail to follow through with making the needed change (Alexandrova & Hartland, 2021), which is a common mistake of new authors. (Keep in mind, however, that disagreements among reviewers may be a sign that your intent is unclear. Think about the possibility of a broader question—What's causing the confusion?—and revise accordingly.)

The editor also may have additional questions or comments for you to address. Some of the questions may be content related and others may involve formatting issues. Editors often request revisions of tables and figures or the addition of tables and figures to supplement the text. For research reports, editors may ask you to use headings within the manuscript that are consistent with the journal's research report format. Do not consider requests from the editor as optional. Follow what you are asked to do, remembering the requested changes will only make your manuscript better.

When you complete your revisions, ask someone else to read through the manuscript again and use the original submission checklist to be sure that you haven't overlooked anything.

Respond: The editor will want to know how you responded to the editor's and reviewers' comments. Follow the format for author responses that is required by the journal. Most editors will ask you to enter your changes directly into the text. Silvia (2015) classifies possible responses to peer-review comments as *change, resist,* or *punt. Change,* where you make the requested revision, is the most common. You should make changes requested by the reviewers unless you have a good reason not to make them. Be sure that's the case, instead of you just not liking the fact that your words were changed. *Resist* refers to a situation in which you disagree with reviewers, who, after all, aren't infallible. If you believe that there is a sound reason not to make a revision or address a comment, provide the rationale, preferably evidence-based, to the editor. *Punt* should be used rarely and only for minor issues. For example, if a reviewer suggests adding a figure that seem to have little value, you can note why you didn't make the additions, but add that the change could be made if the editor wishes.

You'll either summarize your changes in a letter or document, or sometimes a publication or editor will want you to summarize the changes in a table. For the latter approach, copy each comment into the document, then add your response immediately below it. Table 8.2 shows an example of how to organize your summary of manuscript revisions as a table. Note that the location of each revision within the revised manuscript is indicated.

Q *I have been struggling with revisions to a paper. They seem unclear. I was so excited, but now I'm completely bogged down. What should I do?*

A Reach out to your editor if you're struggling with revisions. Some may be willing to provide some guidance, and others may match you with a writing mentor if there is a topic or manuscript they believe is particularly noteworthy. Or better yet, seek out a writing mentor of your own: A published colleague might be willing to help you.

After you're finished with your revisions, you're ready to resubmit your work to the editor or through the editorial management system. Make every effort to adhere to the due date the editor requests for the revisions. Quickly returning a revised manuscript means it will be fresher in the editor's mind (Silvia, 2015). If you know you can't make the deadline, notify the editor as soon as possible. Identify the date when you will resubmit the manuscript—and then honor that deadline.

Editors are working with many issues of journals at any one time. Your manuscript might have been tentatively scheduled (assuming that revisions are accomplished and the article can be accepted) for a certain issue. Journal issues and article "line-ups" are scheduled months in advance for production reasons. Journals may also have themes or special focus issues that a certain article would fit with. If you miss the window for such an issue, you may see a delay in publication. Courtesy and ongoing communication are keys for effectively managing author and editor workloads as well as for maintaining positive working relationships.

With your revised manuscript, include a cover letter (or a note in the body of an email) that tells the editor how you organized any revisions and any major areas that you did not change because you disagreed with a reviewer. Also put the title of your manuscript and your assigned manuscript number (if given one) in the subject line of the email. If you are using an electronic submission system, follow the instructions for uploading your manuscript.

If you made major revisions to your manuscript or were asked to resubmit, you might have to go back through a second peer review and additional editing. Second-round reviews usually occur if more substantive changes were made, including major revisions in the structure, length, organization, style, or research and scientific content.

TABLE 8.2 Organizing Manuscript Revisions Using a Table Format

Requested Revision	Revision Made
Explain why you chose to use multiple regression (page 8, 3rd paragraph).	Added rationale for using this test (page 8, 4th paragraph).
Create a separate section titled "Sample and Setting." (page 5, 3rd paragraph).	Change made (page 5, 5th paragraph).
Add a section on Jones's research to the background section (page 3, 3rd paragraph).	Section not added because of word count constraints and because Smith, whose study is already cited, found similar results in a more recent study.
Suggest moving signs and symptoms from text to a table (page 5, 2nd paragraph).	Created table (page 5).

> **Confidence Booster**
>
> I (Patricia Gonce Morton) was thrilled when my first manuscript was accepted for publication. Yes, I needed to revise, but I was willing to do so and carefully followed all the comments from the reviewers and editor. That first acceptance gave me the confidence to continue writing. Over the course of my career, I have published more than 60 journal articles. One of the best ways I learned to write for a journal was to serve as a reviewer. The process of critiquing a manuscript really helped me understand how to write. I also gained the confidence, under the guidance of a mentor, to publish books. I am proud that I have completed six editions of one book and two editions of another. As my mentor said, once the printer's ink gets in your blood, you can't stop writing for publication.

Author Review

After your manuscript is accepted, the publisher will edit it to fit the publication's style and tone and return it to you for review before or after it is formatted for publication. There will often be questions, or "queries" for you. For example, the editor may ask for clarification about a point or to explain a particular term (Saver & Cullen, 2021). The queries will usually be in the manuscript (either in a different color or via comment boxes in Microsoft Word), and you'll typically respond to them in the manuscript as well. You also should check to ensure no inadvertent errors were introduced in the editing process. (Learn more about queries and the author review step in Chapter 1.)

As with the peer reviews, seeing these editorial changes can be a shock. However, the people who edit your manuscript are experts in what they do and are most familiar with the style and tone of the journal and readers' preferences. They respect you as a content expert, so respect them as editorial experts. Try not to change their edits unless clinical errors have been introduced or your intent has been changed. Once again, it's important to meet your deadline for review.

If you believe that your manuscript has been unfairly edited, contact your editor immediately to express your concerns in a kind, calm, and rational manner. By maintaining professional composure, communication channels will likely remain open for a productive dialogue and resolution of the issues.

Q *My manuscript was accepted a year ago. Today, I got the edited version back with a request to return in two days. Isn't this unreasonable?*

A Ideally, you should have one to three weeks to review the edited article. Preferably, you will be told when your article is scheduled or when you can expect it back for review so that you have some notice. However, journal schedules change, or a topic can suddenly become a hot issue. You will be a hero to your editor if you can turn around your article quickly. However, don't be discouraged if your scheduled article gets "held over" at the last minute. This delay can happen for a variety of reasons and has little to do with the quality of your article or the editor's desire to publish it. Page proofs (PDFs of an article that show how it will appear when published) are much more time sensitive because this step occurs close to the time when the publication needs to be sent to the printer (or posted online). If you're asked to return page proofs in 24 to 48 hours, make sure you do so.

Q *When my article is sent to me for a final review after it has been formatted as it will appear in the journal, can I make changes?*

A After an article is formatted and you see it (usually as a PDF), it's essentially ready for publication. You should correct only typos, formatting issues (e.g., the items in a table are not lined up correctly), or clinical errors that might have been introduced during the editing process. Not all journals have authors review the formatted version of the article.

Publication

Most journals now have the capacity to publish articles online before they appear in the print journal, commonly referred to as "online first" or "published ahead of print." A significant advantage of early online publication is that information can get out into the professional community sooner—this is of particular importance in the case of cutting-edge research.

When the article is made available online, it is considered published because it typically receives a DOI number, which registers the article with the DOI Foundation. This registration step means you cannot make changes to the article, although, of course, corrections can be noted. The article may or may not be subsequently published in the print version of the journal. Open-access journals also consider manuscripts published once they are posted online.

Publication is a time to celebrate, but occasionally the celebration is marred by an error that slipped through all the reviews and ended up in the published product. Always notify the editor of any errors. Provide specific information about where in the article the error appears and the exact correct wording.

The type of error will determine the editor's actions. If you omitted some nonessential information, for example, no action may be needed. However, if you catch a more serious problem, such a mathematical error or an error of fact, the editor will want to address it. A correction notice is usually posted online, along with a new version of the article (ICMJE, 2024). Past versions are then archived. For print publications, the editor publishes an erratum notice in the next issue, along with the link for the corrected articles that are available online.

No one likes to see a publishing error, but handling the situation quickly and professionally can minimize negative effects.

Be Persistent

Everyone who writes started somewhere. To get off to a good start, carefully adhere to the journal's author guidelines when you submit your manuscript. Use the reviewers' and editors' comments to your advantage—to get your manuscript ready for acceptance. Don't be discouraged; be positive and persistent.

As Hawkey notes:

> Writing is an exacting and exciting activity. Although frequently difficult to get started, it can become addictive with practice. Nursing is in great need of a new generation of challenging authors who are prepared to shake off the shackles of caution and timidity in so many current publications. Writing is a weapon of empowerment as well as a medium for communicating ideas. (2001, p. 66)

Write Now!

1. Identify a journal in which you are interested in publishing and review its submission guidelines and some past articles. This step will help you understand what topics are more likely to be accepted.

2. To learn more about peer review, visit Elsevier's reviewers' resource information page (https://www.elsevier.com/reviewers).

3. Pick out your favorite two journals and identify topics for possible development and submission. Set a deadline and start writing!

References

Agarwal, A., Arafa, M., Avidor-Reiss, T., Hamoda, T. A.-A. A.-M. T., Shah, R. (2023). Citation errors in scientific research and publications: Causes, consequences, and remedies. *World Journal of Men's Health, 41*(3), 461–465. https://doi.org/10.5534/wjmh.230001

Alexandrova, A. N., & Hartland, G. V. (2021). Revising manuscripts: Trying to make everyone happy. *Journal of Physical Chemistry, 125*(33), 18087–18088. https://doi.org/10.1021/acs.jpcc.1c07069

American Psychological Association. (2020). *Publication manual of the American Psychological Association* (7th ed.). https://doi.org/10.1037/0000165-000

Author Services. (n.d.). *Article submission and peer review.* Taylor & Francis Group. https://authorservices.taylorandfrancis.com/wp-content/uploads/2021/03/Research_Submission_and_peer_review.pdf

Balch, C. M., McMasters, K. M., Klimberg, S., Pawlik, T. M., Posner, M. C., Roh, M., Tanabe, K. K., Whippen, D., & Ikoma, N. (2018). Steps to getting your manuscript published in a high-quality medical journal. *Annals of Surgical Oncology, 25*(4), 850–855. https://doi.org/10.1245/s10434-017-6320-6

Chicca, J., & Shellenbarger, T. (2020). Revising it right: Five steps to help you get your work published. *Nurse Author & Editor, 30*(1), 1–9. https://doi.org/10.1111/j.1750-4910.2020.tb00003.x

Chicca, J., & Shellenbarger, T. (2023). Crafting a meaningful peer review. *Nurse Author & Editor, 33*(1-2), 13–17. https://doi.org/10.1111/nae2.12053

Conn, V. S. (2022). Revising manuscripts to address reviewer requests for additional content [Editorial]. *Western Journal of Nursing Research, 44*(4), 355. https://doi.org/10.1177/0193945920956597

Council of Science Editors Editorial Policy Committee. (2023). *CSE's recommendations for promoting integrity in scientific journal publications.* https://www.councilscienceeditors.org/recommendations-for-promoting-integrity-in-scientific-journal-publications

CRediT. (n.d.). *Contributor Roles Taxonomy.* https://credit.niso.org/

Fisher, P. G., Goodman, D. M., & Long, S. S. (2017). Getting published: A primer on manuscript writing and the editorial process. *The Journal of Pediatrics, 185,* 241–244. https://doi.org/10.1016/j.jpeds.2017.02.067

Hawkey, M. (2001). Joys, frustrations and concerns of a journal peer reviewer. *Journal of Nursing Management, 9*(2), 65–66. https://doi.org/10.1046/j.1365-2834.2001.00259.x

International Committee of Medical Journal Editors. (2024). *Recommendations for the conduct, reporting, editing, and publication of scholarly work in medical journals.* http://www.icmje.org/recommendations

International Society for Medical Publication Professionals. (2023, Nov. 1). International Society for Medical Publication Professionals (ISMPP) position statement and call to action on artificial intelligence. *Current Medical Research and Opinion.* https://doi.org/10.1080/03007995.2023.2273139

Iwaz, J. (2022). Before you click "submit," be your own first reviewer. *Science Editing, 10*(1), 105–108. https://doi.org/10.6087/kcse.288

JAMA Network Editors. (2020). *AMA manual of style: A guide for authors and editors* (11th ed.). Oxford University Press. https://doi.org/10.1093/jama/9780190246556.001.0001

Mikhail, J. N. (2021). Prevent rejection of your manuscript—read the author guidelines! [Editorial]. *Journal of Trauma Nursing, 28*(3), 145–148. https://doi.org/10.1097/JTN.0000000000000582

Morton, P. G. (2013). Publishing in professional journals, part II: Writing the manuscript. *AACN Advanced Critical Care, 24*(4), 370–374. https://doi.org/10.1097/NCI.0b013e3182a92670

Morton, P. G. (2020). Why was my manuscript rejected? *Journal of Professional Nursing, 36,* 1–4. https://doi.org/10.1016/j.profnurs.2020.02.006

Morton, P.G. (2022). Why oh why won't you revise your manuscript? [Editorial]. *Journal of Professional Nursing, 39,* A3–A4. https://doi.org/10.1016/j.profnurs.2022.02.001

National Institutes of Health Office of the Director. (2023). *Conduct of research in the intramural research program at NIH* (8th ed.). National Institutes of Health. https://oir.nih.gov/system/files/media/file/2023-08/guidelines-conduct_research.pdf

ORCID. (n.d.). *About ORCID.* https://info.orcid.org/what-is-orcid

Pierson, C. A. (2016). The four R's of revising and resubmitting a manuscript [Editorial]. *Journal of the American Association of Nurse Practitioners, 28*(8), 408–409. https://doi.org/10.1002/2327-6924.12399

Saver, C. (2006). Decisions and revisions. *AORN Journal, 84*(2), 183–184, 188. https://doi.org/10.1016/S0001-2092(06)60487-0

Saver, C. (2023, April 14). Use keywords to help readers find your work. *The Writing Mind.* https://www.myamericannurse.com/use-keywords-to-help-readers-find-your-work/

Saver, C., & Cullen, J. (2021). Two sides of editorial queries: Editors and authors. *Nurse Author & Editor, 31*(1), 5–9. https://doi.org/10.1111/nae2.14

Seals, D. R. (2023). Publishing particulars: Part 3. General writing tips, editing, and responding to peer review. *American Journal of Physiology: Regulatory, Integrative and Comparative Physiology, 324,* R409–R424. https://doi.org/10.1152/ajpregu.00270.2022

Sempokuya, T., McDonald, N., & Bilal, M. (2022). How to be a great peer reviewer [Editorial]. *ACG Case Reports Journal, 9*(12), e00932. https://doi.org/10.14309/crj.0000000000000932

Shah, J. (2015). An author's guide to submission, revision, and rejection. *RCS Annals, 97*(8), 546–548. https://doi.org/10.1308/rcsann.2015.0046

Silvia, P. J. (2015). *Write it up: Practical strategies for writing and publishing journal articles.* American Psychological Association.

Su'a, B., MacFater, W. S., & Hill, A. G. (2017). How to write a paper: Revising your manuscript. *ANZ Journal of Surgery, 87*(3), 195–197. https://doi.org/10.1111/ans.13847

World Association of Medical Editors. (2023). *Chatbots, generative AI, and scholarly manuscripts.* https://wame.org/page3.php?id=106

Zinsser, W. (2013). *Writing to learn.* Harper Paperbacks.

Writing a Peer Review

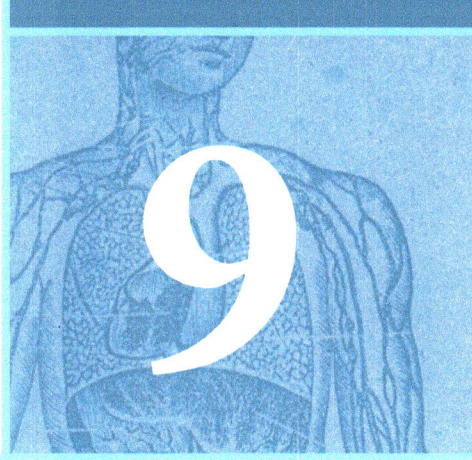

–Cindy L. Munro, PhD, RN, ANP-BC, FAAN, FAANP

> *"I love science. I hate supposition, superstition, exaggeration and falsified data. Show me the research, show me the results, show me the conclusions—and then show me some qualified peer reviews of all that."*
> –Claire Scovell LaZebnik

WHAT YOU'LL LEARN IN THIS CHAPTER

- Peer reviewers are important contributors to the publication process.
- Being a peer reviewer has many benefits and is a skill that can be learned.
- Preparing a review is easier if you go about it systematically.
- A well-done review provides objective, honest, constructive, and specific comments to authors and editors.

Amazingly, peer review of scientific journals dates back to the 1600s (Berenbaum, 2023). Peer reviewers have a crucial role in the publication process. Think of them as watchdogs; they help ensure that published clinical and research articles, which guide nursing practice, are accurate, timely, and useful to readers.

Whether or not you're a published author, consider becoming a peer reviewer. Editors of scholarly journals often depend on peer reviewers for assistance in evaluating and improving manuscripts. Peer reviewer comments influence the editor's decision about whether to accept or reject a manuscript, and they provide recommendations about changes required before acceptance.

This chapter gives you the information you need to know to feel confident about serving as a peer reviewer, including the role and responsibilities of reviewers and the steps to follow in conducting a review. Don't stop reading if you're an author who has no plans to become a reviewer. Understanding the perspective of a peer reviewer helps you anticipate potential questions in your manuscript and makes you a better writer.

Roles and Responsibilities of Peer Reviewers

Editors decide what articles will be published in their journals, and the decision-making process differs among journals. Scholarly or academic journals have traditionally required manuscripts to undergo peer review, and many clinical and other types of journals now require the same. Other types of writing, such as magazines and book reviews, typically don't require peer review.

Although the value of peer review has been debated, the process allows the manuscript to receive what the International Committee of Medical Journal Editors (ICMJE, 2024) refers to as "a fair hearing" among the scientific community.

Peer reviewers act as advisors to the editor, and the editor carefully considers their comments, concerns, and recommendations in making a final decision about the fate of a manuscript. Peer reviewers are expected to be unbiased and good communicators (Tennant & Ross-Hellauer, 2020). As a peer reviewer, your most important role is to help the editor evaluate a manuscript's quality, relevance, and importance.

Peer reviewers provide feedback to authors as well. Editors vary in how they make peer reviewer comments available to authors. Some editors provide the full text of original reviewer comments, whereas other editors prepare a summary of the reviews for the authors. Comments and suggestions made by peer reviewers help authors improve the content of the manuscript and improve the readers' understanding of journal articles.

Benefits of Being a Peer Reviewer

Most journal peer reviewers serve as volunteers, and payment for reviews is not common. Even so, being a peer reviewer benefits the nursing profession and your career (Dance, 2022).

As a peer reviewer, your expert knowledge helps to improve the quality and accuracy of the articles published, strengthening the entire nursing profession. Your critique enables journals to provide trustworthy and useful information for nursing practice, and you provide helpful, objective feedback to authors. If you're an author who expects peer reviewers to be available for your manuscripts, or a clinician who values high-quality information in nursing practice, you should be prepared to contribute to the publications process as a peer reviewer.

Selection as a peer reviewer for a highly respected journal is a recognition of your expertise, which can enhance your career. List peer-review activities on your curriculum vitae or resume to document your service to the profession. Preparing peer reviews hones your ability to critique, and your own writing will benefit from your suggestions to others about how to improve content and clarity of presentation.

Peer-Review Panel

There are many types of expertise—for example, clinical, procedural, methodological, statistical, health system—and very few people are experts in every area. Multiple peer reviewers with various areas of expertise are assigned to the same manuscript so that editors can adequately evaluate the manuscript as a whole. Each reviewer has expert knowledge important to assessing that manuscript. For example, a manuscript on a research study of an intervention to improve vaccination rates in older adults might include a panel composed of reviewers with expertise in research methodology, vaccine hesitancy, and care of older adults. The editor can then read each peer review and evaluate the manuscript from multiple perspectives.

The number of reviewers assigned to each manuscript differs among journals, but two to four reviewers per manuscript is most common.

How to Become a Peer Reviewer

Editors use a variety of methods to identify potential peer reviewers. Your publications or presentations demonstrate that you are an expert in a topic, so many editors search publication databases (e.g., PubMed and the Cumulative Index of Nursing and Allied Health Literature [CINAHL]) and specialty conference proceedings to find new reviewers. Editors value diverse perspectives and strive to minimize bias in editorial processes; they may also recruit reviewers from underrepresented groups (Pickler et al., 2021). Some editors permit authors to suggest names of potential reviewers, usually when only a small number of experts have knowledge of the information.

Most journals maintain a list of qualified individuals who have expressed interest in serving as peer reviewers. If the editor invites you to register in the journal's reviewer database, do so. When you register, you'll be asked to identify in what content and methodological areas you are an expert. Choose carefully, as editors will use these categories to match your expertise to submitted manuscripts for review assignments. It's better to choose fewer categories where you have in-depth expertise, rather than many categories where you have less depth of knowledge. (Note: If you become a regular peer reviewer, be sure to update your areas of expertise as needed [Chicca & Shellenbarger, 2023].) Be certain that all your information is correct, complete, and reflects your true abilities. Don't be dismayed if you do not immediately receive an invitation to perform a peer review; it may be some time before a submitted manuscript matches your qualifications as a reviewer.

Q *What if I want to be a peer reviewer, but no one has contacted me?*

A You don't have to wait for an editor to "discover" you; you can volunteer. Connect with editors at professional conferences or by email to let them know you're interested in volunteering as a peer reviewer. Briefly describe your expertise and why you think you are a good match for the journal. And be sure to provide a curriculum vitae or resume documenting your experience and accomplishments.

Considering an Invitation

You'll typically receive an invitation to be a peer reviewer by email. The invitation will give you some information about the manuscript (usually the title and abstract or a description of the article). The full manuscript is usually provided only after you have agreed to review. The invitation will also provide the timeline for submitting your review. Although journals vary in the time allotted for peer review, two to three weeks is a common deadline. You'll be asked to reply, either accepting or declining the invitation, within a relatively short deadline; if you cannot serve, the editor will need to quickly invite others.

Consider two questions when deciding whether to accept the invitation:

- **Do I have the expertise to do a comprehensive and fair evaluation of the submission?** To answer this question, read the abstract or description included in the invitation to determine whether you have the expertise needed to fairly evaluate the paper. Is the topic something you know a lot about? Is there a particular aspect that aligns with your interests and experience? Remember that you don't have to be an expert in every aspect of the topic. If you don't think your expertise is a good match, decline the invitation. If you aren't clear about why the editor thought you would be the right expert to review the submission, you can ask for clarification before you accept or decline.

- **Can I return the review within the time allotted?** Consider realistically whether you can meet the requested deadline. Delays on your part will extend the entire length of the review process, which will be frustrating for both editors and authors. If it's unlikely you can complete the review on time, you should promptly decline.

Editors will appreciate your honesty if you cannot take on a review assignment, and it will not deter them from inviting you in the future.

Preparing to Be a Peer Reviewer

As you prepare to be a good peer reviewer, establish ground rules for your behavior. Strive to be objective, honest, constructive, and specific. Be respectful and compassionate in composing your final comments—commit to writing reviews that you would want to receive if you were the manuscript's author. Keep in mind that unfair and insensitive peer review can harm an author's mental health and well-being (Bressington et al., 2022). Respectful communication is a highly valued reviewer attribute (Smith & Jackson, 2022).

Being *objective* demands that you focus on the manuscript you are reviewing and consider its own merits. Make a commitment to give every manuscript a fair chance and to keep your review fact-based. Objective peer reviewers do not make assumptions about the author, do not let perceptions about the authors influence their judgment, and do not make any hostile, personal, or derogatory comments about the author.

Do your best to be *honest* in your evaluation, identifying both the positive and negative aspects of the manuscript. As you review, it may be tempting to think, "If I had tackled the problem this manuscript describes, I would have done things differently." You need to focus instead on what the author reports. The author's approach might be an acceptable alternative to how you would have done things. If you think the work is flawed, say so, but resist the impulse to redesign a project that has already been completed or suggest revisions that can't be accomplished without time travel.

Q *What resources can I use to prepare myself to be a peer reviewer?*

A No matter where you fall on the continuum of peer-reviewer expertise (reviewing your first or 101st article), consider tapping into resources available to help peer reviewers improve their skills. These include:

- The Committee on Publication Ethics (COPE; www.publicationethics.org)
- Enhancing the QUAlity and Transparency Of health Research (EQUATOR) Peer Reviewing Research Toolkit; https://www.equator-network.org/toolkits/peer-reviewing-research)
- Web of Science Academy Introduction to Peer Review (https://clarivate.com/web-of-science-academy)
- Sense about Science peer-review workshops (https://senseaboutscience.org/activities/peer-review-the-nuts-and-bolts-2)
- Online tutorials from journals and publishers, such as those from Elsevier (https://researcheracademy.elsevier.com/navigating-peer-review/certified-peer-reviewer-course) and Wiley (https://authorservices.wiley.com/Reviewers/journal-reviewers/becoming-a-reviewer.html/peer-review-training.html).
- Workshops at professional conferences

Make your comments *constructive* and *specific*. Providing constructive comments doesn't mean ignoring problems, but where possible, offer potential suggestions for correcting the deficiencies. The more specific your comments are, the more helpful they will be to editors in evaluating the manuscript and to the author in improving it. In the following example, most authors would find the revised comment to be more helpful than the original.

Original comment: Add more information about the study sample.

Revised comment: Additional information about the demographics and clinical conditions of the study sample should be presented to help readers better evaluate the outcomes of the intervention; it is also critical to replication of the study or to adoption of the intervention in clinical practice. A table presenting the age, sex, and ethnicity of the total sample, intervention group, and control group would help readers see whether groups were equivalent and whether the sample was representative of the types of patients in their own institution (which might affect translation to practice in an institution). Were other common health problems present that might have affected the results, and were they similar in both the intervention and control groups?

Ethics of Peer Review

Ethics in peer review are just as important as ethics in nursing practice. The COPE Council's Ethical Guidelines for Peer Reviewers (2019) provides a good overview of ethical principles related to peer review.

As a peer reviewer, you will see unpublished material that is entrusted to you with an ethical obligation for confidentiality. Never share a manuscript you are reviewing with anyone (ICMJE, 2024). In addition:

- Never use information you obtain during peer review for your own (or anyone else's) advantage, or against anyone.
- Do not reveal any details from the manuscripts before the journal releases the information, and do not discuss peer-review details with anyone (COPE Council, 2019; ICMJE, 2024).

Journal policies regarding the use of artificial intelligence (AI programs, e.g., ChatGPT) in preparing peer reviews differ widely and are still evolving; some journals do not allow any use of AI, and others place specific limits on how it may be used (Flanagin et al., 2023). Entering the text of an author's manuscript to a public AI program raises serious confidentiality concerns and is generally prohibited. You should check with the editor before using AI to assist in preparing your review (ICMJE, 2024).

Types of Peer Review

Although the process can vary slightly from journal to journal, this section describes the basics of peer review. Journals have different approaches to anonymity of authors and reviewers during the peer-review process. The most common approaches are double-anonymous, single-anonymous, and open review (COPE Council, 2019; JAMA Network Editors, 2020; Sense about Science, 2021).

Double-Anonymous

In a *double-anonymous review* (sometimes called double-blind or double-masked), which is the most traditional approach, neither reviewers nor authors know each other's identities. Any information that could identify the author is removed from the manuscript that is sent to reviewers, and the author's name is not revealed to reviewers. Conversely, authors are not told names of the peer reviewers, and reviewers must be careful not to inadvertently or intentionally reveal who they are to authors. Double-anonymous review is designed to minimize any positive or negative bias reviewers might have if they know the author's identity, to encourage frank critique of the manuscript, and to maintain the editor's control over the review process by preventing authors from directly engaging (or challenging) reviewers.

Single-Anonymous

In *single-anonymous reviews* (sometimes called single-blind or single-masked), information that identifies the author is permitted so reviewers can include an assessment of the author's qualifications and past accomplishments in evaluating a submission; the identities of the peer reviewers are not shared with the author. Single-anonymous review is often used in evaluating requests for funding, where details about the investigator and environment are critical to the appraisal of the project, but it's not commonly used in peer review of journal manuscripts.

Open

An *open review* is just what the name implies: Reviewers know authors' identities, and authors know who the reviewers are. Reviewers may be asked to sign the review, and some journals publish comments by the reviewers alongside the author's paper. Proponents of open review believe it holds reviewers more accountable for their remarks than the anonymous-review process does. Journals may select open review to promote intellectual exchange and discussion between authors, reviewers, and readers. Open review is uncommon in nursing publications, however.

As a peer reviewer, you'll want to know the level of anonymity that governs the review process for the journals you serve. You can usually find this information in the author guidelines and reviewer guidelines that the editor will send you, or you can find it on the journal's website.

How to Conduct a Peer Review

You have received and accepted your first invitation to be a peer reviewer. Now what? First, mark the due date on your calendar and plan adequate time to complete the review. Reviewers spend an average of five to six hours to review one scientific manuscript (Kelly et al., 2014), but the time required will vary depending on the complexity of the manuscript and the reviewer's expertise and experience. Next, read the journal's instructions to reviewers and familiarize yourself with any review forms the journal requires. Many journals now use online editorial management systems; if you'll need to submit your review electronically, test your username, password, and ability to access the system, and complete any training needed to learn how to navigate the system. Now you're ready to begin.

> **Confidence Booster**
>
> "I never thought of myself as an 'expert.' Then one day I received an email from the editor of a national nursing journal. She had found my name because I spoke on repair of ruptured aortic aneurysms at my specialty association's national meeting and wanted me to review a manuscript on aortic aneurysms. I wasn't sure if I could do it, so I asked for the guidelines. They seemed clear enough, and I had the time, so I did the review. Several months later, I saw the article in print! Even though I couldn't tell anyone I was the reviewer, I felt proud. I did a couple more reviews, and the next thing I knew I was writing my own article. And ... it was published!"
>
> –*A published nurse author*

Complete an Initial Read

After providing you with reviewer instructions and information on accessing the online editorial management system, the editor will give you access to the full manuscript in an electronic file. Begin by reading the manuscript straight through, from start to finish. Your goal in this first reading is to get a general impression of the manuscript; you don't need to take any notes or write any comments at this point. As you read, consider the writing style, tone, and readability of the manuscript. Is it written similarly to recent articles that the journal has published? Do you think it fits with what the journal's readers expect? Assess the overall presentation and readability of the manuscript. Focus on the ideas being presented; if accepted, the manuscript will undergo copyediting to address errors in language or grammar.

On rare occasions, as you read through the full manuscript, you may discover that there is some reason you should not be a peer reviewer for this particular manuscript. For example, you may realize that you provided consultation on an earlier draft. If you think you have potential conflicting interests, or any other concerns about your ability to review the manuscript objectively and honestly, seek advice from the editor. If at any time during the review you have ethical concerns about the manuscript (e.g., it has substantial similarity to a published article, or you suspect misconduct may have occurred), you should immediately tell the editor. The editor will investigate the situation; even if you think you can identify the author, you should not personally investigate.

Critique Each Section

Now, return to the manuscript and use a systematic approach to critiquing specific sections. As a rule, manuscripts of any type have three broad sections: an *introduction* that provides background information, a *body* that has specific information the author wants to convey, and a *discussion*. Use these broad headings for the overall organization of your notes about the manuscript.

These three sections will differ depending upon the type of article. For example, research articles usually have a background section, a methods section, a presentation of results, and a discussion. The format for how-to clinical articles and for case studies varies from journal to journal. In your notes, add subheadings for the section titles specified by the journal to your main sections of introduction, body, and discussion.

Start with the introduction and leave the abstract for last. You'll be better able to judge how accurately the abstract portrays the manuscript if you complete your critique of the introduction, body, and discussion beforehand. As you read each section carefully, make three groups of notes about each section: *positives*, *problems*, and *potential improvements*.

Here are examples of questions you might ask as you take notes on each section of the manuscript.

Introduction. The introduction should prepare the reader to understand the body of the manuscript.

- Does the background set the stage for the rest of the story?
- Does everything in the introduction relate to what comes after?
- Is there any unrelated or unneeded information?
- Is the literature current and concisely synthesized so that the importance of what has already happened is clear?
- Is the purpose of the manuscript clear?

Body. The body of the manuscript should be the main focus of the article; it is the section where the author conveys new information.

- Is the body complete and understandable to the reader? Tailor your assessment to the specific subheadings of the journal.
- If included, do the figures and tables help you to understand the manuscript?
- Are figures and tables clear, and is all the information necessary?

For articles that describe activities the author conducted, such as research, quality improvement projects, or case studies, ask the following:

- Is it clear why the activities were done and what the expected outcomes were?
- Are the concepts and variables identified and defined?
- Is it clear what was done, and how?
- Were the methods described appropriate to the clinical or research problem, and are the reliability and validity of the methods discussed?

For how-to manuscripts, ask the following:

- Are the procedures and underlying rationales clearly presented and completely explained?
- Are indications and contraindications stated?

After you have answered the questions about what was done and how it was done, proceed to review what happened next.

- How were decisions made about whether the activities were successful or not?
- Were statistical methods used, and if so, were they appropriate for the data?
- Are the clinical or research results understandable?
- Is the body of the manuscript aligned with what you expected to find based on the introduction?

Discussion. The discussion should summarize the major points of the manuscript and put the new information in context.

- Is the new information placed in the context of what is already known?
- Are the conclusions valid?
- Are limitations identified and discussed in enough detail?
- Are the implications for clinical practice discussed?

References. Now that you have reviewed the article, turn to the references.

- Are they current and appropriate?
- Are there too few or too many?
- Are any important references missing?

Depending on the journal, the editor might tell you that you should evaluate a manuscript based on specific reporting guidelines that have been developed by a national consortium. This occurs more commonly with research or quality improvement manuscripts. Reporting guidelines for many study types can be accessed through the EQUATOR (Enhancing the QUAlity and Transparency Of health Research) Network at www.equator-network.org. For example, CONSORT (CONsolidated Standards of Reporting Trials) guidelines used for reporting randomized clinical trials, and SQUIRE (Standards for QUality Improvement Reporting Excellence) 2.0 guidelines for reporting quality improvement projects are both available on the EQUATOR Network website.

Complete a Final Read

After your step-by-step review of the positives, problems, and potential improvements in each section, return to a more general assessment. Based on your initial reading and your detailed review of each section, is the manuscript likely to be of interest to the journal's readers? Does it address an important topic? Does it provide new information? Is it well reasoned, well written, and well organized? Are there any ethical issues?

You began your journey with this manuscript by reading the title and abstract in the invitation to review. Return there to finish your notes about the manuscript. Ask the following:

- Does the information in the abstract match what the journal requires in an abstract?
- Does the information in the abstract match the rest of the manuscript?
- Does the title accurately describe the content, and would the title help you find this content if you were searching for it?
- Does the abstract convey the "so what" factor—why the information is important to nurses? (Chicca & Shellenbarger, 2023)

You're now ready to use the notes you've taken on the positives, problems, and potential improvements for each section to write your review.

Write Your Review

Begin with an opening paragraph that gives a short, two- to three-sentence synopsis of the manuscript. Then, give your overall opinion of the manuscript, based on the notes from the general assessment you did following the step-by-step review of sections.

Summarize the major positive aspects. State the most important problems you've identified, how serious you think they are, and whether it's possible for the author to fix them. Major problems that cannot be fixed are fatal flaws—be objective and honest in identifying them and explaining why you think they are unfixable.

Here is an example of how a well-written review starts:

> This manuscript reports results of an intervention to improve management of pain in mechanically ventilated children. The manuscript is likely to be of high interest to the journal's international readership, and the topic is well matched to the journal.
>
> While the manuscript is generally well done, I have several major concerns. First, the researchers do not carefully explain the limitations of the pre- and post-test design used. Second, there are instances in which literature central to the manuscript is not correctly or completely cited; I believe this is a critical problem that must be addressed in a revision of the manuscript. Third, additional information about the intervention will be crucial to readers. Fourth, the discussion should include alternative explanations for the findings.

Next, summarize your notes for each section of the manuscript; you can present your positives, problems, and possible improvements as bullet lists under each section heading. Address any suggested changes to improve figures and tables.

Before you submit your review, read it carefully—and check for spelling and grammar errors. The author may receive your comments exactly as you wrote them. The written comments should be consistent with the ground rules for peer-reviewer behavior—objective, honest, constructive, and specific.

Submit Your Review

You are now ready to submit your review. The written critique you've prepared is submitted as your comments to the author. Don't put recommendations about acceptance or rejection in the comments to the author; remember that the editor may share these comments in their entirety with the author. Some journals will also ask you to give a numerical score for each section of the manuscript and for the manuscript overall; in that case, the journal will provide information about how to use their scoring system.

Q *After reviewing the manuscript, I have some comments for the editor that I don't want to be shared with the author. What's the best way for me to send these?*

A In addition to the comments to be shared with the author, you may provide confidential comments to the editor; these confidential comments will not be shared with the author. You do not need to repeat anything you have already written in the comments to the author, as the editor already has those. If the journal uses an electronic process for reviews, there is usually an area for submission of confidential comments to the editor. If not, you can simply email the editor confidential comments that expand on your impressions or specific concerns. Be sure to note in the email that you do not want the comments shared with the author.

You should indicate your recommendation regarding publication. Please remember that this is a recommendation; the editor's final decision will incorporate feedback from all reviewers and may differ from your recommendation. You can include your recommendation in the confidential comments to the editor. Publication recommendations are usually given in one of these categories:

- **Accepted.** No modifications are needed. This is the rare case of a perfect manuscript with not a single problem identified or suggestion for improvement. The manuscript will still undergo editing before publication, and the author will need to respond to editorial queries.

- **Accepted Pending Revision.** A few improvements are suggested, but the changes are not essential. (This may also be called a *conditional acceptance*.)

- **Revise and Resubmit.** More substantial revisions are needed. (Some journals will split this recommendation into "minor revisions" and major revisions." Other journals combine conditional acceptance and revise into "accepted pending satisfactory completions of revisions" or "revisions needed before a publication decision can be made.")

- **Rejection.** The manuscript has fatal flaws, or the problems are too extensive to be fixed by a revision.

Instead of writing a peer review, some editors have you complete a review form that asks you to respond to questions. Instead of yes or no, you might be asked to respond based on a rating scale.

Sample questions include the following:

- Is the information relevant for the readers of the journal?
- Does the manuscript provide new information or insights?
- Is the information accurate?
- Is the information current?
- Is the information complete?
- Is the manuscript well written and organized?
- Are figures and tables clear and useful?
- Are references included as needed?
- Are key references missing?
- Are the clinical applications of the manuscript described clearly?

Additional questions for a research study might include these:

- Does the introduction and background identify the problem and review the literature sufficiently?
- Are the methods appropriate for the research question, and are they explained?
- Are the results clearly presented in the text or supporting tables or figures?
- Does the discussion section explain why the results are important and where they fit in the literature?
- Are study limitations included?

You also will usually have a space to provide general comments.

Feedback

It's always helpful to receive feedback to improve your performance as a peer reviewer. After the editor has made a decision about the manuscript, the other peer reviewers' comments may be shared with you. You can see how congruent your assessment of positives, problems, and possible improvements was to the other reviewers, and learn from positives and problems they identified that you might have missed. If your comments differ from theirs, however, do not assume that you did not do a good review. Reviewer comments routinely differ when their areas of expertise are different, and editors welcome a variety of perspectives to inform editorial decisions.

You can also ask the editor to provide you with feedback; some journals provide reviewers with annual evaluations of their performance. Journals may have mentoring programs for new reviewers as well. The most positive evidence of your peer-review skills is an invitation to do another review!

Write Now!

1. List three topic areas where you are an expert and provide evidence of your expertise in each area (e.g., certifications, presentations, publications, clinical experiences).
2. Contact the editor of a journal that publishes articles in your areas of expertise and ask about serving as a peer reviewer.

References

Berenbaum, M. R. (2023). On peer review—Then, now, and soon to be? [Editorial]. *Proceedings of the National Academy of Science of the United States of America, 120*(11), e2302593120. https://doi.org/10.1073/pnas.2302593120

Bressington, D., Thompson, D. R., Jones, M., & Gray, R. (2022). Conducting a sensitive, constructive and ethical peer review. *Nursing Open, 9*(4), 1930–1932. https://doi.org/10.1002/nop2.944

Chicca, J., & Shellenbarger, T. (2023). Crafting a meaningful nursing peer review. *Nurse Author & Editor, 33*(1-2), 13–17. https://doi.org/10.1111/nae2.12053

Committee on Publication Ethics Council. (2019). *Ethical guidelines for peer reviewers*. https://doi.org/10.24318/cope.2019.1.9

Dance, A. (2022). Why early-career researchers should step up to the peer-review plate. *Nature, 602*(7895), 169–171. https://doi.org/10.1038/d41586-022-00216-1

Flanagin, A., Kendall-Taylor, J., & Bibbins-Domingo, K. (2023). Guidance for authors, peer reviewers, and editors on use of AI, language models, and chatbots. *JAMA, 330*(8), 702–703. https://doi.org/10.1001/jama.2023.12500

International Committee of Medical Journal Editors. (2024). *Recommendations for the conduct, reporting, editing, and publication of scholarly work in medical journals.* http://www.icmje.org/recommendations/

JAMA Network Editors. (2020). *AMA manual of style: A guide for authors and editors* (11th ed.). Oxford University Press.

Kelly, J., Sadeghieh, T., & Adeli, K. (2014). Peer review in scientific publications: Benefits, critiques, & a survival guide. *Electronic Journal of the International Federation of Clinical Chemistry and Laboratory Medicine (eIFCC), 25*(3), 227–243. https://www.ncbi.nlm.nih.gov/pmc/articles/PMC4975196/

Pickler, R. H., Munro, C. L., & Likis, F. E. (2021). Addressing racism in editorial practices. *Nurse Author & Editor, 30*(4), 38–40. https://doi.org/10.1111/nae2.11

Sense about Science. (2021). *Peer review: The nuts and bolts.* https://senseaboutscience.org/activities/peer-review-the-nuts-and-bolts-2/

Smith G. D., & Jackson, D. (2022). Integrity and trust in research and publication: The crucial role of peer review. *Journal of Advanced Nursing, 78*(11), e135–e136. https://doi.org/10.1111/jan.15438

Tennant, J. P., & Ross-Hellauer, T. (2020). The limitations to our understanding of peer review. *Research Integrity and Peer Review, 5*(6). https://doi.org/10.1186/s41073-020-00092-1

Publishing for Global Authors

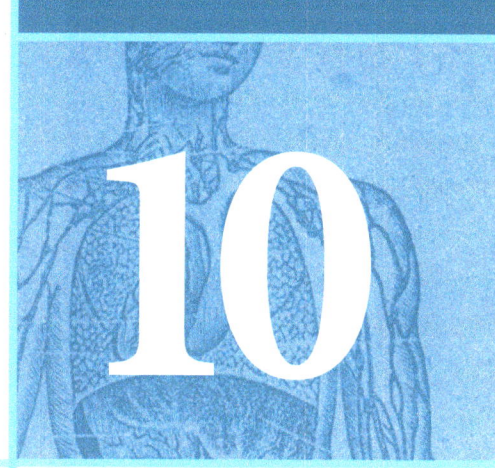

–Susan Gennaro, PhD, RN, FAAN

"Writing and learning and thinking are the same process."
–William Zinsser

WHAT YOU'LL LEARN IN THIS CHAPTER

- Global authors face unique challenges in selecting appropriate journals and in understanding ethical international standards.

- Language barriers are challenging for authors and editors alike. They not only prolong the time for dissemination but also incur costs for authors, who must obtain language assistance, and for editors, who must invest more time into the manuscript.

- Advances in technology can help authors whose first language is not English.

In the global world of the 21st century, we can communicate easily across geographic boundaries and time zones using everything from phone calls and text messages to virtual group meetings. Although time and space no longer curtail our ability to communicate, global authors for whom English is a second language still face publication barriers (Akst, 2020).

Most articles in the sciences are published in English, and English competence has become a professional prerequisite for academics, even though proficiency in English brings costs that native English speakers do not face. These costs include additional time needed to read, comprehend, and write as well as monetary costs for editing support (Lenharo, 2023). In this chapter, you'll learn the implications of English as the language of science, the barriers to publication for non-native English-speaking authors, and strategies for breaking down those barriers.

English and Science

English is currently the language of science just as Greek, Arabic, and Latin were historically the language of science (Drubin & Kellogg, 2012). The number of scientific articles disseminated in English continues to increase in English-speaking countries, such as the United States. English has been adopted by the scientific community in the European Union; increased numbers of journals globally now publish in English, and there is a global increase in the number of students learning English as a second language. Overall, 98% of peer-reviewed science is written in English (Steigerwald et al., 2022).

There are excellent reasons to have one common language for science, such as the ability to build global scientific communities (Di Bietti & Ferraras, 2016; Steigerwald et al., 2022). Non-native English-speaking nurse scientists are urged to publish in English to ensure their work is more accessible to the global community, so that global collaboration and dissemination are advanced (Yanbing et al., 2021). However, the costs to non-Native English speakers pose a threat to scientific advancement by potentially prolonging the time it takes for non-native English speakers to disseminate scientific advancements. Therefore, it's vital that we all work together (scientists, editors, and reviewers) to enhance one language publication while also facilitating publication for non-native English speakers and using the new advances in technology that are increasingly available.

Q *How did English come to be accepted as a global language of science? It doesn't seem fair.*

A World War II hastened the transformation of English as the common language of science because some of the victor nations (notably, England and the United States) were English-speaking. Some non-English-speaking countries with strong backgrounds in science (such as Germany) had longer recovery periods. The growth of computers and computerized databases in English-speaking countries in the latter half of the 20th century helped spur the growth of English. Is it fair? No. But it is a reality of getting your research published.

One difficulty for non-native English speakers in getting published it that too many journal reviewers (and some editors) have difficulty reading a manuscript for the quality of its *science*—not the quality of its *language*. Instead of focusing on the science, they are too easily distracted by grammatical issues resulting from writing English as a second language. However, just as there are global standards for conducting research, there are global standards for communicating research results, and some of these are fairly simple for non-native English speakers to incorporate (Kojima & Popiel, 2022). Grammatical problems with language should not be the focus of peer review because they can be addressed in the publication process by copy editors.

Logic, clarity, and sound scientific arguments may also be influenced by culture and may create unique challenges for non-native English-speaking authors (Weaver & Jackson, 2011). These too can be addressed through the editorial and publication process. However, problems with the actual science of a manuscript are less easily fixed and exist irrespective of language and culture. The good news is that published articles by non-native English speakers do not differ significantly in linguistic complexity from articles by native English speakers (Lu et al., 2019), so if your research is sound and you use the tools to improve writing quality that are readily available while you write, you should be successful in being published in English journals.

Whether the fact that English is the language of science in the 21st century is positive or negative for the future development of science has been much discussed (Flowerdew, 2022), but the dominance of English as the language of science isn't likely to change anytime soon. Certainly, reviewers and editors need to do more to support non-native English-speaking authors, but you can also improve your publication success rate by understanding the global barriers you can control. You might find your work rejected by English-language journals for any of the following reasons:

- Misinterpreting a journal's mission or submitting your paper to the wrong journal
- Language barriers
- Value differences in the scientific newsworthiness or significance of your research
- Lack of a common understanding of scientific rigor and methodology
- Technology barriers such as outdated versions of word-processing programs, making it difficult for editors and authors to exchange files

Fortunately, it's possible to overcome these barriers, including helping you as an author and editors of English-language journals understand some of the differences inherent to global authors and their work.

Fitting Your Work to a Journal's Mission

It has become increasingly easy for an international author to submit a paper to a journal in another country. Author guidelines that clearly state a journal's preferences regarding manuscript style and length are readily available online, and most journal editors are easily accessible by email. You can read the author guidelines to find the types of topics of interest to the editor and then simply send an email to inquire about possible publication. (Learn more about email queries in Chapter 3.) Most manuscripts are now submitted either by email or through electronic editorial management systems.

However, you won't get to manuscript submission unless you do some upfront research and consider how the mission of a journal fits with your topic.

Upfront research includes examining the global literature. Cheung (2010) reports that non-native English-speaking authors find that reading previous issues of the journal to which they plan to submit before starting their own manuscripts is a particularly helpful tool. Li and Flowerdew (2020) suggest that *textual mentorship* (reading other articles on your topic) and examining the structure and content of these articles is a necessary step because it provides information about the science as well as helping with paragraph formation and logical flow, which may differ depending on the language in which an article is written.

Develop excellent search strategies for finding the right articles; look for databases that yield references of a global nature and develop a thorough understanding of the global state of knowledge for a topic. (Learn more about databases in Chapter 4.) This research will help you cast the topic in a global light, making it more likely to be published. There's an added benefit: You'll learn about journals that might previously have been outside your scope of reading.

Q *There have been no articles published on my topic of interest in my country, although research has been done on this topic in other countries. Would a manuscript on this topic be of interest to an international journal?*

A Publishing articles on knowledge that is already widely accepted globally might be of interest to journals in that specific country but are generally not of interest to global journals.

You'll usually find the journal's mission printed in its first few pages and on its website. For example, the mission of the *Journal of Nursing Scholarship* is

> ...to advance knowledge to improve the health of the world's people. We are therefore, most interested in receiving manuscripts that provide new knowledge designed to improve nursing practice globally. (*Journal of Nursing Scholarship*, n.d., para. 1)

That mission tells you what would—and would not—interest that journal's readers. Take a look at some examples.

> Compassion fatigue in Japanese nurses
>
> Conflict resolution and burnout in nurses in Iran

The mission refers to "...the health of the *world's* people" and "...designed to improve nursing practice *globally.*" Both sample topics seem to address regional, not global, issues, so they might not be a good fit.

However, if the manuscript on compassion fatigue in Japanese nurses provides new information about compassion fatigue and how to decrease it that could be used by nurses in other countries, the article is much more likely to be published in the *Journal of Nursing Scholarship* than if the study provides knowledge that can be used only in a specific population. Similarly, burnout is a global problem, but it would be important that information about conflict resolution and burnout address global knowledge, not simply the situation in a particular country, so that it would be of interest to nurses in the 103 countries where the *Journal of Nursing Scholarship* is read.

Authors not only need to know about the mission of a journal but must also consider its quality. The advent of open-access journals has created many more avenues for publishing scientific work, but not all journals are of equal quality. It may be difficult for global authors to assess the global reputation of a specific journal, but bibliometric indices (which help determine the impact of a particular journal), circulation numbers, and information about the electronic databases in which journals are indexed are all measures of quality.

Although journal impact factors are not the only measure of quality, it's an important indicator as to whether your manuscript is being published in an English language journal that other scientists actually read (Baron, 2012). Ensuring that your work is being published in a journal that is indexed in electronic databases such as MEDLINE or the Cumulative Index to Nursing and Allied Health Literature (CINAHL) makes your work accessible to other researchers—if others can't find your work, the impact of that work will be severely limited. (Learn more about selecting a journal in Chapter 3.)

Q *I keep getting emails from journal editors asking me to submit my work to their journal. It makes sense to me to submit to a journal that wants to publish the work of scientists for whom English is not a first language. Is there any disadvantage in publishing in one of the journals that has contacted me?*

A Check if the journal is listed in reputable indices such as CINAHL or Web of Science, which lists the *impact factor* (a measure of the number of times articles in a specific journal are cited by others based on the number of articles published by the journal). Another reliable source is the Directory of Nursing Journals (https://nursingeditors.com/journals-directory), a vetted list from the International Academy of Nurse Editors and the publication *Nurse Author & Editor*.

If a journal to which you would like to submit is listed, you are likely safe to proceed. Not being listed doesn't mean the journal isn't high quality, but it signals that you should be cautious and explore a bit more. Ask about the number of subscribers, or, in the case of online journals, the frequency of article viewings; the peer-review process; and the organization funding the journal. Note that it takes a few issues before a new journal can be indexed.

Be cautious if a journal does not appear to be indexed in any reputable databases. It could be a sign of a *predatory journal*, which expects authors to pay to have their articles published; these journals are usually of poor quality and put self-interest ahead of scholarship (InterAcademy Partnership, 2022). Not only do predatory publishers fail to ensure publication standards are met but they also fail to guarantee that your work will be widely disseminated. See Chapter 3 for more information about predatory journals.

Writing in a Second Language

For authors who use English as a second language, the burden of needing to read as well as to write in English is a barrier in global dissemination of knowledge.

An important strategy for overcoming this barrier is to avoid writing first in your native language and then translating to English (Svavasdottir, 2008). Writing in English from the start supports clarity of the flow of ideas, and the syntax and the construction of your points are more likely to be understood by an English-speaking audience. For authors who use English as a second language, language nuances and stylistic differences—more than grammatical differences—can result in authors not making effective arguments. Cho (2009) found that discourse levels (such as organization and formation of paragraphs) was more important than grammar in whether or not an article was published.

Poor word choice can be distracting to reviewers and impede their understanding of the science in an article. Some examples of inappropriate word choices include essence of life (quality of life), conscious consent (informed consent), and initial prevention (primary prevention; Rezaei-Adaryani, 2012). Compare your word choices with those used in your references, and have a native English speaker who is familiar with word choices read your manuscript to avoid problems.

Here are some tips that can help non-native English-speaking authors improve their writing (European Association of Science Editors, 2018; Nature Reviews Bioengineering, 2023; O'Moore-Klopf, 2017):

- Avoid extremely long paragraphs and very short sentences that don't provide enough information. For example, a statement such as, "Cognitive function was assessed," should include the tool used to assess function and who did the assessment.

- Don't omit articles (a, an, the) in front of words. For example, "Testing for degree of mothers' commitment showed..." should be "Testing for the degree of mothers' commitment..."

- Be sure your subject (topic of the sentence) and the verb (action of the sentence) match. For example, "Participants (subject) completes (verb) a survey..." should be "Participants complete a survey..."

- Use the right verb tense. The main ones you need to know are present, past, and future. For example, "The nurse takes (present tense) the patient to the operating room," "The nurse took (past tense) the patient to the operating room," and "The nurse will take (future tense) the patient to the operating room."

- Use English scientific terms and avoid idioms and colloquial expressions that may be common in your native language but not in English.

- Don't use too many acronyms and keep the language simple and clear. You want to explain key concepts, but not overwhelm readers.

- Be aware of literal translations from one language into English, which can often be wrong (referred to as "false friends"). For example, in Italian, "terrificante" means "terrible" not "terrific," and "incidente" means "car crash" not "incident.

You can learn more about writing effectively in Chapter 6, but you also may want to seek the expertise of an editor who specializes in working on manuscripts by non-native English-speaking authors. However, be aware that although translation and language editing services are more common than ever, it's difficult to ensure that authors are getting quality for cost. You might find that working with universities and English-speaking friends helps you achieve a higher-quality manuscript before you send it for translation.

Many publishers and several international publishing companies offer translation and language editing services. Unfortunately, these services can be very costly, superficial, and at times inaccurate (Akst, 2020). Before choosing a service, ask if the translator or language editor has expertise in your topic area, so that nuances of language do not become problematic. You also should ask how long it takes for the service and what the fee is. Reviews from others who have used the service are probably the most helpful in selecting a translator or editor. Some web-based translation services also are available, but as with all translation services, the expertise of the translator in terms of knowledge of the language and the science affects quality.

You can search online for possible translation and language editing options by entering the phrase "English language editing services" into the search engine.

Another option to improve communication in scientific writing is to include scientists who are native English speakers as part of your research team. It's not always possible to have a native English speaker who is geographically close, but with current technology, it has become increasingly possible to belong to a scientific community that is not geographically bound. Finally, spend some time exploring technology options.

Using Technology to Improve Scholarly Writing

Recent advances in technology, especially in artificial intelligence (AI), have yielded tools that can help authors who are non-native English speakers. Chat-GPT, for example, can help with language translation, as well as checking for spelling and grammar errors, and can improve logical flow and consistency (Lyon, 2023). Other AI tools that can help with grammar and some basic writing skills include Grammarly (https://www.grammarly.com) and Rytr.me (https://rytr.me). Just as spell-check in Microsoft Word is widely accepted as a useful tool to avoid spelling errors, these other tools, which are more economical and more available than many editing services, can be equally helpful in avoiding grammatical errors and in improving the flow and organization of manuscripts.

Q *I have had no luck publishing in English-language journals. Reviewers do not mention language issues in discussing my manuscripts, but they often speak about idea flow. I am not sure what they mean.*

A There are cultural differences in logic and how ideas are presented to make a scientific case. Try reading a lot of different articles from the journal in which you plan to submit and outlining how logical flow is developed. Use this outline of logical flow in developing your own outline for your manuscript. Reading for style, use of subheadings, and length is also helpful in developing a polished manuscript.

AI programs such as Consensus and ChatGPT can be helpful in conducting and organizing literature searches, thereby decreasing time spent in article preparation (Misra & Chandwar, 2023). Although AI tools can be useful for creating initial drafts of some parts of a manuscript (such as the methods section), you must check the output carefully for accuracy. Using AI tools to generate full manuscripts isn't practical because they can't be relied upon to provide accurate content (Misra & Chandwar, 2023). Another issue is that the AI tool doesn't ensure that content is original, so plagiarism becomes a real threat. (Publishers routinely check for plagiarism, which makes it unlikely your article will be accepted for publication.) Keep in mind that AI tools cannot be listed as authors because they can't take responsibility for the submitted manuscript (Committee on

> **Tips for Authors**
>
> Here are some tips for non-native English-speaking authors:
>
> - Choose the journal where you would like your article published. Before and while you write, review several articles from that journal to get a sense of style, flow, and word choice. Following the same general style of subheadings, length, and flow will help you write an article that is more recognizable (and, therefore, more easily reviewed) by reviewers and editors.
>
> - Work with colleagues who are native English speakers to develop an outline for the manuscript. Often, there are cultural differences when presenting scientific arguments. Native English speakers can help to ensure the points that need to be made are placed in the manuscript in a way that is understandable to English-speaking readers and that points are made with a proper degree of forcefulness to ensure that they are understood by the global scientific community.
>
> - Set your word-processing-program preferences to English so that you can use the spell-check and grammar-check features.
>
> - Ask for peer review from others before you submit your article, especially if you can obtain peer review from native English speakers.
>
> - Check with the editor whether the journal provides any additional support to authors who have English as a second language.
>
> - Find grammatical help.
>
> - Use language-editing services if they are available to you. Be sure to evaluate carefully before selecting a service.
>
> - Use artificial intelligence tools for help with article quality including grammar, spelling, organization, and logic flow.

Publication Ethics, 2023; International Committee of Medical Journal Editors [ICMJE], 2024). In addition, journals usually require that you disclose if you used AI technology (such as using large language models for data collection) in producing the manuscript (ICMJE, 2024).

Other factors that authors writing in a second language need to consider are value differences, scientific rigor and methodology, and ethics.

Understanding Global Value Differences

Significance in research is the understanding of the real meaning of a research study. Defining significance means getting beyond the simple facts and understanding *why* the research is important and what potential impact it could have. Globally, nurses are conducting significant research, but explaining that significance is often challenging. Cultures can see these values differently. A nurse from China might see a different relevance than a journal editor or peer reviewer from the United States. Until one can understand what an English-language journal audience finds relevant, this value difference can cause a barrier to publishing for global authors.

Try supporting the significance of the study you're writing about by explaining how global leaders—such as the World Health Organization or the National Academy of Medicine—have framed the topic. Understanding it in global terms can help a reviewer understand the significance of a problem that might not be common in the geographic area where they live.

In a study of editors, Flowerdew (2001) found that *parochialism* (viewing your topic too narrowly in your geographical area) was a barrier for multilingual scientists that kept them from getting published. If you don't describe the significance of your work beyond your local context, peer reviewers will likely not find the work you do to be significant. To combat parochialism, define the global significance from conceptualization of your research project, long before you've thought of where you'll publish. Communicate with international colleagues with an interest in a similar area of research and examine how your study will fit into the needs of the global community (Fazel, 2013).

These international conversations are key components in developing quality research projects and help ensure that the significance of a study is framed so that multiple communities understand its value.

Q *What specific help do journals provide to authors with English as a second language?*

A Resources vary by journal. For example, the *Journal of Nursing Scholarship* has a list of writing resources available on its website, including those available through the journal's publisher. Journals often work closely with editorial board members around the globe to identify local resources, and some have global pools of reviewers who are also helpful in reading for science, not language. Other journals can spend additional editing resources on particularly promising manuscripts before they are resubmitted for further review.

Scientific Rigor and Methodology

Another difference stemming from global cultures can be how scientific methodology is communicated. There are globally accepted conventions for how scientific studies are best communicated, and ensuring that your study contains all the relevant pieces with enough detail helps reviewers and editors to adequately evaluate your work (Simon et al., 2020). If the global "gold standards" for research methods and data analysis aren't used, reviewers often raise questions about the adequacy of a manuscript (Kaplan, 2001).

In nursing, the areas of scientific rigor most likely to be omitted are:

- Information in support of sample size and sample selection
- Information about how design is most appropriate to answer research questions
- Information about the validity and reliability of data collection methods (quantitative studies) or the trustworthiness of data collection and analysis (qualitative studies)

To ensure reviewers understand the rigor of your study, include specific information that justifies sample size and sample selection and provides information about the rigor of the methodology and the appropriateness of the design to answer the research question. (See Chapter 14 for more information on writing a research article.)

Ethics in Publishing for Writers With English as a Second Language

Ethics in publication do have some cultural determinants, so it's helpful for authors to periodically read the guidelines of the Committee on Publication Ethics (n.d.; http://publicationethics.org/resources/guidelines). Although there is universal agreement about the dishonesty of falsifying data, an area that might be a more significant ethical consideration for authors with English as a second language is duplicate publication.

Almost all journals have access to software that provides information on how much of a manuscript is word-for-word the same as other online sources. Writers for whom English is a second language might find that duplicating the language of other scientists in their field improves clarity. However, too often words are copied, and the source of these words is not identified. If authors are going to use the words of others, they need to use quotation marks and adequately reference these words. If an editor finds duplication between a submitted work and the work of others in a manuscript, that manuscript is likely to be rejected, and the ethics of the author are likely to be questioned. (Learn more about publishing ethics in Chapter 11.)

Pathway to Success

Communication within the scientific community is key for the success of global authors. When English is your second language, you can help ensure your manuscript's success by building a team of scientists with different strengths and abilities, including facility with different languages. After your study begins, pay attention to what journals might be a good fit for dissemination of your findings.

> ### Confidence Booster
>
> In all disciplines, the numbers of manuscripts from non-native English speakers being submitted and being published is rising. Your manuscript might be one of those rising numbers; taking into account the concepts in this chapter will increase the likelihood of your success.

When you begin writing a manuscript, use some of the tips in this chapter to help you through the process. Research and submit your work to journals where editors and reviewers are likely to understand the importance of global scientific diversity.

The need for non-native English speakers to publish in English-language journals isn't likely to change soon. Just remember that persistence is a necessary attribute for all authors who ultimately succeed in being published (Uzener, 2008). When English is your second language, that same persistence can result in the satisfaction of seeing your name in print and sharing your information with the world.

Write Now!

1. Identify a topic for a current article. Then go online and identify global publications on this topic.
2. For your next upcoming project, identify global scientists who could help you plan the project so that global considerations are met.

References

Akst, J. (2020, March 10). Publishing in English presents challenges for international authors. *The Scientist*. https://www.the-scientist.com/news-opinion/publishing-in-english-presents-challenges-for-international-authors-67241

Baron, T. H. (2012). ABC's of writing medical papers in English. *Korean Journal of Radiology, 13*(Suppl 1), S1–S11. https://doi.org/10.3348/kjr.2012.13.S1.S1

Cheung, Y. L. (2010). First publications in refereed English journals: Difficulties, coping strategies, and recommendations for student training. *System, 38*(1), 134–141. https://doi.org/10.1016/j.system.2009.12.012

Cho, D. S. (2009). Science journal paper writing in an EFL context: The case of Korea. *English for Specific Purposes, 28*(4), 230–239. https://doi.org/10.1016/j.esp.2009.06.002

Committee on Publication Ethics. (n.d.). *Guidelines*. http://publicationethics.org/resources/guidelines

Committee on Publication Ethics. (2023). *Authorship and AI tools: COPE position statement*. https://publicationethics.org/cope-position-statements/ai-author

Di Bitetti, M. S., & Ferreras, J. A. (2016). Publish (in English) or perish: The effect on citation rates of using languages other than English in scientific publications. *Ambio, 46*(1), 121–127. https://doi.org/10.1007/s13280-016-0820-7

Drubin, D, G., & Kellogg, D. R. (2012). English as the universal language of science: Opportunities and challenges. *Molecular Biology of the Cell, 23*(8), 1399. https://doi.org/10.1091/mbc.E12-02-0108

European Association of Science Editors. (2018). EASE guidelines for authors and translators of scientific articles published in English. *European Science Editing, 44*(4), e1–e6. https://doi.org/10.20316/ESE.2018.44.e1

Fazel, I. (2013). Writing for journal publication: An overview of NNES challenges and strategies. *Pan-Pacific Association of Applied Linguistics, 17*(1), 95–114. https://files.eric.ed.gov/fulltext/EJ1026109.pdf

Flowerdew, J. (2001). Attitudes of journal editors to nonnative speaker contributions. *TESOL Quarterly, 35*(1), 121–150. https://doi.org/10.2307/3587862

Flowerdew, J. (2022). Models of English for research publication. Purposes. *World Englishes, 41*(4), 571–583. https://doi.org/10.1111/weng.12606

InterAcademy Partnership. (2022). *Combatting predatory academic journals and conferences* [Summary report]. https://palast.ps/sites/default/files/inline-files/2.%20Summary%20report%20-%20English.pdf

International Committee of Medical Journal Editors. (2024). *Recommendations for the conduct, reporting, editing, and publication of scholarly work in medical journals*. http://www.icmje.org/recommendations

Journal of Nursing Scholarship. (n.d.). *Author guidelines*. https://sigmapubs.onlinelibrary.wiley.com/hub/journal/15475069/about/forauthors

Kaplan, R. B. (2001). English—The accidental language of science? In U. Aamon (Ed.), *The dominance of English as a language of science: Effects on other languages and language communities* (pp. 9–20). Mouton de Gruyter. https://doi.org/10.1515/9783110869484.3

Kojima, R., & Popiel, H. (2022). Using guidelines to improve scientific writing: Tips on use of correct verb tenses for non-native English speaking researchers. *Journal Korean Medical Science, 37*(29). https://doi.org/10.3346/jkms.2022.37.e226

Lenharo, M. (2023). The true cost of science's language barrier for non-native English speakers. *Nature, 619*(7971), 678–679. https://doi.org/10.1038/d41586-023-02320-2

Li, Y., & Flowerdew, J. (2020). Teaching English for research publication purposes (ERPP): A review of language teachers/pedagogical initiatives. *English for Specific Purposes, 59*, 29–241. https://doi.org/10.1016/j.esp.2020.03.002

Lu, C., Bu, Y., Dong, X., Wang, J., Ding, Y., Lariviere, V., Sugimoto, C. R., Paul, L., Zhang, C. (2019). Analyzing linguistic complexity and scientific impact. *Journal of Informetrics, 13*(3), 817–829. https://doi.org/10.1016/j.joi.2019.07.004

Lyon, D. (2023). Artificial intelligence for oncology nursing authors: Potential utility and concerns about large language model chatbots [Editorial]. *Oncology Nursing Forum, 50*(3), 276–277. https://doi.org/10.1188/23.ONF.276-277

Misra, D. P., & Chandwar, K. (2023). ChatGPT, artificial intelligence and scientific writing: What authors, peer reviewers and editors should know. *Journal of the Royal College of Physicians Edinburgh, 53*(2), 90–93. https://doi.org/10.1177/14782715231181023

Nature Reviews Bioengineering. (2023). Overcoming the language barrier in science communication [Editorial]. *Nat Rev Bioeng, 1*, 305. https://doi.org/10.1038/s44222-023-00073-1

O'Moore-Klopf, K. (2017). *Working with authors who are non-native English speakers* [PowerPoint Slides].

Rezaei-Adaryani, M. (2012). Letters to the editor: Advice for non-English authors writing for international nursing journals. *International Nursing Review, 59*(1), 4. https://doi.org/10.1111/j.1466-7657.2011.00972.x

Simon, E. L., Osei-Ampofo, M., Wachira, B. W., & Kwan, J. (2020). Getting accepted—Successful writing for scientific publication low- and middle-income countries. *African Journal of Emergency Medicine, 10*(Suppl 2), S154–S157. https://doi.org/10.1016/j.afjem.2020.06.006

Steigerwald, E., Ramirez-Castaneda, V., Brandt, D. Y. C., Baldi, A., Shapiro, J. T., Bowker, L., & Tarvin, R. D. (2022). Overcoming language barriers in Academia: Machine translation tools and a vision for a multilingual future. *Bioscience, 72*(10), 988–998. https://doi.org/10.1093/biosci/biac062

Svavasdottir, E. (2008, July). *Publication for authors with English as a second language* [Paper presentation]. Sigma Theta Tau 19th International Research Congress, Singapore.

Uzener, S. (2008). Multilingual scholars' participation in core/global academic communities: A literature review. *Journal of English for Academic Purposes, 7*(4), 250–263. https://doi.org/10.1016/j.jeap.2008.10.007

Weaver, R., & Jackson, D. (2011). Evaluating an academic writing program for nursing students who have English as a second language. *Contemporary Nurse, 38*(1-2), 130–138. https://doi.org/10.5172/conu.2011.38.1-2.130

Yanbing, S., Hua, L., Chao, L., Fenglan, W., & Zhiguang, D. (2021). The state of nursing research from 2000 to 2019: A global analysis. *Journal of Advanced Nursing, 77*(1) 162–175. https://doi.org/10.1111/jan.14564

Legal and Ethical Issues

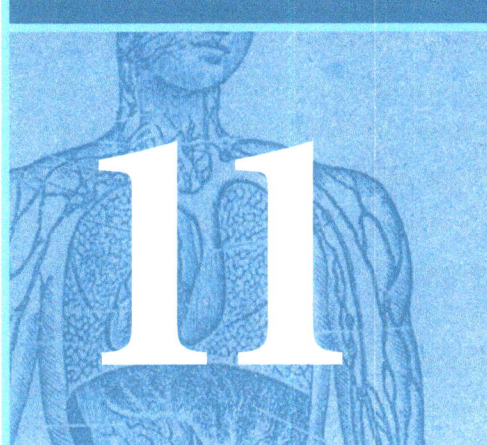

–Nancy J. Brent, JD, MS, RN

"Write what should not be forgotten."
–Isabel Allende

WHAT YOU'LL LEARN IN THIS CHAPTER

- When using another's work in your work, you need to obtain the proper permission.
- When you write, don't plagiarize, and be wary of text recycling.
- Maintain the privacy and confidentiality of patient information.
- Always adhere to publishing ethics.

Writing an article, chapter, or textbook and then seeing your work in print is an exciting experience. Although not nearly as exciting, you also must be aware of legal and ethical issues related to writing, just as you are aware of legal and ethical issues in your daily practice (e.g., ethical issues surrounding end-of-life care). The most important legal concern for an author is compliance with United States copyright law. Ethically, consistency with established principles for writers also is essential. In some cases, such as confidentiality and plagiarism, legal and ethical issues overlap.

This chapter gives you an overview of copyright law and selected ethical issues you need to know to make your writing experience as easy as possible, while keeping a steady eye on your legal and ethical responsibilities.

Copyright and Permissions

New—and even experienced—authors often have questions about copyright. Although copyright law can be complex, some basic information will help you sort out what you need to know.

What Is a Copyright?

Generally, a *copyright* is a type of intellectual property that protects original works of authorship as soon as the author fixes the work in a tangible form of expression (US Copyright Office, n.d.-a, n.d.-b). This legal protection allows a creator of a work of art, literature, or written work the right to control how that work is used (Fishman, 2024). Creators can be authors, photographers, artists, poets, and even nurse researchers. The US Copyright Act of 1976 protects

This chapter is not intended to be legal (or other) specific advice. Readers needing specific advice should seek guidance from a professional.

artwork, photographs, novels, sculptures, computer software, magazine articles, book chapters, songs, and more. Remember that copyright refers to works that are in print, online, or in any other format.

Establishing a copyright grants the author certain rights. Those rights have been defined as the legal right to an author, composer, playwright, or distributor to exclusive publication, production, sale, or distribution of a literary, musical, dramatic, or artistic work (The Free Dictionary, n.d.). In other words, these rights protect your work from unauthorized use, including duplication rights (copying the work), economic rights (selling the rights, receiving royalties), and rewriting or adapting the copyrighted work in some way (Fishman, 2024).

A copyright protects a work against *infringement*, which occurs when someone uses the work without the expressed permission of the creator, such as incorporating a table from a copyrighted article into another article without the permission of the copyright holder.

The United States Copyright Act does not protect everything. For example, concepts, ideas, systems, or methods of doing something are not protected (US Copyright Office, n.d.-a, n.d.-b). For writers, however, the Act protects what is important: the words with which a writer expresses ideas and facts (Fishman, 2024).

How Do I Obtain a Copyright?

In most cases, you don't need to file for copyright after your work is created. In short, a work is protected after it is written down, typed into a computer, or dictated.

Q *Do I need to copyright my work before I submit it to a publisher for publication?*

A No. If your work is accepted for publication with a journal, magazine, website, or book publisher, your publisher will have you sign a transfer of copyright from you to the publisher, but you do not need to formally obtain copyright ahead of time. Obtaining copyright beforehand can cause problems with any required agreement you'll be asked to sign and possibly any pay you might receive.

Q *My publishing contract says that my article is "work made for hire" and that the publisher owns the copyright. Can I reuse any of the material?*

A *Work made for hire* is work that the publisher has contracted from you. Upon completion and acceptance of your work, the publisher owns it—and can, in fact, edit it, repurpose it, and even republish it. Depending on the type of work, writers may earn more for creating this sort of content because they can't reuse it. The bottom line is that writers who enter into this type of arrangement will not retain the copyright, and they will have to contact the publisher to obtain permission to reuse the material.

In some instances, creators of a copyrighted work might want to independently register their work with the Copyright Office (US Copyright Office, n.d.-a), for example, when authors want to make the public aware that they are the holder of the copyright. This might be the case if, for instance, the author developed an innovative nursing practice model. Registration can take place with the use of hard copy forms or through the US Copyright Office's online Registration Portal at https://www.copyright.gov/registration (user login required).

Registration of the work also opens the door to allowing attorney's fees and statutory money damages under the Act if the work is infringed upon and the creator decides to sue.

Do I Need a Copyright Notice on My Work?

A copyright notice on any work is optional for works created after March 1, 1989 (US Copyright Office, 2021a, 2021b), but many authors include a notice, especially when distributing their material to an audience during a presentation or to the public under other circumstances (e.g., in a blog).

The copyright notice consists of three elements and can be used in any of the following forms (US Copyright Office, 2021a, 2021b):

Copyright 2023 Mary Thompson.

Copr. 2023 Mary Thompson.

© 2023 Mary Thompson.

Unfortunately, some people erroneously believe that if a work is online, it's in the public domain, but that isn't true. In fact, materials online, whether in the form of a blog, an article, or research findings, are protected by copyright law. The Digital Millennium Copyright Act was passed by Congress in 1988, which addresses copyright issues in the digital world (Hall, 2023). It established, among other things, safe harbors for internet providers and procedures for the identification and removal of online material that is an infringement of a copyright owner's exclusive rights.

Q *What are copyright rules related to social media?*

A Copyright law applies to social media. When you upload material to Facebook, for example, you retain the copyright to your material and grant Meta, Facebook's parent company, a license to use and to display it. You can learn more about your intellectual property rights and responsibilities when using Facebook by reviewing its "Terms of Service" at facebook.com/terms.php and its "Intellectual Property" page (https://transparency.fb.com/policies/community-standards/).

X (previously Twitter) and other social media apps also are regulated by copyright law through the application of Title II of the Digital Millennium Copyright Act. X's help center (https://help.twitter.com/en/rules-and-policies/copyright-policy) contains information related to copyright, including what to do if someone posts something that infringes on your copyright.

You can usually find copyright information for a social media app on its website. For instance, Instagram's help center answers common copyright questions at https://help.instagram.com/126382350847838.

The world of social media changes quickly, so be aware of copyright issues for any tools that you use.

In short, you must obtain permission for text, artwork, photographs, figures, and any other created content, whether online or in print. If you're unsure if material is copyrighted, you should assume that work published after March 1, 1989, is protected under the Copyright Act.

Individual copyright holders and publishers may specify how the permission should be listed. Publishers always include a copyright notice on the copyright page of a book or a journal, such as Copyright © 2024 by Sigma Theta Tau International.

Q *How do I find the publisher of a book or an article?*

A For a book, look on the copyright page, which follows the title page in the front of the book. In the case of a journal or magazine, this information might be located near the table of contents page for a specific issue, on the inside of the front or back cover of the journal, or online at the publication's website.

Q *I recently used photos for a presentation that I found on the internet under a Creative Commons license. These were OK to use, right?*

A Not necessarily. Creative Commons is a nonprofit organization that gives individuals and organizations a way to grant copyright permission for their creative work. The creator can choose from six licenses, each with a different degree of restriction. The most permissive is CC BY ("attribution"), which allows others to distribute, remix, adapt, and build upon the work, even commercially, as long as they credit the author for the original creation. The most restrictive is CC BY-NC-ND ("attribution-noncommercial-no derivatives"), which allows others to download a work and share it with others as long as they credit the author, don't change the work in any way, and don't use it commercially. Creative Commons also offers a public domain option, which means there is no restriction on use of the work; the author has essentially "opted out" of copyright protection (Creative Commons, n.d.-a).

Each type of permission is associated with an icon (license button) that is then used with the work (see Figure 11.1). Creative Commons provides a tool to help creators choose the license that best fits their needs. Although not required, using the tool allows creators to obtain a license button embedded with a code that facilitates attribution of the work.

FIGURE 11.1 An example of a Creative Commons license button. (Attribution – NonCommerical – ShareAlike).

Many publishing houses and authors also state an additional caveat to the reader—a warning that serves as another way to alert the reader that the work is copyrighted and should not be infringed upon. An example of such a caveat is:

> No part of this work may be reproduced, distributed, or transmitted in any form or by any means, electronic or mechanical, including photocopying, recording, or stored in a database or retrieval system, without the express permission in writing of _____.

Copyright and Publishing

After you sell or release your work to a publisher, you may be able to retain your copyright. However, in most cases, you'll be asked to transfer the copyright of your work to the publisher. To do this, you must guarantee the publisher—in writing—that you have the right to transfer that copyright in its entirety. The two types of copyright transfer are *exclusive* and *assignment/all rights transfer* (Fishman, 2024).

An *exclusive* copyright transfer occurs when one or more rights of the copyright holder are transferred while others are retained (Fishman, 2024). For example, you may transfer to *American Nurse Journal* the exclusive right to publish your article on a new treatment option *for the first time* in the United States and Canada but retain the right to republish that article as one of the chapters in your doctoral thesis. *American Nurse Journal* owns the specific right to publish the article; you, as the author, retain remaining rights, such as republishing or creating a derivative work, not transferred to the journal (Fishman, 2024).

In contrast, an *assignment* or *all rights transfer* occurs when you, as the copyright owner, transfer all your rights of the copyright to a single publisher (Fishman, 2024). The publisher then owns all rights of the copyright; you, as the author, no longer hold any of the rights of the copyright. This is the more typical arrangement in nursing publications, including books.

Regardless of the type of transfer, the holder of the copyright can exercise its options with the manuscript in print form or electronic form. As a result, the journal publishing your article can print it in its journal or on its online publication.

Q *How long does copyright protection last?*

A Copyright protection doesn't last forever; the copyright exists for the life of the author plus 70 years. There are many exceptions and caveats to the rule, but the copyright could outlive you. Copyright is considered an asset and can even be assigned to your heirs as part of your estate.

Some authors are hesitant to relinquish copyright to a publisher because they don't understand why the publisher needs it. Consider that the publisher provides services such as editing, designing, production, distribution, marketing, and sales. The copyright protects the publisher's assets. In addition, the copyright transfer usually includes a statement that the author's name will always be associated with the work.

Copyright addendums to the publisher-author agreement exist to help authors retain certain rights to their works. The Scholars Copyright Addendum Engine helps authors generate a PDF form online that you can attach to a journal publishers' copyright agreement to ensure you retain certain rights (Creative Commons, n.d.-b). However, know that addendums are not typically used in nursing publishing, so you may meet with resistance from the publisher.

Some publishers also will license the copyright over a period of time, such as the life of the book. When the book is out of print, you might be able to request that your copyright be returned to you if you'd like to republish the book or repurpose the content.

Journals that are open access typically allow the author to retain copyright, although authors may still need to sign a contract giving the publisher the right to publish the work. Usually the work is then published under one of the more permissive Creative Commons licenses; the publisher may designate which options an author can choose from. (See Chapter 3 for more information about open access and copyright.)

As an author, before signing a transfer of copyright, you might want to have it reviewed by a nurse attorney, or another attorney with a concentrated practice in intellectual property.

Your informed choice about what right or rights you want to be associated with your original work is important. For example, is a more restricted access to your work through a copyright important to you, or would you prefer your work be more accessible, such as signing with Creative Commons? A useful reference is "Copyright, Creative Commons, and Confusion" (Harrington, 2020).

Noncompete Clauses

Publishing original works can result in financial benefits for publishers. Publishers also want to decrease any competition with these works. As a result, some publishing houses request authors not only transfer copyright rights to them but also include in the publishing agreement a *covenant not to compete* (CNC). These covenants can be quite broad and may last as long as the length of the copyright the publisher owns once it is transferred from the author (Schofield & Walker, 2018).

Challenges by authors to covenants not to compete in the publishing agreements are not common. As a result, publishers can craft a CNC to benefit their specific interests. Read any CNC carefully. If you are not comfortable with the CNC, negotiate with the publisher to make it more balanced (Schofield & Walker, 2018). Although you want your work to be widely disseminated—an objective shared with the publisher as well—you don't want to foreclose future publishing opportunities (Schofield & Walker, 2018). Also important is the "choice of laws" clause in your publishing agreement. The clause indicates which state law will be used if there is a challenge to the CNC or to any other provision of the publishing agreement.

If you think you are not able to handle negotiations in obtaining a more balanced CNC, consult with a nurse attorney, or another attorney whose practice is in intellectual property law.

Permissions and Citations

What happens when you're writing, and you want to use and credit copyrighted material from another work? The most common form of attributing copyright ownership in a writing product is through a citation of the material. A citation should include the author's name, the date of publication, the name of the work, the city where published, the publisher's name, and specific page numbers. The permission of the author or publisher is not needed when citing another's work this way. (Learn more about citations in Chapter 4.)

If, however, a large part of another's work is needed, or you want to include something extensive into your commentary, such as a form developed by another nurse researcher, then you must obtain the permission of the original author to include the material.

To do so, contact the copyright owner. If the owner is a publisher, you can check its website for a permission request section where such requests are handled automatically. If you can't find the information, contact the publisher by email and ask for the permissions department.

In most cases, publishers either have specific online forms on their websites that are used to grant permission to reprint portions of an article or a table, or the website directs authors to the Copyright Clearance Center (https://marketplace.copyright.com/rs-ui-web/mp), where authors complete an online request (a free account is required). The publisher normally provides clear directions as to how the credit for the requested content must appear in your article. You'll be notified by email whether your permission request has been granted or denied. Be sure to save the notification as evidence that you have obtained permission.

If the publisher does not have an automated system for permission requests, simply send a request that includes the specific information, as shown in Example 11.1 (data are fictional).

If the owner is an individual, you must contact the person and obtain written permission. You might be able to find their contact information in the written document (e.g., professor of nursing, University of ABC), or you might have to find the person through public sources. One such resource is the University of Texas searchable database, WATCH (Writers, Artists and Their Copyright Holders) website (https://norman.hrc.utexas.edu/watch; Fishman, 2024). Of course, you can also simply search for the author on a major search engine such as Google. In today's highly connected world, chances are you will be able to find the person.

Here are some other things to remember about permissions:

- The publisher might have restrictions on how the permitted use occurs. For instance, it might grant permission only for a first edition of a textbook, or permission might not extend to electronic forms of the textbook.

- The publisher might charge a fee for use of the material. Check the author guidelines or ask your editor about who is responsible for the fee—usually it's the author.

- Publishers who are members of STM (a trade association for academic and professional publishers) and have signed onto the STM Permissions Guidelines do not charge for certain items (e.g., three figures, tables, or images) if the new work will be reproduced in the journal or book of another publisher that also is part of STM (STM, 2022). However, you may still need to clear your request via email or the Copyright Clearance Center. Signatory STM Publishers include the American Association of Critical-Care Nurses, Elsevier, SAGE, and Wolters Kluwer Health/Lippincott Williams & Wilkins (STM, 2023).

- Individuals who own copyrighted material may use their own forms for granting permission to use their work. Many aspects of these forms are similar to those used by publishing companies.

Subject line:
Permission request for *Nursing Today* ← *Immediately state the purpose of your communication.*

I am requesting permission to use Figure 1, Nurses Entering the Workforce, which appeared in the February 2024 issue (Volume 3, Number 1) of *Nursing Today*. ← *Give complete citation information.*

The figure will be included in an article I am writing on orienting new nurses for the journal *Where Nursing Is Headed*. Attribution will be included. ← *Explain how the information will be used.* / *Note that you plan to credit the original source.*

If you agree to extend permission, please print, sign, scan, and return this note to me via email. If you cannot scan, please clearly indicate permission in your email reply.

If you have any questions, I can be reached at 212-398-4866 or j.brown@somewhere.com. ← *Give multiple ways you can be reached.*

Sincerely,
Jane Brown, MSN, CCRN

I/we hereby grant *Where Nursing Is Headed* permission to reprint and adapt Figure 1, Nurses Entering the Workforce, which appeared in the February 2024 issue (Volume 3, Number 1) of *Nursing Today*.

Please insert any preferred credit line:

Approved (print and sign name)/date:

This is an example of what you might have the person granting permission sign.

Some publishers want the source to be referenced in a specific way, for example: From Nursing Today, *February 2024. Copyright* Name of Publisher. *All Rights Reserved.*

You may not always receive a signed permission form. In that case, save the email in your files; the publisher will want to see documentation that shows you have permission for the reprint.

EXAMPLE 11.1 Sample permission email text.

It's best to start with the publication's website to learn about permission requirements. These are usually found in one of the drop-down menus at the top of the site.

Fair Use and Public Domain

Two major exceptions to the requirement of obtaining permission to use another's work in one's own include the *fair use doctrine*, and those works considered to be in the *public domain*.

The *fair use doctrine* identifies various purposes for which the reproduction of a work can be considered fair. Included in the list are news reporting, teaching, research, criticism, and comment (US Copyright Office, n.d.-a).

The fair use doctrine also describes four factors that a court considers in determining whether a use is fair:

- The purpose and character of the use, including whether the reproduction is commercial or for a nonprofit educational purpose
- The nature of the copyrighted work
- The amount and substantiality of the portion used in relation to the copyrighted work as a whole
- The effect of the use on the potential market for, or value of, the copyrighted work

Fair use is usually a short excerpt of a work with proper citation of the source. It can be difficult to determine what is and is not fair use, so always obtain permission from the copyright holder if you are unsure whether the copyrighted material fits into this doctrine.

Q *It's considered fair use as long as it's fewer than 500 words, right?*

A The "500-word rule" is a common misconception regarding fair use. In fact, a short sentence could be considered an infringement if it were so important that it would preclude anyone from referencing or purchasing the original work. Song lyrics, movie lines, and poetry are also problematic from a fair use standpoint. Avoid their use when possible—and when in doubt, request permission.

A second exception to the requirements of obtaining permission is the *public domain doctrine*, which states that any work not protected by copyright is in the public domain (Fishman, 2023). Public domain works include any works for which the copyright is lost, has expired, or was not renewed. It also includes anything published or funded by the government. Because there is no copyright protection, the public can use the work in any manner it chooses. You still need to properly cite the work.

Q *My study was funded by the National Institutes of Health (NIH). How does that affect copyright?*

A Investigators who are funded by the NIH must submit an electronic version of their final, peer-reviewed manuscript to the National Library of Medicine's PubMed Central (PMC) upon acceptance for publication. The full text of the article will become publicly available no later than 12 months after publication in a journal (NIH, 2022). Many other funding agencies also require or request authors to submit the accepted but not yet published article based on research they have funded to a repository where it can be accessed at no charge. (See Chapter 3 for more information about open access.)

There are several ways to identify works in the public domain. Most governmental publications are public domain works. If so, the publication states that the work is a public domain publication and can be reproduced and copied without permission, but it must be properly cited.

Nongovernmental publications in the public domain can be found in many sources, including The Public Domain Review (https://publicdomainreview.org). A comprehensive resource is Stephen Fishman's (2023) *The Public Domain: How to Find and Use Copyright-Free Writings, Music and More*.

Ethics of Publishing

Ethics can be defined as "the discipline dealing with what is good and bad and with moral duty and obligation" (Merriam-Webster, n.d.-a). Ethical principles govern every aspect of researching, writing, and publishing your original work. Two ethical areas of concern are authorship and conflicts of interest.

Authorship

Although the concept of authorship sounds straightforward, in the real world of publishing, it is not. Authorship makes explicit both the credit and the responsibility for the content of published articles (International Committee of Medical Journal Editors [ICMJE], 2024; World Association of Medical Editors [WAME], 2007).

Authorship should include all those who have made a substantial contribution to the article (ICMJE, 2024) and present an honest account of what took place during the development of the article, chapter, or research. ICMJE (2024 recommends that authors meet these four criteria:

- "Substantial contributions to the conception or design of the work; or the acquisition, analysis, or interpretation of data for the work; AND
- Drafting the work or reviewing it critically for important intellectual content; AND
- Final approval of the version to be published; AND
- Agreement to be accountable for all aspects of the work in ensuring that questions related to the accuracy or integrity of any part of the work are appropriately investigated and resolved."

However, the ICMJE criteria have been found lacking in specificity for the first two items. An International Society for Medical Publication Professionals (ISMPP) task force developed four categories for authorship criteria (Carfagno et al., 2022, p. 866). Note that authors can contribute to any one of them.

- **Concept and design:** Development or substantial modification of research idea, study design, methodology protocol, statistical analysis plan, or a combination of these activities; OR
- **Data acquisition:** Significant contribution of data (quality and quantity) to the final analyses; OR
- **Data analysis:** Performance of the data analysis and assurance of the integrity of the data and statistical analyses; OR
- **Data interpretation:** Derivation of conclusions, placement of results into context, or identification of knowledge gaps for future exploration."

Chatbots (such as ChatGPT) are not considered authors because they can't be responsible for the accuracy, integrity, and originality of the work (ICMJE, 2024). However, authors need to disclose whether they used artificial intelligence (AI) technology (such as large language models) in producing the manuscript (ICMJE, 2024; ISMPP, 2023; WAME, 2023).

There are three main ways a person or persons can falsely state authorship (Elsevier, 2022; Herron, 2023). The first is *gift authorship*: listing names of individuals who make no discernable contribution; for instance, a researcher lists the name of their department head, even though that person didn't substantially contribute to the manuscript. The second is *guest authorship*: adding a well-known researcher who wasn't involved in the study in an effort to enhance the manuscript's credibility. The third is *ghost authorship*: leaving out the names of those individuals who contribute substantially but are not listed..

Those who do not meet the criteria for authorship but contributed to the manuscript should be acknowledged instead of listed as an author. Examples of actions where an acknowledgement would be appropriate include funding acquisition; supervision of a research group or general administrative support; and writing assistance, such as technical editing, language editing, and proofreading (ICMJE, 2024).

Q *Who is a corresponding author?*

A Although all authors involved in a work take responsibility for the accuracy and integrity of a completed manuscript, the corresponding author handles correspondence with the editor and publisher, and with issues that might arise after the work is published. This author's name usually appears on the published work as the corresponding author, with a statement that any questions be directed to that individual. You should choose a corresponding author before writing begins.

If you're working with others to develop and write the results of your research, or to draft an article for publication, avoid potential authorship issues by discussing the issues of credit for the work *before* you begin, and then documenting your decisions in writing. For example, who will be the lead author? How will the authors be listed? Who, if anyone, needs to be acknowledged for their help with the finished product, even though they are not contributing to the actual writing? All authors should agree that there will be no gifting of authorship or any type of ghost authorship. If you have any doubt about who should or should not be listed as an author on your manuscript, consult with your editor. (See Chapter 1 for more information about team writing and author order.)

Some publications ask authors to list the contributions of each author for a manuscript; these may then be listed in the published article. Categories of contributions typically reflect the four ICMJE authorship criteria.

Conflicts of Interest

In the world of publishing, a *conflict of interest* exists when a divergence occurs between an individual author or authors' interests (competing interests) and their responsibilities to scientific and publishing activities, so that a reasonable reader may question whether the authors published product—for example, chapter, blog, or article—was motivated by that competing interest (ICMJE, 2024; WAME, 2009). Conflicts can be personal, financial, commercial, political, religious, or academic (ICMJE, 2024; WAME, 2009). Of these, financial relationships are the easiest to identify and include employment, consultancies, stock ownership, and paid honoraria (ICMJE, 2024).

For example, you are writing an article on a new model of nursing that has gained wide acceptance. You detail its many accomplishments in terms of staff morale and patient care. You do not disclose to the publisher, however, that you received financial support for developing the model. When this fact is discovered, the entire article, your credibility, and the publisher's integrity are brought into question.

It's essential, then, to declare a conflict of interest—or even a *possible* conflict of interest—to the publisher when submitting an article for publication. Most, if not all, publishers require this written declaration and have a form—often called a conflict of interest or disclosure statement—for the author to fill out with the submitted article.

A general rule is helpful here: If you're in doubt about a conflict, declare it. The editor or publisher can then decide whether it truly is a conflict and how to proceed with the article.

If a conflict of interest exists, its presence doesn't necessarily mean that the article, or manuscript (for a book) will not be accepted and published. Depending on the conflict, the publisher may simply note it when the work is published so that the information is transparent to the reader. Publishers must be careful to avoid even the appearance of presenting biased information without disclosure. Typically, statements related to conflict of interest include sources that financially supported the work (e.g., a research study funded by a pharmaceutical company) and the role of the sponsor in any aspect of the study (ICMJE, 2024).

If there is no conflict of interest, many publications routinely state that in the published materials.

Confidentiality and Privacy

Often when nurses publish an article, a book chapter, or a textbook, the contents deal with patient information or patient care issues that illustrate the theory or information presented. As a result, one overriding legal *and* ethical practice that a nurse author must adhere to is maintaining the privacy and confidentiality of the patient information presented in the written manuscript. Both privacy and confidentiality must be safeguarded because an invasion of privacy and a breach of confidentiality are two separate legal and ethical concepts.

Invasion of Privacy

An *invasion of privacy* can occur when one intrudes upon an individual's private life (Legal Dictionary, n.d.). When it comes to publishing, this could occur in several ways. One way is if you include in your article the patient's name or likeness (photograph) for your commercial advantage (the selling of the text) without the patient's consent.

Another example is if the patient's information meets the requirements for a public disclosure about private facts of the individual. In this type of invasion of privacy, the following must apply to the information disclosed (Legal Dictionary, n.d.):

- Private, truthful information is made public (e.g., your published book contains private facts about a patient).
- The information is not of public concern or interest.
- The information released would offend any reasonable person if published or widely disseminated.

You can avoid these allegations by simply obtaining the written permission of patients to include their information or likeness in your written article. Patients may provide you with full information or ask that certain information not be used. They also may request that you not use their real name and that some of the facts about the illness or treatment discussed in the manuscript be changed to further safeguard privacy.

Protecting a patient's privacy is in keeping with a nurse's ethical obligations (Fowler, 2015), and being a nurse author does not eliminate this ethical obligation. If consent can't be obtained from the patient or relative, it is essential to try to obtain informed consent from a legal representative of the patient (e.g., the executor of their estate) or seek permission from an institutional review board.

Some publishers have developed patient permission forms for you to download, but others do not since requirements vary between jurisdictions and organizations (Elsevier, n.d.). You can develop your own form based on those in a formbook such as *Publishing Forms and Contracts* by Roy Kaufman (2008) or consult with a nurse attorney or another attorney in your state who can develop a form for your use.

If you have any questions about protecting patient privacy that aren't covered in the author guidelines, contact the editor.

> **Confidence Booster**
>
> You may be feeling overwhelmed by all the information in this chapter. Know that the editor of the publication is a good resource for answering questions. Take a break with this confidence booster.
>
> Did you know that the late author Toni Morrison, a Nobel Prize and Pulitzer Prize winning writer, novelist, editor, and professor, was in her thirties and a professor at Howard University when she joined a writing group and began her first story about a young African American girl who wished she had blue eyes? That story later became the novel *The Bluest Eye*, which was published in 1970, when Morrison was 39 (Biography, 2021).

Breach of Confidentiality

The protection of patient information shared within a patient–healthcare provider relationship is a unique protection that requires the healthcare provider, including a nurse, not to share the information with a third party unless the consent of the patient is obtained. Although there are exceptions to that overall mandate (e.g., in an emergency, when there is a danger to the patient or to others), the nurse is obligated—again both legally and ethically (Fowler, 2015)—to maintain the confidentiality of the information shared.

Legally, this protection lies in state laws on patient privacy, including state mental health codes and patient privacy laws. If confidentiality is breached, the patient can sue for a breach of confidentiality *and* an invasion of privacy.

As in the case of protecting patient privacy, you can avoid allegations of a breach of confidentiality by obtaining the written permission of patients to use information obtained during their care and treatment. Changing some of the facts or circumstances about the patient can help further ensure confidentiality.

If you are developing a hypothetical case study based on your experiences with multiple patients, you do *not* need to obtain permission because you should not be providing the level of detail needed to identify a particular person. Too often, nurses veer from including real-life experiences for fear of violating confidentiality. However, the true-life experiences are often what drives home a point to a reader. One helpful resource, DeJong's article "Case Studies: Strategies to Protect Patient Privacy" (2012) is an easy-to-follow guide that will help you write case studies while protecting patient privacy.

State laws that protect patient confidentiality often require that specific content be included in a written release by a patient. As an author, you need to review any law in your state for required forms and use them as you write your manuscript. You can also seek a consultation with a nurse attorney, or another attorney whose practice includes confidentiality issues, to identify and obtain copies of those forms.

Some publishers require that forms related to privacy and confidentiality be submitted with the manuscript. Others require authors to state that they obtained consent, but do not collect the signed forms because of the security needed to store this sensitive material and potential legal liability related to privacy laws (Barbour & Committee on Publication Ethics, 2016; Elsevier, n.d.). Keep a copy of any forms you submit.

Avoiding Misconduct

Conducting and publishing research in nursing is an essential part of nursing practice. Indeed, findings from such research have improved clinical outcomes for many patients. When the results of a research project are published, it is vital that the publication is honest, clear, accurate, complete, and balanced; avoid misleading, selective, or ambiguous reporting (Wager & Kleinert, 2012).

Be careful not to condone, participate in, or allow any conduct that compromises your research project and that violates any ethical codes, including the "Code of Ethics for Nurses With Interpretive Statements" (American Nurses Association, 2015) and the "Association for Institutional Research [AIR] Statement of Ethical Principles" (AIR, 2019). Examples of violations related to publishing include not crediting proper authorship of the research study, not maintaining the confidentiality of research participant data, and not being transparent about conflicts of interest.

The Office of Research Integrity (n.d.) notes that research misconduct involves fabrication, falsification, or plagiarism in conducting research and reporting its results.

Plagiarism

Plagiarism, described as dishonest and reprehensible, is not illegal in and of itself, but it raises legal and ethical issues (Anderson, 2016). For example, plagiarism that involves substantial copyright infringement can result in civil or criminal liability (Anderson, 2016). Even without "substantial" infringement, plagiarism is still serious and may result in equally frightening legal ramifications.

In essence, plagiarism is literary theft (Merriam-Webster, n.d.-b), and occurs when one takes another's work, copyrighted or not, and passes it off as their own (Fishman, 2024). Those who steal only works in the public domain are not infringing on a copyright because the Copyright Act provides an exception for works in the public domain. However, in addition to the breach of ethics, there are always potential additional legal consequences to plagiarizing another's work.

For example, when you submit an article for consideration for publication, you often must *warrant* (guarantee) that the work is original. If it's not but you say it is, the publisher or owner can file a breach of contract action or a case alleging fraud against you. In the world of academics, plagiarizing another's work can result in loss of a job (if a teacher) or ramifications from violating a student code of conduct (e.g., probation, dismissal from the program). In the world of publishing, such a breach clearly results in a loss of integrity and honesty that follows authors for the rest of their professional career. In fact, most publishers now routinely use software programs to check for possible plagiarism before sending the manuscript for peer review.

If you used any AI-generated text in preparing your article, check it with other sources to ensure it's accurate, free of plagiarism, and appropriately referenced (Holleywood, 2023). You can use a free plagiarism checking tool such as Scibbr (https://www.scribbr.com/plagiarism-checker), but know that these tools aren't foolproof. As noted earlier, disclose any use of AI when you submit the article.

You may have heard the terms *redundant* or *duplicate publishing*, where an author reports all or a substantial portion of information that appeared elsewhere in a different work (JAMA Network Editors, 2020). This is sometimes referred to as *self-plagiarism* (American Psychological Association, 2020). Although not plagiarism, *salami slicing*, where an author breaks up a study that could be reported as whole into multiple articles, should be avoided because readers can get a distorted view of the significance of the findings (Gennaro, 2021).

Terms such as duplicate publishing and self-plagiarism are imprecise and confusing. In addition, sometimes it is appropriate to reuse information; for example, an author might want to use portions of a literature review from a grant proposal in an article (Hall et al., 2021a). Text recycling is a more helpful term.

Text Recycling

Text recycling is defined by the Text Recycling Research Project (TRRP) as when an author reuses textual material in a new writing that is "identical" or "substantively equivalent in form and content" to its source, is not marked by quotations in the second writing, and at least one of the authors of the second writing is also an author of the prior document (Hall et al., 2021a). Text recycling can be professionally appropriate, ethical, legal, and desirable for clear communication. But it can also be inappropriate, illegal, and unethical, depending on the context of the recycling (Hall et al., 2021a).

Context can be evaluated within the four categories of text recycling identified by TRRP (Hall et al., 2021a, 2021b; Moskovitz, 2021):

- *Developmental recycling* is reuse of material that has not been published, such as content from a poster in a journal article. This is acceptable in most situations.

- *Generative recycling* is the reuse of portions of a previously published work in a new work that makes an original intellectual contribution distinct from the original source. For example, an author may reuse a description of a research method. Whether this is acceptable depends on the specifics of the case, such as the amount of material reused and transparency with editors and readers.

- *Adaptive publication* is the republication of all or the central part of the work, but the work has been modified to fit another context such as a different target audience. An example is reusing material from a published journal article in a blog or magazine article on the same topic. This is acceptable only if the author obtains permission from the copyright holder (usually the publisher of the original work) and is transparent with editors and readers.

- *Duplicate publication* is the publication of a work that is the same in genre, content, and intended audience as the originally published work—for example, making only superficial changes in a published article before submitting it to another journal. This practice is considered unethical and illegal in almost all situations.

TRRP developed a flowchart to help illustrate these four situations (Figure 11.2).

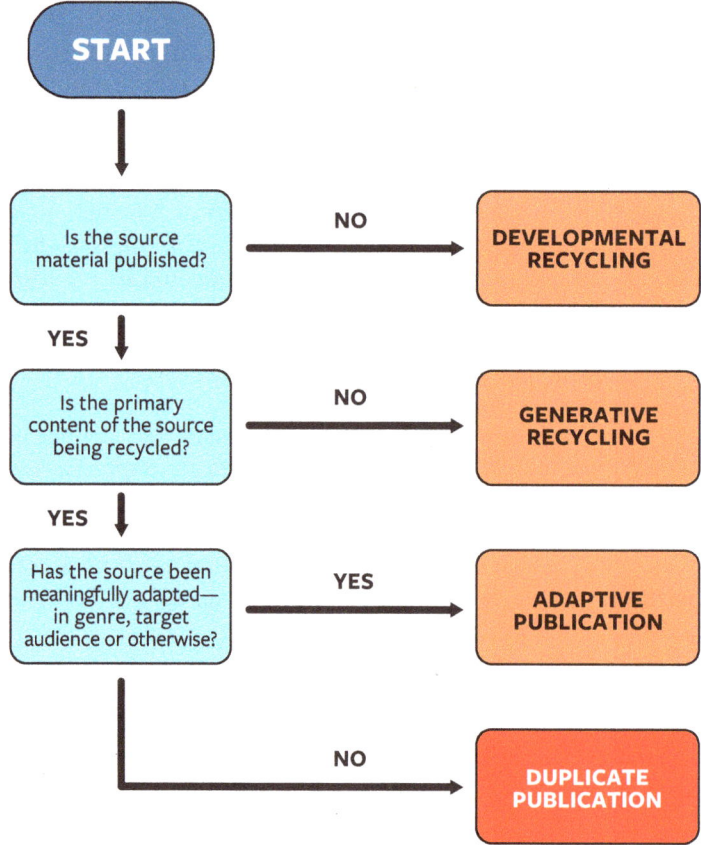

FIGURE 11.2 Categories of text recycling (Hall et al., 2021a). Reprinted with permission.

Learn more about text recycling in relation to copyright and fair use by reading a white paper on the topic (Hansen & Moskovitz, 2021). You might also want to review an article on text recycling for editors that provides greater detail for each recycling category (Hall et al., 2021a).

TRRP provides text recycling best practices for researchers, although they apply to all authors (2021). The best practices include the following:

- Authors should recycle text when consistency of language is needed for accurate communication, such as describing methods that are common across multiple studies. Permission may be needed if the text reused is substantial.
- Authors may recycle text if the recycled material is accurate and appropriate for the new work and doesn't infringe on copyright or violate publisher policies.
- Authors should not recycle text in ways that may mislead editors and readers about the novelty of the new work.
- Authors should be transparent with editors and readers about the use of recycled text.

Q *If I sign the copyright transfer, may I still write another article on the same topic?*

A The transfer of the copyright does not mean you can't write another article about the same topic. However, if you are referring to results or key information previously published, be sure to reference the earlier work.

You need to be careful when using your own work in a subsequent article, book chapter, or research, especially when you have signed a copyright transfer agreement for the original work that was published. A good risk-management approach for avoiding unethical and/or illegal situations is, first and foremost, to disclose to the editor any previous dissemination of your material in another form. That includes an article in another journal, a conference presentation, or material posted online (Roig, 2015). Yes, you can publish for other journals with other audiences on the same topic, but you must have a new focus and new information. Cite the previously published article on the topic and get permission to use content from Article 1 in Article 2, if you are using information from that publication.

Keep in mind that, depending on the level of publishing misconduct, the editor will issue a retraction for your work, which will damage your reputation.

Q *How do I handle the methodology section when reporting on different aspects of a research project in different journal articles?*

A Possible options include asking permission from the publisher of Article 1 to reuse the text (crediting the original source and noting permission granted) or referring the reader to Article 1 for the methodology. The publication's author guidelines may address this situation, or you can consult with the editor.

Errors in Your Published Work

If after your article is published you discover you made an error, you have an ethical responsibility to notify the editor immediately. If it's a significant error, the journal will prepare and publish as soon as possible after the publication date a *corrigendum* or an *erratum*. This notice will be published in any version of the work, whether in print or online.

Generally, your original work is not changed. Rather, the publisher alerts readers to a correction in the publishing record and not the publishing history (Daly, 2019). The publication's website often includes a policy on how it handles corrections.

Resources to learn more about corrections to your published work include the Committee on Publication Ethics (https://publicationethics.org) and the International Association of Scientific, Technical and Medical Publishers (https://www.stm-assoc.org).

Satisfaction in Print

You have learned about several legal and ethical issues related to protecting your own work and the work of others. Be sure you review the publication's author guidelines related to these areas. Follow these guidelines and the suggestions in this chapter (and consult with your editor when in doubt) to navigate the publishing waters. There are many challenges to publishing an original work, but after those challenges are met and you see your work in print or online, it is indeed worth all the effort.

Write Now!

1. Practice writing a permission email to a journal, requesting the use of a figure from an article.
2. Compare and contrast ethical and legal considerations in the authors guidelines for three nursing journals.
3. Explore resources at the Text Recycling Research Project website (https://textrecycling.org).

References

American Nurses Association. (2015). *Code of ethics for nurses with interpretive statements.* https://www.nursingworld.org/practice-policy/nursing-excellence/ethics/code-of-ethics-for-nurses/

American Psychological Association. (2020). *Publication manual of the American Psychological Association* (7th ed.). https://doi.org/10.1037/0000165-000

Anderson, R. (2016, Aug. 17). The difference between copyright infringement and plagiarism—and why it matters/peer to peer review. *Library Journal.* https://www.libraryjournal.com/story/the-difference-between-copyright-infringement-and-plagiarism-and-why-it-matters-peet-to-peer-review

Association for Institutional Research (2019). *AIR Statement of Ethical Principles.* https://www.airweb.org/ir-data-professional-overview/statement-of-ethical-principles

Barbour, V., & Committee on Publication Ethics. (2016). *Journal's best practices for ensuring consent for publishing medical case reports: Guidance from COPE.* https://doi.org/10.24318/cope.2019.1.6

Biography. (2021, May 6). *Toni Morrison.* https://www.biography.com/authors-writers/toni-morrison

Carfagno, M. L., Schweers, S. A., Whann, E. A., Hodgson, M. B., Mittleman, K. D., Nastasee, S. A., Sorgenfrei, T., Kodukulla, M. I., & for The International Society for Medical Publication Professionals Authorship Task Force. (2022). Building consensus on author selection practices for industry-sponsored research: Recommendations from an expert task force of medical publication professionals. *Current Medical Research and Opinion, 38*(6), 863–870. https://doi.org/10.1080/03007995.2022.2050111

Creative Commons (n.d.-a). *About the licenses.* https://creativecommons.org/licenses

Creative Commons. (n.d.-b). *Scholars copyright addendum engine.* https://labs.creativecommons.org/scholars

Daly, P. J. (2019, Nov. 8). What authors need to know about errata, expressions of concern, and retractions. *Wolters Kluwer.* https://www.wolterskluwer.com/en/expert-insights/authors-errata-expressions-of-concern-retractions

DeJong, M. J. (2012). Case studies: Strategies to protect patient privacy. *Nurse Author & Editor, 22*(4), 1–3. https://doi.org/10.1111/j.1750-4910.2012.tb00136.x

Elsevier. (n.d.) *Patient consent.* https://www.elsevier.com/about/policies-and-standards/patient-consent?trial=true

Elsevier. (2022). *Legal guide for editors concerning ethics issues.* https://www.elsevier.com/editor/perk/legal-guide-for-editors

Fishman, S. (2023). *The public domain: How to find and use copyright-free writings, music and more* (10th ed.). Nolo.

Fishman, S. (2024). *The copyright handbook: What every writer needs to know* (15th ed.). Nolo.

Fowler, M. (Ed.). (2015). *Guide to the code of ethics for nurses with interpretive statements: Development, interpretation and application* (2nd ed.). American Nurses Association.

The Free Dictionary. (n.d.). *Copyright.* https:/www.thefreedictionary.com/copyright

Gennaro, S. (2021). Text recycling and salami slicing. *Journal of Nursing Scholarship, 53*(5), 531–532. https://doi.org/10.1111/jnu.12700

Hall, A. (2023, June 19). *The ultimate guide to digital millennium copyright act.* Copyright.com. https://www.copyrighted.com/blog/dmca-guide

Hall, S., Moskovitz, C., & Permberton, M. (2021a). *Understanding text recycling: A guide for editors.* Text Recycling Research Project. https://textrecycling.org/files/2021/06/Understanding-Text-Recycling_A-Guide-for-Editors-V.1.pdf

Hall, S., Moskovitz, C., & Permberton, M. (2021b). *Understanding text recycling: A guide for researchers.* Text Recycling Research Project. https://textrecycling.org/files/2021/06/Understanding-Text-Recycling_A-Guide-for-Researchers-V.1.pdf

Hansen, D., & Moskovitz, C. (2021). *Text recycling in research writing: U.S. copyright law and fair use.* [White paper]. Text Recycling Research Project. https://textrecycling.org/files/2021/05/TRRP-White-Paper-Text-Recycling-in-Research-Writing-U.S.-Copyright-Law-and-Fair-Use.pdf

Harrington, R. (2020, April 20). Copyright, creative commons, and confusion. *The Scholarly Kitchen.* https://scholarlykitchen.sspnet.org/2020/04/20/copyright-creative-commons-and-confusion/

Herron, C. R. (2023). Best practices to guide decisions of authorshihp and author order in a research manuscript. *AMWA Journal, 38*(4), 38–41. https://doi.org/10.55752/amwa.2023.250

Holleywood, C. (2023, November 14). Recommendations for ethical use of AI chatbots in publications. *The Publication Plan.* https://thepublicationplan.com/2023/11/14/recommendations-for-ethical-use-of-ai-chatbots-in-publications/

International Committee of Medical Journal Editors. (2024). *Recommendations for the conduct, reporting, editing, and publication of scholarly work in medical journals.* http://www.icmje.org/recommendations

International Society for Medical Publication Professionals. (2024). International Society for Medical Publication Professionals (ISMPP) position statement and call to action on artificial intelligence. *Current Medical Research and Opinion, 40*(1), 9–10. https://doi.org/10.1080/03007995.2023.2273139

JAMA Network Editors. (2020). *AMA manual of style: A guide for authors and editors* (11th ed.). Oxford University Press.

Kaufman, R. (2008). *Publishing forms and contracts.* Oxford University Press.

Legal Dictionary. (n.d.). *Invasion of privacy.* https://legaldictionary.net/invasion-of-privacy/

Merriam-Webster. (n.d.-a). *Ethics.* https://www.merriam-webster.com/dictionary/ethics

Merriam-Webster. (n.d.-b). *Plagiarize.* https://www.merriam-webster.com/dictionary/plagiarize

Moskovitz, C. (2021). Standardizing terminology for text recycling in research writing. *Learned Publishing, 34*(3), 370–378. https://onlinelibrary.wiley.com/doi/10.1002/leap.1372

National Institutes of Health. (2022). *Public access policy.* https://publicaccess.nih.gov

Office of Research Integrity. (n.d.). *Definition of research misconduct.* https://ori.hhs.gov/definition-research-misconduct

Roig, M. (2015). *Avoiding plagiarism, self-plagiarism, and other questionable practices: A guide to ethical writing.* Office of Research Integrity. https://ori.hhs.gov/sites/default/files/plagiarism.pdf

Schofield, B. L., & Walker, R. K. (Eds.). (2018). *Understanding and negotiating book publisher contracts.* Authors Alliance. https://authorsalliance.org/wp-content/uploads/2018/10/20181003_AuthorsAllianceGuidePublicationContracts.pdf

STM. (2022). STM permissions guidelines. https://www.stm-assoc.org/2022_01_27_STM_Permission_Guidelines_2022.pdf

STM. (2023). Signatories to STM permissions guidelines as of 8 June 2023. https://www.stm-assoc.org/intellectual-property/permissions/permissions-guidelines/

Text Recycling Research Project. (2021). Text recycling: Best practices for researchers. https://textrecycling.org/resources/best-practices-for-researchers/

US Copyright Office. (n.d.-a). Chapter 1: Subject matter of scope of copyright. In *Copyright Law of the United States.* https://copyright.gov/title17/92chap1.html#102

US Copyright Office. (n.d.-b). *What is copyright?* https://www.copyright.gov/what-is-copyright/

US Copyright Office. (2021a). *Compendium of US Copyright Office practices* (3rd ed.). Chapter 2200 Section 2204. https://www.copyright.gov/comp3/chapter2200.html

US Copyright Office. (2021b). *Copyright notice.* https://copyright.gov/circs/circ03.pdf

Wager, E., & Kleinert, S. (2012). Responsible research publication: International standards for authors. In T. Mayer & N. Steneck (Eds.), *Promoting research integrity in a global environment* (pp 311–319). World Scientific.

World Association of Medical Editors. (2007). *Authorship.* http://wame.org/authorship

World Association of Medical Editors. (2009). *Conflict of interest in peer-reviewed medical journals.* http://wame.org/conflict-of-interest-in-peer-reviewed-medical-journals

World Association of Medical Editors. (2023). *Chatbots, generative AI, and scholarly manuscripts.* https://wame.org/page3.php?id=106

Promoting Your Work

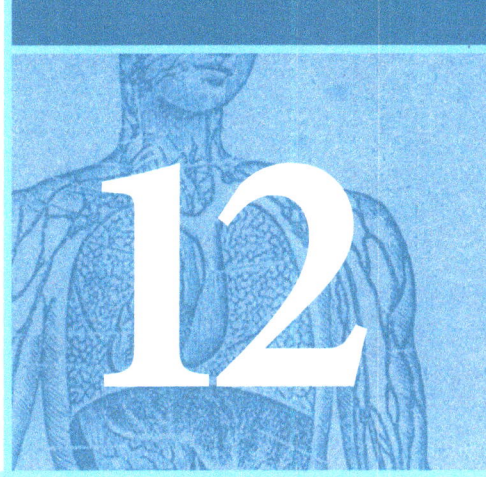

–Timothy Landers, PhD, RN, APRN-CNP, CIC, FAAN
–Stephanie J. Schulte, MLIS

WHAT YOU'LL LEARN IN THIS CHAPTER

- Using a few key steps can help increase the visibility of your work and its impact on practice.
- Applying these steps strategically can increase the reach of your publications.
- Several tools are used to measure how often a work is referenced, cited, adopted, and used.

*"Not all marketing people are writers,
but all writers must learn to be marketers."*
–Joanne Kraft

You've worked hard at writing, editing, and revising your manuscript, and that effort pays off with a publication in print or online. You may think it's time to pat yourself on the back for a job well done and take it easy. But by pushing yourself to take just a few more steps, you can ensure your work has a much wider impact than a single journal or website. As a nurse, you might be uncomfortable with self-promotion, yet promoting your published work is an important part of disseminating your findings to others in the profession—and beyond.

Your Responsibility

You have the largest role to play in helping your findings reach the right audience with the right message. It has been shown that it can take more than a decade for research findings to impact clinical practice (Hanney et al., 2015; Morris et al., 2011). By developing a plan to promote your published work, your writing can have an impact more quickly and be disseminated more rapidly to frontline caregivers, so practice can be based on the latest evidence. Sharing your work with a wide audience is also important for your organization, funders and sponsors, and those who participated in your project. In addition, achieving a wider impact helps advance your career and obtain funding for future projects.

Most successful authors have a plan to distribute their writing to the right people as quickly as possible. In essence, they have a marketing plan. Many think of marketing only in terms of products or services, but it's not just for new cars and investment consulting. Marketing enables you to accomplish your dissemination goals, whether that's letting critical care nurses know about the latest suctioning technique, informing first-time mothers of a new strategy for breastfeeding, or increasing public awareness about patient safety efforts.

Start thinking about marketing even as you write. For instance, a title that reflects key points of the article is essential to attract readers; this and a well-written abstract help optimize search engine results for those seeking information related to your topic. (See Chapter 5 to learn more about writing titles and abstracts.) But the title and abstract are only part of the overall marketing plan you'll need to create. The plan will pay off by making sure that the hard work you have done preparing and writing your work has the biggest impact on fellow nurses and improves patient care.

In creating a marketing plan, think about what groups might be interested in your findings and the key messages for each group. Keep in mind that people reading your work will likely come with different interests and ideas about why your writing is important to them.

Confidence Booster

Remember that the real reason for promoting your work is to share your important message(s) with as many people as possible. Nurses are among the most trusted health professions; patients, families, and other healthcare colleagues—including your fellow nurses—are interested in what you have to say!

Summarizing Your Work

Using plain language (or lay) summaries, graphical abstracts, and video abstracts can help you sum up your work in a way that readers can easily understand.

Plain Language Summaries

Like the abstract you write for a formal journal article or manuscript, a *plain language summary* (PLS) is an overview of your work, but it's written in non-technical language. As you write, it might be helpful to think about how you would summarize your writing for a friend or family member. However, keep in mind that you need to consider the literacy level of your target audience. (For more information about literacy, see Chapter 23.) Some journals now require authors write a PLS for publication with the article.

A PLS should address enough specifics—including the who, what, how, and why of a topic—so people interested in your work can get a glimpse into what you did and why it is important. Dormer and colleagues (2022) developed a guide for writing a PLS for scientific publications. Here is a brief overview of the approach:

Who Might Be Interested in Your Work?

These questions can help you identify who would benefit from knowing about your work.

- **Researchers and academicians:** How do your findings contribute to science and help advance knowledge about nursing and nursing practice? What are the next steps in addressing the problem you have studied? What issues or barriers did you encounter and how did you overcome them?

- **Nurses and other healthcare professionals:** What are the implications of your writing for practice? Is your work ready for wide adoption, or is additional work needed?

- **Other professions:** How might an attorney use your work when learning about the standard of care? Would dentists, veterinarians, or hospital engineers want to learn about your idea to try in their profession?

- **Industry and manufacturers:** What new ideas could be of interest in developing or testing new medical products or supplies? Does your work highlight a gap in current products and services?

- **Patients and caregivers:** How does your work help patients better understand their health or treatment options? Do your results include specific steps that patients and families can take to improve their health or ideas they can discuss with their healthcare team?

- **General public:** Does your work relate to an emerging and important item from the news? How can it relate to current events?

- **Policymakers:** How could your work be used to change regulations or payment mechanisms? What does your writing mean for people developing these policies?

Step 1: Consider the rationale and scope. Consider why the PLS is being created, plans for where it will be published, and resources that will be required for its creation.

Step 2: Identify your target audience. This helps determine the audience's needs and, therefore, what should be included.

Step 3: Consider dissemination channels. The channel (e.g., social media platform) will affect content and format. Check journal and conference requirements related to PLSs.

Step 4: Identify your key stakeholders for co-creation. You want to involve members of your target audience so content is relevant.

Step 5: Write. As you write, consider factors such as reading level and ways to engage readers (see Chapter 23 for more information about reading level and writing for a general audience). If possible, test your PLS with your target audience to obtain feedback.

Step 5: Disseminate. Those positioned to disseminate the PLS include the journal that published it, you, your organization, patients, advocacy groups, and healthcare providers. Outlets include social media and websites. As part of dissemination, reference the scientific manuscript and provide a link to it.

The guide was developed with input from those experienced with PLS and patient involvement, as well as members of the general public. You can download the guide at https://pemsuite.org/How-to-Guides/WG5.pdf.

Graphical Abstracts

Building on your plain language summary, *graphical abstracts* (sometimes called visual abstracts) are overviews of the work and draw readers to want to read more. As the name implies, a graphical abstract uses graphics to highlight your work. Elements of a graphical abstract include the following:

- The background or setting for your work
- The methods used
- Results or implications of your work
- Name and affiliation
- Contact information

Pick images that are eye-catching and support the information. Keep the text short—bullet points are better than long sentences. Simplicity and clarity are the key concepts to keep in mind. Several online resources can help with creating an exciting and impactful graphical abstract:

- **Canva** (www.canva.com): a web-based graphical design tool
- **Piktochart** (https://piktochart.com): includes infographic templates and tips
- **Easelly** (https://easel.ly): guides you through the steps of visually conveying highlights of your work
- **Venngage** (https://venngage.com): easy-to-use steps help create informative and well-designed graphics

When using these tools, be sure to check whether the final graphics can be used without purchasing a license. However, even without a license, these tools can give you ideas to spark your development of a graphical abstract. (You can learn more about creating these abstracts in Chapter 5.)

Video Abstracts

A *video abstract* is a short presentation of your article that tells viewers why they should want to read it (McGrath & Brandon, 2016). Video abstracts can be used for any type of article, not just research reports. These are exciting "snippets" of the research and a great chance to highlight your work.

Many publishers offer the opportunity to develop and produce a video abstract and have resources available to authors. In the case of journals, video abstracts are typically submitted after an article has been accepted for publication.

Here are a few tips for making a video abstract, which can be created on your tablet or smartphone (BMJ Author Hub, n.d.; Taylor & Francis, n.d.; Wolters Kluwer/Lippincott Williams & Wilkins, n.d.):

- Check the publication's requirements related to file size and format and submission requirements

- Try to use a microphone, although if you have a very quiet spot, this might not be necessary.
- Consider the setting. You don't want a distracting background; on the other hand, a plain wall doesn't add to the look of your video. Be sure to have enough light, but don't stand in front of a window.
- Keep it short (recommendations range from 2 minutes and 20 seconds to 3–5 minutes).
- Think about the key points you want to convey. For example, why is your research important, how do your evidence-based improvement findings affect current knowledge, or how can your quality improvement project be implemented in practice.
- Don't read from a script. Instead, write down bullet points you want to cover. Speak naturally (and with enthusiasm) to the camera.
- Consider a few images (such as figures on a PowerPoint slide), but these aren't essential for the video to be successful.
- Include a call to action: What do you want people to do after watching the video?
- Do a test run to ensure everything is working properly and you are satisfied with your delivery. You don't want to be too close or too far away from the camera.
- Become familiar with the editing features on your camera. These can help strengthen the look of your video.

Video abstracts are a great opportunity to highlight your work. Although their impact has not been well documented, one study found that they result in increased views of a research article and may increase citations (Bonnevie et al., 2023).

Plain language summaries, graphical abstracts, and video abstracts, which can be shared online, increase the accessibility of your work to a much broader, general audience who may not otherwise be exposed to it.

Using Online Outlets

Social media has revolutionized the way we communicate in our personal and work lives. In today's world, most of us use Facebook, X, LinkedIn, Instagram, or other social media sites to share important happenings in our lives. Just as these can be used to help create a personal network, they also provide avenues for promoting our writing. As Susan Gennaro, editor of the *Journal of Nursing Scholarship*, writes, "It is clear that social media is a powerful tool to help your research be disseminated as widely as possible and to connect with communities of interest in new ways" (2015, p. 377).

Social media options include your personal accounts and accounts the publisher may have. The popularity of various social media outlets changes over time, with new options coming on the scene, so be aware of these changing preferences. When using social media, it's important to offer additional content or commentary instead of simply posting links to other sources. Consider giving your followers a reason to react to your post and share it with others. Using keywords or *hashtags* (the # symbol, followed by the keywords) will make content more accessible and increase its reach, especially if you reference professional associations, organizations, or other commentators in your posts. Using images can also draw attention to posts and increase visibility.

Here are examples of posts that will grab a user's attention:

- New study questions what we know about the pandemic
- Team of nurse researchers helping to keep kids fit. Find out more
- The same old hospital problem with a new solution

In addition to general social media sites, you'll want to engage in scientific social networking through freely available websites where researchers can both present and promote their publications and presentations. Some of these sites are shown in Table 12.1. Benefits of using these sites include wider dissemination of research to both academic and public communities and discovering new collaborators for future work by identifying common research interests.

TABLE 12.1 Comparing Academic Social Media Sites

Site	Description	Major Functions	Altmetrics Integration
Academia.edu https://www.academia.edu	Article-sharing platform to "accelerate the world's research"	Create personal research profile Share links or upload full-text articles Follow other researchers on the platform Read feed of articles from areas of interest or researchers being followed View analytics related to readers of your published works in last 30 or 60 days Create online feedback session to gather comments from followers on paper in progress Access a detailed help section	Allows linking of profile to wide variety of online social networks, including Facebook, X, Instagram, LinkedIn, and ORCID Impact scores of publications only available through premium subscription
Google Scholar Citations https://scholar.google.com/citations	Platform for tracking citations to author's scholarly work	Semi-automatically create profile based on spelling of name during setup Track citations to individual publications Access automatic calculation of personal h-index Manually add additional articles not found Produce public profile discoverable in Google Scholar search	Traditional citation metrics only
Kudos https://www.growkudos.com	A platform built to explain, share, and measure the impact of scholarship	Semi-automatically create profile using DOI or words from title Provide layperson summary explanations of research papers Share easily through connections with Facebook, X, and LinkedIn Gather usage analytics such as views on Kudos, click-throughs, downloads; Altmetric data including tweets, Mendeley readers, and Google+ posts Link articles to publisher site or other repository for full-text access	Fully integrated with most major altmetrics-connected sites such as Altmetric, ORCID, and CrossRef, as well as traditional citation metrics in Web of Science

continues

TABLE 12.1 Comparing Academic Social Media Sites *(continued)*

Site	Description	Major Functions	Altmetrics Integration
ResearchGate https://www.researchgate.net	A collaboration platform for sharing articles, connecting with other researchers, and seeking feedback from around the world	Create profile and add articles via a click-through verification process Receive suggestions of projects and publications based on your research interests and skills View career opportunities based on profile Quickly view profiles of others who have cited your papers Ask questions of the community and gather feedback Upload and share full text of publications via drag-and-drop (if permitted per the publication's copyright agreement) Add comments to citations within the platform	Not integrated into other common social media platforms such as Facebook and X Networking is housed within the ResearchGate platform Articles findable in Google search

Q *How can I make it more likely that my article will come up in an online search?*

A *Search engine optimization*, or SEO, is a tool for improving the likelihood that your article is found through an online search. Most publishers provide tips to make sure your results come up at the top of the page. Here are a few (UCLA Library, 2023; Burns & Butcher, 2023; Wiley, n.d.):

- Make the title descriptive and put keywords and phrases related to your topic within the first 65 characters of the title.
- Use keywords in your abstract, headings, and other content areas such as tables.
- Don't overdo keywords because search engines may then "un-index" your article.
- Use keywords that are popular on Google Trends (https://trends.google.com/trends).
- Provide captions for figures and tables.
- Use accurate words to describe the contents of your article. Medical Subject Headings (MeSH terms) and CINAHL subject headings are a great way to start. (See Chapter 4 for more information about MeSH.)
- Keep authors' names and initials consistent from one publication to another and include authors' Open Researcher and Contributor ID (discussed later in this chapter).
- Provide links to related articles and resources and link to your article across your social media and other networking sites, especially those that are commonly cited. Encourage colleagues to link to your article.

By using these tips, you can help to be sure that readers who are interested in your topic find your work as efficiently as possible.

For faculty who need to track their research impact for reappointment, promotion, and tenure purposes, some sites produce alternative metrics (*altmetrics*) that can be used to help quantify interest in the research. Some platforms integrate functionality that tracks online activity on common social media outlets, such as X, LinkedIn, and Facebook, and calculates metrics automatically based on activity.

Even if you aren't a faculty member, you'll still want to know how widely your work is being disseminated, and free online tools can help you with that.

Q *My colleague says I need to look into author-level metrics. What are those, and how are they helpful?*

A Author-level metrics measure the productivity and dissemination reach of authors. For example, the *h-index* measures productivity and scientific impact, looking at a researcher's most cited articles and the number of citations they have received in other people's publications. You can access your h-index on Web of Science, Scopus, and Google Scholar Citations (Hirsch, 2005; UIC University Library, 2023). Go to http://researchguides.uic.edu/c.php?g=252299&p=1683205 to learn more.

You can also set up a Google Alert (https://www.google.com/alerts) for your name or the name of a key part of your article. This enables you to receive an automatic email when a search engine finds a reference to your work. You can set how often you want to be updated: as it happens, once a day, or once a week.

A number of academic social sites are available, making it difficult to know which is best suited to your needs. You'll want to understand the site's features and what it can achieve for a researcher, as all sites require some initial front-end setup that can take from several minutes to several hours, depending on the site functionality and the researcher's desire to create a complete profile. Table 12.1 provides a comparison of some of the tools available and how they are integrated into altmetrics. You may want to start with two or three sites that will help you reach your intended audience—an experienced nurse colleague or librarian can help pick out which sites would be the most relevant.

Other Online Outlets

Although social media is probably the fastest and easiest way to disseminate your work, you can also turn to the following:

- **Blog:** A "print" or video blog provides a regular outlet where you can share your work. Keep in mind, however, that blogs require a significant time commitment; you should blog at least a few times a week. If your hospital or organization has an internal or external blog, you may contact the system administrators for the blog to ask if you can submit a posting. Organizations are often happy to include your research and highlight your work.

- **LinkedIn:** A detailed profile on LinkedIn provides social media opportunities and the ability to disseminate information about yourself and your work by posting links to your articles and adding videos, slides, or audio recordings. Be sure to include a professional photo of yourself to enhance the likelihood people will read your profile. Those who plan conferences can quickly find what they need to ask you to speak at an event. Of course, you can also create a website, but many are finding that LinkedIn is sufficient for their professional needs.

- **ORCID:** By registering in Open Researcher and Contributor ID (ORCID), you become part of a database of researchers (ORCID, n.d.). You'll receive a unique identification number, which helps keep your work associated with you; this can be especially important if you have changed your name during your career (e.g., because of a change in marital status) or if others have a name similar to yours. ORCID also facilitates your ability to share your work with others and to identify possible collaborators. Be sure to keep your ORCID account current with your list of publications.

It takes a bit of time to get started on these outlets, but the payoff is well worth it.

Copyright Considerations

One caveat when uploading documents to any online platform is copyright. The copyright agreement signed by the author (or usually the lead author on behalf of all authors in the case of multi-authored works) governs whether authors can legally share a version of the publication on these sites or elsewhere, such as a university-supported institutional repository. Additionally, each platform has its own terms of use that typically require that authors have the right to upload articles.

Read the copyright agreement carefully before signing, and look for information about article sharing on scholarly collaborative networks. The author guidelines may have information about what a publisher allows to be shared. Many publishers support the article-sharing guidelines from STM (2015, 2022), an international association of academic and professional publishers, but this doesn't grant a license to systematically distribute articles. If a publisher's copyright agreement does not include article sharing, you may be able to negotiate this right via an addendum to the initial copyright agreement. The Scholarly Publishing and Academic Resources Coalition (SPARC), a member-based organization of primarily academic and research libraries, works to provide broader access to research works and provides a sample addendum authors can use (http://sparcopen.org/wp-content/uploads/2016/01/Access-Reuse_Addendum.pdf). You can learn more about copyright in Chapter 11. If your research was federally funded, know that as of 2026, articles related to the research must be freely available upon publication (Office of Science and Technology Policy, 2022). This new guidance for federally funded research also requires that peer-reviewed publications be made available without an embargo (or waiting time between publication and open access).

Q *I'm getting a lot of email invitations to present at conferences. Many of these aren't from my home country and come from professional-sounding groups I haven't heard of before. How do I know if these are real and if I should follow up?*

A An unfortunate trend has been the emergence of fake or predatory conferences. Like the predatory journals discussed in Chapter 3, these conferences have little to no peer review and charge large travel or presentation fees. Although it can be tempting to think about travelling to exotic locations and fulfilling requirements to disseminate your work quickly, doing so can be an expensive waste of time and money, because you may pay a registration fee and your travel costs only to arrive to find few people attending your session (Cleary et al., 2016; InterAcademy Partnership, 2022). Even worse, the companies operating these conferences may direct you to predatory journals.

If you don't know the name of the conference organizer, do your homework. Other red flags that may indicate a predatory conference include an invitation that doesn't relate to your field of research, one that starts with a compliment about requesting your "gracious presence" or "outstanding expertise," and the presence of grammatical errors.

One of the best ways to identify predatory conferences and publishers is to ask a trusted nurse colleague, faculty member, or knowledgeable librarian. Most importantly, remember the adage: If something sounds too good to be true, it probably is.

Keep in mind that a conference may be low quality and not predatory. A report from the InterAcademy Partnership (2022) describes the spectrum from quality (low risk) to fraudulent (high risk) and provides indicators for each. These markers can help identify best options for presenting your work.

Working With Publishers

Like authors, editors and publishers have an interest in making sure that your writing reaches as broad an audience as possible; this includes promoting your work through the publication's social media, and, depending on the nature of the work, media releases. Most publishers have tips and guidelines for interacting with the media and promoting your work.

Some publishers hold webinars, host podcasts or online chats with authors who can discuss their work, or will post slides summarizing your findings on the journal's website so that it's easier for others to present your findings while crediting your work. Others may be willing to post a video of you discussing your work on the journal's YouTube channel. If not, you might want to consider posting a video abstract yourself.

Note that publishers may provide (for a fee) services such as creating interactive visuals or even a multimedia program related to your work for posting.

Q *What are resources that can help me with promoting my work?*

A Many publishers' resources for authors cover this topic—and provide other useful information as well. Here are a few:

- Elsevier Author Tools & Resources (https://beta.elsevier.com/researcher/author/tools-and-resources?trial=true#3-promotion)
- Lippincott Journals: Author Resources (https://www.wolterskluwer.com/en/solutions/lippincott-journals/author-resources)
- Springer Nature: Maximize Your Visibility (https://www.springernature.com/gp/researchers/publication-promotion)
- Taylor & Francis Group: Research Impact (https://authorservices.taylorandfrancis.com/resources/research-impact-ebook)

Working With Media Outlets

If you feel your work is applicable to a general audience, contact the communications department in your organization. You want them to have information about you and your areas of expertise for when they receive media inquiries for interviews. They can also help you craft a media release for research findings. Keep in mind, however, that to justify a media release, your findings need to be something that would entice the general public.

A media release isn't just for when you publish study results. It can be used to promote your expertise when the time is right. For example, when an enterovirus outbreak sent children to several hospitals, the organization where one of the chapter authors worked sent a media release about prevention, something of keen interest to the public (see Example 12.1).

Each type of media has different needs for information and can help tell your story in a different way. For example, a television reporter often seeks compelling video or an on-camera expert quote for a short broadcast story, while a newspaper or magazine writer may want to cover your work in a way that provides additional background context to another story.

Media requests usually happen soon after a release is sent out but can also occur months later, as your topic becomes newsworthy. Keep in mind that the news cycle is influenced by what is happening in the rest of the world.

What Makes a Great Media Release?

A well-written media or press release can help spread the word about your publication to a wider audience. A media release is a brief, one-page summary of your work and its importance to the field that is meant to grab the attention of busy reporters and editors. Wynne (2016) says the ingredients for a successful media release are simple: headline, opening sentence, body (what is the story and why does it matter?), and contact information.

If you work at a small facility, you might not have someone who can write a media release, but here is how you can do it yourself:

- Use an attention-getting headline: This is the most important feature (Hayes, 2016; Kraus, 2023; Wynne, 2016). For example, if you were a reporter, which of the following headlines would make you want to read more?

    Hand Washing Prevents Spread of Enterovirus

    or

    It's All About the Soap: Hand Washing, Not Alcohol Rubs, Recommended to Prevent Spread of Enterovirus

- Include the following information as succinctly as possible; many reporters receive hundreds of media releases, and you want yours to stand out. You might want to think about it as three short paragraphs:

1. An introduction/summary of your publication (starting with a powerful first sentence that encapsulates the key points or findings of the study; otherwise, reporters' eyes will glaze over)

2. Background on the methods (a brief explanation of what was done) and findings (a bit more detail to support what was in your first sentence)

3. A concluding paragraph with the reason the topic is important (the "So what?" of the findings.)

- Include your full professional title, relevant degrees, and contact information including email, text, and phone for both you and the media experts at your organization. (Note: Don't overdo the degrees and certifications, just list what is relevant.)

- Provide information about your organization. (You will need to clear this with your organization before sending. Most have a standard statement that they use.)

You can also include one or two interesting visuals or videos to spark interest. Be brief; a typical media release is no more than 300 to 500 words (Kraus, 2023). Ask others to read your release, then email it to reporters at media outlets you think would be a good fit for your information.

[Contact information for media personnel and the expert]

It's all about the soap: Hand washing, not alcohol rubs, recommended to prevent spread of enterovirus ⟵ Attention-getting title and opening

In recent years, alcohol-based antiviral rubs have become the go-to for hand hygiene and combating illness. With perfumed scents and cutesy carriers, they're even considered "chichi" among trendy tweens.

However, an expert at The Ohio State University says that such rubs are no help against the recent outbreak of enterovirus EV-D68, which has sent children to hospitals in several Midwestern states. ⟵ Ties the information provided to the news

Timothy F. Landers, associate professor in the College of Nursing at The Ohio State University, is a hand-hygiene researcher. He recommends washing hands with soap and water for at least 15 seconds to help prevent the spread of enterovirus. ⟵ Key information, succinctly stated

"The goal of soap is to remove the oils and the virus from the hands, not to kill the virus," Landers said. ⟵ Quote for media outlets without the resources to conduct interviews

Landers operates a hand-hygiene center and lab at the College of Nursing and focuses on infection prevention efforts. ⟵ Establishes expertise; note lack of alphabet soup of credentials

He also recommends practicing proper cough etiquette, staying home if you have symptoms, drying hands with paper towels, and using a paper towel when turning the sink on and off. Additionally, focus on areas between fingers and the tips of fingers while washing, as these are often forgotten and can come in contact with germs.

Landers recommends liquid soap, as opposed to bar soap, which can harbor bacteria.

"One of the best things we can do to stay healthy is what we learned as kids—wash our hands!"

NOTE TO REPORTERS, ASSIGNMENT EDITORS: Landers operates a lab at the College of Nursing in which members of the media can have their hands tested for bacteria—excellent visuals are available. ⟵ Offer of visuals

About The Ohio State University College of Nursing ⟵ About the organization
The Ohio State University College of Nursing is the world's preeminent college; known for accomplishing what is considered impossible through its transformational leadership and innovation in nursing and health, evidence-based practice, and unsurpassed wellness. As part of the largest health science campus in the US, the College of Nursing offers seven innovative academic programs. The college's graduate nursing programs are among the top 5% in the country, according to *U.S. News and World Report*.

EXAMPLE 12.1 Sample media release.

The news cycle evolves rapidly, so respond quickly to media requests before you miss the chance to share your message. Prepare for the interview by identifying the two or three main points you want to make and thinking about how you will answer questions you might receive (American Association for the Advancement of Science [AAAS], n.d.). The AAAS offers these tips to help you succeed in an interview:

- State the most important information and provide backup.
- Keep your responses brief but be sure to provide enough so the reporter can get quotes that can be used in the article.
- Don't talk too much and don't get off track.
- Speak in lay terms; you can't assume the reporter will know medical jargon.
- Try to use metaphors or analogies to create images that emphasize your points.
- If you don't understand the question, ask for clarification.
- Be clear when you are offering an opinion instead of stating facts.
- If you don't know the answer, say so, and then offer to find out.
- Be honest.
- Try to make your final comment one that is clear, concise, and emphasizes your main point.

Confidence Booster

When a reporter or editor from a magazine, television, or other media outlet contacts you, it's normal to feel a little nervous. After all, we want to make sure we get our message—and our facts—right. Keep in mind that journalists are professionally motivated to report correct information in their stories and reports, so we are all on the same page. Most reporters will have some knowledge about the story they are covering, but using straightforward language, and not technical jargon, will help them do their job of covering your story. It turns out that the same approach and language that we use with our patients goes a long way.

Respond promptly to any follow-up requests for additional information. Email or text a quick thank-you after the article or news story appears, so the reporter keeps you in mind for future opportunities.

The Essentials for Promoting Your Work

If you don't do anything else to promote your work, at least follow these essential guidelines:

- Craft your title and abstract for search-engine optimization.
- Create at least one research profile on an academic social media site and post your articles there, if copyright agreement permits.
- Post information about your published work on your own social media accounts. Keep the entries short and provide a link.
- Ask staff in the communications department of your organization if they will post the information on the organization's social media outlets.
- Add the publication to your curriculum vitae and to your research profiles (e.g., ORCID).
- Share the news about your publication with the nursing school you attended so it can be listed in newsletters and other publications.
- Network with others at conferences you attend, so you can share your work. It's also a great way to identify potential research collaborators.
- Present your own work at conferences. (See Chapter 17 for more information.)
- Include your contact information in slide presentations, handouts, and other materials, and add your latest article to the signature line of your email.
- Share your publication with two or three people who you think will be interested and see if they are willing to promote it through their own social media outlets.

Extending Your Influence

A marketing plan helps you effectively reach out to different audiences with the messages you want to share. For major projects, professional marketing and communication firms can develop a detailed plan, but for the most part, you are the one who must take responsibility for disseminating your work. In addition to the ideas in this chapter, you might want to download the free book *The 30-Day Impact Challenge*, by Stacy Konkiel (n.d.), a treasure trove of valuable strategies.

Above all, shove aside excuses like, "I don't have enough time," and make a commitment today to extend your influence by promoting your work. Doing so will help you make a difference in people's lives—the ultimate goal of every nurse.

Write Now!

1. Identify two or three target audiences for your work, then describe the top two points of interest for each group.
2. Write three social media messages for a publication (ideally, your own!) and review them with a friend or colleague.
3. Make a list of potential magazines or news outlets for your work.

References

American Association for the Advancement of Science. (n.d.). *Media interview tips*. http://www.aaas.org/sites/default/files/AAAS_Media_Tips.pdf

BMJ Author Hub. (n.d.). *Video abstracts*. https://authors.bmj.com/writing-and-formatting/video-abstracts/

Bonnevie, T., Repel, A., Gravier, F.-E., Ladner, J., Sibert, L., Muir, J.-F., Cuvelier, A., & Fischer, M.-O. (2023). Video abstracts are associated with an increase in research reports citations, views and social attention: A cross-sectional study. *Scientometrics, 128*, 3001–3015. https://doi.org/10.1007/s11192-023-04675-9

Burns, P., & Butcher, B. (2023). How to get your writing found: Why medical writers and academics need to use search engine optimization. *Medical Writing, 32*(4), 56–58.

Cleary, M., Sayer, J., & Kornhaber, R. (2016). Conference presentations: Tips, tricks and traps. *Nurse Author & Editor, 26*(3), 1-10. https://doi.org/10.1111/j.1750-4910.2016.tb00227.x

Dormer, L., Schindler, T., Williams, L. A., Lobban, D., Khawaja, S., Hunn, A., Ubilla, D. L., Sargeant I., & Hamoir, A.-M. (2022). A practical 'how-to' guide to plain language summaries (PLS) of peer-reviewed scientific publications: Results of a multi-stakeholder initiative utilizing co-creation methodology. *Research Involvement and Engagement, 8*(23). https://doi.org/10.1186/s40900-022-00358-6

Gennaro, S. (2015). Scientists and social media. *Journal of Nursing Scholarship, 47*(5), 377–378. https://doi.org/10.1111/jnu.12161

Hanney, S. R., Castle-Clarke, S., Grant, J., Guthrie, S., Henshall, C., Mestre-Ferrandiz, J., Pistollato, M., Pollitt, A., Sussex, J., & Wooding, S. (2015). How long does biomedical research take? Studying the time taken between biomedical and health research and its translation into products, policy, and practice. *Health Research Policy and Systems, 13*(1). https://doi.org/10.1186/1478-4505-13-1

Hayes, N. (2016). Journalists' advice on how to write press releases they'll actually read. *MarketingProfs*. http://www.marketingprofs.com/articles/2016/30604/journalists-advice-on-how-to-write-press-releases-theyll-actually-read

Hirsch, J. E. (2005). An index to quantify an individual's scientific research output. *Proceedings of the National Academy of Sciences of the United States of America, 102*(46), 16569–16572. https://doi.org/10.1073/pnas.0507655102

InterAcademy Partnership. (2022). *Combatting predatory academic journals and conferences*. [Summary report]. https://palast.ps/sites/default/files/inline-files/2.%20Summary%20report%20-%20English.pdf

Konkiel, S. (n.d.). *The 30-day impact challenge: The ultimate guide to raising the profile of your research*. http://blog.impactstory.org/wp-content/uploads/2015/01/impact_challenge_ebook_links.pdf

Kraus, A. R. (2023, Nov. 13). What makes a good press release: 15 ways to stand out. *Fit Small Business*. https://fitsmallbusiness.com/what-makes-a-good-press-release/

McGrath, J. M., & Brandon, D. (2016). Video abstracts: A fun, easy way to capture your audience: Try it! [Letter]. *Advances in Neonatal Care, 16*(1), 1–12. https://doi.org/10.1097/ANC.0000000000000271

Morris, Z. S., Wooding, S., & Grant, J. (2011). The answer is 17 years, what is the question: Understanding time lags in translational research. *Journal of the Royal Society of Medicine, 104*(12), 510–520. https://doi.org/10.1258/jrsm.2011.110180

Office of Science and Technology Policy, Executive Office of the President. (2022). *Ensuring free, immediate, and equitable access to federally funded research*. http://whitehouse.gov/wp-content/uploads/2022/08/08-2022-OSTP-Public-Access-Memo.pdf

Open Researcher and Contributor ID. (n.d.). *About ORCID.* http://orcid.org/about/what-is-orcid/mission

STM. (2015). *STM consultation on article sharing.* http://www.stm-assoc.org/stm-consultations/scn-consultation-2015

STM. (2022). *STM permissions guidelines.* https://www.stm-assoc.org/2022_01_27_STM_Permission_Guidelines_2022.pdf

Taylor & Francis. (n.d.). Creating a video abstract for your research. *Author Services.* https://authorservices.taylorandfrancis.com/research-impact/creating-a-video-abstract-for-your-research/

UCLA Library. (2023). *Research visibility.* https://guides.library.ucla.edu/seo/author

UIC University Library. (2023, Feb. 9). *Measuring your impact: Impact factor, citation analysis, and other metrics: Citation analysis.* http://researchguides.uic.edu/c.php?g=252299&p=1683205

Wiley. (n.d.). *Search engine optimization (SEO) for your article.* https://authorservices.wiley.com/author-resources/Journal-Authors/Prepare/writing-for-seo.html

Wolters Kluwer/Lippincott Williams & Wilkins. (n.d.). *Journal toolkit: How to create a video abstract.* https://journals.lww.com/jgpt/Documents/LWW_Toolkit_-_How_to_Create_a_Video_Abstract.pdf

Wynne, R. (2016, June 13). How to write a press release. *Forbes.* http://www.forbes.com/sites/robertwynne/2016/06/13/how-to-write-a-press-release/#44ceba92505e

Part II
Tips for Writing Different Types of Articles

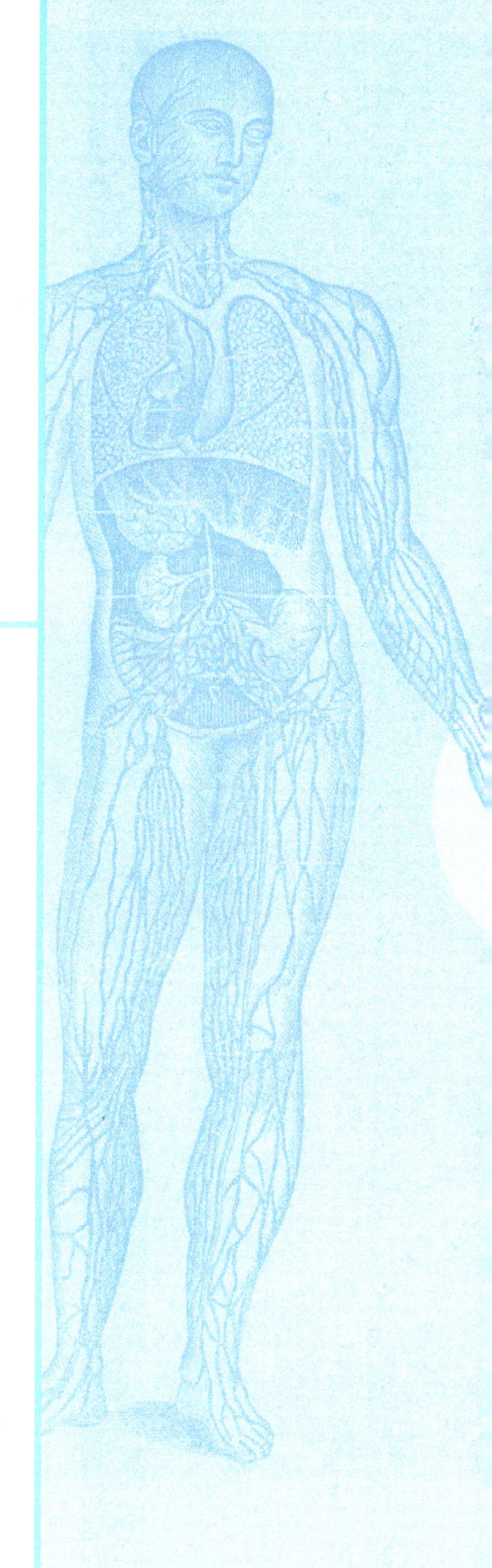

13	Writing the Clinical Article	187
14	Writing the Research Report	199
15	Writing the Review Article	215
16	Reporting the Quality Improvement or Evidence-Based Practice Project	231
17	Writing for Presentations	241
18	From Student Project or Dissertation to Publication	255
19	Writing a Continuing Professional Development Activity	267
20	Writing the Nursing Narrative	283
21	Think Outside the Journal: Alternative Publication Options	297
22	Writing a Book or Book Chapter	307
23	Writing for a General Audience	319

Writing the Clinical Article

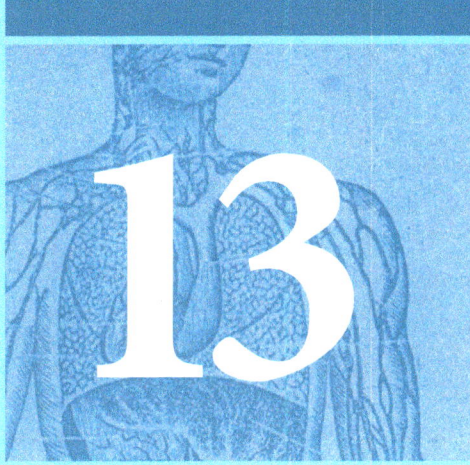

– Cheryl L. Mee, MSN, MBA, RN, FAAN
– Fidelindo Lim, DNP, CCRN, FAAN

> *"If it reads nice and easy, chances are it took hard work.
> If it's wordy and complicated, chances are it was very easy to write."*
> –William Zinsser

WHAT YOU'LL LEARN IN THIS CHAPTER

- It's essential to take sufficient time to plan before writing a clinical manuscript.
- You should gather more information than you think you need on your topic.
- Multiple manuscript edits are essential to good writing.
- Developing a time schedule for researching, preparing, and writing your article will help you stay on task and on track.

Because you're likely most familiar with clinical articles, they make a great starting point for you to start your professional writing. Clinical articles are read by nurses in nearly all specialties and settings and are published in many types of nursing journals. Formats can vary from journal to journal, but underlying all clinical articles is a discussion of a disease or health issue affecting a patient population. Clinical articles not only help nurses understand a particular disease or health concern but also place the topic in a context that helps readers understand how their patient population might present, how the illness might progress, what assessments and interventions should be considered, and how the patient may be treated, along with potential complications and outcomes.

Many clinical articles also include patient education and medication information (either a medication summary or an in-depth review), depending on the journal or author/editor preferences. Ultimately, a well-written clinical article will paint a picture for the nurse reader of a patient's presentation and progression, focused assessment, and comprehensive plan of care, helping the reader better comprehend patient needs and nursing care considerations so they can provide better care for patients and improve outcomes.

This chapter will help you craft an effective clinical article. First, however, let's look at how a clinical article differs from a research article.

Clinical and Research Articles

Clinical articles target the nurse clinician: a nurse in any clinical practice setting who wants useful takeaway information that can be readily applied to day-to-day practice. Clinical articles focus on patients, their clinical presentation, and plan of care options that might be considered. These articles can include opinions from expert clinicians, key evidence, and information on typical procedures and therapies, as well as innovations to consider now and those on the horizon.

Research articles (also called scholarly" or "academic" articles) are geared toward nurses in research and academia. This is not to say that researchers don't read clinical articles or that clinicians don't read research articles; that is indeed not the case. Many nurse researchers are also practicing clinicians, and clinicians read research articles on current practice and new practice evidence.

However, compared with clinical articles, research articles typically include a more in-depth review of the literature, contain more information related to the data collection process and new research, and focus more on the science of nursing and less on the clinical, hands-on application of the content or expert clinical commentary. Research articles are written to build the science and literature base of the profession, share new research and insights, and encourage more research related to the topic.

Q *I'm not sure I have the experience to write a clinical article, but I think I should try. Do you have any advice for me?*

A Unfortunately, some nurses shy away from writing because they believe they don't have enough expertise or credentials in an area—that they aren't good enough or knowledgeable enough. This lack of confidence holds nurses back from writing when, in fact, they can develop a well-done, well-researched clinical article that journal editors value for their publication. If editors waited for only the top experts and gurus in a field to write, we would have little nursing literature with few perspectives.

Additionally, some nurses hesitate to write clinical articles because they assume the topic is already well covered in the nursing literature. Others believe their perspectives on the topic are nothing new. Journal editors look for journal articles on topics with fresh clinical perspectives from nurses who provide care and improve outcomes. A special case study or your perspective on caring for a specific patient population can be the catalyst for a new clinical article.

With the profession's focus on evidence-based practice, the line between clinical and research articles has blurred as clinical articles include more data and evidence, and research articles include more discussion of the clinical application to practice. Some overlap exists, but in general, clinical articles are more immediately relevant to practicing clinicians.

Writing Process

Nurses should write clinical articles to share their expertise and knowledge in a subject or specialty. Don't be deterred by imagined barriers. For example, you don't have to be *the* specialty expert to write a clinical article on a topic in your clinical setting with which you are familiar.

Writing a strong clinical article is within your grasp if you consider a step-by-step approach (Redulla, 2022), such as this:

1. Develop a clinical topic and focus.
2. Select a journal to target for submission.
3. Send a query email to the journal.
4. Choose an appropriate format.
5. Gather information.
6. Prepare to write.
7. Write using authoritative and active voice.
8. Edit your manuscript.
9. Submit.

Here is a closer look at each step.

Develop a Clinical Topic and Focus

Think about clinical articles you found helpful. They usually don't cover too much: The focus is tight, and although the topic is well covered, the article is not too long. Journal articles aren't like textbook chapters; they are typically more focused. So instead of writing on a general, broad topic, such as "diabetes in the home care patient," narrow your topic to "patient teaching and continuous blood glucose monitoring for the home care patient with diabetes."

Exploring the current literature in your area of interest will help you develop and refine topics. As you review the information, consider what new perspective you can bring to an article. You also might brainstorm for a possible topic by asking yourself, "What in my clinical practice bothers me that I can address in an article?"

Keeping a tight focus prevents you from writing too much on a broad topic and helps you maintain better control of manuscript length. It's important to match the length of the manuscript to the suggested manuscript length in the journal's author guidelines. It's a natural tendency to believe that more is better, but a concise article is preferred.

Q *I know I'd like to write, but I'm not sure what to write about. Where do I start?*

A Consider writing in content areas where you have a passion. Think about patient care experiences you found interesting and particularly rewarding. Use your passion from your work to fuel your topic idea list. The process might take some time, and passion helps you continue through the process. Selecting a topic takes time and energy, so this step can be a roadblock for some new authors. In most cases you'll find that this step is more time-consuming than you expected. After developing a topic idea, review recent clinical articles on the topic to understand what has been covered most recently. Take the time to delve into the literature, and work to develop and refine your topic focus. Think of your audience and what they will find relevant. Define the aspects of your experience that were important to you, and you'll lay a strong foundation that keeps you energized as you work through the project. (Learn more about identifying a topic in Chapter 2.)

Obtain feedback on your topic from colleagues. Ask them what they might look for in a journal article on the topic. Getting various perspectives can help you develop ideas for key content areas to cover and help confirm your content outline.

As you develop the topic, list four to six main content areas or headings and populate them with key points. As you gather resources and references on the topic, refine this list (remembering to keep it focused) and add some sub-bullets. Keep this outline fluid as you brainstorm what to cover and what not to cover (content that deviates from the article's focus). Later you'll use the outline as a guide when writing to keep yourself from drifting off topic. The following is an excerpt of what might have been the initial outline for a published clinical article (Jones et al., 2023):

Compassionate Care for People with Cancer and Opioid Use Disorder

    Caring for Mr. Wright

    Medication Treatment for Opioid Use Disorder (OUD)

    Reducing Harm

    Treating Pain and OUD

    Coprescribing Analgesia

    Death with Dignity

Use the list of key topics in your query letter (an email to the editor asking if there is interest in a topic) to describe the proposed content of your article. A query with specifics makes an impression on an editor and helps them come to a decision more quickly. Another benefit of a query letter is that the editor may guide you in developing an article that better meets the journal's needs but varies from your original proposal: Your topic might be modified instead of rejected. Even when ideas are accepted, editors may work with you to further refine the topic for their journal. (Learn more about queries in Chapter 3.)

Select a Journal to Target for Submission

Chapter 3 discusses selecting a journal in detail. Once you have identified the journal, review its aims, scope, mission (or purpose statement), and read at least three to four recent issues so that you have a good understanding of expectations for any submitted article. Remember that the editor is the gatekeeper of the content. So, if you are working toward the same goal as the editor in developing the manuscript, you will have a stronger chance of manuscript acceptance.

Choose an Appropriate Format

Clinical articles can cover a broad array of topics relevant to the area of clinical practice and may cover key topic themes such as practice issues, leadership, technology, and more. Although formats for clinical articles can vary, some elements are standard, particularly for articles that discuss a specific disease state. Depending on the topic and the journal, other formats might include case studies, "how to" articles,

> **All About Columns**
>
> A good place to target your topic might be a journal's columns, also called *departments*. Columns, which are typically shorter than feature articles, run regularly in multiple issues throughout the year. These pieces are intentionally developed to be shorter reads that mix with longer feature articles in a journal issue. The topic changes, but the theme remains the same. For example, some nursing journals have a regularly occurring legal column with changing topics each month, such as "Informed Consent" or "Malpractice Insurance." Note that columns are highly focused and have a limited word count.
>
> Columns may have a regular author, but in many cases, they are open to any author with a good topic idea. Editors are often challenged to develop topics for columns because they are published frequently. They look for new "takes" on common topics. For example, a regularly occurring column on documentation might be a good place for you to write about your work with electronic health records and incident documentation. Follow word counts carefully and be concise in your writing. If you can come up with an innovative way to write about these "evergreen" topics, editors may find the idea a good fit.

and articles that answer frequently asked questions about a particular topic such as palliative care. Formats can be combined; for example, a case study may be used to illustrate key assessment findings in an article on neonatal abstinence syndrome.

Before choosing a format, refer to the journal's author guidelines. Your review of past issues will also give you insights into what might work best for your article. (Refer to Chapter 5 for more information about formats and organizing an article.)

Case studies

Case studies may be developed from real-life cases with the patient's identity concealed. Concealing identity in a real case study report can be difficult, so you should seek patient permission if there is any chance that the patient identity could be identified via the text (refer to Chapter 11 for more information). Case studies also can be fictional, but they should be based on real-life cases. You might pull together a fictional case study based on your experience of caring for multiple patients. This method helps you demonstrate various aspects of patient care; for example, a fictional case might emphasize multiple potential complications and nursing interventions at various points in time.

The case study serves as an example that enables readers to take the pieces of the clinical article and fit them into a patient scenario, helping them better understand the content. Case studies encourage readers to visualize a real patient, which brings the article to life. Readers can relate to the case study, and the knowledge they gain from reading the article becomes more memorable. The case study might be presented first, followed by other sections of the clinical article (pathophysiology, results of key studies, nursing care), or it might be interwoven throughout the article. Here is an example of a case study that opens an article on acute kidney injury (Lim & Li, 2023):

> Kay Dempsey,* a 70-year-old woman, arrives by ambulance at the emergency department (ED) after being found lethargic, pale, and diaphoretic in the nursing home where she lives. Her medical history includes hypertension, hyperlipidemia, type 2 diabetes, heart failure (HF), and kidney stones. On admission, her vital signs are blood pressure (BP) 86/40 mmHg, heart rate (HR) 136 beats per minute (bpm), respiratory rate (RR) 30 breaths per minute, oxygen saturation 94% on 6 L of oxygen by nasal cannula, and temperature 101.4° F (38.5° C). In addition, she has +1 edema of her lower extremities.
>
> Abnormal findings from Ms. Dempsey's initial basic metabolic panel (BMP) include blood urea nitrogen (BUN) 35 mg/dL (normal: 8–23 mg/dL), serum creatinine (SCr) 1.6 mg/dL (normal: 0.6–1.2 mg/dL), potassium 5.2 mEq/L (normal: 3.5–5 mEq/L), and glucose 224 mg/dL (normal: 70–110 mg/dL).
>
> Notable findings from the complete blood count (CBC) upon admission include white blood cells 24,000/mm3 (normal: 4,500–11,000/mm3), hemoglobin 10 g/dL (normal: 12–14 g/dL), and hematocrit 30% (normal: 36–44%). Arterial blood gasses show Ms. Dempsey's pH 7.30 (normal: 7.35–7.45), PaO2 116 mmHg (normal: 80–100 mmHg), PaCO2 30 mmHg (normal: 35–45 mmHg), and HCO3 16 mEq/L (normal: 22–26 mEq/L). Her serum lactate is 5.4 mmol/L (normal: 0.6–2.2 mmol/L).

Elements of Clinical Articles

A nursing journal clinical article might include all or some of the following elements. Always read recent issues to see how these are handled in the journal that you are targeting.

- **Etiology:** The cause or the origin of the disease, focusing on the most common ones. The detail included in this section varies from journal to journal.

- **Incidence:** The frequency at which a disease presents in a population. *Prevalence*, which is similar, is the number of cases present at a point in time.

- **Health disparities:** Includes relevant disparities that readers need to know. In discussing race and ethnicity, keep in mind that they are considered "social constructs, without scientific or biological meaning" (Flanagin et al., 2021). In 2021, the *Journal of the American Medical Association* published an editorial outlining details that should be included in manuscripts when reporting on race and ethnicity (Flanagin et al., 2021).

- **Pathophysiology:** The changes in physiology that occur with the disease. This section elaborates on the etiology and helps the reader better understand the disease process. Note that some journals may use artwork and design elements to provide a visual representation. If the journal you are writing for uses art for pathophysiology, you might consider including suggestions for artwork. If you use art from another source, obtain permission from the copyright holder. (Chapter 11 covers permissions in detail, and Chapter 7 provides information about graphics.) Refer to the journal's author guidelines for more details on artwork and permissions.

- **Clinical presentation:** What signs and symptoms the patient might present that are pieces of the nursing assessment. When reporting lab results, indicate normal ranges.

- **Differential diagnosis:** Especially important for nurse practitioners because it provides clinical information about similar diseases or illnesses and how they differ.

- **Diagnostics:** The diagnostic tests, along with normal and abnormal values, that are relevant to the topic.

- **Treatment:** Treatment includes medications, surgery, and other interventions. Journals handle this content differently. Some might include detailed tables and charts on various medications, dose, and key nursing considerations.

- **Nursing implications:** Consider nursing implications throughout the article. Be sure to cover all areas of the nursing process, including key assessment data and cues, priorities in care, interventions, and various outcomes. Discuss components of critical thinking and decision-making that are important as you care for the patient. Some editors call this the "So what?" Be sure the reader understands the application to their practice. Does the reader take away information that is relevant to patient care and readily applicable to practice? Some journals want nursing implications presented in one section of the article, while others want them integrated throughout the text.

- **Patient education:** Some journals include a patient education handout written at a specified grade level. Others might only include a short section on important patient education considerations.

- **Prevention:** Note that prevention might be wrapped into the patient education section; include prevention of complications.

- **Case studies:** A realistic case study may be woven through the manuscript, describing a patient and including presentation and progression through the illness and response to care. This is a great way to help nurse readers understand the topic, as it presents an unfolding image of a patient whom the nurse might care for.

In the ambulance, Ms. Dempsey received a 500 mL bolus of 0.9% normal saline without improvement in her vital signs. A physical exam in the ED reveals a weeping Stage 4 sacral pressure injury. Following sepsis protocol, the ED physician initiates 30 mL/kg of normal saline and consulted the intensivist.

*Name is fictitious.

This case study then continues with a discussion of the common causes and pathophysiology of acute kidney injury, gerontologic considerations, diagnosis, and collaborative management. The case study method helps to pull the reader into the "real-life story" of a patient and their care.

How-to articles

How-to articles may focus on skills, procedures, interventions, or processes. For example, how-to topics from past issues of *Nursing* include heart failure management, personal protective equipment for antineoplastic safety, approaches for managing neuropsychiatric symptoms of dementia, and preventing transfusion-associated circulatory overload. These articles usually follow a progression of steps; carefully review each journal's published how-to articles to determine the best fit for your topic.

To ensure how-to articles have the most value for practicing nurses, don't make them a step-by-step guide that you might find in product-use literature. Keep the focus on important aspects for the nurse that surround the use of the product, such as teaching tips, key infection prevention practices, psychosocial considerations, and valuable nursing assessment, intervention, and evaluation details pertinent to the topic. The writer's role is to help the reader understand the concept with clear, concise writing.

How-to articles may look simple to write, but depending on the topic, they take a great deal of effort along with a tremendous attention to details. Eliminating extra text and keeping your writing focused is key. Photos or artwork may accompany this type of writing, along with carefully edited descriptions of the figures.

Gather Information

Even if you are well versed in a topic area, gather more resources than you think you need, including articles and books in nursing. Also look at the literature in other disciplines, such as medicine, psychology, social work, and pharmacy. For example, in the article titled "Compassionate Care for People with Cancer and Opioid Use Disorder," published in the *American Journal of Nursing*, the author refers to literature not only from nursing, but also from medicine, psychiatry, palliative care, social work, the Cochrane database, textbooks, and governmental reports (Jones et al., 2023).

Reading a great deal on the subject in a wide array of literature immerses you in the topic; when you start writing, it will come more quickly and naturally. You might want to keep all your sources in a folder that you can easily access for reading and reviewing if you prefer print. Some authors prefer paper they can easily write on and prioritize; others prefer digital copies, which can be stored in reference management systems such as Mendeley, RefWorks, and Zotero. The reference librarian at your institution can assist you in using these programs. (Chapter 4 also has more details on reference management systems, as well as tips for researching your topic.)

Don't forget to read current lay literature on the topic such as the health section of leading newspapers to get a perspective on what the public is reading. Lay press articles may include interesting anecdotes, scenarios, and statistics gleaned from primary sources. Always seek out primary sources and reference them if they are included in your manuscript.

Q *What is a primary source?*

A The *primary source* is the original article that an article, as a secondary source, is citing. Use primary sources in your article.

For example, if *The New York Times* quotes statistics from the CDC pertinent to your manuscript, refer to the CDC original document and cite the CDC as the source. (You can usually download government documents at the agency's website.) Verify that the information in the original source matches what was reported in the secondary source. The author of the secondary source may have misinterpreted information in the primary source; in that case, you would not want to repeat the error. Note that using information from government websites is considered "public domain," and no permission for use is required, although it must be properly referenced.

It's a good idea to read all the articles and information you gather once as an overview, without worrying about highlighting or taking notes. This gives you overall baseline knowledge of the recent literature. Then read them a second time, highlighting key areas and making notes in the margins for the manuscript (or making notes in the electronic copies).

Reread the content a few times. As you read, think about the clinical applications of the content to your work experience and how you can use *your* experiences in practice in your writing. This combination of knowing the literature well and connecting this knowledge to your clinical experiences is an important factor in developing a strong manuscript. Start to develop a list of key aspects of patient care that you want to be sure to emphasize for the reader. This helps you create an original manuscript based on your experience combined with current evidence—the ideal article.

Prepare to Write

Notice that a lot of effort is spent on preparing to write—selecting a topic, focus, and journal; gathering information; and immersing yourself in the literature. If you do your homework and prepare well, the writing process should be easier and quicker. Start by paying careful attention to the author guidelines for your target journal. It's important to follow these guidelines closely to be sure your final manuscript adheres to all specifications. Remember that an editor reads and writes all day long and will immediately identify manuscripts that don't adhere to the guidelines. First impressions really count! A polished manuscript shows you did your homework.

Some authors start writing in the middle of the manuscript, not worrying about grammar and punctuation but rather focusing on getting the main points, ideas, and key elements into the first draft They then add areas such as an introduction and conclusion later. Other authors convert their outlines to content. For example, they list the main headings for the article, such as "Introduction" and "Pathophysiology" followed by the bullet points under each heading. These authors then fill out each section, adding more information and reorganizing as needed. They continue writing until the manuscript starts to take shape, referring to the outline as a guide to stay on track. Find what works best for you, but certainly following an outline can be particularly helpful for new writers.

A helpful hint: Don't cut and paste from other documents when writing, even if your intention is to rewrite the information and use it only as a reference or "idea holder" in the manuscript. You can accidentally plagiarize the content by not eliminating the content as planned. Your writing *must* be your own unless you are quoting another source; in that case, cite the source as a reference.

First-time writers can seek out an experienced co-author to collaborate on a writing project. You may find a writing mentor and collaborator among your current and former nursing faculty or at your place of work. (Refer to Chapter 1 for more information about collaborative writing.)

Q *Is it acceptable to use artificial intelligence (AI) technology, such as large language models, chatbots, or image creators in developing a clinical article?*

A Check the journal's author guidelines for details on authorship and publication ethics related to AI. Journals typically require disclosure of any use of AI tools in producing the article, including collecting and analyzing data, producing images, and developing content. The Committee on Publication Ethics (COPE, 2023) states unequivocally that AI tools such as ChatGPT cannot be listed as an author. The International Committee of Medical Journal Editors (ICMJE) recommendations (2024) also note that chatbots are not considered authors. In addition, ICMJE notes that any use of AI should be described in the appropriate section of the manuscript. When using generative AI tools, remember that they "cannot reliably detect between fact and fiction," so check information carefully (Harrington, 2023, p. 281).

Write Using Authoritative and Active Voice

Writing from clinical experience and writing for a clinical journal requires you to be authoritative in your writing. Getting your perspective and experiences on patient care into the manuscript helps the nurse reader visualize that care experience. Remember that for clinical articles, it's acceptable to put yourself into the writing: Your experience and knowledge in the area are valuable, so you can be authoritative, speak about your interpretations, and voice an opinion, as appropriate.

> ### A Word About References
>
> Carefully cite appropriate statements with references according to the journal's author guidelines. Guidelines and formats vary. Two common reference styles are the American Medical Association (AMA) and the American Psychological Association (APA). It's important to note that many journals use a modified style that takes pieces of one style and then tailors it to editorial team preferences and feedback from journal readers.
>
> Cite relevant references from recent years. Many journals prefer references from within the past five years. That doesn't mean you can't use older references; just be selective. For example, when writing about pressure injuries, the groundbreaking work by Barbara J. Braden on predicting pressure injuries may be relevant, and many articles on this topic are older than five years. Be sure that older references are relevant and look for more up-to-date information that augments the findings. As you work on your manuscript, continue to check for new relevant literature at least monthly, so you incorporate the most recent literature.
>
> Don't reference every line of clinical article content. Too much referencing is difficult to read and not necessary. Much information in clinical articles can be considered common knowledge, and a source isn't necessary. Use your best judgment, keeping in mind that statistics and specific recommendations from practice guidelines should be referenced, and ultimately the writing must be your own. Mix referenced content with your own experience and knowledge, balancing a blend of referenced and original material in the article. If you are ever in doubt about whether material needs to be referenced, take that as a sign that you should probably include a source.

Traditionally, we learn to make much of our documentation as healthcare providers objective and to state only the facts. This is important from a legal and a clinical perspective, but we often carry this concept into our professional writing. Nurses may be uncomfortable with authoritative writing because we are familiar with writing objectively in our daily work. Think back on some of your favorite articles, though. The authors might not have only described what happened but included their perspectives as well. Do comply with the journal style and with the kinds of writing you find in current issues of your targeted journal, but don't be shy. Be bold and state what you have experienced in practice. What editors are looking for in clinical articles is not just a statement of the facts, but experience and confidence that makes for strong, compelling writing. Editors and readers can sense that strength and authority in your writing, which makes for more interesting reading.

Active voice adds to this concept and speaks directly to the reader. See Chapter 6 for more information, but here is a simple example:

Passive voice: The patient was assessed by the registered nurse shortly after admission.

In passive voice, the subject receives the action. The patient is the subject and is being acted upon (assessed). The word "by" is a tip-off that the sentence is in passive voice.

Active voice: The registered nurse assessed the patient shortly after admission.

The registered nurse is the subject of the sentence and does the action.

An important difference between active and passive voice is that active voice uses fewer words. Think about active voice as speaking directly to the nurse reader in straightforward language. Visualize a straight line from the author to the reader in the communication (see Figure 13.1). Passive voice, on the other hand, is less direct. Imagine passive voice as circling around the issue instead of moving in a shorter, straight line. Passive voice takes the longer, indirect path to describe the concept and uses more words.

Active writing brings you and your clinical experience into the article and helps readers connect with you. Think of it as painting a picture. The reader can see the patient-nurse interaction and imagine the clinical care. Again, consider some of your favorite reading material. You like it because you can feel and see the story in your mind. In good writing—even in professional publications—you can use active voice to tell a story and describe care. Note that in more formal articles, reporting research for example, writing in active voice improves the abstract, the introduction, and the discussion sections that reflect on

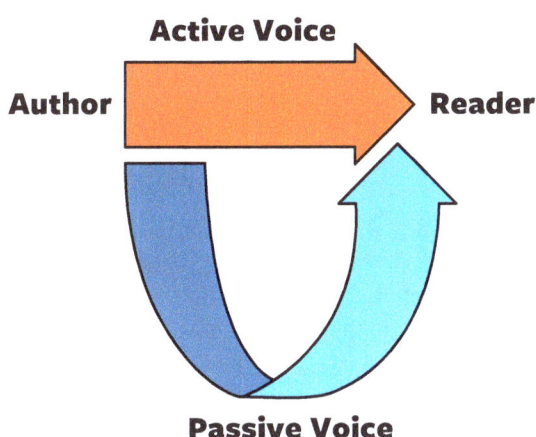

FIGURE 13.1 Active voice speaks directly to the reader about an issue. Passive voice is indirect and circuitous.

the relevance and interpretation of the results, but passive voice may be used in other sections, such as methodology.

Finally, the last step is usually to write the lead paragraph and title. After you have a well-developed manuscript, the lead paragraph and title should be easier to write. Try to add a value proposition. What benefit will readers get from the article? Why should they read the article, and why should they care about the topic? Include this information in the title if possible. If not, work this information into the first paragraph and the abstract. In many cases the editorial team will modify titles and leads, but sending in a manuscript that is well polished can make a difference. Example 13.1 shows a couple article titles with what might have been their original titles.

Edit Your Manuscript

Editing polishes your manuscript. After reading and editing the manuscript for flow and organization, start to dig, read, and edit *every word*. You can probably eliminate at least one or two unnecessary words in many sentences. Again, think back to the editor reading multiple manuscripts. If you can eliminate 200 to 300 words and say the same thing, your writing is more concise. Eliminating extra words improves the manuscript, and a tighter, shorter manuscript gets the editor's attention. Editors notice a well-edited manuscript after reading just a few sentences.

Shorter is better because the reader gets through the same material with less time and fewer words. Added unnecessary words can cause reader fatigue. Readers will find the work more interesting and inviting because they are not working as hard to glean the information. Continue this process—honing and rewriting sentences—for a few rounds.

Read your manuscript aloud, and you'll immediately hear the extra words and problem sentences. Or have someone read your manuscript out loud to you. You might be surprised at the writing problems you hear that you didn't recognize in your earlier edits. A minimum of three edits is a good target. You'll likely get bored from reading the same information multiple times, but it's worth the effort because your manuscript becomes more polished. Appendix A has an editing checklist you may find helpful.

Seek feedback from experts and non-experts on your work. Have someone who knows the topic well, such as a well-respected colleague, critique and edit your manuscript. Provide an electronic and a hard copy (so they have a choice of how to submit their comments), and instruct your reviewers to provide valuable constructive feedback. Tell them that you appreciate their critique to help improve the manuscript and that you don't want them to just be polite and say that the work is good—you want a critical review with comments and suggestions for edits.

Possible original title: Managing Patients With Dementia

Improved title: The ABCD Approach for Managing Neuropsychiatric Symptoms of Dementia (Siple, 2023)

Possible original title: Debriefings on Moral Distress

Improved title: Impact of Case Review Debriefings on Moral Distress of Extracorporeal Membrane Oxygenation Nurses (Griggs et al., 2023)

EXAMPLE 13.1 Original versus improved manuscript titles.

> **Getting Good Feedback**
>
> Here are a few questions you might ask colleagues to address when they review your manuscript:
>
> - Is the clinical content valuable and accurate?
> - Is content missing?
> - Does the content flow well, or are there gaps?
> - Is it organized?
> - Is the work current and relevant?
> - Can you comment and make suggestions for edits?
> - Would you want to read this in a journal? If not, why?

Non-experts who will be reading the article also can provide valuable insights. For instance, someone less experienced in the specialty can help you identify missing pieces and provide feedback as to the level of content. They can comment on the flow and their understanding of the article or identify if you made leaps that skipped over essential information. You as the writer take the feedback from colleagues and consider what to change and what to keep, but critical reviews help you hone the manuscript.

Long uninterrupted text is difficult to read (and boring), so be sure to use subheads throughout the manuscript. A subhead breaks up the text and defines a section of the article. It also acts as a step for the reader when skimming an article. Reading a 4,000-word article with 10 subheads helps the reader understand the organization of the article better than the same article with only three subheads. Not having sufficient subheads leaves long narrative sections, which can cause reader fatigue.

Use other elements such as charts, graphs, tables, figures, bulleted lists, or boxes with text. These elements attract readers' eyes as they skim the journal, which makes them popular with editors. They also may cut down the length of the narrative in the manuscript. For example, a clinical article with 3,500 words can be shortened if a section covering common medications, their drug classes, and related nursing considerations were pulled from the narrative running text and listed in a table. (Learn more about these elements in Chapter 7.) Scan the journal you are targeting to see how these elements appear. Your use of graphic elements gets an editor's attention and is a sign of an experienced writer.

Submit

When you have finished your article, you're ready to submit. Be sure to follow the author guidelines, which contain detailed information about how to prepare your manuscript and graphics, ancillary documents to include (such as a cover letter, a title page, and copyright agreements from authors), and where to submit the files. In many cases, you will be submitting to an online editorial management system. Chapter 8 provides detailed information about the submission process.

Setting a Timeline

Allow time for each step in writing a clinical article. A timeline can help you stay on track, and as you complete each step you can get satisfaction in knowing you are progressing. As you can see, the preparation phase can take some time. Topic and focus development may take two weeks, journal investigation and gathering and reviewing literature another two to three weeks, query and planning the content another two weeks, and so on. If you skip steps, you might get frustrated because you are not primed to write. Not preparing may hinder your success.

> **Confidence Booster**
>
> You followed the journal's author guidelines; put a lot of time, energy, and passion into your work; and submitted your manuscript. After the editor sends the manuscript through the review process, you receive an email requesting revisions. You're frustrated because you already did your very best in writing the manuscript!
>
> Don't give up: Make the revisions. The editor liked your manuscript enough to invest time in it and send it for review. But the editor and peer reviewers may have made recommendations that will improve the manuscript. Change your feeling of defeat into recognition of the comments as a gift. The editorial suggestions will most likely make your final article better.
>
> Some nurse writers stop here and give up, but don't. You have a high chance of acceptance if you make the suggested edits and revisions.

As you write, use your bulleted topic outline to plan your writing. Give yourself a week, for example, to write a set number of words for each bullet on the outline, based on the total suggested manuscript length in the author guidelines. Break up the time to write each section; don't plan to write for eight hours straight. Some prolific writers can write all day, and they do it well, but many novice writers get fatigued after a short time (an hour or two at most), so plan breaks and achievable goals. Walking away and thinking about the work brings a fresh perspective and new ideas for writing and keeps the creative juices flowing. Moving away from your desk, walking, and thinking about patients helps with recall of anecdotes about real patient care that can enhance the manuscript. Connecting your experience with patients to the clinical content on paper can make a big difference in your finished work.

Remember: You are not just writing clinical facts. You want to write an interesting piece that draws in readers and holds their attention. Crafting and editing take time.

Keep It Simple

Now you know the steps for writing a clinical article. Using these steps can help you work through the process and keep your writing simple and straightforward. You'll soon find you have a finished manuscript ready to submit.

Write Now!

1. List one or two possible ideas for a clinical article.
2. Look for a prototype article format that fits your topic of choice.
3. Identify one or two target journals, review the author guidelines, and start writing.

References

Committee on Publication Ethics (COPE). (2023). *Authorship and AI tools.* https://publicationethics.org/cope-position-statements/ai-author

Flanagin, A., Frey, T., Christiansen, S. L., & AMA Manual of Style Committee. (2021). Updated guidance on the reporting of race and ethnicity in medical and science journals. *JAMA, 326*(7), 621–627. https://doi.org/10.1001/jama.2021.13304

Griggs, S., Hampton, D., Edward, J., & McFarlin, J. (2023). Impact of case review debriefings on moral distress of extracorporeal membrane oxygenation nurses. *Critical Care Nurse, 43*(3), 12–18. https://doi.org/10.4037/ccn2023870

Harrington, L. (2023). ChatGPT is trending: Trust but verify. *AACN Advanced Critical Care, 34*(4), 280–286. https://doi.org/10.4037/aacnacc2023129

International Committee of Medical Journal Editors. (2024). *Recommendations for the conduct, reporting, editing, and publication of scholarly work in medical journals.* http://www.icmje.org/recommendations

Jones, K. F., Broglio, K., Ho, J. J., & Rosa, W. E. (2023). Compassionate care for people with cancer and opioid use disorder. *American Journal of Nursing, 123*(8), 56–61. https://doi.org/10.1097/01.NAJ.0000947480.74410.06

Lim, F., & Li, A. (2023). Acute kidney injury: A nursing challenge. *American Nurse Journal, 18*(6), 6–12. https://doi.org/10.51256/ANJ062306

Redulla, R. (2022). Writing clinical articles: A step-by-step guide for nurses. *American Nurse Journal, 17*(5), 24–26.

Siple A. (2023). The ABCD approach for managing neuropsychiatric symptoms of dementia. *Nursing, 53*(8), 24–28. https://doi.org/10.1097/01.NURSE.0000942784.14340.1f

Zinsser, W. (2016). *On writing well: The classic guide to writing nonfiction* (30th anniversary ed.). HarperCollins Publishers.

Writing the Research Report

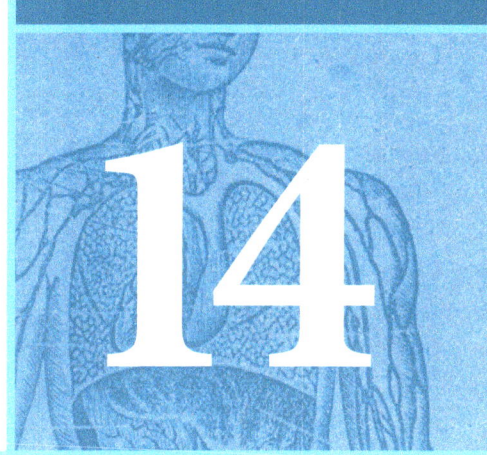

–Patricia Gonce Morton, PhD, RN, ACNP-BC, FAAN

> *"Keep a small can of WD-40 on your desk—away from any open flames—to remind yourself that if you don't write daily, you will get rusty."*
> –George Singleton

With the increased complexity of healthcare and the need to solve patient care problems based on evidence, nurses more than ever are conducting research studies to contribute to the evidence that guides practice. The results of these studies must be disseminated. Publishing the results of research in journals is an excellent way to ensure that evidence is disseminated and readily available to guide practice. Multiple opportunities exist for nurses to publish their findings in journals intended for nurses or other healthcare professionals, as well as in basic science and social science journals.

This chapter describes how to write articles based on quantitative, qualitative, or mixed-methods research. You'll learn how to report your original research so that systematic reviewers and those conducting replications can include your study in future reviews. Keep in mind that articles need to be written clearly using accepted standards of research reporting so readers can evaluate the quality of the findings and their relevance for current clinical practice.

Anatomy of a Research Article

Typically, a report of quantitative research includes these elements:

- Title
- Keywords
- Abstract
- Introduction

The author wishes to acknowledge with gratitude Shaké Ketefian and Richard W. Redman, who wrote and revised this chapter in previous editions of this book.

WHAT YOU'LL LEARN IN THIS CHAPTER

- A research report typically includes an abstract, introduction, literature review, methods, results, and discussion.
- Quantitative research is an approach to studying phenomena that can be categorized, rank ordered, or counted in units of measure.
- Qualitative research is an interpretive, naturalistic approach to study phenomena that can be observed but not measured.
- Mixed-methods research combines quantitative and qualitative methods to answer a research question.

- Literature Review
- Research Questions or Hypotheses
- Methods
- Results
- Discussion
- Conclusion

An easy way to remember the main sections of the article is IMRAD—Introduction, Methods, Results, and Discussion (Aga & Nissar, 2022; Ozcakar et al., 2022).

Not all journals use this exact organizing framework, so be sure to read the author guidelines for the journal you've targeted. Read some recent issues, too, so you'll have a good sense of how to present your report. Find an article based on a research design similar to yours and use it as an example when formatting your manuscript. The article you select doesn't have to be on the same topic as yours.

Check the author guidelines for the format the journal uses and any reporting structure requirements. For example, some journals require that randomized controlled trials be reported according to Consolidated Standards of Reporting Trials (CONSORT) guidelines (Butcher et al., 2022; Schulz et al., 2010;). You can go to www.consort-statement.org to access the guidelines. (A list of guidelines for reporting results is in Appendix D.)

Reporting Quantitative Studies

Quantitative research is a structured and systematic means to investigate phenomena from a variety of sources by gathering quantifiable data to formulate facts and patterns and generate knowledge and new understandings of the phenomena. Here is a closer look at the key components of reports of quantitative studies.

Title

The title is an important selling point for your article. A succinct, clearly written, and informative title attracts readers (Aga & Nissar, 2022; Ozcakar et al., 2022; Seals, 2023). Keep in mind that abstracting and indexing services also rely on an informative and accurate title to extract keywords for cross-referencing. Good titles are succinct, contain the most important descriptors of the study, capture readers' attention, and don't include abbreviations or jargon. (See Chapter 5 for more tips on writing a strong title.)

Keywords

You may need to list keywords for your article when you submit your manuscript. The right keywords are essential to help others who are searching various indexes and databases for articles relevant to their work (American Psychological Association [APA], 2020). The selected keywords should be specific, representing the main topics of the manuscript. MEDLINE uses Medical Subject Headings (also known as MeSH) terms for indexing, so consider using these terms for your keywords. The National Library of Medicine provides two resources to help you select MeSH terms—MeSH On Demand (https://www.nlm.nih.gov/oet/ed/mesh/meshondemand.html) and MeSH Browser (https://www.nlm.nih.gov/mesh/mbinfo.html).

Abstract

If the title captured readers' attention, they are likely to scrutinize the abstract next to determine their level of interest in reading the research report. The abstract offers an initial impression of the significance of the research and the rigor used to conduct the study. Provide enough information in the abstract to communicate the highlights of your study and to spark the reader's interest to learn more about it (Seals, 2023). Be sure the information in the abstract is consistent with the information in the article. For example, the purpose statement in the abstract should be the same as the purpose statement in the article. In addition, the conclusions in the abstract must be supported by the data in the article.

Some journals prefer abstracts organized by headings. Others want abstracts without headings. Be sure to follow the journal's author guidelines, including any word limitation. When headings are required, the most common requested format is background, purpose, methods, results, and conclusion. Within that format, tell readers what you did, why you did it, how you did it, what you found, and what it means (Aga & Nissar, 2022; PLOS, n.d.) After reviewing your abstract, the reader should have a clear picture of what will follow in the article.

In writing the following abstract from "Burnout Among Academic Nursing Faculty" (Zangaro et al., 2023), the authors complied with the guidelines from the *Journal of Professional Nursing*. Note the brevity and precision with which the authors communicate the essential features of their work.

Background: Nurse faculty burnout is a growing concern in the United States. There are limited studies exploring the level of burnout in nursing faculty.

Purpose: The purpose of the study was to assess the prevalence of burnout among nurse faculty in undergraduate and graduate programs and its relationship with specific demographic and organizational variables.

Methods: A descriptive cross-sectional research design was employed to examine the level of burnout of nursing faculty. An internet-based survey was administered to nursing faculty in over 1000 schools of nursing in the United States. Burnout was measured using the Oldenburg Burnout Inventory.

Results: A total of 3556 surveys were returned. Among all participants, most of the sample exhibited moderate levels of burnout, exhaustion, and disengagement. Based on the findings from the OBI, a moderate/high exhaustion level was reported in 85.5% of participants, while disengagement was moderate/high in 84.9%, and overall burnout was at moderate/high levels in 85.2% of the nursing faculty.

Conclusions: The nation's nurse faculty population is experiencing a moderate to high level of burnout, exhaustion, and disengagement. Academic nursing leaders are encouraged to identify ways and take action to reduce faculty burnout and promote faculty wellness and resilience.

Note: Copyright Elsevier 2023.

Learn more about abstracts in Chapter 5.

Introduction

Your introduction sets the stage for your research report and explains why the study was important to conduct. The introduction clearly answers the "Who cares?" question and helps the reader understand the scope and significance of the problem you have selected to study. After reading the introduction, the reader should be convinced that the problem you have chosen to study is important and there is a true need for research to address the problem (Seals, 2023).

The introduction establishes the importance of your study by answering these questions:

- What is the research problem?
- What is the incidence of the problem?
- Why is the study important?
- What is the magnitude of the problem?
- Who experiences this problem?
- How extensive is the problem?
- What barriers have prevented solving the problem?

A Model for Writing Abstracts

Jennifer L. Greer, PhD, developed the OJISH model for writing abstracts. This model is based on the work of Swales, Feak, and other researchers who have identified common rhetorical "moves" in research abstracts. "Moves" are formulaic phrases or sentences (e.g., "little is known about" or "few studies have addressed") that are identified through discourse or text analysis as strategic language a writer uses to advance the story to the next phase (Greer & Wingo, 2017).

OJISH prompts the writer to work through five moves in quick succession, using a 10-minute timed writing exercise followed by a 10-minute pair-share feedback session. (You do not have to have someone to work on this with you, although the feedback is useful.) Each of the five moves is part of the OJISH mnemonic:

- **O**utline a pressing problem in the field.
- **J**ustify a new study with a gap in the literature.
- **I**ntroduce the purpose of the proposed or present study.
- **S**ummarize the methodology (briefly).
- **H**ighlight the major findings (interpreted, not raw, results).

Here's an example of an introduction from Hamlin et al., 2023:

> Despite efforts to improve early detection of deterioration in patients' condition, a large proportion of hospitalized patients continue to experience delays in intervention, which can lead to serious adverse events such as unplanned intensive care unit admission or death. Up to 80% of serious adverse events are preceded by clinical signs of instability 24 hours or more before the event. In addition to monitoring of vital signs, early indicators of deterioration can be identified through physical assessment and purposeful and frequent surveillance of patients.

Note: Copyright American Association of Critical-Care Nurses, 2023.

Note how the authors provide a short section on the incidence, the groups affected, and the significance of the problem for patients. The introduction provides an excellent transition into the next section of a research article, the literature review.

Literature Review

The literature review (sometimes called review of the literature) serves to place the reported research in context of past studies. It provides the reader with a synopsis of what is known about each variable in your study, what is not known, and how your study fills the gap. An excellent way to organize the literature review is to use each of your study variables as a subheading. Within the review, be sure to present the theoretical definition of each variable. The review should offer the reader a concise synthesis of the findings from previous studies, not an extensive summary of one study after another with all the details of the investigation (Morton, 2017b; Ozcakar et al., 2022).

If the literature review convinces the reader that the answer to your research question is known, readers will wonder why you conducted the study. Instead, after reading the review, the reader should have a clear understanding of the gap in knowledge that your study addresses.

Either within or after the literature review, you may include a summary of the theoretical or conceptual framework that influenced the direction of the study. Often, a theoretical or conceptual framework is used as a guide for selecting, logically developing, and understanding the different, yet interconnected, variables for your study. A figure showing the relationships among the variables may be helpful.

The literature review and theoretical framework provide the basis for the research questions or research hypotheses, which should be included next in the research report. Make certain that the research questions or hypotheses are stated the same as they were written in the abstract. Use consistent terms for all the variables.

> **Q** *Why do I need a literature review? Shouldn't those in my field already know what's being published?*
>
> **A** All empirical research needs to present a literature review to locate, study, and analyze what has been done before in the area of your interest. It's critical to the development of science—each time we conduct a study, we build on and extend what is known to date; in turn, those who come after us will use our work as the foundation for their own research; in this sense, each time we carry out research it serves as a bridge to the past, and will in turn serve as a bridge to future research by later generations.

Here are more tips for writing the literature review:

- Rely on paraphrasing authors' ideas and your own syntheses rather than listing quotations from others or simply describing them in a few sentences.
- Illuminate the variables and relationships that are central to your study.

Preparing to Write the Research Article

You can prepare to write your article even as you begin your research. For example, as you analyze and synthesize the literature, you'll be making comparisons of the reports and the perspectives that particular authors show. Start thinking about how what you are reading fits into the different sections of the research report. For example, you might find some items useful in the introduction of your paper, others for the literature review, and still others might help you frame the theoretical rationale for your study or help shape the methodological approach you take. You'll be writing about all these in your manuscript, so this preparation will serve you well.

- Synthesize the outcomes of previous research. Detailed information about each study is not needed.
- Include what is known and identify gaps, making the case for your own study.
- Organize the review by the variables in your study and show the relationships among the variables, because research is primarily about establishing relationships.
- Discuss the theoretical rationale that supports your own approach. You might use a framework that is well known in the field, an aspect of which you tested in your study, or one that you formulated in view of what you synthesized from the knowledge that is known.
- Conclude the review with a paragraph or more summarizing the highlights of the section and the gap in knowledge. The readers should have a clear understanding of the knowledge void that you are addressing with your study.
- After the concluding paragraph, clearly state the research questions or hypotheses. Make certain they are the same as those stated in the abstract.

Don't make the literature review too long; keep it focused on what is relevant to your specific research topic. If you're new to the process, read the literature review of experienced investigators and see examples of literature reviews in your targeted journal. When you have a draft, ask a colleague or a mentor to read it and provide constructive suggestions for improvement.

After reading the literature review, the reader should have a clear understanding of why your study was needed, the key findings of the previously conducted studies, the variables you are investigating, the relationship of any of those variables to each other or to a theoretical or conceptual framework, and the research questions or hypotheses that you will be testing.

Research Questions or Hypotheses

Next in the research report, clearly tell readers the research questions or hypotheses. Make certain these questions or hypotheses are the same as presented in the abstract and that they show a clear link to the gap in the literature. Within the questions or hypotheses, explicitly state the variables you selected to investigate, using the same names as the variable headings included in literature review. It's imperative that you also use the same name for a variable throughout the remainder of the research report. For example, if in the research question or hypothesis you name the variable "resilience," at other times don't call it "endurance." If the research question or hypothesis indicates you are measuring "factors," tell the reader the names of the variables that constitute the factors.

Q *How can I improve my ability to write a research article?*

A Sharpening your analytical skills makes you a better writer. Try this exercise: Identify two research articles from a journal on a topic of interest to you, published in the same year by different authors. Read the significance, literature review, and theoretical rationale sections. Compare and contrast the approaches the authors took. Consider how successful they were in conveying to you as the reader their grasp of the issues, how they analyzed and synthesized the work of different authors, and how they presented their theoretical rationale to justify their study. Ask questions such as:

- Were the variables theoretically defined?
- Was the research problem clearly stated?
- Has the author included a theoretical framework or rationale that provides justification for the study hypotheses or research questions?
- Does the information set the tone for the rest of the article?
- Do I understand the gap in the literature that the reported research will address?
- Am I interested in reading more?

Then apply what you've learned to your own writing.

Methods

The methods section offers the reader a road map of the steps you used to answer the research questions. The methods section should answer the questions (Aga & Nissar, 2022):

- What was done?
- When was it done?
- Where was it done?
- How was it done?

A well-written methods section meticulously describes each step of your journey. That description will be used by others to judge the quality and validity of the study or to replicate the study. Adhere to the author guidelines of your targeted journal when writing the methods section. Most often the journal will require the use of sub-headings.

Typically, the methods section of a research article includes these elements:

- Design
- Sample
- Setting
- Procedures
- Ethics
- Instruments
- Data analyses

Design: Quantitative research designs include descriptive, correlational, quasi-experimental, and experimental. The design must be appropriate to answer the research question (Roe-Prior, 2023). For example, you cannot ask a cause-effect research question and use a descriptive or correlational design to answer it. Explain your design in specific terms. For instance, if you used a quasi-experimental design, clarify whether it was a posttest only or both pretest and posttest. Also, note the number of comparison groups and any number of variations in quasi-experimental designs. This information prepares the reader for what follows.

Sample: Explain the inclusion and exclusion criteria you used to select subjects. Inform the reader of the sampling method you employed. Was it a random, systematic, stratified, cluster, convenience, quota, purposive, or snowball technique (Roe-Prior, 2023)? Describe how subjects were recruited. Were they contacted by email or face-to-face, and how often were they contacted? Tell the reader how you determined the sample size, because you must have an adequate sample size to answer the research questions. Did you conduct a power analysis? Did you use a guideline for the number of subjects per variable? Clarify the number of subjects invited and the actual number who participated. This response rate is usually reported as a percentage.

Setting: Describe the setting where the research was conducted, such as rural or urban, community health setting or inpatient hospital units, or a different country. Provide details as to the type of institution or organization so readers can better put the study in context. For instance, were the primary care clinics where you studied patients with diabetes located in rural settings or in large cities? These details help readers evaluate the relevance of your work to settings or samples of interest to them.

Procedures: In this section of the research report, provide detailed information so that others can replicate your study. Describe the specific steps you took during the research process to ensure the internal validity of the study, such as how you controlled potential extraneous variables and what you did to ensure consistency in obtaining data and administering treatment to all subjects. If your study has an experimental design, describe the nature of the intervention in this section. If you used research assistants, discuss how they were trained; offer any relevant information, such as their qualifications for performing the task; and provide data to show that their coding/scoring or administration of interventions and instruments are comparable to each other and to yours. Tell the reader when the study took place. Readers need to know the age of your data.

Ethics: Describe the safeguards you used to protect the subjects from harm and to ensure their rights. Explain how participant consent was obtained and how the anonymity of subjects was maintained or not (Roe-Prior, 2023). All studies involving human subjects must be reviewed and approved by the relevant institutional review boards (IRBs). IRB review is required by the Department of Health and Human Services (DHHS) and differs from any administrative or collegial reviews that may occur either to improve the quality of the project or to secure access to research subjects. The researcher never has the right to determine that a study is exempt from IRB review; that decision can only be made by the IRB or its designee (Oermann et al., 2021). If students are the subjects, explain how you avoided coercion of students to participate in your study and how you allayed their fears of retaliation if they did not participate.

Instruments: The reader needs to know that the instruments were appropriate for measuring the study variables for your subjects. For example, if you are studying the variable "confidence," then you need

Reporting the Research Instrument

Here are some key characteristics of the instrument that you need to describe in the research report:

Purpose
- Indicate the variable the instrument was designed to measure.
- Explain the type of subjects the instrument was tested on previously.
- Tell the reader your rationale for selecting the instrument.

Structure
- Describe the total number of items and domains, and the level of data the instrument will generate.
- Discuss how the questions are answered, such as a Likert scale or open-ended responses.
- Provide the total score and the possible range of scores and their meaning.
- Indicate any modifications that you made and their possible effects on the psychometric properties.

Reliability and Validity
- Explain how the developers of the instrument established its validity and reliability as well as the types of subjects the instrument(s) has been used with to date. It is not adequate to merely state that the instruments have adequate psychometric properties. You must discuss the reliability and validity of the instruments.
- Report your reliability data based on use of the instrument with your subjects.

Procedure
- Inform the reader who developed the instrument and indicate that you obtained permission to use it.
- Offer a citation to give the reader a source for information about the instrument and its development.
- Describe how the instrument was distributed to the subjects.
- Explain if the instrument was self-administered, paper and pencil, or online.

to use an instrument designed to measure that variable. If you employ an instrument intended to measure "self-assurance," it may be inappropriate unless your theoretical definition of "confidence" and "self-assurance" are the same. Remember that a study is only as good as the measures you use. If you used several instruments, consider providing a table to present complex information concisely.

If you used your own tool, keep in mind that development of a research instrument is a long and rigorous process including analysis of the literature, concept definition, item development, and testing of the reliability and validity of the instrument. Often, novice investigators underestimate the importance of these steps and create an instrument with little or no testing of its reliability and validity. In these situations, the data gathered from the instrument cannot be used to draw any conclusions. Such studies risk rejection by an editor.

Data analyses: Organize this section of the research report using your research questions or hypotheses. Include these specifics:

- How the measures were scored, coded, and used
- Whether analyses treated data as continuous or categorical variables
- Whether you used instrument subscales or a single, total measure
- What level of data is generated from your instruments and what statistical procedures you used for testing each hypothesis or each research question

The type of data being collected depends on the research question and the type of measurement being used, which in turn determine the types of statistical tests that you can use to analyze the data. Describe the statistical test used for each question or hypothesis and the software program used for the data analysis. Include the level of statistical significance that was set for the study. Be aware that if you used the wrong statistical tests to analyze the data, your manuscript is likely to be rejected (Dwivedi, 2022). (You can access a list of statistical abbreviations in Appendix E.)

> **Confidence Booster**
>
> Like some nurses, you may view statistics with trepidation. Few nurse researchers cast themselves in the role of statistical experts, although that number is increasing.
>
> Instead, they've learned from taking classes, reading books, and working with mentors. Most importantly, these nurses know they are part of a team that includes statisticians who can help with data analysis. Ask another researcher for suggestions. Above all, don't let your fear of statistics hold you back from conducting research. In time, you'll feel more confident in using and interpreting statistics.

Results

The results section starts with a text summary or a table displaying demographic data about the subjects and the response rate (Aga & Nissar, 2022). Indicate how many subjects began in the study, the number who dropped out, and the final number used for data analysis.

Q *My advisor says I've included too much data in my article. What do you recommend to better present the information?*

A If you have too much detail, consider creating tables and figures. This approach allows you to present your information clearly and concisely. There's no need to repeat tabular information in your running text. Just provide the highlights in your text and refer your readers to the table. Some journals will permit appendices of additional tables online.

Use the research questions as the organizing framework for the remainder of the results section of the report. The results section concentrates on reporting the findings, but the explanation of these findings does not appear until the discussion section of the research report. Present findings in text, tables, and/or figures. Text is good for easily explained data and to highlight the most important findings. Tables and figures provide a more detailed display of data and are a succinct way to show patterns, trends, and comparisons; a table is often a helpful tool for the demographics of your study population. Tables summarizing descriptive information about your variables—including means, standard deviations, and other relevant descriptive numbers—are helpful. Readers also expect to see tables that display the results of statistical tests. Create figures that draw the reader's eye to the most critical parts for rapid interpretation of the information (Seals, 2023). When creating tables and figures make certain to cite each table and figure in the text by its sequential number (Ozcakar et al., 2022).

Use these tips when creating tables and figures:

- Follow the author guidelines for tables and figures to determine if they should be embedded in the text or appear at the end of the manuscript, if the journal allows color or only black and white, and if there is a limit to their number.

- Use titles for the tables and figures that clearly describe their contents, such as the statistical test used to analyze the displayed data.

- Place titles at the top for tables and at the bottom for figures.

- Be sure that each table or figure stands alone, augments what is in the text, and has clear labels for all parts.

- Use the same number of places after the decimal point when reporting figures.

- Define all abbreviations either within the table or figure or in a legend at the bottom of the table or figure, even if the abbreviations have been defined within the text of the report.

- Indicate probability levels and units of measurement (in table or footnote).

- Obtain permission for all adapted tables or figures.

See Chapter 7 for more information about graphics and tables.

When reporting the results, indicate if the findings were statistically significant (Dwivedi, 2022). For some studies, it may be important to note clinical significance in addition to statistical significance. For example, in a clinical trial of a new medication, the potassium level of patients may be closely tracked. If the mean potassium level for the control group was 5.2 mmol/L and the mean potassium level for the experimental group was 6.1 mmol/L, the difference may not be statistically significant. However, a potassium level of 6.1 mmol/L is considered life threatening, whereas a level of 5.2 mmol/L is considered the

> **Reporting Demographics**
>
> Many journals and funding organizations (including the National Institutes of Health) now have guidelines related to reporting sex, gender, race, ethnicity, age, and socioeconomic conditions that you need to adhere to. For example, guidance from the *AMA Manual of Style* Committee (Flanagin et al., 2021) notes that the methods section should include who identified participant race and ethnicity and the source of the classifications used (e.g., self-report, electronic health record). The article also should note the reason race and ethnicity categories were collected, and racial and ethnic categories should be listed in alphabetical order in tables of results. Sensitivity related to demographics is important for all sections of your research report. Use inclusive, bias-free language and tap into resources such as the Sex and Gender Equity in Research (SAGER) guidelines (Heidari et al., 2016). (Learn more about bias-free language in Chapter 6.)

upper limit of normal. In this case, the difference is not statistically significant but is certainly clinically significant.

A common mistake made in the results section is a discussion of relationships among the variables that were never delineated in any of the research questions. For example, researchers sometimes report if the outcomes of the study were different based on sex or age. If these relationships between the study variables and sex or age were not part of a research question, then the information should not appear in the results section. This approach is called a "fishing expedition" and often indicates the researcher is desperately looking for significant findings (Bar-Zeev, 2018).

Discussion

The purpose of the discussion section is to interpret your results and explain their implications for the area of scientific study. It pulls together the entire article (Angelini, 2023). An effective discussion is one that synthesizes the contributions made by the researchers toward the advancement of knowledge in general and the field of research in particular. After reading the discussion, readers should know how the findings compare with previous research and how to apply the findings (Aga & Nissar, 2022).

Like the results section, the discussion can be organized by the research questions. Do not merely repeat the results in the discussion section (Behzadi & Gajdacs, 2021). Talk about the findings, then offer possible explanations for them. Explain the meaning of your findings to the reader. Conjecture why you found what you did. Several elements should be part of the discussion section (APA, 2020; Seals, 2023).

Summary of findings: Begin by stating support or non-support for your hypotheses. You need to discuss both significant and nonsignificant findings. Sometimes researchers fail to explain their nonsignificant findings because they perceive these as less interesting. An explanation of nonsignificant findings is just as important as a discussion of significant findings. Speculate on the reason for your results (Seals, 2023).

Context: If you used a conceptual or theoretical framework to guide your study, tie your results to the framework. Do your results support existing conceptions and theories? Or do they indicate a different view of the phenomena studied?

Comparison: Relate your findings to the literature you synthesized in the literature review section of the research report. Are your findings consistent with previous studies, or do they refute them (Busse & August, 2021)? Do not introduce literature in the discussion section that was not part of the literature review section. Researchers sometimes make a mistake of saying in the literature review that very little research has been done previously on the topic and then in the discussion section compare their results to many previous studies.

Interpretation: One of the greatest challenges is to explain the results when they didn't support your hypotheses or expected findings. A common mistake is to say the findings were "almost significant" and then discuss them as if they were significant. If one group's score is higher than another but the difference is not statistically significant, you cannot conclude that the action or intervention with the higher score is better. If one group had higher scores than another group, you can only discuss the effectiveness of the intervention if the difference was statistically significant. Otherwise, you need to explain why the intervention was ineffective.

When your findings aren't what you expect, avoid the mistake of saying the results would have been significant if the sample was larger or if the instruments had better reliability or validity. You have no way of knowing if that statement is true. Instead, offer the reader an explanation for what you did find, not what you hoped to find.

Another common mistake in the discussion section is to make conclusions without the supporting results. Sometimes researchers offer grandiose conclusions that go beyond what the data indicate. For example, if your survey revealed that one hospital in your region is "very satisfied" with your nursing program's graduates, you cannot say that employers throughout the state are "satisfied" with the quality of the graduates and are eager to hire them. Keep discussion and conclusions consistent with the results.

Critique: In addition to summarizing the strengths of your study, summarize its limitations, such as the subjects being from one area of the country (these features may limit the generalizability of your results). Point out the limitation of a poor response rate, which markedly limits the generalizability of your findings. You should also include next steps for further research that will build on your research findings. Be specific. Instead of stating "more research is needed," give examples of what types of studies are needed.

Speculation on implications: Write about the implications of your findings for research, education, practice, or policy (Angelini, 2023). Ask questions such as: How do your findings affect practice? What specific recommendations can be drawn? Ibrahim and Dimick (2018) suggest considering how the study affects the four Ps: patients, providers, payers, and policymakers.

Conclusion

End the research report with a concise conclusion. Avoid rehashing what you have already written, and don't introduce new information or ideas. Instead, recap the main take-home message for readers. Emphasize what new findings have been added to the literature and what are future perspectives in the field of study. Focus on what you want the reader to remember (Aga & Nissar, 2022).

Reporting Qualitative Studies

Another major approach to the conduct of nursing research is the use of qualitative methods. *Qualitative research* is a systematic scientific inquiry that is primarily exploratory; it offers understanding and insights to a problem and helps to develop ideas or hypotheses that might be used in quantitative research. Qualitative research provides an understanding of the rationale for underlying behavior and decisions which can lead to theory development (Ancker et al., 2021). This type of research seeks to build a holistic, largely narrative description that informs the researcher's understanding of a social or cultural phenomenon. It also offers approaches for taking a deeper dive into a problem in a way that quantitative data or numbers can't always capture (Chicca, 2020).

Qualitative research enables the researcher to study issues in depth and detail without being limited by predetermined categories of analysis. In contrast, quantitative research is concerned with measurement and numbers, while qualitative research is focused on understandings and words. Quantitative research is based on the value of control; qualitative research values openness and flexibility. The quantitative researcher assumes an objective, rather detached stance, while the qualitative researcher is a key instrument intimately involved with the data collection and analysis (Denzin & Lincoln, 2017).

The following abstract from a published qualitative study, "Experiences of Thriving Nursing Students," illustrates qualitative research (Mentag, 2022). The emphasis on understanding the meanings of the lived experiences of thriving undergraduate nursing students from their perspective and identifying themes are hallmarks of the qualitative approach.

> **Background:** As the demand for qualified nurses increases, nursing education prepares students for the complex healthcare setting. Nursing education focuses on academic success measures, including licensure examination passage, graduation rates, and grade point average. Though these outcomes are important, they fail to capture the complexities of student success, resulting in a fragmented approach in nursing programs. Thriving, the conceptual framework for this study, is a phenomenon within higher education that expands on the traditional measures of success and integrates cognitive and psychological aspects of the college experience.
>
> **Purpose:** This study aimed to understand the meanings of the lived experiences of thriving undergraduate nursing students.

Method: Guided by interpretive phenomenology, semi-structured interviews were conducted with eight participants who were deemed as thriving, according to the Thriving Quotient. These participants were undergraduate students from two baccalaureate nursing programs.

Results: Five themes emerged from the data analysis: professors' investment in students, partnerships with peers, success through hardships, greater purpose, and finding a balance.

Conclusion: The study's findings add to the unique understanding of thriving among nursing students. Furthermore, the results support the call for an expansive view of success to effectively prepare students for the nursing profession.

Note: Copyright Elsevier, 2022.

Writing the Qualitative Report

The research report for qualitative studies generally includes the same types of sections as those for quantitative studies described earlier in this chapter. When journal editors evaluate qualitative research manuscripts, they may use the Consolidated Criteria for Reporting Qualitative Research (COREQ) checklist (Tong et al., 2007) or the Standards for Reporting QUalitative Research (SQUIRE 2.0; O'Brien et al., 2014; Ogrinc et al., 2015).

Sometimes the order of presentation in a qualitative report differs from the quantitative report to reflect the traditions of qualitative research. For example, the qualitative research report may begin with the introduction and purpose and move right into a description of the methods rather than starting with a detailed literature review of prior research and theory. A literature review at the outset may be too prescriptive or constraining in setting the stage for certain types of qualitative methods.

While an explanation of reliability and validity are essential components of quantitative research reports, an explanation of the trustworthiness of data is an important part of many types of qualitative research reports. *Trustworthiness* refers to criteria for the rigor of a study and informs the reader that the reported results and conclusions are sound. Trustworthiness is the degree of confidence a reader can have in the data, interpretation, and methods used to ensure a quality study (Connelly, 2016; Polit & Beck, 2020; Stahl & King, 2020). Lincoln and Guba (1985) outlined four criteria for trustworthiness: credibility, dependability, transferability, and confirmability.

- *Credibility* refers to the confidence in the accuracy of the research study and the truth of the findings.
- *Dependability* is the extent to which the study could be repeated by other researchers and the findings would be consistent.
- *Transferability* implies that the findings have applicability in other settings and contexts.
- *Confirmability* means that the findings are derived from the participants' responses and do not show any bias or personal motivation of the researchers.

In the research report, identify strategies used to address the elements of trustworthiness such as audit trails, member checking, and vivid descriptions (Chicca, 2020).

As with reporting quantitative research, follow a set structure to make it easier for the reader to understand the results. The following tips for selected sections of the quantitative research report may help you write the qualitative research report.

Research Questions

- Provide a clear purpose statement. Generally, no hypotheses are tested. Research questions may or may not be needed.

Sample

- Refer to subjects as participants for most qualitative studies.
- Describe the sampling method. Usually it is either purposive, convenience, consecutive, or snowball.
- Explain how participants were selected and contacted.
- Inform the reader if data saturation was achieved. Data saturation determines the number of participants for some qualitative methods.

Method

- Clearly state which of the following methods you used, keeping in mind that each represents a unique approach. This is key; if you simply state that you used some open-ended questions to obtain qualitative data, you are misrepresenting the study, and your manuscript will be rejected.
  - *Phenomenological research* aims to describe a phenomenon by exploring it from the perspective of those who have experienced it.
  - *Grounded theory research* investigates processes, actions, or interactions with the goal of developing a theory grounded in the data, systematically obtained and analyzed using comparative analysis.
  - *Ethnographic research* examines the social interaction of people in an environment to acquire an in-depth insight into the person's views and actions in addition to what they encounter during their day.
  - *Narrative research* focuses on collecting and interpreting information about the lives of individuals as told through their own stories with the goal of exploring the meanings people assign to their experiences.
  - *Historical research* examines and describes events of the past for the purpose of drawing conclusions and making predictions about the future.

Procedure

- Describe the setting/site or any other contextual features.
- State who conducted the interviews and what their relationship was with the participants.
- Discuss what participants knew about the interviewer.
- Supply either a table with the interview questions or a sampling of the questions.
- Indicate if the interviews were audio or visually recorded.

Data Analysis

- Note who transcribed the recordings.
- Explain who and how many coded the data.
- Provide information about any software used to manage the data—name it.
- Describe the process for identifying themes.
- State whether participants reviewed any of the transcripts or generated themes.

Results

- Show the perspectives of the participants, separate from those of the researcher.
- Include direct quotes from the participants. Assign each participant a number, and place the number with the quote so the reader knows if the quotes come from a variety of participants or from just a few.
- Use selected text from documents to illustrate the identified themes.
- Do not report numbers or percentages. For example, avoid saying, "Five of the nine participants agreed with the theme."

Discussion

- Relate the derived themes to previous literature.
- Differentiate the participants' point of view from the researcher's perspective.
- Link the utility or application of the findings to clinical or educational practice.
- Ensure consistency between data, discussion, and conclusions.

Reporting Mixed-Methods Research

Mixed methods, another approach to research, has become more prevalent in nursing. It combines both quantitative and qualitative methods and data in the same study. Mixed-methods research doesn't mean adding a few open-ended questions at the end of a survey (Morton, 2017a). Instead, mixed methods means, for example, that you have implemented a quantitative method such as an experimental study with the elements of phenomenology. *Mixed-methods research* brings together the underpinnings of two different philosophical approaches to answering research questions—a quantitative perspective of control and quantifying with a qualitative perspective of naturalistic inquiry (Wasti et al., 2022).

The blending of the two methods offers a broader understanding of a research topic. For example, in a clinical trial conducted to test an intervention, focus groups might be carried out with a small sample of patients who received the intervention to gain insights on how the patients are experiencing the intervention and whether it might be improved in some way to make it more acceptable. Or, a study to develop an instrument to assess patient behavior might begin with patient interviews to gain insights from their perspective that then could be used to develop items in the instrument that incorporate the patients' own words and unique perspectives.

Mixed-methods research offers advantages over quantitative or qualitative methods alone. It can provide more comprehensive evidence, giving voice to the participants in a way that numbers alone cannot. Mixed-methods research offers the investigator an opportunity to answer different types of research questions that could not be answered by using only quantitative or qualitative methods (Kajamaa et al., 2020).

Use the strategies already discussed to report on this type of research, keeping in mind the principles of clear reporting and linkage to practice.

By now your head might be spinning as you consider all you have read. Table 14.1 will help you better understand quantitative, qualitative, and mixed-methods research by comparing key features of the three.

Spread the Knowledge

Writing a research article or report can be intimidating. It's worth considering what will happen if you don't share your results: What you have learned will languish, depriving researchers, clinicians, and educators the opportunity to benefit from your work. Ultimately those who lose the most are the patients who could gain from what you learned. Take that important final step as a researcher: Share your results.

TABLE 14.1 Comparing Features of Quantitative, Qualitative, and Mixed-Methods Approaches

	Quantitative Research	Qualitative Research	Mixed-Methods Research
Purpose	To look at cause and effect, test hypotheses, make predictions	To explore; to discover, construct, and describe themes	Combines both quantitative and qualitative purposes
Scientific approach	Deductive or "top down"	Inductive or "bottom up"	Both deductive and inductive
Nature of study	Measurement under generally controlled conditions	Observation in natural environment or context	Measurement under more than one condition or context
Type of data	Numeric variables and statistics	Narrative data using semi-structured or unstructured instruments; words or tests'; images	Multiple types of data, both numeric and narrative
Results	Generalizable	Particularistic	Integrated results that may be generalizable
Final report	Statistical report with interpretation and implications for practice or theory	Narrative report with contextual description, categories, or themes, and supporting quotations from respondents	Statistical report with in-depth examination of narrative findings, interpretation and implications for practice or theory

Adapted from Creswell & Creswell (2018); Johnson & Christensen (2019); University of Wisconsin-Madison (n.d.); Wolcott (2009)

Write Now!

1. Read a published research article without reading the abstract. Then, write your own abstract and compare it to the published one.

2. Based on the abstract from the study by Zangaro and colleagues (2023) included in this chapter, formulate one or two research questions and several hypotheses you may wish to test if you were doing this study. Then read the entire article by these authors and see if any of your questions/hypotheses match those of the authors.

3. Read the results section of two research articles and note how the authors have used tables and figures to supplement the article. Critique the two papers in how well they presented their results and the extent to which tables and figures helped you understand what the authors were trying to convey. What would you do differently?

References

Aga, S. S., & Nissar, S. (2022). Essential guide to manuscript writing for academic dummies: An editor's perspective. *Biochemistry Research International, 2022*, 1492058. https://doi.org/10.1155/2022/1492058

American Psychological Association. (2020). *Publication manual of the American Psychological Association* (7th ed.). https://doi.org/10.1037/0000165-000

Ancker, J. S., Benda, N. C., Reddy, M., Unertl, K. M., & Veino, T. (2021). Guidance for publishing qualitative research in informatics. *Journal of the American Medical Informatics Association, 28*(12), 2743–2748. https://doi.org/10.1093/jamia/ocab195

Angelini, D. J. (2023). Delving into the critical components of the discussion section. *Nurse Author & Editor, 33*(3-4), 26–29. https://doi.org/10.1111/nae2.12056

Bar-Zeev, Y. (2018, July 22). ERC is not a grant for "fishing expedition" research. *Enspire.science*. https://zenodo.org/record/1318812

Behzadi, P., & Gajdacs, M. (2021). Writing a strong scientific paper in medicine and the biomedical sciences: a checklist and recommendations for early career researchers. *Biologia Futura, 72*(4), 395–407. https://doi.org/10.1007/s42977-021-00095-z

Busse, C., & August, E. (2021). How to write and publish a research paper for a peer-reviewed journal. *Journal of Cancer Education, 36*(5), 909–913. https://doi.org/10.1007/s13187-020-01751-z

Butcher, N. J., Monsour, A., Mew, E. J., Chan, A., Moher, D., Mayo-Wilson, E., Terwee, C. B., Chee-A-Tow, A., Baba, A., Gavin, F., Grimshaw, J. M., Kelly, L. E., Saeed, L., Thabane, L., Askie, L., Smith, M., Farid-Kapadia, M., Williamson, P. R., Szatmari, P., Tugwell, P., Golub, R. M., Monga, S., Vohra, S., Marlin, S., Ungar, W. J., & Offringa, M. (2022). Guidelines for reporting outcomes in trial reports: The CONSORT-Outcomes 2022 extension. *The Journal of the American Medical Association, 328*(22), 2252–2264. https://doi.org/10.1001/jama.2022.21022

Chicca, J. (2020). Introduction to qualitative nursing research. *American Nurse Journal, 15*(6), 28–32. https://www.myamericannurse.com/introduction-to-qualitative-nursing-research/

Connelly, L. M. (2016). Trustworthiness in qualitative research. *MedSurg Nursing, 25*(6), 435–436.

Creswell, J. W., & Creswell, J. D. (2018). *Research design: Qualitative, quantitative, and mixed methods approaches* (5th ed.). SAGE Publications.

Denzin, N. K., & Lincoln, Y. S. (2017). *The SAGE handbook of qualitative research* (5th ed.). SAGE Publications.

Dwivedi, A.K. (2022). How to write statistical analysis section in medical research. *Journal of Investigative Medicine, 70*(8), 1759–1770. https://doi.org/10.1136/jim-2022-002479

Flanagin, A., Frey, T., Christiansen, S. L., & *AMA Manual of Style* Committee. (2021). Updated guidance on the reporting of race and ethnicity in medical and science journals [Editorial]. *JAMA, 326*(7), 621–627. https://doi.org/10.1001/jama.2021.13304

Greer, J. L., & Wingo, N. P. (2017). "My research article was accepted for publication!" *American Nurse Journal, 12*(1), 37–39. https://www.myamericannurse.com/wp-content/uploads/2016/12/ant1-Abstracts-1213.pdf

Hamlin, S. K., Fontenot, N. M., Hooker, S. I., & Chen, H. M. (2023). Systems-based physical assessments: Earlier detection of clinical deterioration and reduced mortality. *American Journal of Critical Care, 32*(5), 329–337. https://doi.org/10.4037/ajcc2023113

Heidari, S., Babor, T. F., De Castro, P., Tort, S., & Curno, M. (2016). Sex and Gender Equity in Research: Rationale for the SAGER guidelines and recommended use. *Research Integrity and Peer Review, 1*(2). https://doi.org/10.1186/s41073-016-0007-6

Ibrahim, A. M., & Dimick, J. B. (2018). Writing for impact: How to prepare a journal article. In J. Markovac, M. Kleinman, & M. Ebglesbe (Eds.), *Medical and scientific publishing* (pp. 81–92). Elsevier. https://doi.org/10.1016/B978-0-12-809969-8.00009-7

Johnson, R. B., & Christensen, L. (2019). *Educational research: Quantitative, qualitative, and mixed approaches* (7th ed.). Sage Publications.

Kajamaa, A., Mattick, K., & de La Croix, A. (2020). How to… do mixed methods research. *The Clinical Teacher, 17*(3), 267–271. https://doi.org/10.1111/tct.13145

Lincoln, Y. S., & Guba, E. G. (1985). *Naturalistic inquiry*. Sage.

Mentag, N. M. (2022). Experiences of thriving nursing students. *Journal of Professional Nursing, 41,* 166–175. https://doi.org/10.1016/j.profnurs.2022.05.005

Morton, P. G. (2017a). Nursing education research: An editor's view. *Journal of Professional Nursing, 33*(5), 311–312. https://doi.org/10.1016/j.profnurs.2017.08.002

Morton, P. G. (2017b). Strategies for writing a research article: An editor's perspective. *Nurse Author & Editor, 27*(1), 1–9. https://doi.org/10.1111/j.1750-4910.2017.tb00238.x

O'Brien, B. C., Harris, I. B., Beckman, T. J., Reed, D. A., & Cook, D. A. (2014). Standards for reporting qualitative research: A synthesis of recommendations. *Academic Medicine, 89*(9), 1245–1251. https://doi.org/10.1097/ACM.0000000000000388

Oermann, M. H., Barton, A., Yoder-Wise, P. S., Morton, P.G. (2021). Research in nursing education and the institutional review board/ethics committee. *Journal of Professional Nursing, 37*(2), 342–347. https://doi.org/10.1016/j.profnurs.2021.01.003

Ogrinc, G., Davies, L., Goodman, D., Batalden, P., Davidoff, F., & Stevens, D. (2015). SQUIRE 2.0 (Standards for QUality Improvement Reporting Excellence): Revised publication guidelines from a detailed consensus process. *BMJ Quality & Safety, 25,* 986–992. https://doi.org/10.1136/bmjqs-2015-004411

Ozcakar, L., Rizzo, J. R., Franchignoni, F., Negrini, S., & Frontera, W. R. (2022). Let's write a manuscript: A primer with tips and tricks for penning an original article. *American Journal of Physical Medicine & Rehabilitation, 101*(7), 698–701. https://doi.org/10.1097/PHM.0000000000001847

PLOS. (n.d.). *How to write an abstract*. https://plos.org/resource/how-to-write-a-great-abstract/

Polit, D. F., & Beck, C. T. (2020). *Nursing research: Generating and assessing evidence for nursing practice* (11th ed.). Wolters Kluwer.

Roe-Prior, P. (2023). Writing the methods section [Editorial]. *Journal for Nurses in Professional Development, 39*(1), 67–68. https://doi.org/10.1097/NND.0000000000000957

Schulz, K. F., Altman, D. G., Moher, D., & CONSORT Group. (2010). CONSORT 2010 statement: Updated guidelines for reporting parallel group randomized trials. *Annals of Internal Medicine, 152*(11), 726–732. https://doi.org/10.7326/0003-4819-152-11-201006010-00232

Seals, D. R. (2023). Publishing particulars: Part 2. Tips for effective manuscript development. *American Journal of Physiology Regulatory Comparative and Integrative Physiology, 324,* R393–R408. https://doi.org/10.1152/ajpregu.00267.2022

Stahl, N. A., & King, J. R. (2020). Expanding approaches for research: Understanding and using trustworthiness in qualitative research. *Journal of Developmental Education, 44*(1), 26–28.

Tong, A., Sainsbury, P., & Craig, J. (2007). Consolidated criteria for reporting qualitative research (COREQ): A 32-item checklist for interviews and focus groups. *International Journal for Quality in Health Care, 19*(6), 349–357. https://doi.org/10.1093/intqhc/mzm042

University of Wisconsin-Madison. (n.d.). *Nursing resources: Qualitative vs. quantitative*. https://researchguides.library.wisc.edu/c.php?g=861013&p=6170079

Wasti, S. P., Simkhada, P., van Teijlingen, E. R., & Banerjee, I. (2022). The growing importance of mixed-methods research in health. *Nepal Journal of Epidemiology, 12*(1), 1175–1178. https://doi.org/10.3126/nje.v12i1.43633

Wolcott, H. F. (2009). Linking up. In H. F. Wolcott (Ed.), *Writing up qualitative research* (3rd ed., pp. 65–92). SAGE Publications.

Zangaro, G. A., Rosseter, R., Trautman, D., & Leaver, C. (2023). Burnout among academic nursing faculty. *Journal of Professional Nursing, 48,* 54–59. https://doi.org/10.1016/j.profnurs.2023.06.001

Writing the Review Article

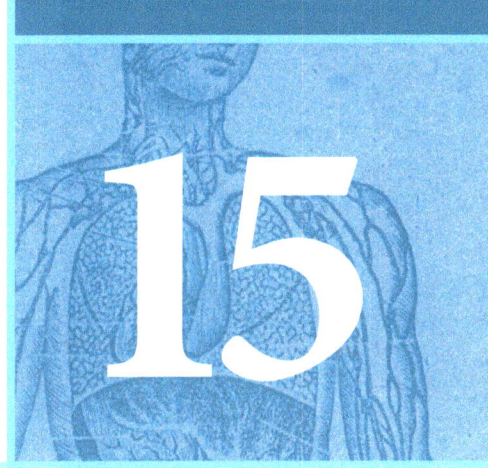

–Lisa Hopp, PhD, RN, FAAN

"It is surely a great criticism of our profession that we have not organized a critical summary, by specialty or subspecialty, adapted periodically, of all relevant randomized control trials."
–Archie Cochrane

WHAT YOU'LL LEARN IN THIS CHAPTER

- Review articles synthesize a large amount of information from previously published literature.

- Literature reviews may facilitate knowledge translation and synthesis.

- Systematic reviews follow a specific structure and explicit methods and rules, which enhances their rigor.

- Scoping reviews provide a map of the breadth of coverage of available studies or literature without critically appraising how well studies were conducted.

- An integrative review integrates findings from both qualitative and quantitative literature.

Reviews are a common and popular type of article because the authors do the hard work of finding a body of literature, analyzing it, and providing a synthesis of the works. Many types of review articles exist, and there has been rapid growth in the methods to guide their conduct. Because so many methodologies have evolved, investigators have tried to organize the reviews into typologies, taxonomies, ecosystems, or families (Grant & Booth, 2009; Munn et al., 2023; Sutton et al., 2019; Tricco et al., 2016). Sutton et al. (2019) found 48 distinct review types as they created families of reviews. Seeking further clarity, investigators at JBI (formerly the Joanna Briggs Institute) are conducting a scoping review to inventory the typologies, taxonomies, and classification schemes for various types of evidence syntheses (Munn et al., 2023).

Because many methods are still evolving, there is a lack of clarity in how authors create their reviews and even what they name them. Indeed, bibliographic databases don't consistently define or index different types of reviews. For example, the Cumulative Index of Nursing and Allied Health Literature (CINAHL) scope notes for "systematic review" include both integrative and systematic reviews and do not include explicit methodologic criteria, whereas MEDLINE MeSH scope notes define systematic review with its well-established methodologic steps. (*Scope notes* are definitions of the search term that you can view when searching for CINAHL headings or Medical Subject Headings [MeSH] terms.) This makes it difficult to easily identify the type of review and to know what to expect when searching bibliographic databases. As an author, you need to align the type and methods of the review with the objectives and questions you ask (Silva et al., 2022). In addition, you need to have adequate training and preparation to use specific methodologies to rigorously conduct the review (Aromataris & Munn, 2020).

Evidence-based practice compels us to use *the best available evidence* with *patient preferences* and *clinical expertise* in the context of *finite resources* to make clinical decisions (Sackett et al., 1996). Each element of this definition has implications for how you might approach writing (or reading) a review article. Knowledge syntheses that are rigorous, comprehensive, reproducible, and transparent are generally superior to individual studies when making decisions for guidelines, policy, and clinical decisions because they are less susceptible to bias (Egger et al., 2022). In this chapter, you'll learn about several types of review articles that vary in their breadth, purpose, methods, rigor, and analysis approach.

Anatomy of a Review Article

The general format of review articles resembles a primary research report:

- Abstract
- Background
- Objectives
- Methods
- Results
- Discussion

Although the various types of reviews share some structure, they are differentiated by their objectives and the methods used to manage bias and analysis. Like primary research, the purpose or questions will drive how you decide what methods best fit the objectives or answer the questions, the type of results you will expect, and how you will analyze and make sense of the results so that you can write the review. Any research project begins with a sense of wanting to know, to solve a problem, or to move the science along. In the context of evidence-based practice, research review articles play different roles. You need to understand those roles so that you pick the correct approach, which will make it easier to write an article based on the results of your review (see Table 15.1).

The different types of reviews have varying levels of methodologic development and international consensus about the best way to do the science. Some review types are newer (rapid reviews), and others are more fully developed (systematic reviews). For example, integrative reviews have a limited number of articles that guide the methodology of developing this type of synthesis, even though they are quite popular in nursing literature. Most authors of integrative reviews rely on one commonly cited article that updated previous methods (Whittemore & Knafl, 2005). Contrast this to the international collaborations of scientists, journals, handbooks, and funding sources committed to other methodologies like systematic reviews.

This chapter focuses on four common types of reviews: literature, systematic, scoping, and integrative.

Q *Is a meta-analysis the same as a systematic review?*

A No. Meta-analysis is a statistical technique for pooling quantitative data. Meta-analysis may be part of a systematic review of quantitative data, or it could be conducted on data that were not gathered through the systematic review process. Similarly, systematic reviews may not include a meta-analysis, either because the data were not appropriate for statistical pooling or it was not the aim of the review. For example, systematic reviews of meaningfulness aim to synthesize qualitative data using words as the data element.

You may also hear the term *network meta-analysis*, which is a method that allows the comparison of multiple interventions simultaneously using both direct comparisons (head-to-head comparisons) and indirect comparisons. For example, the investigator may want to compare the effectiveness of both pharmacologic and nonpharmacologic interventions both as single treatments or combined to manage pain. A traditional meta-analysis can only compare two treatment characteristics in pairwise fashion (e.g., one analgesic versus placebo). Network meta-analysis is more complex and requires the investigator to understand the various "nodes" or interventions and how they connect (Watt & Del Giovane, 2022).

Literature Reviews

Since the advent of formalized systematic and other types of reviews, it is a bit difficult to define the traditional literature review article or to describe its methods. Sutton et al. (2019) include in their "family" or typology of traditional reviews these types: critical reviews, narrative reviews, narrative

TABLE 15.1 Types of Reviews

Type of Review	Definition
Literature review	A general term for a synthesis of a body of work that is usually broad in scope, does not necessarily follow a standardized methodology, and may reflect the biases of the author(s) or the research or opinions included
Scoping review/mapping reviews	A synthesis that aims to map a broad body of evidence that is complex, dispersed across disciplines or areas of study, and used to define where research is and is not; these reviews generally do not attempt to assess risk of bias or credibility (Peters et al., 2020; Silva et al., 2022)
Systematic review	"research synthesis...conducted by [those] with specialized skills who set out to identify and retrieve international evidence that is relevant to a particular question or questions and to appraise and synthesize the results of this search to inform practice, policy and in some cases, further research" (Munn et al., 2018, para. 2)
	"A systematic review attempts to identify, appraise and synthesize all the empirical evidence that meets pre-specified eligibility criteria to answer a specific research question. Researchers conducting systematic reviews use explicit, systematic methods that are selected with a view aimed at minimizing bias, to produce more reliable findings to inform decision making." (Cochrane Library, n.d., para. 2)
Umbrella review/overview of reviews/systematic review of reviews	A summary of existing research syntheses for different types of interventions or phenomena of interest with the same condition, or different outcomes for the same interventions or phenomena of interest with the same condition, or different outcomes for the same intervention or phenomena of interest (Aromataris et al., 2020)
Rapid review	"a form of knowledge synthesis that accelerates the process of conducting a traditional systematic review through streamlining or omitting a variety of methods to produce evidence in a resource-efficient manner" (Hamel et al., 2021, p. 80).
Evidence summary	"synopses that summarize existing international evidence on healthcare interventions or activities, and as with systematic reviews, standardization of methods is a significant marker of quality and reliability" (Munn et al., 2015, Methods, para. 1).
Integrative review	A review that collates and brings together evidence and information from different types of sources that can include quantitative and qualitative empirical evidence, theory, or methodologic evidence (Silva et al., 2022).
	Methods do not include estimates of risk of bias or credibility.

summary, state of the art review, and even integrative synthesis/review. These authors view this set of traditional reviews' purposes to include critical analysis, providing overview, and/or describing, summarizing, and identifying gaps in knowledge. No formal methodologies exist to guide literature reviews, and they generally lack the transparency of other review types that are guided by protocols and structured methods. For example, authors use purposive searches rather than exhaustive approaches, they do not use specific appraisal tools, and they are not explicit about how they extract information from their sources (Sutton et al., 2019). Therefore, many consider traditional literature reviews vulnerable to bias and not suited to guide clinical decision-making (Grant & Booth, 2009). Nonetheless, traditional literature reviews continue to have a place in knowledge translation and synthesis. (Refer to Chapter 14 for information on writing literature reviews as part of a research article.)

When writing a literature review, start with a clear idea of what body of work you wish to review and the objective. Unlike other review types, the format of a traditional review will vary from those that use a standardized approach. The structure will likely include an introduction, objectives or purpose, and perhaps methods, results, and conclusions. Alternatively, the author may organize the review into thematic areas to summarize the key areas in the body of literature and discuss the findings under headings representing these areas.

Like any other review type, the objective will guide your approach to searching and uncovering the literature you will include. Based on the objective, develop inclusion criteria that will guide your search. Your review will be stronger if you explicitly state the databases that you searched and the number of articles you netted relevant to your objectives. For example, you may choose to include a Preferred Reporting Items for Systematic reviews and Meta-Analyses (PRISMA) flow diagram, a tool developed for systematic reviews (Page et al., 2021).

All types of review articles (not just the literature review) generally include a summary table of the key characteristics of the literature informing the review. You'll need to organize a method to extract these key characteristics as you digest each article. Again, the objective of your review will determine the categories of information you include in the summary table. Each row of the table contains information on one citation, the column labels determine the details you identify, and each cell contains the data from each article. Most tables will have columns for the authors and year of publication, purpose and/or type of source (e.g., type of research design, theory development, case study), population/sample, results, conclusions. Younas and Ali (2021) offer the following tips for constructing a summary table:

- Provide detailed information about the frameworks and methods.
- Note strengths and limitations for each included article.
- Briefly summarize the conceptual contribution of each article.
- Develop potential themes while you integrate and interpret the literature.
- Customize the table to suit the review purpose.

Reviews aim to synthesize, so take care to remain within the scope of the literature you reviewed and identify the key concepts and findings in your conclusion. Leave the reader with a balanced view that aligns with your synthesis and provides them with what remains to be known.

Systematic Reviews

Systematic reviews can answer a variety of questions that call for the synthesis of quantitative or qualitative evidence. Organizations like Cochrane and JBI have developed standardized methodologies and analysis strategies for quantitative questions (Aromataris & Munn, 2020; Higgins et al., 2023). JBI has organized quantitative reviews around questions of prevalence, diagnostic tests, etiology and risk, measurement properties, and economic evaluation (Aromataris & Munn, 2020). Although both JBI and Cochrane have published guidance about how to conduct a systematic review of qualitative evidence, the JBI guidance has the longest history. Both organizations publish handbooks with in-depth guidance that you can consult; however, you should seek training in the methodologies to learn more about the research techniques.

Writing a Systematic Review Protocol

Just like you write a proposal before you start a primary research project, you write a protocol before you start a systematic review. The *protocol*, which should be based on a well-defined review question, is your recipe and guide for how you will proceed. You should submit your protocol to an international organization like JBI or Cochrane or a database like PROSPERO (www.crd.york.ac.uk/prospero) before proceeding with the review. These organizations publish protocols once peer reviewers and editors are satisfied the proposed methods are rigorous and will lead to a high-quality systematic review. Feedback from the review of the protocol will help you strengthen your methods before you invest your time and effort in the review. Registration also lets others know your work is in progress, so the review is not duplicated.

Write the protocol in the future tense because it describes what you *will* do to conduct the systematic review. The elements of the protocol will resemble the report you write after your complete the review and follow a standard structure:

- Title (Include "systematic review" and align it with your question.)
- Introduction and background (Note the significance, what is known and unknown, and that a current review on the topic doesn't exist—be sure the latter is true.)

Advancing the Science and Production of Systematic Reviews

Three international organizations, established in the mid-1990s, have advanced the science of systematic review and publish reviews on their websites: Cochrane, the Campbell Collaboration, and JBI.

Cochrane is an international organization with tools for learning how to conduct systematic reviews, including software for review production (RevMan). The Cochrane Library is a collection of databases that includes the Cochrane Database of Systematic Reviews (CDSR) and a registry of controlled trials (CENTRAL) to facilitate searching. Cochrane is recognized for guiding and publishing systematic reviews of effectiveness of interventions and diagnostic tests accuracy, with a focus on the synthesis of randomized and clinical controlled trials. They also strive to provide reviews of research for healthcare and policy requiring other types of evidence. Cochrane review groups focus on a topic area and provide methodologic and editorial support (www.cochrane.org).

The Campbell Collaboration is an international organization concerned with the social sciences such as education, crime and justice, climate, and social welfare. The organization focuses on policy-relevant evidence syntheses. Similar to the Cochrane group, they have coordinating groups that oversee the scientific merit of their publications (www.campbellcollaboration.org).

JBI is an international organization located at the University of Adelaide. It includes a global collaboration of centers and groups that produce systematic reviews and focus on the translation and implementation of evidence. JBI has developed review methods, software tools (SUMMARI) and training, and they publish protocols and reviews in their journals. Since their beginning, the organization has focused on the systematic review of both quantitative and qualitative evidence. They also provide methodologies, tools, training, and publication outlets for evidence implementation and evaluation (https://jbi.global).

- Objectives and review question(s) (Use PICO format [see next bullet] for quantitative reviews and PICo or another appropriate type for qualitative reviews. See tips sidebar for more explanation.)
- Inclusion criteria (This consists of study and publication characteristics.)
    - Population
    - Intervention(s) or phenomenon of interest
    - Comparator(s) or Context
    - Outcome
    - Types of studies
    - Languages and time frame
- Search strategy
    - Information sources (Include what databases, search engines, and grey or fugitive literature you plan to use; see Chapter 4 for more information about grey literature.)
    - Three phases (These are: mining keywords in major databases, database-specific strategy, and reference checking.)
- Retrieval of studies (Note that you plan to use dual reviewers who decide to retrieve an article based on meeting inclusion criteria in the title, abstract, or full text.) and bibliographic management software if used (e.g., EndNote, RefWorks).
- Critical appraisal (Note the use of dual reviewers, include standardized instruments as appendices, and explain how you will resolve reviewer disagreements.)
- Data extraction (Include the number of reviewers, instruments, and how you will resolve reviewer disagreements.)
- Synthesis (Note statistical specifics of meta-analysis or details of narrative synthesis or meta-aggregation, including how you plan to grade the evidence.)

> **Tips for Writing Questions for a Systematic Review**
>
> Like any research project, your review question is critically important because it will influence all your decisions in the review process. Mnemonic devices like "PICO" or "PICo" are useful to help you write unambiguous questions. PICO is the traditional reminder for quantitative systematic reviews of effectiveness questions where: P = population, I = intervention, C = comparator, O = outcome. Systematic reviews of qualitative evidence of meaningfulness use an adapted mnemonic of PICo where P = population, I = phenomenon of interest, Co = context.
>
> Finding the right scope for your project requires a conceptual understanding of factors related to the topic at hand. It's useful to construct a logic or concept map or use an existing framework to help you find the right scope for your question. Finding the right size for your project is a bit like playing an accordion, stretching and squeezing as you consider what you want to know. You may start with a question that has a large scope, then you squeeze it smaller and then stretch it back out just a bit more to find a question that is manageable but remains significant enough to invest your time.
>
> For example, you may begin with a question like: What is the effect of telehealth (I) versus usual face-to-face management (C) on health outcomes (O) in patients in primary care (P)? This question is large in scope because there is no specification of what type of telehealth or who provides it, what specific outcomes are of interest, or what types of primary care patient problems are of interest.
>
> Squeezing the question much smaller, you might write: What is the effect of a 15-minute telephone interview (I) versus a 15-minute in-office visit (C) delivered by a family nurse practitioner on serum glucose stability (O) in pre-diabetic patients (P)? This question is too narrow and would not lead to more expansive knowledge for decision-making.
>
> Stretching the question back out might look like: What is the effect of family nurse practitioners in primary care who provide all types of telehealth care (I) versus usual office visits (C) on hemoglobin A1C stability, patient satisfaction, and knowledge of self-management (O) in patients diagnosed with pre-diabetes or type 2 diabetes (P)? This question will then lead to a specific set of search terms and inclusion criteria that inform decision-making about a significant healthcare problem.

Q *Can artificial intelligence assist authors in the review process?*

A This is a big question as artificial intelligence (AI) disrupts and transforms many elements of our lives. It's difficult to give firm recommendations at this time because the science of AI is changing quickly and is likely to remain fluid. Current AI tools may help with different aspects of the review process. For example, Golan et al. (2023) advise that AI tools can help authors identify themes, trends, and concepts as they develop the background of the review. It can refine the clarity of writing, even help generate images from text descriptions.

Others have studied the ability of AI tools to speed the search process and screen the title and abstract based on inclusion criteria. They caution that while there is promise, the decision to stop searching and the accuracy of the retrieval decision for full text review should be checked by humans for reliability to avoid article selection bias (van Dijk et al., 2023). In addition, a study comparing AI- and human-generated review articles on the same topic found that ChatGPT 4.0 generated a high number of incorrect references (errors in citation information, fabricated references, and references not relevant to the information cited in the text), further supporting the need to check AI's output (Kacena et al., 2024).

Given that transparency is a hallmark of systematic review reporting, it follows that reviewers should transparently represent how they used AI tools throughout the review process (e.g., search, title, and abstract screening; data extraction). The International Committee of Medical Journal Editors recommendations, which many journals follow, state that authors who use AI technology should describe its use in the appropriate section of the manuscript (2024). For example, if AI was used in conducting a literature search, this should be noted in the methods section.

Without doubt, recommendations about how to use AI tools in the review process, regardless of the type of review, will evolve alongside its rapid development and integration into how we achieve best practices.

Writing a Systematic Review Report

In primary research, you collect and analyze the data and then write a research article that is a report of all the elements of the project. Similarly, a systematic review is the report of the secondary research you did to conduct the review.

Your systematic review report will include the same elements as the protocol. Because you will have completed the search, appraisal, extraction, analysis of results, and discussion, you'll need to change the protocol tense from future to past tense. If you changed anything from the protocol, you should acknowledge this. For example, you may have discovered that you needed to clarify inclusion criteria as you made decisions to retrieve articles. Include the protocol citation in your report. Your report should cover the following elements:

Abstract. Like any other report of research, you'll need to write an abstract that contains all the elements of the systematic review. Write the abstract last. (Learn more about writing abstracts in Chapter 5.)

Introduction and background. Use the introduction and background from your protocol, keeping in mind that by the time you are ready to submit a systematic review for peer review, you may need to update the background information. Identify where readers can find the protocol.

Objectives/questions. State your objectives and questions exactly as you did in the protocol. Remember, editors and knowledge users may return to your protocol to make sure you have not varied from what you promised to do.

Methods. You'll need to describe in detail how you obtained the material you chose and how it was analyzed. This provides support for the remainder of the report, so be sure you have a well-thought-out process before beginning the project. The methods section should include several key items. (Tips on how you can conduct the project so that you will have what you need for these items are in parentheses.)

- How you mined the databases (First mine the major databases to find a comprehensive list of keywords/controlled language based on your question and inclusion criteria. In the second phase, search each database separately, using the controlled language, Boolean operators, wild cards, and so on that are specific to the database. Finally, use the reference list of articles that are particularly related to your topic to ensure you haven't missed studies. You may want to use a bibliographic database management tool like EndNote or Mendeley to manage the studies you find, to track duplications, and to retain a record of your findings; learn more about these tools in Chapter 4.)

- Use of dual, independent reviewers who made the decision as to what articles to retrieve for appraisal

- The standardized appraisal instrument the reviewers used

- How a lack of consensus between the two reviewers was resolved (typically through a third reviewer)

- How information was extracted from the publications (Extract the details of the publication and study using the instruments you specified in the protocol. Software systems may automatically generate an evidence table based on the electronic data you extract. If you are completing a meta-analysis, the software will guide you to set up the analysis table. Similarly, if you are synthesizing qualitative evidence, software exists to guide how you extract narrative data for meta-aggregation or other synthesis techniques.)

- How you synthesized the data (Your approach will depend on the type of data you extracted to answer your questions. If you're able to perform a meta-analysis, report the details of the meta-analysis such as the effect size [e.g., odds or risk ratios for dichotomous data, weighted mean difference for continuous data], how you analyzed heterogeneity, any subgroup analysis, and any other details that would be helpful to the reader. If you conducted a meta-aggregation of qualitative data, describe your approach to analysis.)

Results. You need to report *all* the details of the search strategy in two ways: the actual strategy for each database (some journals may not publish these details) and the outcome of the search using a PRISMA flow diagram to transparently represent your article gathering. In this diagram, you'll show how many records you identified, how many you screened after removing duplications, the number of records excluded based on initial screening, number of full-text articles appraised, those excluded and why, and finally, how many you included in the type of synthesis you used (e.g., in a meta-analysis). (Refer to http://www.prisma-statement.org/PRISMAStatement/FlowDiagram).

Q *Is PRISMA a methodologic guide about how to conduct a systematic review?*

A No. While the conduct and reporting of a systematic review are linked, PRISMA is a statement about the minimum items that authors should report to ensure adequate transparency so knowledge users can judge the quality of the review. It's an annotated checklist about what to include in the report. Other comprehensive handbooks exist to guide your actual conduct of the review. Though PRISMA is not an appraisal tool, it can help you know what editors and peer reviewers will look for in your report (Page et al., 2021). You should not make a statement that you followed the PRISMA guidelines to conduct the systematic review because it is about reporting standards; it is not a methodological guide.

Include an evidence table that organizes the essential details of the included studies, and give a narrative synthesis of the types of studies and evidence you included. Provide an overview of the quality of the studies and perhaps a table of individual criteria ratings that represent risks of bias (quantitative studies) or credibility (qualitative studies). Readers need to understand how confident they can be of the science you synthesized.

If you conducted a meta-analysis of quantitative outcomes, you should provide a forest plot or series of plots of the extracted data and the appropriate statistic to pool the data. Most meta-analysis software (JBI's SUMARI, Cochrane's RevMan, Biostat's Comprehensive Meta-Analysis) will allow you to export the figure. Other elements you need to report include a measurement of heterogeneity, the statistical model (fixed, random, or mixed effects), and any sensitivity or subgroup analysis. If the outcome variables were dichotomous, your effect size may be calculated as an absolute risk difference, risk ratio, or odds ratio. If your outcome variables were continuous, the pooled effect size may be measured as standard mean difference or weighted mean difference; you need to supply the particular computational method (e.g., Cohen's d). Make sure to represent the confidence intervals around the point estimates. Interpret the meta-analysis accurately for your readers, including the statistical effect, its direction and the magnitude of these differences, and the relationship to clinical impact (Tufanaru et al., 2020).

If you aggregated qualitative data, you may provide a meta-view of the synthesis, revealing the extracted findings, the categories, and, finally, synthesized statements, as this helps readers understand how you synthesized findings. For example, in a systematic review where one of the questions related to the experience of new mothers with postpartum depression living at home, one of the synthesized findings was "depressed mothers feel unable to control their own lives due to low resilience" (Holopainen & Hakulinen, 2019, p. 1739). Include enough narrative to illustrate the categories and synthesized findings. In the postpartum depression example, the authors synthesized five categories they developed from 47 findings. They provided some illustrations from the articles they included in the review (Holopainen & Hakulinen, 2019). The meta-view and illustrations may best be reserved for an online addendum (Lockwood et al., 2020).

Discussion. This portion of the report is your chance to make sense of your review and identify for readers the "So what?" Include the following:

- Conclusions that can be drawn
- Implications for practice or policy
- Recommendations for next steps in research
- What gaps in knowledge were addressed through this study and what further work may be indicated
- Strengths and limitations of the review

Q *What do I do if I'm writing a quantitative systematic review and the data aren't amenable to a meta-analysis?*

A This is a fairly common problem in nursing literature. Typical reasons that you cannot use statistical pooling via meta-analysis include too much heterogeneity or diversity among the populations studied, the way investigators tested the interventions or the interventions themselves, and the measurement of the outcomes and the results. If you can't use meta-analysis, represent the results as a narrative. Follow guidelines so that you are transparent in how you represent the effects, how you weigh the strength of findings, and how you remain within the boundaries of the science. The Synthesis Without Meta-Analysis (SWiM) guidance provides international advice to augment the PRISMA suite of checklists (Campbell et al., 2020).

Q *What is an "empty review"?*

A *Empty reviews* are systematic reviews where investigators find no studies that are eligible to meet their inclusion or quality criteria. You might find them in the Cochrane Database of Systematic Reviews. Reasons for empty reviews include a lack of study in a new area, narrow questions with very specific inclusion criteria, strict methodologic criteria, or a reluctance to consider lesser study designs despite a desire to represent the "best available evidence" (Yaffe et al., 2012). Empty reviews can be helpful in identifying gaps in knowledge, but realistically, they are quite difficult to get published (Gray, 2021). Sometimes an empty review is unavoidable because of lack of research in an area, but you can limit the likelihood of ending your efforts with one by crafting an effective research question and following methodology guidance developed by groups such as JBI and Cochrane.

Scoping Reviews

Scoping reviews are like systematic reviews in that they follow a structured process and are an increasingly popular type of review. However, they have different purposes and some key differences in methodologies (Munn et al., 2018). Scoping reviews are meant to determine the breadth and coverage of an area of study and to map the body of literature. They are versatile, can clarify key concepts, and can help researchers decide if there is adequate literature available to justify the effort required for a systematic review. They have been used to identify research methods that have been applied in an area and gaps in science as a mechanism to justify new primary research (Arksey & O'Malley, 2006; Peters et al., 2020; Woo et al., 2022).

Arksey and O'Malley (2006) developed the original framework for scoping reviews. They emphasized that scoping reviews need to be transparent and reproducible; the search must be exhaustive and requires iterative attempts as you learn more about the literature. Since this original work, others have developed the methodology further. Levac et al. (2010) clarified and enhanced the original methods, JBI developed methodological guidance, and the PRISMA group developed reporting guidelines (PRISMA-ScR). The stages of a scoping review are (Arksey & O'Malley, 2006; Levac et al., 2010; Peters et al., 2020):

1. Identify the research question (link to the review's purpose).
2. Identify relevant studies (balance feasibility of the search with breadth and comprehensiveness).
3. Select studies (dual reviewers using an iterative team approach with searching).
4. Chart data (numerical and conceptual analysis to characterize trends, gaps to map the topic).
5. Collate, summarize, and report the results.
6. Consult (with key stakeholders involved in knowledge exchange).

Writing a Scoping Review Protocol

Before you write your scoping review protocol, you need to align your purpose with your decision to choose this particular methodology. According to Peters et al. (2020), reasons for conducting a scoping review are:

- As a precursor to a systematic review
- To identify the types of available evidence in a given field
- To identify and analyze knowledge gaps
- To clarify key concepts/definitions in the literature
- To examine how research is conducted on a certain topic or field
- To identify key characteristics or factors related to a concept

Like a systematic review, your protocol should detail the plan for the scoping review. However, understand that these plans may change because of what you find along the way. Your protocol elements should include (see Peters et al., 2020, for full guidance on all phases of a scoping review):

- Title (Include "scoping review" and align it with your question.)
- Introduction and background (Note the significance, what is known and unknown, and that a current review on the topic doesn't exist—be sure the latter is true.)
- Objectives and review question (Use the PCC format [see next bullet].)

- Inclusion criteria (This consists of study and publication characteristics.):
  - **P**opulation/participants
  - **C**oncept
  - **C**ontext
  - Types of studies and other literature
  - Languages and time frame
- Search strategy
  - Information sources (Include what databases, search engines, and grey or fugitive literature you plan to use.)
  - Iterative process based on findings
- Process of selecting sources (Include pilot testing, dual reviewers, title/abstract/full text), and bibliographic management database, if used.)
- Data extraction plan for charting details of studies/evidence (Note that a pilot test was conducted.)
- Analysis of the evidence (This depends on the purpose, type of evidence, and judgment of the investigators.)
- Plan to present the results (For example, this may include a table with frequencies of study designs, populations, characteristics of the evidence, or a diagram representing a map of the findings.)

Writing a Scoping Review Report

Your report should cover the following elements:

Abstract. Include all the key elements of the review, reserving the bulk of abstract for the main results. Write the abstract last.

Introduction/background. This section is similar to that of a systematic review and reflects the background of the protocol, with any updates since you wrote the protocol. Include a discussion of your preliminary search for other scoping reviews to justify the need and significance of review.

Review questions. State the question, explain how the question relates to the purpose, and clarify the elements. For example, a "PCC" question might be: What interventions exist to promote self-care (concept) in patients with moderate-to-severe chronic obstructive pulmonary disease (COPD) (population) living in their own homes or assisted living (context)? This question could relate to an objective that maps all types of self-care interventions to promote symptom management, such as exercise, activities of daily living, dyspnea, and medication use. The breadth of this question becomes evident as you begin to project what areas of the concept may emerge.

Inclusion criteria. These are the criteria you used to guide the search and selection of research for your review. You may need to report how you modified the inclusion criteria as part of the iterative nature of the conduct of a scoping review. In the self-care example, you may have discovered that you needed to expand the definition of self-care interventions to also include strategies that caregivers use to help patients with COPD manage their response to the disease.

Search strategy. Describe the search process as a three-stage process (mining keywords in major databases, database-specific strategy, and reference checking), similar to the systematic review process. However, you'll probably be more expansive in the types of publications (primary literature, systematic reviews, even texts and opinions) as you try to map the entirety of an area of literature. As you conducted the search, you should have used an iterative process as you became more familiar with the body of literature. It's imperative that you use tools to document your search and subsequently report the strategy and output in a transparent and auditable fashion.

Selection of sources. Scoping reviews are, by their nature, broad in scope, which means you may have used a team to work through the findings of your search. Describe your process. For example, did you pilot your predefined inclusion criteria with your team and make adjustments as needed? Like the systematic review, two independent reviewers need to make the decision to retrieve and include a source, and you should document that was done. Report your decision-making process using a PRISMA diagram (see Tricco et al., 2018).

Data extraction/charting. Document how you extracted information from the articles you selected, including whether you piloted your approach. You may include the final extraction form as an appendix or online addendum in your publication, depending on the editor's preference. Record the bibliographic details and the elements that relate to your question (e.g., aim, sample, intervention[s], outcome details and key findings).

Analysis. The goal of a scoping review is to summarize or map rather than synthesize and interpret. Unlike systematic reviews, the approach to analysis in scoping reviews is much less standardized. You may code characteristics in your data extraction tool so you can report counts of occurrences such as study designs, concepts, and outcomes. Aim to be as transparent as you can be and justify your approach.

Presentation of results. If you plan how to present the findings of the review before you begin and refine as you understand the body of literature, your ability to extract, analyze, and then present results will be more methodical. Options for presenting results include tables that could be guided by your PCC question, a conceptual diagram of relationships, and charts of frequencies of concepts. If you consulted with stakeholders throughout the review or at the end of the review, report how you involved them. Your narrative should expand on any representation of the findings with a goal of providing a meaningful summary that reflects your purpose and review question.

Q *How long will it take me to write a review?*

A This is a hard question to answer because it depends on the scope of the review, the tools you have to help you conduct the review, the size of your team, and the complexity of the topic. Some have estimated that a systematic review can take one to two years from start to finish. Because scoping reviews are meant to be broad, they often require a significant time investment. If you have a review team, you can divide and conquer the workload. Rapid reviews have evolved to answer important questions more quickly. The jury remains undecided on if the sacrifice is worth taking shortcuts (Munn et al., 2023).

Integrative Reviews

Integrative reviews are meant to bring together different types of evidence, including empirical and theoretical, into a single synthesis. They may include both research and theory as data sources and are unique in that they often synthesize a wide variety of primary methodologies. While there is systematized and logical development in integrative reviews, they are not systematic reviews.

One can argue that integrative reviews have not had the same degree of methodological development as other reviews (Hopia et al., 2016). Whittemore and Knafl's (2005) guidance is most often referred to as the basis of integrative reviews. When they wrote this guidance, other review types were developing to address some of the reasons that you might consider an integrative review. For example, JBI has developed

> **Confidence Booster**
>
> You may be feeling like writing a review is an overwhelming task. You can do this! Here are some tips:
>
> - Choose the right type of review to meet your purpose.
> - Seek training for specialized review methodologies (Cochrane and JBI offer regular training).
> - Be organized as you plan, carry out, and then write your review.
> - Use software for writing your protocol, tracking your search results, conducting the analysis, and reporting. Some software packages (e.g., Cochrane's RevMan and JBI's SUMARI) can aid much of the review process, including generating statistical analyses.
> - Use a bibliographic database manager like EndNote. You may be able to select a specific reference style guide, and some review software programs allow you to import the citations into the analysis software.
> - Work with a review team to share the workload; you need a review partner anyway for different stages of the review.
> - Keep an appraisal tool for your review type at your side so you know how your review might be judged, and use the appropriate checklist (e.g., PRISMA) to make sure you are meeting all the reporting expectations.
> - Know that reviews can accelerate the translation of knowledge to practice. Think about how you might add a "plain language" summary to help readers understand the essence of your review.

comprehensive approaches to systematically review a wide variety of types of evidence (study designs serving meaningfulness, appropriateness, and feasibility and effectiveness) far beyond traditional RCTs or quasi-experimental designs. However, the integrative review is a type of review that can combine both empirical and theoretical data unlike any of the current systematic review methodologies (Aromataris & Munn, 2020; Whittemore & Knafl, 2005).

Conducting and Writing an Integrative Review

Unlike the other review types discussed in this chapter, the integrative review does not begin with a protocol. However, when you write your article, you'll need to address the following phases you should have used in conducting the review: problem identification, literature search, data evaluation, and data analysis. You'll also need to consider presentation.

Problem identification. Integrative reviews, like all others, require you to identify the problem clearly so that you can, in turn, clearly define variables of interest (including population, healthcare issue, concepts) and the types of evidence or theories considered.

Literature search. Whittemore and Knafl (2005) note that the search should be documented (database[s], keywords), logical, and justified; it may include iterative stages. For example, you may use certain keywords that you originally thought would capture a comprehensive representation of the existing literature, but find additional terms that relate to your topic so that you revise and restart the search. The search may include a "purposive" stage combined with a comprehensive search to reach a particular element of the issue. (A *purposive search* is more focused than a comprehensive search because it aims to uncover literature related to a sub-element of the review question, such as a deeper but narrower dive into the population of interest.)

Data evaluation. Appraising the quality of the primary works in an integrative review is complex because of the breadth of the evidence sources (Whittemore & Knafl, 2005). Describe your approach in enough detail to show that you evaluated the quality of the studies and other literature in a meaningful way.

Data analysis. Evidence sources may vary in the type of data they yield, so explain and justify your approach to analysis and synthesis. Whittemore and Knafl (2005) described a process of data reduction through classifying by subgroups that may be defined by chronology, settings, sample characteristics, or pre-defined concepts. Note how you used these groupings to extract and code the data. Provide data displays (e.g. matrices, graphs, charts, networks) that align with the data-reduction techniques to help readers visualize patterns and find meaning in the data.

Presentation. Your report will probably contain tables or diagrams as well as your narrative synthesis related to your conclusions. Rigor arises from defense of your logic and how you justify conclusions. Include a summary of methodological limitations and implications for practice, policy, and research that remain within the boundaries of the study (Whittemore & Knafl, 2005).

Q *Where can I find guidance for conducting different types of reviews?*

A The organizations committed to the synthesis of evidence have ongoing scientific committees that aim to continuously improve the methodologies of synthesis. Cochrane, Campbell, and JBI produce handbooks to guide synthesis (see reference list). In addition, the journal *Research Synthesis Methods*, the official publication of the Society for Research Synthesis Methodology, has rich sources of methodologic information. Finally, you will find debate about methodological development in the general scientific literature.

Spread Your Knowledge

This chapter has focused on review methods most commonly found in the nursing literature, but there are many other types. You might wish to conduct and write a review but aren't sure what type best fits what you would like to accomplish. Table 15.2 compares some of the key features for three of the reviews discussed in the chapter. Pick the one that meets your purposes and the needs of your knowledge users, conduct the review, and share the results with your colleagues through publication.

TABLE 15.2 Comparing Review Key Features

	Systematic Review (quantitative)	Systematic Review (qualitative)	Scoping Review	Integrative Review
Methodological developers	Cochrane, JBI, and others	Cochrane, JBI, and others	JBI, funded researchers	Whittemore & Knafl, with some development in the general literature
Typical aim	Effectiveness	Meaning	Map	Integrate
Clear objective or research question	PICO or similar form	PICo or similar form	Broadly defined	Broadly defined
Predefined, published protocol	Yes	Yes	Yes	Not usually
Comprehensive, exhaustive, and transparent search	Yes	Yes	Yes, iterative	Iterative, less consistently defined
Dual, independent reviewers for retrieval and appraisal	Yes	Yes	Yes	Sometimes
Documentation of destiny of all retrieved articles	Yes	Yes	Yes	Sometimes
Data extraction tools represented	Yes	Yes	Yes, but iterative	Unclear
Appraisal represented	Yes, often in tabular form or represented as risk of bias	Yes, often in tabular form with appraisal of credibility	No; aim is to map	Unclear
Synthesis methods	Meta-analysis or narrative	Meta-aggregation or meta-ethnography	Summary rather than synthesis	Iterative and dependent on types of evidence
Ratings of evidence strength or certainty	Yes, usually GRADE methods related to certainty of findings	Yes, using standardized methods related to credibility and dependability of findings	No, although there may be a map of study designs found	Not described

Write Now!

1. Find an example of a systematic review, a scoping review, and an integrative review. Compare them to differentiate their purposes, methods, findings, and conclusions.

2. Read a published systematic review without reading the abstract. Then write one, following the elements of a systematic review. Did you find similar conclusions as the investigators who published the review?

3. Find an appraisal tool for one type of review (e.g., find the CASP tool for systematic reviews). Read the review and identify its strengths and weaknesses.

References

Arksey, H., & O'Malley, L. (2006). Scoping studies: Towards a methodological framework. *International Journal of Social Research Methodology, 8*(1), 19–32. https://doi.org/10.1080/1364557032000119616

Aromataris, E., Fernandez, R., Godfrey, C., Holly C., Khalil, H., & Tungpunkom, P. (2020). Chapter 10: Umbrella reviews. In E. Aromataris & Z. Munn (Eds.), *JBI manual for evidence synthesis*. JBI. https://doi.org/10.46658/JBIRM-17-08

Aromataris, E., & Munn, Z. (Eds.). (2020). *JBI manual for evidence synthesis*. JBI. https://doi.org/10.46658/JBIMES-20-01

Campbell, C., McKenzie, J. E., Sowden, A., Katikireddi, S. V., Brennan, S. E., Ellis, S., Hartmann-Boyce, J., Ryan, R., Shepperd, S., Thomas, J., Welch, V., & Thomson, H. (2020). Synthesis without meta-analysis (SWiM) in systematic reviews: Reporting guideline. *BMJ, 368*, l6890. https://doi.org/10.1136/bmj.l6890

CINAHL (2023). *Scope note for "systematic review."* https://web-p-ebscohost-com.rosalindfranklin.idm.oclc.org/ehost/mesh?vid=2&sid=466f67d7-1ac2-48cb-a600-5262ee86bad9%40redis

Cochrane Library. (n.d.). *About Cochrane reviews*. https://www.cochranelibrary.com/about/about-cochrane-reviews

Egger, M., Higgins, J. P. T., & Smith, G. D. (2022). Systematic reviews in health research. In M. Egger, J. P. T Higgins, & G. D. Smit (Eds.), *Systematic reviews in health research*. John Wiley & Sons. http://dx.doi.org/10.1002/9781119099369

Golan, R., Reddy, R., Muthigi, A., & Ramasamy, R. (2023). Artificial intelligence in academic writing: A paradigm-shifting technological advance. *Nature Reviews: Urology, 20*(6), 327–328. https://doi.org/10.1038/s41585-023-00746-x

Grant, M. J., & Booth, A. (2009). A typology of reviews: An analysis of 14 review types and associated methodologies. *Health Information and Libraries Journal, 26*(2), 91–108. https://doi.org/10.1111/j.1471-1842.2009.00848.x

Gray, R. (2021). Empty systematic reviews: Identifying gaps in knowledge or a waste of time and effort? *Nurse Author & Editor, 31*(2), 42–44. https://doi.org/10.1111/nae2.23

Hamel, C., Michaud, A., Thuku, M., Skidmore, B., Stevens, A., Nussbaumer-Streit, B., & Garrity, C. (2021). Defining rapid reviews: A systematic scoping review and thematic analysis of definitions and defining characteristics of rapid reviews. *Journal of Clinical Epidemiology, 129*, 74–85. https://doi.org/10.1016/j.clinepi.2020.09.041

Higgins, J. P. T., Thomas, J., Chandler, J., Cumpston, M., Li, T., Page, M. J., & Welch, V. A. (Eds.). (2023). *Cochrane Handbook for Systematic Reviews of Interventions* (Version 6.4, updated August 2023). https://training.cochrane.org/handbook/current

Holopainen, A., & Hakulinen, T. (2019). New parents' experiences of postpartum depression: A systematic review of qualitative evidence. *JBI Database of Systematic Reviews and Implementation Reports, 17*(9), 1731–1769. https://doi.org/10.11124/JBISRIR-2017-003909

Hopia, H., Latvala, E., & Liimatainen, L. (2016). Reviewing the methodology of an integrative review. *Scandinavian Journal of Caring Sciences, 30*(4), 662–669. https://doi.org/10.1111/scs.12327

International Committee of Medical Journal Editors. (2024). *Recommendations for the conduct, reporting, editing, and publication of scholarly work in medical journals*. http://www.icmje.org/recommendations

Kacena, M. A., Plotkin, L. I., & Fehrenbacher, J. C. (2024). The use of artificial intelligence in writing scientific review articles. *Current Osteoporosis Reports*. https://doi.org/10.1007/s11914-023-00852-0

Levac, D., Colquhoun, H., & O'Brien, K. K. (2010). Scoping studies: Advancing the methodology. *Implementation Science, 5*(69). https://doi.org/10.1186/1748-5908-5-69

Lockwood, C., Porrit, K., Munn, Z., Rittenmeyer, L., Salmond, S., Bjerrum, M., Loveday, H., Carrier, J., & Stannard, D. (2020). Chapter 2: Systematic reviews of qualitative evidence. In E. Aromataris & Z. Munn (Eds.), *JBI manual for evidence synthesis*. JBI. https://doi.org/10.46658/JBIMES-20-03

Munn, Z., Lockwood, C., & Moola, S. (2015). The development and use of evidence summaries for point of care information systems: A streamlined rapid review approach. *Worldviews on Evidence-Based Nursing, 12*(3), 131–138. https://doi.org/10.1111/wvn.12094

Munn, Z., Peters, M., Stern, C., Tufanaru, C., McArthur, A., & Aromataris, E. (2018). Systematic review or scoping review? Guidance for authors when choosing between a systematic or scoping review approach. *BMC Medical Research Methodology, 18*(143). https://doi.org/10.1186/s12874-018-0611-x

Munn, Z., Pollack, D., Barker, T., Stone, J., Stern, C., Aromataris, E., Pearson, A., Strauss, S., Khalil, H., Mustafa, R. A., Tricco, A., & Schunemann; H. J. (2023). The dark side of rapid reviews: A retreat from systematic approaches and the need for clear expectations and reporting. *Annals of Internal Medicine, 176*, 266–267. https://doi.org/10.7326/M22-2603

Page, M. J., McKenzie, J. E., Bossuyt, P. M., & the PRISMA Group. (2021). The PRISMA 2020 statement: An updated guideline for reporting systematic reviews. *BMJ, 372*, 1–9. http://dx.doi.org/10.1136/bmj.n71

Peters, M. D. J., Godfrey, C., McInerney, P., Munn, Z., Tricco, A. C., & Khalil, H. (2020). Scoping reviews (2020 version). In E. Aromataris & Z. Munn (Eds.), *JBI manual for evidence synthesis*. JBI. https://doi.org/10.46658/JBIRM-20-01

Sackett, D. L., Rosenberg, W. C., Muir, J. A., Haynes, R. B., & Richardson, W. S. (1996). Evidence based medicine: What it is and isn't. *British Medical Journal, 312*, 71. https://doi.org/10.1136/bmj.312.7023.71

Silva, A. R., Padiliha, M. I., Petra, S., Silva, V. S. E., Woo, K., Galica, J., Wilson, R., & Luctkar-Flude, M. (2022). Reviews of literature in nursing research: Methodologies, considerations, and defining characteristics. *Advances in Nursing Science, 45*(3), 197–208. http://dx.doi.org/10.1097/ANS.0000000000000418

Sutton, A., Clowes, M., Preston, L., & Booth, A. (2019). Meeting the review family: Exploring review types and associated information retrieval requirements. *Health Information & Libraries Journal, 36*(3), 202–222. http://dx.doi.org/10.1111/hir.12276

Tricco, A. C., Lillie, E., Zarin, W., O'Brien, K. K., Colquhoun, H., Levac, D., Moher, D., Peters, M. D., Horsley, T., Weeks, L., Hempel, S., Akl, E. A., Chang, C., McGowan, J., Stewart, L., Hartling, L., Aldcroft, A., Wilson, M. G., Garritty, C. Lewin, S., Godfrey, C. M., Macdonald, M. T., Langlois, E. V., Soares-Weiser, K., Moriarty, J., Clifford, T., Tuncalp, O., & Straus, S. E. (2018). PRISMA extension for scoping reviews (PRISMA-ScR): Checklist and explanation. *Annals of Internal Medicine, 169*(7), 467–473. https://doi.org/10.7326/M18-0850

Tricco, A. C., Soobiah, C., Antony, J., Cogo, E., MacDonald, H., Lillie, E., Tran, J., D'Souza, J., Hui, W., Perrier, L., Welch, V., Horsley, T., Straus, S. E., & Kastner, M. (2016). A scoping review identifies multiple emerging knowledge synthesis methods, but few studies operationalize the method. *Journal of Clinical Epidemiology, 73*, 19–28. http://dx.doi.org/10.1016/j.jclinepi.2015.08.030

Tufanaru, C., Munn, Z., Aromataris, E., Campbell, J., & Hopp, L. (2020). Chapter 3: Systematic reviews of effectiveness. In E. Aromataris & Z. Munn (Eds.), *JBI manual for evidence synthesis*. JBI. https://doi.org/10.46658/JBIMES-20-04

van Dijk, S. H. B, Brusse-Keizer, M. G. J, Bucsán, C. C., van der Palen, J., Doggen, C. J. M., & Lenferink, A. (2023). Artificial intelligence in systematic reviews: Promising when appropriately used. *BMJ Open, 13*(7), e072254. http://dx.doi.org/10.1136/bmjopen-2023-072254

Watt, J., & Del Giovane, C. D. (2022). Network meta-analysis. In E. Evangelou, A. A. Veroniki (Eds.), *Meta-Research: Methods and protocols* (pp. 187–201). Humana. https://doi.org/10.1007/978-1-0716-1566-9_12

Whittemore, R., & Knafl, K. (2005). The integrative review: Updated methodology. *Journal of Advanced Nursing, 52*(5), 546–553. http://dx.doi.org/10.1111/j.1365-2648.2005.03621.x

Woo, B. F. Y., Tam, W. W. S., Williams, M. Y., Yong, J. Q. Y. O., Cheong, Z. Y., Ong, Y. C., Poon, S. M., Goh, Y. S. (2022). Characteristics, methodological, and reporting quality of scoping reviews published in nursing journals: A systematic review. *Journal of Nursing Scholarship, 55*(4), 874–885. https://doi.org/10.1111/jnu.12861

Yaffe, J., Montgomery, P., Hopewell, S., & Shepard, L. D. (2012). Empty reviews: A description and consideration of Cochrane systematic reviews with no included studies. *PLoS One, 7*(5), e36626. https://doi.org/10.1371/journal.pone.0036626

Younas, A., & Ali, P. (2021). Five tips for developing useful literature summary tables for writing review articles. *Evidence Based Nursing, 24*, 32–34. https://doi.org/10.1136/ebnurs-2021-103417

Reporting the Quality Improvement or Evidence-Based Practice Project

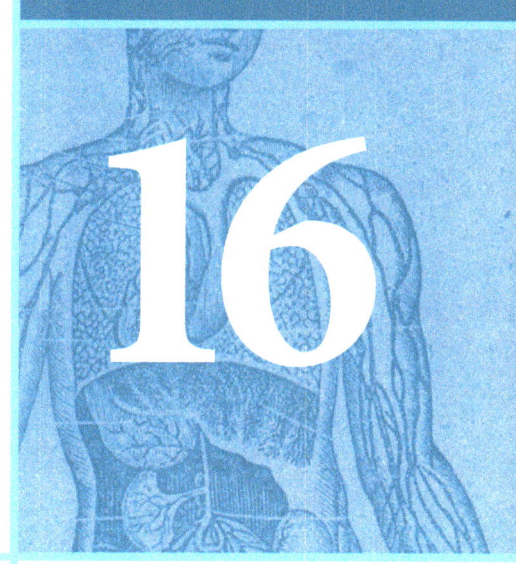

–Jo Rycroft-Malone, OBE, PhD, MSc, BSc (Hons), RN
–Christopher Burton, DPhil, RN

"If you wait for inspiration to write you're not a writer, you're a waiter."
–Dan Poynter

WHAT YOU'LL LEARN IN THIS CHAPTER

- Quality improvement (QI) and evidence-based practice (EBP) projects attempt to demonstrate and evaluate ways in which care, service delivery, or practice can be improved.

- These projects can be just as rigorous as research, but writing about them can be challenging.

- You can strengthen your article about a QI or an EBP project by following guidelines for reporting this type of work.

- Be sure to include enough detail, including the context and implications of your results, to help readers gain insights that might have relevance to their own practice.

Improving care and service delivery is every nurse's and healthcare team's responsibility. Making evidence-informed changes in healthcare practice and service delivery that have the potential to lead to better patient outcomes, better system performance, and better professional development (Connor et al., 2023) is important, yet challenging.

Although quality improvement (QI) and evidence-based practice (EBP) projects have distinguishing features that differ, such as the role that evidence plays and the types of interventions implemented, both have the same goal—providing patients with the best and safest care possible consistently (Dixon-Woods, 2019, The Health Foundation, 2013).

This chapter guides you through how to write articles about QI and EBP projects. Although similar to the process for writing a research article, these projects require the use of unique techniques, such as following reporting guidelines specific to QI projects. Using these techniques helps ensure that readers gain the most from your work and increases the potential for the wider community to learn from your improvement practice and research.

Common Questions About QI and EBP Projects

The answers to a few common questions about writing about QI and EBP projects will help prepare you to write.

What Is the Difference Between a QI or EBP Project and a Research Study?

Some people say that QI and EBP projects are not as rigorous as a full-scale research study, but this is not necessarily the case. All types of projects—research, QI, or EBP—can be conducted with more or less rigor. In fact, the quality and safety movement has been championing the need for more rigorous methods and transparent reporting.

Others say that QI and EBP projects tend to be local and focused on particular patient populations; however, you probably have read reports of research studies that have been conducted in a particular context with a specific patient group. And you only need to read articles in the journal *BMJ Quality and Safety* to see that many quality projects can be large scale and fully funded by external agencies.

The one characteristic that differentiates QI and EBP projects from research projects is that they are consistently concerned with attempting to demonstrate and evaluate ways in which care, service delivery, or practice can be improved. These projects may be local, and some may be small scale, but they should be no less rigorously conducted than traditional research.

What Are the Challenges of Writing About Quality Improvement Work?

Quality improvement is a complex and multifactorial process (for an example, see Storkholm et al., 2019). Consequently, improvement interventions are like recipes—they rarely rely on one ingredient. It's likely that you'll have used a number of different strategies and interventions to effect change at different organizational levels, including with coworkers and managers, and potentially with patients and family caregivers. Unpacking the active ingredients, how they relate to each other, and how much of each is required presents considerable methodological and design challenges. A good article on QI will make sense of the active ingredients, carefully describing the reality of what was done, why, with whom, and with what impact.

Who Reads About Improvement?

Four main groups seek information about improvement projects. *Clinical nurses* who are developing their own projects or improving the safety, reliability, quality, and effectiveness of clinical practice might be particularly interested in rich, practical insights that could have relevance for their own work. *Project staff*, including individuals with improvement as part of their everyday work and those who have been assigned to support particular projects, will be interested to know what approaches or techniques seem to be helpful in delivering a successful improvement project. *Policymakers* have an interest in how findings from improvement projects might be more broadly applied. *Researchers* will be interested in what theoretical perspectives have been used and how the methodologies used to evaluate the impacts of projects have generated new insights.

The publication where you choose to publish your work will have a target readership, which should guide the style and content of your writing. Although your work may most often appear in nursing publications, remember that there is now interest in learning whether knowledge of "what works" in improvement can be transferred to other professional fields, potentially extending your readership. Follow these steps to increase the reach of your report:

- Understand the needs of the audiences you are writing for: What will they be interested in knowing about and why?
- Within the constraints of your chosen medium, adopt as rich and descriptive a writing style as possible without being overly wordy.
- Include information on both the theory and practice of QI, including any lessons learned.
- Pay attention to the use of jargon, avoiding it when possible and clarifying it when necessary.
- Tease out the findings that may have relevance for a non-nursing audience.

Researchers are increasingly adopting a more collaborative approach to the design and conduct of improvement studies (Graham et al., 2022; Jones et al., 2019), which is thought to increase the likelihood the findings will be used. In this spirit, consider consulting with key stakeholders from your target audience to see how you might increase the impact of your writing.

Start Writing

There are minimal standards for reporting on research about implementation, where the subject matter is concerned with closing the gap between what we "know" and what is practiced (Pinnock et al., 2017).

One commonly used set of standards for the QI project is the "Standards for QUality Improvement Reporting Excellence (SQUIRE) 2.0" (Goodman et al., 2016; Ogrinc et al., 2016). These guidelines provide a framework for sharing the knowledge acquired through both the practice and research of implementing improvement interventions, systematically and in detail. They are useful because they encourage you to clarify your thinking, verify your observations, and justify your inferences. The "Standards for QUality Improvement Reporting Excellence in Education (SQUIRE-EDU)," which focus on projects related to education, are an extension for the SQUIRE guidelines (Ogrinc et al., 2019).

Q *Are the SQUIRE guidelines the only ones I need to consult?*

A No. Depending on the approach you've taken for your improvement interventions and the requirements of the publication where you are submitting, you might also need to refer to other reporting standards. The Consolidated Standards for Reporting Clinical Trials, or CONSORT (Schulz et al., 2010), apply to randomized clinical trials, and the Consolidated Standards for Reporting Qualitative Research (COREQ) is a 32-item checklist for qualitative research involving interviews and focus groups (Tong et al., 2007). In 2013, EBP Process Quality Assessment (EPQA) guidelines were released (Ching Lee et al., 2013), and in 2021 the Evidence-Based Practice Dissemination Guide (Dean & Gallagher-Ford, 2021) was published. These guidelines can be used to help guide, evaluate, and publish EBP projects. Appendix D lists guidelines you may find helpful.

The following sections draw primarily on the SQUIRE 2.0 framework with additions from the Evidence-Based Practice Dissemination Guide (Dean & Gallagher-Ford, 2021) to help guide you through the issues that are important to consider when writing your article. Another resource is a template for publishing an evidence-based practice project, which you can find in the book by Dang and colleagues (2021) listed in the references.

Title

Busy readers need to understand the heart of your article quickly. They will use your title and abstract to make decisions about the relevance and importance of your paper. Titles should contain keywords that provide signposts for your article so those searching the literature can easily find it and understand how it's similar to or different from other articles. SQUIRE points to the three components of a title that will provide clear reference points for the reader:

How quality is considered within the study. Quality can be considered in different ways, including patient safety, clinical effectiveness, patient-centeredness, timeliness, efficiency, and equity of care. In addition, the way that improvement work in nursing is organized and practiced can reflect different traditions such as:

- Evidence-based practice (Melnyk & Fineout-Overholt., 2019)
- Quality improvement (The Health Foundation, 2013)
- Practice development (Dewing et al., 2021)
- Implementation and co-production (Graham et al., 2022)

Where possible, including one of these terms or phrases in the title to describe your approach will be a helpful signpost for readers.

The aims of the intervention. The title should provide a clear focus for the improvement or evidence-based practice activity. For example, were you attempting to change a process of care such as a patient's length of stay? Or were you focused on the reliability of care processes rather than a change in the process itself? You might be also interested in impacts for patients, staff, and other stakeholders.

The specifics of the study methods used in the improvement work. The methods that researchers use to evaluate improvement initiatives are broad. Providing some details in the title that show the methods used in your project will help orient readers to your article early on.

Example 16.1 shows an effective title.

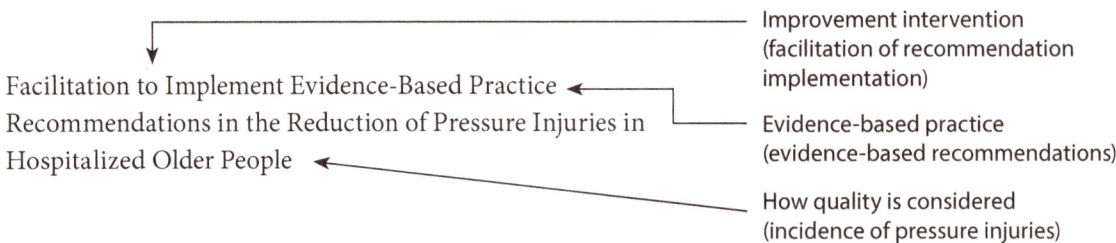

EXAMPLE 16.1 An effective title.

Abstract

Most publications require an abstract, which is a summary of your study. It's important to follow the publication's author guidelines because different publications have different requirements, but abstracts typically include several sections: a *background* that sets out the challenge and aim of your improvement; the *methods*, including interventions used in improvement and evaluation; your *findings* (e.g., outcomes and impact); and the *conclusions* and *implications for practice*. It's usually best to write the abstract after the main article is nearly final because by then you have a much clearer idea about what issues are significant. However, some authors find writing the abstract first a useful way to summarize the planned content of the article (Learn more about writing abstracts in Chapters 5 and 14.)

Introduction

In this section, explain to the reader why you undertook the project and why it was important. Include a summary of current knowledge about the problem you tackled and a detailed description of the context(s) in which the project took place. This will require you to report on the existing evidence about the topic (including, as appropriate, literature focused on policy, practice, and research) and to draw on your knowledge of the locality.

Your introduction should answer the following questions:

- **What is currently known about the topic?** For example, if the focus of your article is on a project to improve the care of peripheral intravenous lines, introduce what the policy, practice, and research evidence shows about best practice in this area and how others have previously improved practice or service delivery.

- **What prompted the need to attend to this issue?** For instance, was there an incident or safety event that identified the need for an intervention around the care of peripheral intravenous lines?

- **What is the gap or current practice or problem you are attempting to improve?** For example, "An audit of documentation found that information about why peripheral intravenous lines were being inserted and subsequently managed was poorly recorded." Clearly articulate the gap between what is currently happening in practice and what the evidence tells us about what should be happening—this is the *improvement gap*.

- **What is the improvement-related question?** After you've identified the gap, clearly and specifically state the main and secondary questions you were addressing within the project. Include what you were expecting to see change and how.

- **What is the context of improvement?** The implementation of improvement interventions is contingent upon the context in which they are being implemented, so a detailed description of the context is vital. This is described in the SQUIRE guidelines as the "environment ... meaningful to the success, failure and unexpected consequences of the intervention" (Ogrinc et al., 2016, "Context" section). It's not enough to describe just the physical context; readers must understand the details of the structures, processes, people, and patterns of care of the setting(s) in which the project took place. In the earlier title example of implementing an evidence-based approach to reducing pressure injuries, factors such as nurse-to-patient ratios and the profile of patient comorbidities might mediate successful implementation and should be highlighted to readers.

- **What theory and/or framework guided your project?** Describe how the evidence-based practice theory or framework was used to plan, implement, and evaluate the project.

After the introduction, you should continue with a discussion of methods used.

Methods

The reader needs to understand the decisions you made in designing your QI or EBP project. This should include a consideration of any ethical issues that you felt were relevant, the setting in which you were working, the interventions or strategies you selected (and why), how you planned to study improvement, the measurement of effects, and the analysis of data. When describing the design used to address the quality issue, differentiate between improvement *activity* (e.g., EBP in infection control and prevention) and improvement *interventions* (e.g., training and education). The SQUIRE guidelines provide a useful framework for doing this and for writing an effective methods section. You may find the Standards for Reporting Implementation Studies (StaRI) useful for this too (Pinnock et al., 2017).

Ethical issues. These include any changes in clinical practice that might have implications for patients, family caregivers, staff, and other professionals and, therefore, warrant critical review from an ethical perspective. If you sought approval from an ethics review committee or institutional review board for your work, make that explicit. However, simply stating that ethical review was obtained tells the reader little about the potential ethical issues that you faced in the study. Specific issues you might want to discuss include the following:

- **The protection of patients' well-being:** Was there any risk that care could be compromised through the project?
- **The protection of staff:** What support was provided to ensure members of nursing staff were prepared for any changes?
- **Clinical governance:** Were any changes sanctioned by the appropriate organizational care committees?

State how you addressed these concerns—for example, by obtaining consent from participants.

Context (setting). Your description of the study setting needs to include more than geography. You should also note those aspects of the context that were anticipated to influence improvement. The following example of a study related to improving infection prevention and control illustrates how to write about setting.

Example of a poor description of setting:
Implementation of a new infection prevention and control guideline was evaluated in an acute care unit.

Example of a good description of setting:
Implementation of a new evidence-based infection prevention and control guideline was evaluated on a 16-bed acute care medical unit. In the most recent hospital audit, the unit's performance was in the upper quartile. The staffing profile and levels were consistent with national recommendations, with consistent and strong unit leadership. The unit was part of a regional quality improvement collaborative with a strong ethos of multidisciplinary working and service development.

Staff had been involved in a range of evidence-based practice and quality improvement initiatives over the previous three years, including process mapping, audit and feedback, and networking. There was also a culture of evaluation in the unit and hospital.

This profile of organizational experience and external evaluation indicated that the quality of baseline clinical practice would provide a credible context for testing guideline implementation.

In this example, the reader is pointed to aspects of the history of organizational change, baseline performance, and experience with improvement, all of which were anticipated to positively influence the effects of guideline implementation.

> **Confidence Booster**
>
> If you're writing an article for the first time, consider asking someone who has been published before to help you. In the case of a QI article, tap into the expertise of stakeholders who were involved in the original project. You might want to include one or two of them as coauthors. Just be sure that you decide up front who will be the lead author and what responsibilities each author will have. You might also ask a trusted friend or mentor for encouragement as you move through the different stages of writing.

Intervention(s). Quality improvement work can include two types of interventions:

- The new nursing practice or intervention that you have implemented as part of your quality improvement project—for example, promoting infection control practice.
- The implementation interventions that you have used to support staff in their use of the new nursing practice or intervention—for example, champions who have a specific role in promoting appropriate infection control in clinical practice (Williams et al., 2016).

Fully describe both, considering the following questions:

- What are the component parts of the intervention? Who completed the activities, and how were they prepared and supported? What would another team need to know to be able to reproduce what you did in their own work?
- What was your justification for selecting the intervention? You might make links to your analysis of previous work and theory outlined in the introduction section, but pay attention to their fit with the local contexts where your improvement work was completed.

It's important to include a description of how a practice and/or implementation or improvement intervention was modified or tailored to the local context.

The following provides an example of how using SQUIRE guidelines adds meaning when writing the intervention section (as well as other sections) of your article:

Non-SQUIRE Guidelines: The new dietetic referral system included a nutritional screening assessment, which was completed by ward staff as the basis for prioritizing patients. Referrals were then coded as urgent, important, or routine, and managed by the service administration staff.

SQUIRE Guidelines: The new referral system included a screening assessment (see Table 3), which registered nurses completed as the basis for prioritizing patients. The nurses coded referrals as urgent, important, or routine. Service administration staff then managed the referrals. All registered nursing staff completed two hours of education on how to complete the screening assessment, which included a test of reliability (threshold 90%). To promote successful implementation:

- A working group (which included members of the unit team who would be completing the screening) developed the assessment.
- The screening assessment was embedded within the electronic health record for all patients admitted to the unit.

Implementation Taxonomy

A good strategy when writing about your implementation intervention is to use words from a published taxonomy such as the Cochrane Effective Practice and Organisation of Care Review Group (2011) taxonomy, which includes four major types of interventions (see Table 16.1).

TABLE 16.1 Types of Implementation Interventions

Types of Interventions	Examples
Professional	Distribution of educational materials, local consensus processes, audit and feedback, reminders
Financial	Fee-for-service, incentives
Organizational	Revision of professional roles, skill mix change, patient involvement, changing documentation systems
Regulatory	Management of patient complaints, peer review

Monthly audits of the timely completion of screening, referrals, and patient outcomes were provided and shared with staff to support ongoing review and development of this quality assessment.

Study of the intervention. Your improvement project will be expected to have several consequences, or effects, for different stakeholders. You need to collect data, including the administration of relevant measures, to determine the impacts of the intervention. These effects may relate to individual impacts (e.g., changing thinking, changing behavior), care processes (e.g., length of stay), and patient outcomes (e.g., quality of care).

The following points will help you comprehensively describe the study effects:

- How will you know that your interventions have been implemented sufficiently? You may consider how many different intervention components are delivered within the study (dosage).
- You'll have a good idea as to how you anticipate the intervention working. Is there a chain of events or certain changes that your intervention will cause? Does your guiding theory/framework help with anticipating how interventions might work? If so, consider what data you could collect to test whether these changes are taking place.
- Does the overall study design reflect anticipation of these potential changes? What are the most important outcomes that you want to consider? You should consider what strengths your study design has to support any assertions about the effects of your intervention that you might want to make.
- Your study will not have happened in a vacuum. Were there any events, either within the project or in the wider organization, that might influence your findings?

Once you have described how the project was done, the next step is to describe the measures for evaluation.

Measures (methods of evaluation). Report the quality of any measures used within the study, paying attention to issues of validity and reliability. If you used standardized measures, have they been evaluated in previous studies? If you are relying on local data, such as clinical performance, how have you ensured that these data are credible? You may also want to describe any education in data-collection techniques that members of project staff have completed as part of your project.

Analysis. Finally, your analysis section needs to provide an overview of how your data were managed and analyzed. How have quantitative data been summarized, and how has variation between key variables been assessed? You can summarize qualitative data using appropriate codes, which you can in turn link through overarching themes that have the potential to explain what occurred within your project.

Results

Your results section should include two key sections: the nature of the setting and the improvement intervention, and changes in processes of care and patient outcomes.

Check the author guidelines for the publication you are targeting for more information on how different types of data should be presented. The following provides an indication of what you might like to include in each of these sections:

- Revisiting your description of the study setting in light of your experiences of the study will highlight those elements that provided an important context for it. For example, how did the relationships between leadership, staffing, and resources affect buy-in to the project? This information provides a useful reference for findings related to the actual course of the intervention, the degree of success of implementation, and any lessons learned.
- In addition to summarizing impacts on processes and patient outcomes, pay attention to any unexpected findings. Inevitably, focusing attention on one aspect of clinical care in an improvement project means you're paying less attention to something else. Carefully describe any adverse events or unintended consequences (positive or negative) that others might want to watch out for.

It's not enough to simply report your results; you need to put them in context for the reader, which helps with both understanding and the potential for their transferability to different contexts.

Discussion

The discussion section of the article gives you the opportunity to put the findings of your project into a wider context, highlight some of the successes and challenges of your project and its evaluation, and consider the implications of your work.

Follow these tips to ensure your discussion section is effective:

- Give the reader a short digest of the main findings of the project related to answering your original question before going on to discuss how these findings fit with the broader literature. Try to boil down your findings to three or four main points; you can then also share these points through social media, such as X or via video blogs (vlogs), to encourage wider dissemination of your findings. (See Chapter 12 for more information on how to promote your work.)

- Focus most of the discussion section on how the findings of your project relate to existing literature. Don't look for evidence that simply supports your findings; also look for evidence that might contradict what you have found. Such a discussion is helpful for readers to consider the relevance of your findings. Using tables or figures to summarize and compare previous work to your own work can be helpful as presentation tools.

- Reflect on whether the study went as planned and achieved the outcomes you expected. If not, explain to the reader why you think this might have happened. For example, often things don't go to plan because something happened that you weren't able to predict at the outset (e.g., a change in leadership); describe the unexpected event and how it could influence what you (or others) might do differently in the future.

- Discuss how you think the findings from your work add to the existing body of evidence and, where appropriate, theory. It could be you added to the evidence for a particular issue, such as frequency of dressing changes for a peripheral intravenous line, or you might have learned more about how a particular intervention, such as audit or feedback, was used to improve management of a clinical issue.

- Consider the limitations of the project, such as issues about the way that data were collected, tools used for data collection, sample selection, funder constraints, and the design of the project. Clearly describe them so others can make an informed judgment about the transferability, generalizability, credibility, and trustworthiness of your findings.

Now that you have discussed your findings, you are ready to complete the article by summarizing conclusions and implications.

Conclusion and Implications

Finish the article with clear and data-driven conclusions and implications that have broad, rather than local, applicability. First, highlight what you believe to be the lessons learned, including what the next steps for investigation might be. Point out specific questions, challenges, and potential methods/approaches.

Second, describe the implications that arise from your work, including implications for policy, practice or service delivery, research, and management. Consider implications for the following (although not all may apply): unit based, organization wide, other systems or organizations, and other settings, such as different countries and different communities within your country. Readers will want to consider the relevance for their own settings, so it's useful to think about the type of information that could help others in their research and practice.

Remember to include a note at the end of the article about any sources of funding that supported the work and the role of that source in conducting the project. For example, "This project was funded by [insert name of organization]; the organization had no role in the design or conduct of the study."

Disseminating Your Work

Every day, nurses are conducting QI and EBP projects designed to improve processes and interventions that will help achieve better patient outcomes. By taking time to share the results of these projects you're involved in, you can ensure your knowledge spreads beyond your organization to benefit patients in other settings.

Strengthening Your Article

The SQUIRE guidelines provide a good starting point to help you structure the writing about a quality improvement (QI) project, but they aren't the only considerations.

How you or your team have approached the design of the project and how you have chosen to evaluate the project will reflect some fundamental beliefs about what QI and evidence-based practice (EBP) are and how they should be studied. If you're writing up the project for a more academic audience, you may want to pay particular attention to a theory of change and fidelity.

Theory of change. Using theory, which explains how and why improvement approach or interventions work, that has evolved through observation and testing, provides an opportunity to design a quality improvement initiative that has a greater chance of success. Similarly, the use of theory in guiding evaluations of improvement initiatives will be helpful in better understanding mediating factors (see Davidoff et al. [2015] and Rycroft-Malone & Bucknall [2010] for an in-depth consideration). Therefore, when writing articles about your QI or EBP project, it's important to fully describe how theory might have been used, and, if appropriate, how theory was advanced or tested through use. If you didn't explicitly use theory in the project, you could refer to theory in the discussion section of your article. This will help contextualize your work for readers in a wider evidence base and enhance the potential for theoretical transferability of the findings.

Fidelity. The practical world of improvement is often messy: Evidence can be contested, problems may emerge over time, and planned activities need tailoring to meet challenges that emerge in the field. A key question to help you consider fidelity is: To what degree did what you planned actually happen? What components of your intervention changed, and why? This builds on the SQUIRE guidelines, which require you to include information about how any formative evaluation would be used to modify the interventions that you studied.

Write Now!

1. Think about a QI or EBP project that you have either led or been involved in: Write an outline for an article, including subheadings and sample text for each section. Think about how you might involve other relevant stakeholders in this planning process.

2. Go to different journals and find different types of articles that report QI or EBP projects. Use the framework described in this chapter to assess the articles: What are some of the common missing elements from the articles you find? How would you improve them?

References

Ching Lee, M., Johnson, K. L., Newhouse, R. P., & Warren, J. I. (2013). Evidence-based practice process quality assessment: EPQA guidelines. *Worldviews on Evidence-Based Nursing, 10*(3), 140–149. https://doi.org/10.1111/j.1741-6787.2012.00264.x

Cochrane Effective Practice and Organisation of Care Review Group. (2011). *Data collection checklist*. Institute of Population Health, University of Ottawa. https://methods.cochrane.org/sites/methods.cochrane.org.bias/files/public/uploads/EPOC%20Data%20Collection%20Checklist.pdf

Connor, L., Dean, J. McNett M., Tydings D. M., Shrout, A., Gorsuch P. F., Hole, A., Moore, L., Brown, R., Melnyk, B. M., & Gallagher-Ford, L. (2023). Evidence-based practice improves patient outcomes and healthcare system return on investment: Findings from a scoping review. *Worldviews on Evidence-Based Nursing, 20*(1), 6–15. https://doi.org/10.1111/wvn.12621

Dang, D., Dearholt, S. L., Bissett, K., Ascenzi, J., & Whalen, M. (2021). *Johns Hopkins evidence-based practice for nurses and allied healthcare professionals: Model and guidelines* (4th ed.). Sigma Theta Tau International.

Davidoff, F., Dixon-Woods, M., Leviton, L., & Michie, S. (2015). De-mystifying theory and its use in improvement. *BMJ Quality and Safety, 24*(3), 228–238. http://dx.doi.org/10.1136/bmjqs-2014-003627

Dean, J., & Gallagher-Ford, L. (2021). Evidence-based practice: A new dissemination guide [Editorial]. *Worldviews on Evidence-Based Nursing, 18*(1), 4–7. https://doi.org/10.1111/wvn.12489

Dewing, J., McCormack, B., & McCance, T. (Eds.). (2021). *Person-centred nursing research: Methodology, methods and outcomes*. Springer.

Dixon-Woods, M., (2019) How to improve healthcare improvement—an essay by Mary Dixon-Woods. *BMJ, 367*, l5514. https://doi.org/10.1136/bmj.l5514

Goodman, D., Ogrinc, G., Davies, L., Ross Baker, G., Barnsteiner, J., Foster, T. C., Gali, K., Hilden, J., Horwitz, L., Kaplan, H. C., Leis, J., Matulis, J. C., Michie, S., Miltner, R., Neily, J., Nelson, W. A., Niedner, M., Oliver, B., Rutman, L., Thomson, R., & Thor, J. (2016). Explanation and elaboration of the SQUIRE (Standards for Quality Improvement Reporting Excellence) Guidelines, V.2.0: Examples of SQUIRE elements in the healthcare improvement literature. *BMJ Quality and Safety, 25*(12), e7. https://doi.org/10.1136/bmjqs-2015-004480

Graham, I. D., Rycroft-Malone, J., Kothari, A., & McCutcheon, C. (Eds.). (2022). *Research coproduction in healthcare*. Wiley-Blackwell.

The Health Foundation. (2013). *Quality improvement made simple: What everyone should know about health care quality improvement*. https://www.health.org.uk/sites/default/files/QualityImprovementMadeSimple.pdf

Jones, B., Vaux, E., & Olsson-Brown, A. (2019). How to get started in quality improvement. *BMJ, 364*, k5408. https://doi.org/10.1136/bmj.k5437

Melnyk, B. M., & Fineout-Overholt, E. (Eds.). (2019). *Evidence-based practice in nursing & healthcare: A guide to best practice* (4th ed.). Lippincott Williams & Wilkins.

Ogrinc, G., Armstrong, G. E., Dolansky, M. A., Singh, M. K., Davies, L. (2019). SQUIRE-EDU (Standards for Quality Improvement Reporting Excellence in Education: Publication guidelines for educational improvement. *Academic Medicine, 94*(10), 1461–1470. https://doi.org/10.1097/ACM.0000000000002750

Ogrinc, G., Davies, L., Goodman, D., Batalden, P., Davidoff, F., & Stevens, D. (2016). SQUIRE 2.0 (Standards for QUality Improvement Reporting Excellence): Revised publication guidelines from a detailed consensus process. *BMJ Quality & Safety, 25*(12), 986–992. https://doi.org/10.1136/bmjqs-2015-004411

Pinnock, H., Barwick, M., Carpenter, C. R., Eldridge, S., Grandes, G., Griffiths, C. J., Rycroft-Malone, J., Meissner, P., Murray, E., Patel, A., Sheikh, A., & Taylor, S. J. C. (2017). Standards for Reporting Implementation Studies (StaRI) statement. *BMJ, 356*, i6795. https://doi.org/10.1136/bmj.i6795

Rycroft-Malone, J., & Bucknall, T. (2010). *Models and frameworks for implementing evidence-based practice: Linking evidence to action*. Wiley-Blackwell.

Schulz, K. F., Altman, D. G., Moher, D., & CONSORT Group. (2010). CONSORT 2010 statement: Updated guidelines for reporting parallel group randomized trials. *Annals of Internal Medicine, 152*(11), 726–732. https://doi.org/10.7326/0003-4819-152-11-201006010-00232

Storkholm, M. H., Mazzocato, P., & Savage, C. (2019). Make it complicated: A qualitative study utilizing a complexity framework to explain quality improvement in health care. *BMC Health Services Research, 19*, 842. https://doi.org/10.1186/s12913-019-4705-x

Tong, A., Sainsbury, P., & Craig, J. (2007). Consolidated criteria for reporting qualitative research (COREQ): A 32-item checklist for interviews and focus groups. *International Journal of Quality in Health Care, 19*(6), 349–357. https://doi.org/10.1093/intqhc/mzm042

Williams, L., Rycroft-Malone, J., & Burton, C. (2016). Implementing best practice in infection prevention and control. A realist evaluation of the role of intermediaries. *International Journal of Nursing Studies, 60*, 156–167. https://doi.org/10.1016/j.ijnurstu.2016.04.012

Writing for Presentations

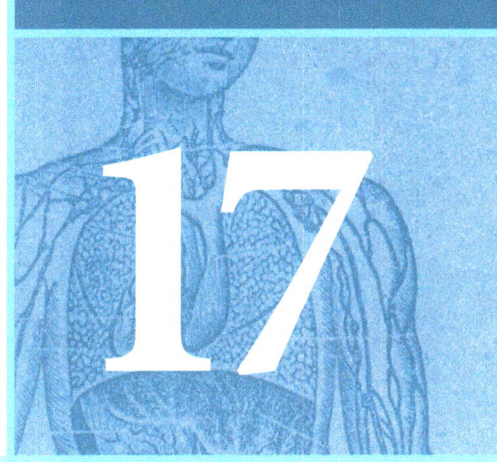

–Rose O. Sherman, EdD, RN, NEA-BC, FAAN

> *"If you want to be a writer, you must do two things above all others: read a lot and write a lot. There is no way around these two things that I am aware of, no shortcut."*
> –Stephen King

WHAT YOU'LL LEARN IN THIS CHAPTER

- Following the call for abstracts improves the chance your submission will be accepted.
- Use the abstract as a guide when developing a poster or presentation.
- Limit content in posters and presentations so the focus remains on your key points.
- Don't let your enthusiasm fade; write your journal article when you return from the conference.

Most of us attend professional conferences in our specialty areas of interest throughout our careers. Whether that interest is medical/surgical nursing, nurse management, or being an educator, conferences can be valuable ways to communicate with colleagues, meet collaborators, and share your research. The organizers of these conferences depend on nurses like you, who are either creating innovative new programs or doing research, to submit their work for presentation. New nursing knowledge is disseminated across the discipline through researchers like you at conferences and in publications. Equally valuable is the real-time feedback that you receive during a conference about the work that you have done.

This chapter focuses on writing for presentations, whether it's presenting a poster or a live lecture, so you can share your work with others. You'll learn how to craft an effective abstract so your presentation is more likely to be accepted for a conference, how to create an effective poster, and how you can turn your presentation into a journal article.

All About Abstracts

An *abstract* is a brief, informative summary of the major content that you plan to present in your podium or poster presentation to give the reviewer a snapshot of your work. (See Chapter 5 for information about abstracts for publication.) Completed work is generally preferred, but some conferences allow you to submit work in progress. Conference abstracts are often limited to as few as 250 words, so brevity and clarity are vital. Happell (2007) suggests that well-constructed abstracts should answer the following questions:

- **Why** was this work important, and what were the issues and problems?
- **Where** was your setting, and what population did you use?

- **How** did you design your research, initiative, or educational program?
- **What** were the outcomes, findings, and lessons learned?
- **What now,** and how should others use this information?

How Should I Review a Call for Abstracts?

If you're a member of a professional association or group, you will probably receive in an email or regular mail, or see published in the association's journal, what is often described as a *call for abstracts* well in advance of the conference itself. This call is an invitation to submit an abstract for conference presentation. Most conference organizers receive more abstracts—particularly for podium presentations—than they have speaker slots. The selection process is often quite competitive. Carefully review the call for abstracts guidelines to put yourself in the best possible position.

Legitimate professional conferences use the process just described to solicit and evaluate abstracts. Unfortunately, you may receive invitations to present at conferences that are predatory. *Predatory conferences* claim to be scholarly but are instead focused on financial gain versus quality scholarship (InterAcademy Partnership, 2022). They are organized by groups outside the mainstream of professional organizations you are familiar with. The quality of work presented at these conferences is usually not peer-reviewed, and presenters are selected based on their willingness to pay registration fees and travel expenses.

To avoid predatory conferences, keep in mind that legitimate professional conferences generally issue a call for abstracts and don't issue invitations to selected individuals. If you are unsure about a conference, always double-check its legitimacy with your colleagues and by using tools like the checklist available at Think. Check. Attend. (https://thinkcheckattend.org). The checklist includes questions you should ask before submitting an abstract, such as:

- Are you aware of the society or the association organizing the conference?
- Have you or your colleagues attended this conference before?
- Is there clear information about the timeline and the agenda for the conference?
- Is the editorial committee listed on the website and, if so, have you heard of them?

Negative answers to these questions should make you cautious about proceeding. Of course, conferences can be low quality, but not predatory (InterAcademy Partnership, 2022). For example, the conference might lack focus, or the organization may be poor. Even though not predatory, you want to avoid these conferences. Watch for signs such as misspellings and grammatical errors and planned topic areas that are too broad in scope. Again, one of the best checks is whether you or a colleague has attended the conference before and found it to be helpful.

Once you decide a conference is legitimate and of high quality, you're ready to review the call for abstracts. Example 17.1 is a sample call for abstracts for a national conference.

Barker and Phillips (2021) recommend that you target your work to the right conference. This is a key step because many professional conferences have themes or focus areas. Conference organizers are looking for presentations that are a good fit with the theme of the conference, and with the educational needs and interests of those attending the conference. As you review a call for abstracts, consider the following questions:

- Is this a conference I would enjoy attending?
- Can I align my work to the conference theme and tracks?
- Who are the attendees, and will they be interested in this work?
- Will I be able to attend this conference, with or without funding?
- How long is the presentation, and is that enough time for me to present my work?
- If I have done this work as part of a team, can we all present, or are there restrictions on the number of presenters?
- Do I have the resources to have a poster designed to the conference specifications?
- When and how will I learn whether the abstract has been accepted?
- Can I meet all the required deadlines for abstract submission?

International Nursing Administration Research Conference (INARC)
Call for Abstracts—Podium and Poster Presentations

Implementing Innovation Across the Health Care Continuum ← Conference theme that your abstract should be aligned to

Bi-Annual Conference

The Villanova University College of Nursing and the Association for Leadership Science in Nursing (ALSN) will be co-providing this year's International Nursing Administration Research Conference (INARC). This conference serves as a prominent vehicle for nursing educators, executives, administrators, and researchers from all over the United States and Canada to strengthen their roles through learning, sharing, and networking with professional colleagues. This is a call for abstracts for both podium and poster presentations. ← Along with the name of the sponsoring organization, indicates whom the conference is targeting

We encourage the submission of abstracts of work that has not been published in a peer-reviewed journal or presented at another national meeting. Topics can include any area of health services scholarly practice changes and research, nursing administration, or health care delivery systems. Of particular interest are presentations that describe the implementation of research findings to improve quality, safety, and cost outcomes in nursing care settings. ← List of possible topics

There are two presentation options. Podium presentations are 45 minutes in length and 10 minutes of this time should be left for questions. Poster presentations are scheduled from 5:00 p.m. to 8:00 p.m., during the Wednesday evening reception. Authors will have the opportunity to discuss materials and distribute handouts related to their work. The size of posters can be no larger than 4 feet high by 6 feet wide and must be capable of being hung. ← Length of presentation and poster specifications

All fees, expenses and arrangements associated with attending the conference are the responsibility of presenter(s). Presenters are prohibited from marketing commercial products and/or services through either poster or podium presentations. The speaker guidelines are included in this announcement. The deadline for abstract submission is month/day/year. ← Financial/ethical responsibilities
← Deadline

Abstract Content
← Word limit
The Abstract is limited to no more than 250 words (excluding author names and affiliation) and should include the following: ← Format of abstract

    Title of the Podium or Poster Presentation
    One Learner Objective with Measurable Outcomes
    Purpose of the Project
    Background and Significance of the Project
    Approach or Method Used
    Major Outcomes
    Conclusions and Recommendations

You will also be asked to include a brief biography for each presenter, specifying the contact information for the lead presenter. All abstracts should be submitted electronically to the conference website. Presenters will be notified of abstract selection by month/day/year. ← How to submit
← When acceptance will be communicated

Reprinted with permission from College of Nursing Villanova University Continuing Education in Nursing and Healthcare.

EXAMPLE 17.1 Sample call for abstracts for a national conference.

Q *May I submit my abstract to different conferences at the same time so that I have a better chance of being accepted?*

A Unlike journal article submissions, where you must clearly be rejected by one journal before submitting to the next, presenters often submit similar abstracts to more than one professional conference in similar time frames. Submissions to some conferences may require verification that the work is original and has not been presented at other conferences. When your abstract is selected for presentation, you will be given a short time frame to accept or decline. After you accept, you have made a professional commitment and should plan to attend despite other opportunities that may be offered. It's discouraging to conference planners when speakers who are on the program cancel just before the event. This behavior is considered unprofessional, and your future abstracts may not be selected for conference presentation.

Podium or Poster?

Most calls for abstracts offer you an option of submitting for a *podium presentation* (a presentation in a meeting room or in a presentation session), or a *poster presentation* (in which you present a storyboard of information on your poster).

Sometimes you can submit for both. If you are turned down for the podium presentation, you may be offered a poster presentation slot. Although podium presentations are often considered more prestigious, poster presentations have several major advantages.

If you are a novice at presenting your work, posters are a great way to get started and receive feedback. If you're new to the conference or organization, you can meet the audience at poster sessions and sit in on podium presentations to gain insight into how other presenters showcase their work. If your work is still in progress, a poster session provides a forum for getting feedback and suggestions from other professionals.

For most professional conferences, a limited number of abstracts are usually selected for oral presentation. Podium presentations are often part of a menu of concurrent sessions offered during a specific time frame. Although not all conference participants will hear about your presentation, your abstract will often be published in a conference proceedings book, professional association journal, or placed on a conference website available to a broader audience than conference participants. In contrast, most conferences have scheduled times when all participants can attend the poster session. Contact hours are frequently awarded, and attendance is often excellent. Many professional groups also archive posters on their websites so even those not able to attend the conference can view them. Potentially, with the poster, your work can reach more attendees, and you have more opportunity to discuss your work and network with interested participants (Redulla, 2021).

Writing Effective Abstracts

Remember that several different audiences will see your abstract (Beckett, 2021). The first audience will be the expert reviewers who select the abstracts that best meet the conference's objectives. The second audience includes the conference attendees who use abstracts to guide their decisions about which presentations to attend or posters to view. A third but less obvious audience consists of journal editors who comb conference pages searching for an interesting work that could be expanded into a journal article. Keep in mind that you need to sell your topic and your expertise and experience to boost the likelihood that your abstract will be accepted among all the others submitted (Innocent, 2024). Here are some tips for making sure that your abstract stands out in a crowd.

Consider the Audience

Will the conference audience be members of a specialty association, a cross-section of the nursing profession, or interdisciplinary professionals? Is the conference targeted to local, state, national, or international participants? Knowing the answers to these questions will help you to write a more effective abstract that will appeal to the conference audience (Beckett, 2021).

Create an Immediate Impression

The title is the first thing a busy reviewer will see on your abstract, and it can create an immediate impression. Try to make your title descriptive and compelling, and be sure that it connects to the conference's theme.

For example, say that you are a neonatal nurse and want to submit a presentation for a National Association of Neonatal Nurses' annual conference focused on parenting. Your project is a kangaroo parenting intervention that you implemented in your NICU. Consider the following two titles:

> Kangaroo Parenting Intervention in a Neonatal ICU
>
> or
>
> Healthy Neonate Parenting: What We Can Learn From Kangaroos

The first title tells what your work is about, but the second title is more likely to capture the attention of your reviewers because it is both interesting and makes an immediate connection to the conference theme: parenting.

Follow the Guidelines

Like author guidelines for journal articles, the call for abstracts usually clearly specifies the sections to be included in the abstract. The sample call for abstracts from earlier in this chapter is a common outline for presentations involving evidence-based innovations. However, the sections in a call for *research abstracts* would be different and commonly include:

- Background and significance
- Aims of the study
- Methods
- Results
- Discussion and implications

Succinctly presenting all the information required in the abstract within the required word count can be challenging, but it is very important. Fonts and font sizes are often specified, and you must follow these guidelines. Many organizations have an online submission process, which typically includes the presenter's information, objectives, and an abstract. It's best to type all the components in a Microsoft Word document, carefully review it (including running a spell- and grammar-check), and then cut and paste pieces as appropriate into the online submission form. With online submission systems, you might not receive a final copy of what you have submitted, so remember to keep a copy for your records.

No matter how you submit your abstract, having someone else review your work for clarity, grammar, and spelling is also a good idea. Try to avoid common abstract mistakes (see sidebar).

Avoiding Common Mistakes for Abstract Submission

Submitting for a conference podium or poster presentation and then receiving a letter notifying you that your abstract was not accepted can be frustrating. Even experienced presenters sometimes receive denials, but you can increase the odds of acceptance of your abstract by avoiding these common mistakes:

- The abstract doesn't make a clear link to the conference theme.
- The abstract has grammatical and spelling errors.
- A generic abstract is developed for submission to multiple conferences without tailoring the presentation to the audience.
- The conference abstract guidelines aren't followed (e.g., too short, too long, or lacks objectives or outcomes).
- The content of the abstract contains too much material to reasonably deliver in the time allotted for the presentation.
- The aims, objectives, and content of the presentation are not clear to the reviewers.
- The innovation or research is not presented in a manner that would be interesting, or it does not provide new information for the target audience.
- The learning objectives are poorly written, with no action verbs. (See Chapter 19 for tips on writing objectives.)
- The abstract fails to convey what the implications are for the profession.

Abstract Review

Abstracts are sometimes *reviewed anonymously*: that is, the reviewer doesn't know the presenter or the institution where the work was done (this is also referred to as a blind review). Example 17.2 shows a typical scoring sheet given to reviewers of abstracts.

Abstract reviewers are given specific guidelines that reference the call for abstracts, so careful adherence

NURSING CONFERENCE

Abstract Review Scoring Criteria
Abstract # _____ Abstract Title: _____
Reviewer: _____
Rating: NA= not applicable 1= poor 2= fair 3= good 4= very good 5= excellent

Criteria	Comments	Rating
The submitted abstract:		
The topic of the presentation is relevant to the conference theme.		
The content is evidence-based.		
Outcomes for the study/project are clearly addressed in the abstract.		
The implications for other settings are described.		
The topic will be of interest to the target audience.		
The abstract is clear and followed the guidelines outlined in the call for abstracts.		
The presenters have experience with presentations to similar audiences.		
Total score		

EXAMPLE 17.2 Sample scoring sheet for abstract reviewers.

to the guidelines is important. As reviewers look at your abstract, they will ask themselves the following questions:

- Is this topic timely, and does it address an important problem?
- Does the author appear to have knowledge and expertise on this topic?
- Will the content in this abstract be well presented?
- Would I want to hear this presentation?
- Will this be of interest to our target audience?

Now that you understand how to submit an abstract, it's time to apply that information to a practical example.

Case Example

Let's look at a case example. You are the director of nursing professional practice in a large academic medical center in the Northeast. For two consecutive years in the post-COVID-19 environment, nurse engagement scores dropped in your medical center, and participation in professional governance initiatives was low. Last year, your hospital received grant funding from a local foundation to implement a strengths-based professional practice program to improve staff engagement. You coordinated the program, which involved a strengths-based assessment for each professional staff nurse, an educational workshop, and two follow-up coaching sessions. The project had positive outcomes on several measurable dimensions, including improvements in professional governance participation, nurse satisfaction, and engagement. In reviewing the literature on strengths-based development for professional nurses, you noted that little had been written on using strengths-based development to improve engagement and participation in shared governance initiatives.

You recently received a call for abstracts from the ANCC Pathways to Excellence Conference®. Your medical center has achieved Pathway designation, so you decide this is an excellent opportunity to showcase this work. Topic areas of interest outlined in the abstract include the following: shared decision-making and leadership, safety and quality, nurse well-being, and professional development. Your project addresses both nurse well-being and professional development.

ANCC Pathway to Excellence Conference objectives:

1. Examine the positive impact of shared governance, effective leadership, interprofessional partnerships, and inclusivity that exemplify workplace excellence.

2. Evaluate evidence-based practice, research, quality, and safety initiatives.

3. Assess nurse-driven and organizational initiatives to foster a culture of health and safeguard clinician and community well-being.

4. Demonstrate the values of lifelong learning and nurse empowerment on organizational outcomes.

The call for abstracts asks for the following:

- Title of the abstract
- Desired type of session (concurrent session or poster), with a first and second choice listed
- Objectives of the presentation (behaviorally stated, reflective of the content, no more than three)
- Description of the content of the presentation (not to exceed 150 words)

With these guidelines in mind, you prepare the following first draft for your colleagues and chief nursing officer to review. You ask them to think of themselves as part of an expert panel appointed to review abstracts for this conference.

Draft 1

Title: Implementation of a Strengths-Based Development Program

Session Preference: Concurrent Session

Objectives:
1. Present an overview of a strengths-based development program.
2. Discuss program outcomes.
3. Identify the implications for other organizations.

Description of Content:

This presentation will describe a strengths-based development program for registered nurses conducted as a significant initiative at All-Star Hospital. This program received grant funding from a local foundation. Eight hundred registered nurses from different clinical areas took the Gallup StrengthsFinder assessment, attended a one-day development program, and received two follow-up coaching sessions. The program was highly rated by staff, improved staff engagement and participation in professional practice councils, and had excellent unit-based outcomes. In this program, we will discuss our experiences developing the program and our lessons learned. We will show a short video that illustrates the response of nurses to the program through follow-up interviews. We will discuss the outcome evaluations, review engagement and practice council participation improvements, and make recommendations for other organizations.

Your colleagues offer some excellent suggestions. They point out that although the abstract follows most of the guidelines (you failed to indicate your first and second choices), it does not appear innovative nor capture the excitement or impact that this project generated at All-Star Hospital.

Draft 2 – After review and input from colleagues

Title: Leveraging Nurses' Strengths to Improve Engagement, Nurse Well-Being, and Patient Outcomes

Session Preference: First Choice–Concurrent Session; Second Choice–Poster Session

Objectives:
1. Identify the critical need to improve nurse engagement in their work and shared decision-making.
2. Describe an innovative, strengths-based professional development program.
3. Present program outcomes and implications for other settings.

Description of Content:

Nurse engagement in their work is a critical challenge in today's healthcare environment. Evidence-based strategies for improving engagement and participation in shared governance efforts are rarely discussed in the nursing literature, and most agencies struggle with low engagement scores. This presentation will highlight an innovative strengths-based development program using the Gallup StrengthsFinder assessment. The program was designed to help nurses identify their top five strengths/talent themes from their strength-finders assessment; we then used coaching to assist staff in leveraging their strengths in practice for greater professional effectiveness.

The program, which 800 nurses completed, included using the Gallup StrengthsFinder assessment, an educational program on using strengths in practice, and two individual follow-up coaching sessions. The project outcomes included a significant increase in nurse engagement, a decrease in nurse turnover and absenteeism, and increased patient satisfaction. Lessons learned and implications for other organizations will be discussed.

The second draft does a much more effective job of capturing the significance of your innovative program, beginning with the program title. The content description meets the 150-word limit but still offers the reader a comprehensive overview of what you will cover.

Presenting Your Work

It is always exciting to receive an email or letter informing you that your work has been accepted for presentation. When you receive notice of acceptance, you will also usually receive speaker or poster presenter guidelines. Use these guidelines when developing your presentation. Your abstract should serve as your guide for your poster or podium session content.

Redulla (2021) observed that many presenters attempt to cover too much content in their presentations. You have likely had this same experience when you attended conference sessions. The great American architect Ludwig Mies van der Rohe is well known for his quote, "Less is more." This is good advice for presenters. When tempted to share every detail of your research or project, remember that you generally will not have the poster space or podium time to do this.

Designing an Effective Podium Presentation

Whether you have extensive experience speaking in public or you are brand new to presentations, effective planning is a key for success. You might have only 20 to 30 minutes to present. As you design your presentation, consider two to three major areas that you would like to cover. These should be the most important points for the audience.

Q *What if my computer breaks down at the conference before my podium presentation?*

A Always carry a copy of your presentation on a flash (thumb) drive, email a copy to yourself, and, if you are able, upload it to a cloud storage platform. That way, you will always have a backup. For larger conferences, the conference hosts will often ask you to send your presentation ahead of time so that it can be preloaded onto one computer. This avoids changing the computer for every speaker. Even when the host takes responsibility for preloading your presentation, have your backups as an added precaution. Most experienced presenters also suggest that you bring a printout of your presentation in case the technology fails and you need to present without your slides.

If you are presenting on an innovation—such as the strengths-based development program addressed earlier in this chapter—you might decide to divide your presentation into three sections:

1. The need for the innovation
2. The innovation
3. The outcomes and implications

If you plan to use Microsoft PowerPoint slides, consider that most presenters spend between two and three minutes on each slide; be sure to leave about five to ten minutes for questions and discussion. Avoid using embedded video or other bells and whistles unless you are an expert on solving audiovisual problems. The focus should be on your content. Many conferences today require you to use their presentation template as part of their branding.

After you design your presentation, practice it several times, ideally in front of an audience of your peers, who can give you feedback. Effective podium presentations end on time, so ensure your content does not exceed the time frame given for your session. Otherwise, you might appear disorganized to the audience.

Know that you may be asked to agree to present virtually if the conference is moved from a live date due to circumstances such as a pandemic or natural disaster. In this case, you would deliver your presentation via a videoconferencing platform such as Zoom or submit your slides with taped comments, but it's still important to practice ahead of time.

Q *Do I need handouts?*

A Some attendees will be interested in taking back information about your work to their settings. Many conferences allow you to submit handouts for participants, which are included on the conference app or website. Make sure to submit your materials by conference deadlines. If you have business cards, take them with you and offer to allow participants to download your presentation via a QR code or email your presentation to anyone who requests it.

Creating a Professional Poster Presentation

Redulla (2021) reinforces the importance of starting early and developing a timeline after your poster abstract has been accepted. Review the poster guidelines for your conference before you start your poster. The guidelines will specify the poster size and how it will be displayed: for example, posted with pushpins on a large corkboard or placed on a table. Tabletop posters should be created so they are freestanding; don't rely on the meeting organizers to supply an easel. The allowable poster size for conferences varies widely and will affect how much information you can place on the poster.

Before jumping into design, spend time considering what you want to convey. Think of the poster as the story of your study or project. You want it to deliver key information and build to a conclusion that resonates with conference participants. Organize the information so that the poster tells your story in an easy-to-follow format.

Many healthcare agencies and universities have graphic design resources to help you with the poster design, but some don't. Fortunately, there are many online resources to help you design your poster; Case Western Reserve University has a list of some of these (https://researchguides.case.edu/posterdesign/resources). You can readily access steps on how to create a poster from schools and hospitals, such as the University of North Carolina (https://gradschool.unc.edu/academics/resources/postertips.html) and Duke University Medical Center (https://guides.mclibrary.duke.edu/gettingpublished/posters). Some conference organizations have templates all presenters are asked to use.

Weaver-Moore et al. (2001) surveyed nurses with poster presentation experience. Their findings indicate that the following were important poster components:

- Simplicity
- Readability
- Interesting graphics

Participants in the study reported that limiting the amount of information shared was the most common challenge in poster preparation.

Posters should be visually attractive. In a study of nurses, aesthetics—such as overall visual appeal, color, organization, and layout—had the most influence on whether a conference participant would view a poster (Siedlecki, 2017). Participants then considered relevance, primarily by reading the poster's title.

Q *What are ideas for organizing my poster?*

A One easy way is to base poster headings on the type of content (Berg & Hicks, 2017). For research posters, use background and problem, purpose, sample, methods, results, conclusions, and implications. For clinical presentations, use background/problem, purpose, summary of what is known, steps in developing the solution or strategy, outcomes, and implications. For project posters, use background/problem, purpose, sample and setting, strategies, results, and implications. For evidence-based practice projects, Becket (2021) recommends you cover several key areas: background/significance, spirit of inquiry/clinical inquiry; PICO(T) question (population, intervention, comparison group or current practice, outcomes, time frame [if applicable]); search strategy; appraisal, evaluation, and synthesis tables; change recommendation; implementation plan, outcomes, and measurement plan; and dissemination. Becket provides a template you can use as a guide.

For all types, you do not have to cover each item as a separate heading; that may get too wordy. Focus on the key points of what you did and your results. You can always provide a handout of additional information.

Figure 17.1 illustrates a standard layout for a research poster that can help ensure your poster stands out among a sea of others.

You can use Microsoft Word, Excel, PowerPoint, InDesign, Canva, or Adobe InDesign to create your poster. (Excel is particularly useful for creating data charts.) Remember to consider that what might seem readable on the computer screen may be too small when enlarged to poster size. Some larger organizations have templates you can use as a starting point. Another option is to search online for templates and examples (request permission before using any material with a copyright).

First make a rough layout of the poster on graph paper or with a computer software program to get an idea where to place the title, text, and any graphics, such as tables or illustrations. It may be helpful to divide the poster into three columns and consider what would go into each column. Conference participants stroll rows of posters, so consider how to make yours stand out from the crowd.

Consider several factors as you create your poster, keeping in mind that you need to follow any conference guidelines and to proofread the final poster carefully.

Title: The title should succinctly state what the poster is about, and the most important information should be in the top part of the poster rather than the bottom. Use upper and lower case, rather than all capital letters, which are harder to read (Berg & Hicks, 2017; UCLA Library, 2022).

Color: Color can help gain viewers' attention, but remember that some attendees may be color blind, so have difficulty distinguishing between red and green (Carter et al., 2024; Berg & Hicks, 2017). Limit yourself to two to three colors. Be sure the colors have significant contrast, even when using different shades of the same color (Thiebes, 2022). Usually cool colors (blue, green) work better than warm (red, orange, yellow) ones.

Graphics: You may want to add a few graphics, such as images or icons, to draw attention to key points and improve overall visual appeal. You can find these online (e.g., the Noun Project: https://thenounproject.com and Vector Stock: www.vectorstock.com), but be sure to obtain permission if images have a copyright. Tables and figures also can help break up text.

Word count: Rossi et al. (2020) recommend limiting word count to about 150 to 250 words, with no

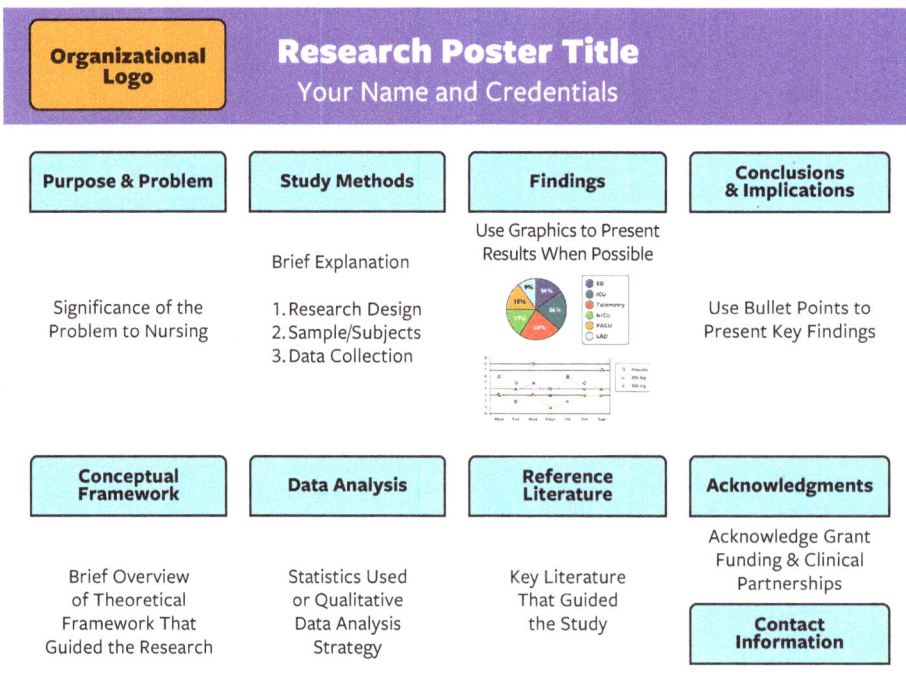

FIGURE 17.1 This example shows a common way to organize a poster.

more than two to three graphs. Others allow for more words, such as 400 to 600 (Baker, 2017). (The appropriate number of words will be partly based on the size of the poster.) Limiting the word count can be challenging, but the point is that you don't want to fill up every inch of the poster with text or images, which makes it hard for the viewer to absorb the information. It's been recommended to use 40% graphics, 30% text, and 30% white space (Long & Beck, 2017). Use bullet points rather than lots of solid text to facilitate reading.

Fonts: Avoid fancy fonts that can be difficult to read; instead use standards such as Arial, Times New Roman, Rockwell, Georgia, and Baskerville (Baker, 2017; Carter et al., 2024; Redulla, 2021). It's best to avoid using more than two or three different fonts. You'll also want to consider font size. Farrington (2018) suggests the title be as large as 85 points; other recommendations include at least 50 points (UCLA Library, 2022) and at least 72 points (Baker, 2017). Long and Beck (2017) suggest 48 points for section headings and 36 points for section text, while Baker (2017) suggests at least 54 points for subtitles, 30 or more points for text, and 20 points or more for subtext. In general, the title should be readable from 15 to 20 feet away, with most of the text readable from 5 to 6 feet (Berg & Hicks, 2017).

Contact information and handouts: Include your contact information for those who would like more information. You may also want to create a QR code (www.qrcode-monkey.com) to make it easy for attendees to obtain a copy of your poster or access additional information (Innocent, 2024). Consider making handouts of your poster to distribute to those who would like to take information back with them to their work area.

Ideally, the poster should be on one sheet of paper. You will need to work with a copy center to enlarge and print the poster, or your organization may print it for you. If you need to assemble your poster in pieces, be sure to use glue or Velcro to attach materials securely.

Consider how you will transport your poster to the conference. Most presenters prefer to hand-carry their posters in a poster canister or portfolio because hotel delivery can be unreliable. Do not put the poster in your checked baggage. You may want to carry tape, stickpins, and scissors in case these aren't readily available on site (Berg & Hicks, 2017).

> **About ePosters**
>
> Many organizations have moved to electronic poster presentation sessions. Most ePoster guidelines require you to use PowerPoint templates, which can be easily downloaded from sites like PosterSession.com. The same design rules for traditional posters apply to ePosters. With onsite ePoster sessions, you may be given a specific timeslot that your poster will be on an LCD screen and have a submission charge to cover the cost of the LCD rental screens. Much like you would with a physical poster, you will stand next to the screen to answer questions about your project. A disadvantage to these sessions is that your poster may only be on display for 30 minutes during a two-hour poster session, giving you less time to present your work to attendees.
>
> Some conferences have ePoster galleries where attendees can access posters through a conference app or website. With these conferences, live participation is usually not expected, and your poster becomes part of an ePoster gallery. You may be asked to record a short presentation to accompany your slides.

Most conferences designate time for attendees to speak with poster presenters. It can be hard to watch as people pass your poster by, but remember that attendees have limited time and must choose based on their interests. Stand to one side so you don't block your poster and dress professionally (Berg & Hicks, 2017). When people stop by and ask you about your poster, beware of inundating them with too many details. Rossi et al. (2020) recommend speaking no longer than one minute, because you don't yet know their specific area of interest and how much detail they are seeking. Ask open-ended questions and base your subsequent discussion on their responses. Remember to thank people for their interest before they move on. This is an ideal time to build your network.

From Conference Presentation to Article

After presenting your work at a professional conference, consider taking the next step and converting the conference presentation into an article. Doing so allows a broader audience (those who didn't attend the conference) to learn from your work and allows you to contribute to a body of evidence that can help in improving care (Melnyk, 2016). Your podium or poster presentation can serve as a beginning outline of what you will cover in a journal article (Saver, 2021).

Q *Is it acceptable to write an article related to the presentation before I present it at the conference?*

A If your presentation is related to research, then it's usually best to wait until after the conference because some organizations specify that the information must not have been published elsewhere beforehand. If you have written an article on your podium or poster presentation, be sure to reference it in the materials you present at the conference. In some situations, you might have signed over the copyright for the material. You will want to seek permission from a publisher before providing handouts of a specific article at a conference.

You might want to initially consider the journals of interest to the target audience who attended the conference. Often, journal editors attend specialty conferences and are in the exhibition hall booths of their publishers. This is a good time to personally query an editor about any interest in your topic. A strong advantage to presenting your work at a professional conference is that you learn from attendees the aspects of your work that particularly resonate with your audience. This can provide you with a better lens of how to present your work in a journal article so it will be informative and interesting as well as provide clear implications for the profession.

Often, your presentation abstract itself will provide you with a great working outline for your article, beginning with your title, which could serve as an article title or header. The objectives you used for your presentation can serve as an overview of what you plan to present in the article. Your methods, findings, and recommendations will serve as the body of the journal article. Figures or tables that you used in your presentation can make great visuals to illustrate your work in an article. Professional implications were probably a key part of your poster or podium presentation and will provide important summary content in your article.

Above all, don't let your enthusiasm from the conference fade before you begin work on your article. Melnyk (2016) recommends setting a goal of

> **Confidence Booster**
>
> Sally Elliot is a critical care educator in a community hospital. She developed an innovative game to help her new critical care nurses remember key concepts. She used this game in her hospital with great success and presented a poster at the American Association of Critical-Care Nursing, National Teaching Institute (NTI). Other critical care educators were intrigued with her results and encouraged her to write about it. Sally had never envisioned herself as an author. She is enrolled in a master's program in education and decided to ask one of her faculty for help taking the next step. The faculty member is delighted to assist her. She gives Sally suggestions for an article outline based on her poster presentation and offers to critique the article after it is written. As she begins to develop her article, Sally is surprised at her own passion as she explains her work in the article. Her article is accepted for publication in an education journal's "Teaching Tips" section. Sally feels a great sense of pride. Although she felt like a novice beginning this process, she took a risk and wrote the article.

submitting a manuscript within 90 days of a presentation, but even if you can't meet that ambitious goal, don't give up. Just remember that the closer to the time of the presentation you write the article, the easier it will be because the information will be fresh in your mind.

Saver (2022) offers seven steps to successfully converting your poster to a publication:

1. **Form a writing team,** especially if your work is collaborative.
2. **Find a publication outlet,** for example, a journal, newsletter, or blogsite.
3. **Query the editor** of the publication to assess interest in your work. (This is usually done by email; check the author guidelines and refer to Chapter 3 for more information about writing a query.)
4. **Organize the content,** following the publication's author guidelines.
5. **Widen the breadth** by including more comprehensive content than was included on the poster.

6. **Look back at previous issues** of your target publication, paying attention to article structure and tone.
7. **Start now** and don't lose the momentum while the material is fresh on your mind.

Write Now!

1. Pick one of the resources for creating a poster mentioned in this chapter and review what it offers.
2. Visit the website of a professional organization in your specialty area and look for the date of the next conference and when the call for abstracts will be posted.
3. Plan to submit an abstract for a poster or podium presentation using the information presented in this chapter.

References

Baker, D. (2017). *Posters: Improving your research posters*. Oxford University.

Barker, E., & Phillips, V. (2021). Creating conference posters: Structure, form and content. *Journal of Perioperative Nursing, 31*(7-8), 296–299. https://doi.org/10.1177/1750458921996254

Beckett, C. D. (2021). Dissemination of evidence-based practice projects: Key strategies for successful poster presentations. *Worldviews on Evidence-Based Nursing, 18*(3), 158–160. https://doi.org/10.1111/wvn.12502

Berg, J., & Hicks, R. (2017). Successful design and delivery of a professional poster. *Journal of the American Association of Nurse Practitioners, 29*(8), 461–469. https://doi.org/10.1002/2327-6924.12478

Carter, J. B., Ekanayake, J. Venort T., Vought, K., Nobel, S., & Watson, A. (2024). *Marking an effective virtual scientific poster presentation*. IFAS Extension, University of Florida. https://doi.org/10.32473/edis-AE592-2024

Farrington, M. (2018). Sharing knowledge through poster presentations. [Editorial]. *Head and Neck Nursing, 36*(1), 4–6. https://www.sohnnurse.com/assets/docs/Sharing%20Knowledge%20Through%20Poster%20Presentations-Editorial.pdf

Happell, B. (2007). Hitting the target! A no tears approach to writing an abstract for a conference presentation. *International Journal of Mental Health Nursing, 16*(6), 447–452. https://doi.org/10.1111/j.1447-0349.2007.00501.x

Innocent, K. (2024). How to get started presenting at conferences. *Nursing 2024, 54*(2), 38–43. https://doi.org/10.1097/01.NURSE.0000995588.06386.24

InterAcademy Partnership. (2022). *Combatting predatory academic journals and conferences. Summary report*. https://palast.ps/sites/default/files/inline-files/2.%20Summary%20report%20-%20English.pdf

Long, T. L., & Beck, C. T. (2017). *Writing in nursing: A brief guide*. Oxford University Press.

Melnyk, B. (2016). Disseminating evidence by turning presentations into publications: Key strategies for success. *World Views on Evidence-Based Nursing, 13*(4), 259–260. https://doi.org/10.1111/wvn.12175

Redulla, R. (2021). Creating a compelling poster. *American Nurse Journal, 16*(6), 14–17. https://www.myamericannurse.com/wp-content/uploads/2021/04/an6-Poster-512.pdf

Rossi, T., Slattery, F., & Richter, K. (2020). The evolution of the scientific poster: From eye-sore to eye-catcher. *Medical Writing, 29*(1), 36–40. https://journal.emwa.org/visual-communications/the-evolution-of-the-scientific-poster-from-eye-sore-to-eye-catcher/

Saver, C. (2021, July). Powerful posters. *American Nurse Journal*. https://www.myamericannurse.com/the-writing-mind-powerful-posters/

Saver, C. (2022). From poster to publication: Seven steps to success. *Nurse Author and Editor, 32*(1), 8–10. https://doi.org/10.1111/nae2.34

Siedlecki, S. L. (2017). How to create a poster that attracts an audience. *American Journal of Nursing, 117*(3), 48–54. https://doi.org/10.1097/01.NAJ.0000513287.29624.7e

Thiebes, K. (2022, March 11). Best color palettes for scientific figures and data visualization. *Simplified Science Publishing*. https://www.simplifiedsciencepublishing.com/resources/best-color-palettes-for-scientific-figures-and-data-visualizations

UCLA Library. (2022). *Poster presentations*. https://guides.library.ucla.edu/c.php?g=223540&p=1480858#s-lg-box-4484263

Weaver-Moore, L., Augspurger, P., King, M., & Proffitt, C. (2001). Insights on the poster presentation and presentation process. *Applied Nursing Research, 14*(2), 100–104. https://doi.org/10.1053/apnr.2001.22376

From Student Project or Dissertation to Publication

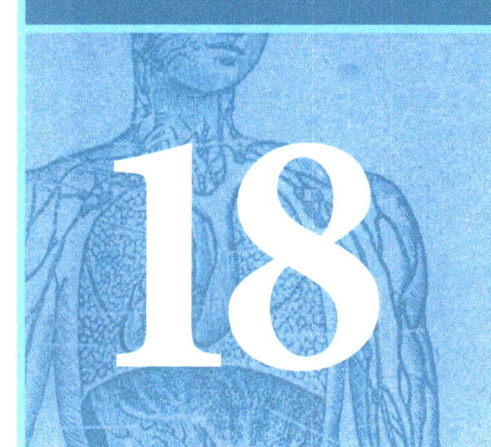

–Deborah Lindell, DNP, MSN, RN, CNE, ANEF, FAAN
–Lorraine Steefel, DNP, RN, CTN-A

*"The secret to editing your work is simple:
You need to become its editor instead of its writer."*
—Zadie Smith

WHAT YOU'LL LEARN IN THIS CHAPTER

- Academic projects can be turned into published articles, but the work must be transformed to emphasize how it contributes new knowledge and to fit with the targeted publication and its readers.

- A framework for adapting your academic work helps in preparing a manuscript for publication.

- Tools such as outlines, reporting guidelines, and the journal's author instructions will enhance the likelihood your article will be accepted for publication.

Have you earned high praise on your academic paper, project, or dissertation? Did your faculty or colleagues suggest or require you submit your work for publication? Or perhaps you wondered, "How can I get this work published?" If so, this chapter is for you. It focuses on how to transform academic projects into manuscripts to submit for publication. (Student presentations also can be turned into articles for publication; see Chapter 17 to learn more.)

Consider the potential benefits of publishing articles based on work you completed as a student. (In this chapter, "student" refers to a current student or a graduate who is converting a student assignment to a manuscript.) Depending on the nature of the work, you may have the opportunity to enhance nursing scholarship, influence policy, and share knowledge that can improve health systems and patient outcomes (Ayala et al., 2022). Your work also may help advance research (Radford et al., 2020). For you individually, demonstrating your expertise through publishing may open other opportunities such as invitations to speak at conferences, review manuscripts, or serve as a consultant on the subject you wrote about (Morton & Nerges, 2020).

How can you reap these benefits? In a perfect world, authors of manuscripts for professional publications focus on publishing from the start, fashioning their words to a target journal. For students, however, the process is usually quite the reverse. The author begins with a completed assignment and revises it to create a publishable manuscript. You're like a gardener who, rather than planting a small, new rosebush where it's supposed to grow, takes a full-grown bush, prunes away the unnecessary parts, calls out its best qualities, and then reshapes it to fit a particular garden spot.

As you modify your completed student project, deciding what should go and what should stay isn't easy, but this reworking is necessary to create a manuscript that will catch the interest of an editor—and readers. Unfortunately, instead of taking the time to rework, many students simply submit the original paper or report, which almost always results in rejection. A more successful approach is to use a framework to guide your process.

Framework Overview

The framework presented here consists of the following:

- Check in with yourself about pursuing publication.
- Write a purpose statement.
- Determine who will be authors.
- Decide on the publication venue.
- Choose the article type.
- Establish a time frame.
- Write the article.
- As you write, apply strategies based on the type of academic work.

Although listed in a sequence, the process is iterative, so expect to go back and forth between items. You can find more details about each of these throughout this book, so here the focus is on the author who is converting a student paper to a manuscript.

Check-in

Before beginning to write, take the time to "check-in" with yourself. Reflecting on a few questions can help you determine if you should pursue publication.

What is my knowledge of the topic? Editors expect authors to have expertise about their topics and to reflect that expertise in their writing. Ask yourself: Do I have a deep understanding of, and experience with, this topic? For example, you may have written an outstanding paper on why nurses should be involved in politics, but do you have experience with politics, and is that experience reflected in your paper? If so, you're ready to move forward with the next check-in question. If not, you might not be qualified to write on this topic for a publication.

Will my manuscript provide new information? What is appropriate, even stellar, for a class assignment may be inappropriate for an article. On the other hand, the findings from these efforts may be of interest to your target readers (Roush, 2020). Converting your prior work into a manuscript calls for broader goals beyond meeting requirements of an assignment or project. Ask yourself: What new information will I contribute to expanding nursing's body of knowledge, enhancing nursing practice, and/or improving health outcomes (Morton & Nerges, 2020)?

If you haven't done so recently, conduct a comprehensive literature review using multiple keywords and search engines such as PubMed, CINAHL, and Google Scholar to build on what you did for your student work. Then, after lots of reading of nursing and (depending on the topic) non-nursing literature, identify what is currently known and where your gaps in knowledge are. Determine if your work can contribute to what already exists, keeping in mind that you might be able to refocus your topic so it better fits with what is needed.

How widely applicable is my work? To answer this question, you need to understand the difference between a quality improvement project or program evaluation, which are often required to complete a doctor of nursing practice (DNP) degree, and

> **Case Study: Converting a Student Paper**
>
> A graduate student in China completed rigorous research that showed significant positive effects of reproductive health education (RHE) for female high school students. At the time in China, nurses and RHE were novel in public schools. The student aimed to publish in an English-language journal with global readership. Her first submission to a journal based in the United States was rejected because the manuscript did not contain knowledge that would be new to readers in this country. The student then researched other journals, reshaped her content to emphasize relevance to countries where school nurses and RHE were not standard practice, and submitted to an English-language journal based in Asia but with a global reach. After review and further revisions, the journal published her manuscript (Su & Lindell, 2016).

research. Quality improvement projects and program evaluations are designed to meet the needs of a specific healthcare setting, so the objectives are based on unit-specific data. The sample size is often small and from one site. These characteristics make them less widely applicable compared to research studies, which are designed to fill a specific gap in knowledge or practice and be generalizable to a broad audience. (Note: If you received institutional review board approval for your project, you'll need to check that the approval allows for dissemination in a journal.)

That's not to say you can never find a publishing home for your completed quality improvement or program evaluation project. Review your findings carefully to determine whether they are relevant to the broader profession. Even if the specific findings are not widely applicable, you may be able to craft an article based on the knowledge you gained in working on the project. For instance, your quality improvement project on making telehealth assessments more effective may morph into an article on best practices for telehealth assessment, based on information you gleaned when you worked on your project.

If your academic work doesn't contribute to the existing literature, it's probably best not to submit a manuscript to a peer-reviewed journal. As Sebach and Shellenbarger (2020, p. 6) succinctly note, "Not every project meets a standard necessary for publication in a journal." However, don't give up! Instead, be creative and consider other options for your academic work. These include non-peer-reviewed print or online venues such as a state nurses association's publication, a blog (e.g., Nursology [https://nursology.net]; Perspectives, which is part of the *American Nurse Journal* website [https://www.myamericannurse.com/category/perspectives]), a news or opinion piece, or a magazine geared to the public. You'll learn more about potential venues later in this chapter.

Am I ready? Be honest with yourself. How good is your writing? A survey that assessed benefits and challenges of submitting manuscripts related to DNP projects to peer-reviewed journals found that quality of scholarly writing is a significant challenge (Ayala et al., 2022). If your writing skills are lacking, consider classes or working with a mentor to improve them before diving into publication. Another aspect of readiness is commitment. Converting your academic work to a manuscript "will involve an element of self-management and organization…" (Radford et al., 2020, p. 792). What are your current employment, academic, and personal commitments? Are

> **Confidence Booster**
>
> If you're feeling overwhelmed by the idea of turning your project into an article for publication and aren't sure where to start, consider the words of author Louis L'Amour: "Start writing, no matter what. The water does not flow until the faucet is turned on."

you ready to commit the time and effort necessary to transform your academic paper into a manuscript for publication?

If your responses to the check-in questions were positive, you're ready move onto the next part of the framework—writing a purpose statement.

Purpose Statement

Once an author has a topic (which you do) the next step is to write a purpose statement. A purpose statement immediately orients the reader to the nature of the article by indicating the aim of the article and how it contributes new or key information related to nursing practice and healthcare. Here are two examples:

> This study examined the effect of active learning strategies (ALSs) during clinical post conference sessions on the clinical judgement (CJ) of undergraduate students (Calcagni et al., 2023, p. 175).

> [T]his study aimed to explore the lived experience of young adults growing up with parents with serious mental illness, including their childhood and young adult experiences (Shestiperov et al., 2024, p. 3).

The purpose statement helps keep you focused on the goals and scope of the manuscript. Review it regularly as you write to ensure the article stays on track (Morton & Nerges, 2020). If you have coauthors, they should be involved in writing the purpose statement.

Authorship

Many manuscripts for publication have more than one author. If faculty or other colleagues were involved in the project, authorship should be discussed as soon as the idea of a manuscript is raised. Here are some questions to consider. (See Chapters 1 and 11 for more about authorship.)

Who is an author? All authors must verify to the journal that they made substantial contributions to the manuscript (Eiswirth & Fry, 2022). What does "substantial" mean? The International Committee of Medical Journal Editors (ICMJE) sought to answer this question with the following criteria (2023):

- "Substantial contributions to the conception or design of the work; or the acquisition, analysis, or interpretation of data for the work; AND
- Drafting the work or reviewing it critically for important intellectual content; AND
- Final approval of the version to be published; AND
- Agreement to be accountable for all aspects of the work in ensuring that questions related to the accuracy or integrity of any part of the work are appropriately investigated and resolved."

The use of "AND" means all four criteria must be met.

For students, authorship requires an open, collegial discussion among the potential authors. Because faculty taught the course for an assignment and provided feedback, or supervised or advised your DNP project, does not mean they qualify to be an author. Before making final decisions on authorship, review your target publication's authorship criteria (found in the author guidelines) and any related policies at your school. If the assignment or project was presented at an event such as a defense, where potential co-authors were present, it's helpful to have initial discussions about whether to prepare a manuscript, what journal to target, and authorship.

What if someone was key to your project but doesn't qualify as an author? You may have noted that some published articles include acknowledgments. This is an opportunity to recognize individuals such as a writing mentor, a statistician, committee members, or study participants.

In what order should authors be listed? The student who completed the academic paper or report should be the first author. Beyond that, determining the sequence for listing authors requires open discussion and, possibly, negotiation. Some disciplines have conventions such as the most senior author being last. Other options include alphabetical order or the degree of contribution by those meeting the criteria for authorship (Roush, 2020).

What are authors' responsibilities? The student, as first author, leads the writing team. When faculty are coauthors, this entails a change of relationship and may require careful navigation. The student author should convene a meeting of the writing team to discuss how each will contribute to the manuscript (Roush, 2020). During the meeting, discuss the strengths and time availability of each author. Typically, the first author will lead the project and have final say on the manuscript. However, if the first author is a novice in writing for publication, a member of the team may assume a role in which they have strong influence on the work. Authors also should agree on the review process before starting the article. In most cases, it works best if the co-authors review sequentially, one at a time (Radford et al., 2020). The important thing is to be coordinated and to have these discussions at the start of the project. Throughout the writing process, the first author maintains regular contact, including scheduling meetings as indicated, with other authors to ensure assignments are completed on time.

Publication Venue

Authors should submit to one publication at a time, and the review process can take several months before you receive a decision. Therefore, it's important to be deliberate about determining your target journal. The first step is to identify several journals that might be interested in your topic. This process takes some detective work and strategic thinking. Start by determining your target audience and the publications they read. If your article has a clinical focus, ask yourself if it's for registered nurses or advanced practice registered nurses (or both), because different journals target different types of practice. You'll also want

---

Confidence Booster

A writing mentor can help you decide whether your prior work is appropriate for publication and guide you through the writing process, thereby boosting your confidence. Your mentor may be one of your coauthors if they have expertise in writing for publication. However, if your coauthors don't have strong writing experience, you can seek a mentor elsewhere, such as a faculty member or a colleague with publishing experience. Should your manuscript be accepted, you can usually acknowledge the mentor's support in your final manuscript.

to consider which specialties would be interested in your topic.

For example, if you want to write about preventing infection during insertion of peripherally inserted central catheter (PICC) lines for nurses who specialize in IV therapy, you might want to target the *Journal of Infusion Nursing*. However, if you want to reach nurses who care for patients with PICC lines as part of their other duties, you might consider a general nursing journal, such as *American Nurse Journal*, the official publication of the American Nurses Association.

Resources to find journals that match with your topic and target audience include references from your academic work, suggestions from colleagues or faculty, and the Directory of Nursing Journals (https://nursingeditors.com/journals-directory), a vetted list from the International Academy of Nurse Editors (INANE) and the publication *Nurse Author & Editor*. (Learn more about selecting a journal in Chapter 3.)

Publishing in a nursing journal helps to build the body of nursing knowledge and reach nurse readers. However, you also can publish in non-nursing journals or popular magazines to spread the word about your scholarly work. If your topic would be suitable for a non-nursing journal, partner with a professional in the targeted discipline to write the article. For instance, you could collaborate with a respiratory therapist on your article about assessing patients' readiness for weaning from mechanical ventilation. Publishing in consumer venues provides the opportunity to show the general public the impact of nurses' work, and, depending on the topic, allow you to reach those who will directly benefit from the information.

Publishing in a range of different venues provides maximum exposure for your work and can lead to other opportunities to disseminate your work. Consider the example of Linda Aiken, professor at the University of Pennsylvania and founding director of the Center for Health Outcomes and Policy Research (Aiken, n.d.). In 2023, Aiken, an international expert of the healthcare workforce and quality of care, was published as first author in a medical journal (*JAMA Health Forum*) and a nursing journal (*Nursing Outlook*) and as a co-author in six other nursing or medical journals (Google Scholar, 2023). In addition, Aiken and Christine Schindler were interviewed in *Good Housekeeping* in 2020 (Rich, 2020). Of course, you need to be sure that each article you publish is different so that you avoid redundant or duplicate publication, which is unethical. (Learn more about this topic in Chapter 11.)

Once you identify journals that publish your content, check sections of the corresponding websites that have titles such as "About" and "Information for Authors." Review aims, scope, and author guidelines. You'll also want to determine the journal's business model. For example, some journals are open access, which makes your article more available to readers. Be sure you understand the nuances for various business models by reading Chapter 3.

Another way to narrow your choices and find the best fit for your topic is to read several of the published articles, noting the types of articles that are included.

Article Type

Types of articles include research reports, integrated or systematic reviews, evidence-based practice, innovations, and case studies. (Learn more about types of articles in Chapter 5.) When choosing, consider the gaps in the current literature, the message you want to convey, and your target readers. For example, in 2020, Davidson and colleagues published a longitudinal analysis of nurse suicide in a special issue of *Worldviews on Evidence-Based Nursing* (Davidson

School Submission Requirements

Does your institution require students to submit (or perhaps you already submitted) your final report to a public database such as ProQuest or (in Ohio) OhioLINK, or to your school's own repository? Check your school's policies and how the editor of the publication you've chosen views such submissions. The editor may be willing to review your manuscript because they expect it to be different from that in the public database, or they may say that if it is posted to a public database, they will reject your manuscript, considering it already published. If the latter, and you haven't uploaded your report, check with your school; you may be able to arrange to delay (or embargo) public posting so that you have time to pursue publication. For example, you can request a delay of six months, one year, or two years for publication in ProQuest (NYU Libraries, 2023).

et al., 2020). In preparing to do this study, which had not been done previously, the researchers found they needed a methodology for identifying the incidence of nurse suicide. Thus, in 2018 they published a report of how they developed and tested the methodology in the *Journal of Nursing Administration* (Davidson et al., 2018).

Another example is that if your purpose is to describe the method of inserting a PICC line, you could write a how-to article, guiding readers through a step-by-step process. If, however, your purpose is to discuss decreasing the delay in the use of PICC lines after insertion, you could write a review of literature that discusses methods nurses use to expedite use of PICC lines. Don't rule out submitting to a journal's regular department or column. These can provide the opportunity to share an innovative strategy for clinical practice, education, or leadership.

Once you've chosen an article type and understand the various options, you're ready to select a target journal. The time for your detective phase is time well spent, laying the groundwork for your manuscript. Read the author guidelines closely and, as you write, follow the guidelines and review sample articles (Howland, 2017).

Time Frame

There are two aspects to timing related to writing for publication—internal and external. *Internal* timing pertains to aspects you can control. For example, you can establish a schedule for your writing project to keep yourself on track. Start with the date you want to submit your article and work backwards to add in key milestones, such as when you will have the content outline completed. Schedule time for writing and commit to it. (Chapter 1 has more ideas for managing your time.)

Q *I've picked my target publication. Now what do I do?*

A Check if the editor of the journal you identified will accept an email inquiry (referred to as a "query") regarding their interest in an article on your topic. The editor's name will be in the front of the journal, or you can find it on the journal's website under "about."

If you identified more than one possible journal, it's usually best to query one editor at a time, allowing three to five days for a response, but many editors believe that sending simultaneous query submissions is acceptable. (However, you should never submit a manuscript to multiple editors at the same time.)

Be professional and succinct in your email. Include a brief description of the proposed article, why the topic is important to the journal's readers, why you are qualified to write the article, a statement that the manuscript has not been published elsewhere, and your contact information. You may also want to include the date it will be ready to submit. It's usually best to avoid stating that the manuscript is from a student work because too many editors have had negative experiences with receiving student papers instead of manuscripts suitable for the journal. However, if relevant, you might mention that you completed the work as part of a dissertation or DNP project, but add that the content would be repurposed to fit the journal's target audience. Do not include a draft of the manuscript (Saver, 2016).

A positive response from an editor may include advice as to what should (or should not) be included in the article and will spur you to write. Even with a positive query, however, publication is not guaranteed. For most journals, the manuscript still must go through peer review. If you receive a negative response, send your query to a different journal. A negative response to your query saves you time because you want to craft your article to fit with the journal that expresses interest in your topic. (See Chapter 3 for more information about queries and a sample query email.)

> ### Confidence Booster
>
> Most authors struggle with demands on their time. Consider this advice from J. K. Rowling: "Be ruthless about protecting writing days, i.e., do not cave in to endless requests to have 'essential' and 'long overdue' meetings on those days. The funny thing is that, although writing has been my actual job for several years now, I still seem to have to fight for time in which to do it. Some people do not seem to grasp that I still have to sit down in peace and write the books, apparently believing that they pop up like mushrooms without my connivance." (as cited in Leibowitz, 2018)

As you plan, keep the timeliness of your topic in mind. For instance, if your school project related to a new health policy or new guidelines for caring for patients with a certain condition, you would want to submit before what is "new" becomes widely disseminated.

External timing pertains to actions by the publication. Although you may hope to have your article in print as soon as possible, the publishing process takes time. If the editor feels your submitted manuscript has potential for the journal, it will be sent to two to three peer reviewers. This process can take six to eight weeks or even a few months. Assuming the reviewers are positive, you'll be asked to revise the manuscript, which sometimes is then sent for a second peer review. Once the article is accepted, the date of publication depends on several factors. Journal editors typically plan several months ahead, although changes are made based on reader priorities. In addition, journals may have themes for each issue, which means your article might need to wait a few months for the applicable theme. All this can take as long as two years, so be patient. Many journals have online editorial dashboards for authors where you can check the status of your manuscript.

Your article may be published online (e-publication), it may be published online and then in later in print, or it may be published in print and online simultaneously. You can list e-publications on your curriculum vitae, and you may have an option of including supplemental files in the e-publication that are not in the print copy. For example, the article on the longitudinal analysis of nurse suicide had several online supplemental tables, including one that showed the availability of data by state (Davidson et al., 2020).

You also may consider publishing your article on a preprint server before or upon submission to a journal. Posting before submission allows you to obtain feedback on your work. Before posting, however, you need to understand the nuances of preprints. If you are interested in this option, consult with an author who has experience with preprints, and read the targeted journal's requirements in this area. Chapter 3 contains more information about preprints.

Write

You've written a purpose statement, chosen a journal and type of article, had a positive response from your editorial query, and have established your timeline. Now it's time to write! As you write, keep in mind that as a student, your purpose was to meet academic requirements and demonstrate your knowledge (Sebach & Shellenbarger, 2020). Now your focus is on the reader and ensuring you are providing real-world content that will help nurses in their practice. Here are tips for success.

Outline. Don't be tempted to skip this step. It's a secret to success for many experienced writers. An outline provides a useful framework for organizing a manuscript (Saver, 2022). Sound organization is key because a poorly organized manuscript may be rejected even when it includes relevant content (Lake, 2020). The author guidelines of the journal often provide required sections and headings for the main manuscript and the abstract. If they do, use them.

The author instructions also may note if you are required to follow reporting guidelines for certain types of articles. For example, if you'll be reporting a quality improvement project, you might be required to use the Standards for QUality Improvement Reporting Excellence (SQUIRE) 2.0 guidelines (Ogrinc et al., 2016). If the project involved education, the Standards for QUality Improvement Reporting Excellence in Education (SQUIRE-EDU) guidelines (Ogrinc et al., 2019) might be required. You can find a list of reporting guidelines in Appendix D. Even if the journal doesn't specify use of these guidelines, you can use them to help organize your article.

Q *What if my journal doesn't provide sections for the manuscript?*

A Possible sections include introduction, background, problem, purpose, questions or objectives, conceptual or theoretical framework, methods, results, discussion (including limitations and recommendations for practice), and conclusions. Sections are determined by topic. For example, a research study on breastfeeding education for mothers who are homeless would likely have a theoretical or conceptual framework, but an article on placement of nasogastric tubes probably would not. You'll also need to provide references, as well as figures, tables, and boxes, which are frequently used to enhance readability.

As you begin to flesh out the sections of your outline, continue to consider how you will transform your academic paper into a manuscript of broader interest. Here is an example.

Topic of original school paper	This paper discusses the benefits of a website to teach nurses about transitional care and discharge planning, as shown by the results of a quality improvement study.
Transformed topic for a clinical journal	This article discusses how to develop a website to teach nurses about transitional care and discharge planning.

Format correctly. If you are revising your original document, rather than starting from scratch, incorporate any revisions based on faculty feedback, then save your document as a new, clean version. Be aware of formatting requirements for the type of article you plan to submit, as noted in the author guidelines. Pay attention to word or page limits and what those numbers include. For example, references and/or tables may not be included in the total. Likewise, adhere to requirements such as the number of words in the title, key words, highlights, and references. If your manuscript is not properly formatted, your article may be rejected or your publication may be delayed (Radford et al., 2020).

Act with integrity. Adhere to legal and ethical principles for publication, including authorship, attribution of sources, use of copyrighted material, and, when indicated, human rights protection. Refer to Chapters 4 and 11, as well as the journal's guidelines. Avoid any content by which your participants could be identified. Complete a plagiarism or similarity check before submitting. The editorial staff will check as well; you don't want to be rejected due to plagiarism, which can be unintended. If you received institutional review board approval for your project, note that in the article, along with strategies for protection of human subjects. The author guidelines and sample articles will help guide what you need to include.

Write thoughtfully. Be sure your manuscript is well organized and flows logically. Check for correct grammar, spelling, sentence structure, and appropriate use of paragraphs. Poor use of English language can be a reason for an editor to reject an article without sending it for peer review (Lake, 2020). See Chapters 5 and 6 for more information. Keep your purpose in mind and ask what readers need to know as opposed to what is nice to know. Write according to the style of the journal—some journals have a more informal style than others. Ask others to review your final draft and provide input.

Persevere. Don't be discouraged if the writing process takes several months. You may need to completely rewrite your paper, but rewriting is essential for success. As author Khaled Hosseini said, "Writing for me is largely about rewriting" (Charney, 2017, para. 6). A writing mentor can help by providing encouragement and feedback during the process.

Include figures and tables. The adage, "A picture speaks a thousand words," applies to manuscripts. In addition to tables with statistical data, boxes with bullets of key points can be helpful to the reader. However, use tables and figures judiciously and coordinate with the narrative to avoid duplicating content. Check the author guidelines for instructions on the number and format of figures and tables. Cite sources and secure permission to use copyrighted material such as a diagram of a theoretical framework. Refer to Chapter 7 for more guidance on figures and tables.

Prepare to submit. Take a few steps before submitting to boost the likelihood of your article being accepted for publication. If applicable, check your manuscript against criteria for reporting your type of article. Be sure your manuscript has no track changes or comments, and have all authors sign off on the final draft. Consider using the proofing checklist in Appendix B. If your article relates to your schoolwork and you are still a student, list your affiliation as the educational institution. If you have graduated, list your employer. Determine who will be the *corresponding author*—the author the editorial staff will communicate with directly.

Cowell and Pierson (2016) identified characteristics of strong manuscripts that had their origins in student work. Review their list and ensure your writing has these characteristics:

- Journal is appropriate for the topic
- Content contributes new, impactful information on the topic
- Manuscript is well-organized and formatted per author guidelines
- References are used selectively and cited per journal guidelines
- Strong scholarly writing is evident, including synthesis of ideas

- Manuscript shows in-depth understanding of the topic
- Implications for nursing practice are clear
- Authorship is purposeful and appropriate
- Authors demonstrate professional and ethical behavior

You'll also need to gather required supplemental documents such as conflict of interest statements and statements confirming that each author meets authorship requirements. The journal often has forms you need to use for this information.

Follow submission instructions. Review the journal's instructions for submission and take time to complete all the steps (Peate, 2020). It's not uncommon for articles to languish in a journal's database because an author didn't submit all the required documentation. In addition, don't submit if you don't intend to follow through on requested revisions (Kennedy et al., 2017). See Chapter 8 for guidance on submissions, rejections, revisions, and resubmissions.

Strategies Based on Past Work

The nature of your student work influences how you adapt it for publication.

Course-Based Paper

Revising a paper written for a specific course assignment often involves putting the content into the format required by the journal. Because your paper likely had a focused (rather than broad) topic and you are a novice writer, consider a shorter type of article such as innovation in practice or a case study. Be clear about implications for nursing, whether clinical practice, education, administration, or policy development. Refer to Chapter 13 for more information about writing a clinical article.

> **Confidence Booster**
>
> Are you a fan of checklists? How about one from editors of nursing journals? For a detailed list of steps to follow and criteria to meet when converting a student paper to manuscript, check out the "School Paper to Manuscript Student Checklist" from the journal *Nurse Author & Editor* (Owens et al., 2020).

Student Project

Projects generally involve quality improvement or program implementation and evaluation initiatives, including those developed to meet DNP requirements. Editors of clinical practice journals welcome "well-executed and well-written quality improvement (QI) projects…or comprehensive and well-synthesized clinical reviews" (Kennedy & Barnsteiner, 2017, p. 7).

Although editors welcome these types of articles, you must still fashion your work to meet the mission and style of the publication and the needs of the readers. The limited word count for a journal (compared to your project report) usually means you'll have to significantly synthesize the background, theoretical framework, literature review, and methods sections. In the discussion, clearly indicate implications for practice. Try to be objective as you rework your project—you want to present the information in the most useful way possible for readers, not share everything that you did as part of the project.

Refer to Chapter 16 for more information about reporting a quality improvement or evidence-based practice project.

Research-Focused Theses and Doctoral Dissertation

Master's research theses and doctoral dissertations are not widely circulated. A particular challenge is that editors of research journals are not likely to accept small-scale or pilot studies. However, it may be possible to convert your work into one or more manuscripts so it can reach a wider audience. Search for a journal that will publish a shorter version of research, such as a brief, or find an outlet that will publish an article based on some aspect of your project (Carter-Templeton, 2015).

Writing a thesis or dissertation demonstrates that you have learned the process of research and can independently conduct a project (Radford et al., 2020). However, for a journal article, you want to convey information that contributes to patient care or helps advance the profession (Lake, 2020). Understanding these different goals helps you determine what you can leave out and what you can present more succinctly.

Here are some tips related to the various sections of the manuscript that will help you develop from your thesis or dissertation. Learn more about writing a research report in Chapter 14.

First paragraph. You probably did not give a lot of thought to the introduction of your student work, but now you need to grab the reader's attention with the first paragraph. Use statistics or trends to depict the problem or topic. Then convey the purpose of the article and indicate the gap in knowledge about nursing practice, healthcare, or health outcomes it intends to address. Think of your article as a story, with the strongest parts of the story being the introduction and discussion (Radford et al., 2020).

Background and literature review. Include the information needed to describe the problem, briefly outline what is known, and identify the gaps in knowledge. This section should support the purpose statement. For your academic work, you likely conducted an extensive literature review to support your knowledge of the topic, but now think about your target audience and journal and ask yourself, "What does the reader already know and what do they need to know?" Remember to update your literature review to include relevant articles published since you completed your work.

Adhere to the journal's word limit, keeping in mind that the reader is primarily interested in your results and conclusions. However, you do need to provide a line of reasoning to guide the reader from what is currently known to how and what you are contributing to an identified gap in knowledge.

The next four sections (problem through framework) may be separate paragraphs in background or have their own headings, depending on the journal. If included in background, use the words for each section at the start of the paragraph so the reader knows what the paragraph is about.

Problem and Purpose. You likely had problem and purpose statements in your student paper. As you write the manuscript, review them to make sure: a) the problem is a succinct statement that flows from the background and indicates the gap in knowledge about the focus of the manuscript, and b) the purpose flows directly from the problem and is reflected throughout the paper.

Questions or objectives. Review other articles in the journal. If the purpose is clear, the questions or objectives may or may not be included. If included, use a sentence to introduce the research/study questions or project objectives and then list them with numbers.

Conceptual or theoretical framework. Was your student thesis or dissertation guided by a theoretical or conceptual framework? If so, including it will strengthen your manuscript because having a theoretical perspective increases the scientific value of research findings (McEwen, 2019). Did you use a nursing theory to guide your study? If so, include it so your work can build on, and advance, nursing's disciplinary knowledge (Littzen-Brown, 2021).

When you include a framework, be clear on how it was applied in your study (Morton & Nerges, 2020). Introduce it in the background section; in the methods section, explain why and how it was used; and in the discussion section, address how the findings align (or not) with the framework and implications for nursing going forward (McEwen, 2019).

Methods. You should not go into the depth of detail that you did in your thesis or dissertation. Keep the description of methods clear and succinct such that another researcher can understand and implement them (Steefel & Saver, 2013). A box with a list of steps in your protocol can save words and provide a clear picture for the reader. If applicable, include institutional review board approval and your permission to use instruments.

Results. Indicate your approaches to statistical analyses, describe your sample, and answer the purpose and/or research questions clearly and accurately. If you had objectives for a project, note whether they were met. Use tables and figures as indicated to supplement (not overwhelm) the text. (See Chapter 7 for more information on graphics.) You'll also want to address issues of power and reliability of the measurement tools. For example, did you do a power analysis to identify the optimal size of your sample? If so, interpret the final size of your sample in this regard. Likewise, if you did reliability tests of your measurement tools, interpret those results as well.

Discussion. The discussion must link back to the introduction. Instead of repeating the results, interpret their meaning for the reader. If possible, compare your sample to the target population to indicate how representative it was (or was not). Compare your results to the literature to highlight ways in which your work supports or extends current knowledge. This is an area where you might need to expand from your thesis or dissertation. For example, you may need to make the implications for practice, education, administration, or policy development, and the recommendations for future research more specific.

Conclusions. Indicate the significance of your work: how it contributes to nursing knowledge and how it can be used to improve nursing practice and/or health outcomes. Stay true to your purpose statement, avoid overreaching, and be clear and succinct. Be sure the abstract, introduction, and conclusions touch all the same points (Houze, 2009). Houze suggests using a highlighter to mark the points made in the abstract, introduction, and conclusion to make sure there is "closure."

Title and abstract. Your student paper or report had a title, and you may have had an abstract. Check them to make sure they reflect any changes made from your student paper to the manuscript, that they adhere to the format and word limit in the author guidelines, and that the title reflects the key topic of the manuscript. It's best to write these two items last to ensure they accurately reflect the content.

References. Be sure your reference list at the end of the article includes everything you have cited in the text. You'll want to cut down the number of references; you don't have to reference every sentence in the article (Steefel & Saver, 2013). If you have several references for a point you are making, select the one or two most valuable to the reader. Avoid long passages from references (even if you cite them) because they interrupt the article's flow. Follow the journal's author guidelines for reference format. Most schools use the American Psychological Association format, but many journals use the American Medical Association format. (See Chapter 4 for a comparison.) The guidelines also may specify the number of references that can be included.

For student projects, theses, and dissertations, consult with your advisor as to which parts of your work are essential for an article and which can be removed or used for another manuscript. If you plan to publish more than one article from your dissertation, be careful to avoid publications with repetitive content.(See Chapter 11 for more information.)

Share Your Knowledge

Transforming your presentation or academic paper, project, or dissertation is a challenge, but it is worth doing. You have already done so much work on a topic you care passionately about. Now it's time to share your knowledge. If you don't tell others about what you have learned, your only reward will be the grade on your transcript or abstract in a conference program. By publishing, you contribute to the body of nursing knowledge and help improve nursing practice and health outcomes. Moreover, your byline provides the personal reward of recognition for your work.

Write Now!

1. Choose one assignment that you're passionate about or did well on and research publications that would be appropriate for an article related to your work.

2. Find out your school's requirements related to sharing work in databases.

References

Aiken, L. (n.d.). *Linda H. Aiken, PhD, RN, FAAN, FRCN.* University of Pennsylvania. https://www.nursing.upenn.edu/details/profiles.php?id=93

Ayala, F. J., DeBoard, E., Waldrop, J., Pereira, K., Oermann, M., & Silva, S. G. (2022). Dissemination of doctor of nursing practice project findings: Benefits and challenges associate with publishing in healthcare journals. *Nursing Outlook, 70*(6), 846–855. https://doi.org/10.1016/j.outlook.2022.07.011

Calcagni L, Lindell D, Weaver, A., & Jackson, M. (2023) Clinical judgment development and assessment in clinical nursing education. *Nurse Educator, 48*(4), 175–181, https://doi.org/10.1097/NNE.0000000000001357

Carter-Templeton, H. (2015). Converting a DNP scholarly project into a manuscript. *Nurse Author & Editor, 25*(1), 1–7. https://doi.org/10.1111/j.1750-4910.2015.tb00195.x

Charney, N. (2017, July 14). Khaled Hosseini: How I write. *Daily Beast.* https://www.thedailybeast.com/khaled-hosseini-how-i-write

Cowell, J. M., & Pierson, C. A. (2016). Helping students get published: Tips from journal editors. *Nurse Author & Editor, 26*(4), 1–8. https://doi.org/10.1111/j.1750-4910.2016.tb00233.x

Davidson, J. E., Proudfoot, J., Lee, K., Terterian, G., & Zisook, S. (2020). A longitudinal analysis of nurse suicide in the United States (2005–2016) with recommendations for action. *Worldviews Evidence-Based Nursing, 17*(1), 6–15. https://doi.org/10.1111/wvn.12419

Davidson, J. E., Stuck, A. R., Zisook, S., & Proudfoot, J. (2018). Testing a strategy to identify incidence of nurse suicide in the United States. *Journal of Nursing Administration, 48*(5), 259–265. https://doi.org/10.1097/NNA.0000000000000610

Eiswirth, E., & Fry, A. (2022) Faculty-student authorship: Opportunities and challenges. *Journal of Professional Nursing, 42*, 106–110. https://doi.org/10.1016/j.profnurs.2022.06.009

Google Scholar. (2023, Oct. 3). *Results of Linda Aiken search*. https://scholar.google.com/scholar?hl=en&as_sdt=0%2C18&q=linda+aiken+2023&btnG=

Houze, R. (2009). Quotes from experts on effective scientific writing. *Eloquent Science*. http://eloquentscience.com/2009/08/quotes-from-experts-on-effective-scientific-writing/

Howland, W. A. (2017). Student manuscripts [Letter to the editor]. *AJN, 117*(10), 13. https://doi.org/10.1097/01.NAJ.0000525854.29698.ee

International Committee of Medical Journal Editors. (2023). *Recommendations for the conduct, reporting, editing, and publication of scholarly work in medical journals*. http://www.icmje.org/recommendations

Kennedy, M. S., & Barnsteiner, J. (2017). A plea to faculty: Rethink student writing assignments [Editorial]. *American Journal of Nursing, 117*(8), 7. https://doi.org/10.1097/01.NAJ.0000521948.22577.6d

Kennedy, M. S., Newland, J. A., & Owens, J. K. (2017). Findings from the INANE survey on student papers submitted to nursing journals. *Journal of Professional Nursing, 33*(3), 175–183. https://doi.org/10.1016/j.profnurs.2016.09.001

Lake, E. T. (2020). Why and how to avoid a desk rejection [Editorial]. *Research in Nursing and Health, 43*(2), 141–142. https://doi.org/10.1002/nur.22016

Leibowitz, G. (2018, Dec. 31). 60 Inspiring quotes to help you achieve your writing goals in 2019. *Inc*. https://www.inc.com/glenn-leibowitz/60-inspiring-quotes-about-writing-from-worlds-greatest-authors.html

Littzen-Brown, C. (2021, Nov. 9) Theory-guided research: What, why, and how? *Nursology*. https://nursology.net/2021/11/09/theory-guided-research-what-why-and-how%ef%bf%bc/

McEwen, M. (2019). Application of theory in nursing research. In M. McEwen & E. Wills (Eds.), *Theoretical basis for nursing* (5th ed., pp. 452–474). Wolters Kluwer.

Morton, P. G., & Nerges, J. (2020). Strategies to turn a graduate school paper into a publishable journal manuscript. *AACN Advanced Critical Care, 31*(4), 371–379. https://doi.org/10.4037/aacnacc2020716

NYU Libraries. (2023). *Publishing your dissertation*. https://guides.nyu.edu/c.php?g=276978&p=1846701

Ogrinc, G., Armstrong, G. E., Dolansky, M.S., Singh, M. K., & Davies, L. (2019). SQUIRE-EDU (Standards for Quality Improvement Reporting Excellence in Education. *Academic Medicine, 94*(10), 1461–1470. https://doi.org/10.1097/ACM.0000000000002750

Ogrinc, G., Davies, L., Goodman, D., Batalden, P. B., Davidoff, F., & Stevens, D. (2016). SQUIRE 2.0 (Standards for QUality Improvement Reporting Excellence): Revised publication guidelines from a detailed consensus process. *BMJ Quality and Safety, 25*(12), 986–992. https://doi.org/10.1136/bmjqs-2015-004411

Owens, J. K., Cowell, J. M., Kennedy, S. M., Newland, J. A., & Pierson, C. A. (2020). School paper to manuscript: Student checklist. *Nurse Author & Editor*. https://onlinelibrary.wiley.com/pb-assets/assets/17504910/Checklist%20pdfs/6-School-Paper-to-Manuscript-Student-Checklist-1599562514443.pdf

Peate, I. (2020). Turning your assignment into an article for British Journal of Nursing. *British Journal of Nursing, 29*(3), 178–180. https://doi.org/10.12968/bjon.2020.29.3.178

Radford, D. R., Seath, R. J. G., Davda, L. S., & Potts, G. (2020). Research dissertation to published paper: The journey to a successful publication. *British Dental Journal, 228*(10), 791–794. https://doi.org/10.1038/s41415-020-1539-1

Rich, G. (2020, Jan. 24). Why are our school nurses disappearing? *Good Housekeeping*. https://www.goodhousekeeping.com/life/parenting/a30520693/school-nurse-shortage/

Roush, K. (2020). *A nurse's step-by-step guide to publishing a dissertation or DNP project*. Sigma.

Saver, C. (2016). Effective queries can save authors time and effort. *Nurse Author & Editor, 26*(3), 1–9. https://doi.org/10.1111/j.1750-4910.2016.tb00225.x

Saver, C. (2022, Feb.). The awesome outline. *American Nurse Journal*. https://www.myamericannurse.com/the-awesome-outline/

Sebach, A. M., & Shellenbarger, T. (2020). Modifications needed: Additional strategies to transform DNP projects into publishable manuscripts. *Nurse Author & Editor, 30*(2), 1–8. https://doi.org/10.1111/j.1750-4910.2020.tb00057.x

Shestiperov, A., Grinstein-Cohen, O., Lindell, D., Irani, E., Kagan, I. (2024). Lived experiences: Growing up with a seriously mentally ill parent. *Journal of Nursing Scholarship*. Advance online publication. https://doi.org/10.1111/jnu.12955

Steefel, L., & Saver, C. (2013). From capstone project manuscript to published article. *American Nurse Journal, 8*(5), 54–56. https://www.myamericannurse.com/from-capstone-project-to-published-article/

Su, J. J., & Lindell, D. (2016). Promoting the menstrual health of adolescent girls in China. *Nursing and Health Sciences, 18*(4), 481–487. https://doi.org/10.1111/nhs.12295

Writing a Continuing Professional Development Activity

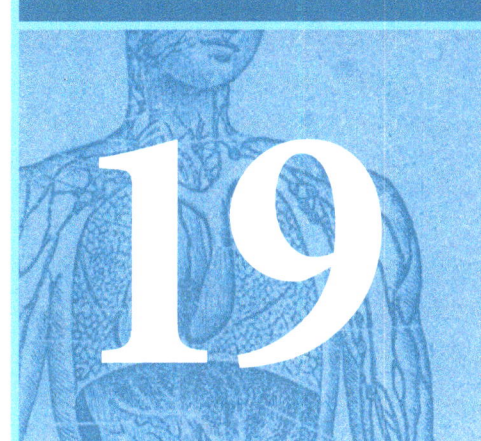

19

–Nadine Salmon, MSN, RN, NPD-BC, IBCLC

> *"Education is the most powerful weapon which you can use to change the world."*
> –Nelson Mandela

WHAT YOU'LL LEARN IN THIS CHAPTER

- Nursing continuing professional development (NCPD) is vital for optimal patient outcomes.

- An NCPD learning activity typically includes a gap analysis, a needs assessment, a goal statement, instructional objectives, an introduction, the narrative, a concluding paragraph, and an exam.

- Interprofessional continuing education (IPCE) learning activities provide opportunities for healthcare professions from two or more professions (e.g., physicians and nurses) to learn how to collaborate effectively together as a team, to improve patient outcomes.

- Interactive teaching-learning strategies such as case studies, exercises, study questions, or self-assessment tools are used to enhance learning.

Why is continuing education (CE) so important? The example of artificial intelligence (AI) helps answer that question. Although AI has been used in healthcare since the early 1970s, only in the last few years have clinicians begun to embrace what it offers. Automating the monitoring and interpretation of vital signs in patients, enhancing clinician-patient interactions, and analyzing diagnostic data are just a few ways AI can be used to improve patient safety, outcomes, and experiences. For instance, the manual process of discharging a patient from an acute care facility is often a laborious task, requiring time, patience, and effective communication between different members of the healthcare team. It's often an inefficient process, fraught with delays and miscommunication. But now there is a growing trend towards using AI to streamline the discharge process; it can partially automate the process by identifying and coordinating discharge activities (Nayak, 2023).

The benefits of AI come with the need for clinicians to understand when and how it can be integrated into workflows to improve processes and patient care. Clinicians also need to understand potential problems, such as bias in the data used to develop AI algorithms. This is where CE comes in. Well-written and evidence-based CE learning activities can prepare clinicians to better incorporate tools such as AI into their practice. From a wider perspective, ongoing education helps clinicians improve their expertise by keeping them up to date with advances in healthcare.

Writing a nursing continuing professional development (NCPD) or an interprofessional continuing education (IPCE) learning activity can be a fun and interesting experience, but it takes commitment and requires patience and persistence to plan, write, and revise your activity to perfection. You may choose to approach a nursing journal or website about developing an NCPD activity,

The author wishes to acknowledge with gratitude Nan Callender-Price, MA, RN, who wrote and co-revised this chapter in the first four editions of this book.

or you may partner with a healthcare professional outside of nursing to develop an IPCE activity. IPCE activities expand your target audience and, depending on the topic, involving those from other professions can increase the effectiveness of the activity. For example, an article on new pharmacologic options for patients with diabetes could be more informative with a pharmacist coauthor.

NCPD or IPCE activities can have multiple delivery options, such as printed in a journal or magazine, usually with an online version; online only, which might include an interactive presentation or a webinar; a video; or a podcast. But no matter what the format, the basic steps remain the same.

Q *Is NCPD the same as CNE?*

A In July 2022, the American Nurses Credentialing Center (ANCC) adopted new standards from the Accreditation Council for Continuing Medical Education (ACCME) and changed the terminology for continuing nursing education (CNE) to nursing continuing professional development (NCPD). You'll still see CNE and even CE used to refer to continuing education for nurses, but NCPD is the preferred terminology.

How to Get Started

Think of writing a learning activity as an adventure, like taking a road trip. You have an idea about where you would like to go, but for a trip to be successful, you have to spend time preparing for it. Preparation is also the first step on your CE journey, which starts with reviewing the author guidelines.

Q *I'm already so busy. Why should I take the time to write an NCPD or IPCE activity?*

A Writing an NCPD or IPCE activity can enhance your career. After it's published, you can add it to your resume or curriculum vitae. The process of writing also reinforces your knowledge and keeps you current on the subject. Many nursing specialty certification boards accept NCPD publications as credit toward contact hours needed for certification or recertification.

Read the Author Guidelines

On your CE journey, just like the journey to writing any kind of article, a publication's author guidelines will guide you, setting the ground rules from which you can begin to plan the learning activity. The guidelines inform you about a publication's word requirements (length), method for writing objectives, reference style, and any required special features, such as a clinical vignette.

Review the guidelines carefully and ask questions before you get started to save time for both you and the editor. You will typically need to submit a gap analysis and needs assessment, your target audience, the topic of the educational activity, a goal, objectives, and expected outcomes. An outline may be requested as well.

About CE Accreditation

Organizations that offer NCPD programs are accredited as providers of NCPD by an accrediting body, such as the ANCC Accreditation Program (part of the ANA Enterprise, and the largest nurse credentialing organization) or as providers of IPCE by the Joint Accreditation for Interprofessional Education. Accreditation by the Joint Accreditation for Interprofessional Education enables organizations to offer CE activities to multiple professionals, such as nurses, nurse practitioners, physicians, physician assistants, pharmacists, psychologists, dietitians, and social workers (Joint Accreditation for Interprofessional Continuing Education, 2023).

Some state nursing organizations can approve NCPD programs, but these organizations are limited by certain restrictions, such as ensuring that more than 50% of the target audience is in their geographical location.

Individual activity approval is also available. ANCC and some state nursing and specialty organizations approve individual NCPD activities, with certain restrictions.

Providers of NCPD must meet specific criteria to maintain their provider status, such as ensuring that programs are of an appropriate length for the contact hours awarded.

Q *Why do CE activities have to be accredited?*

A Requirements vary state to state, but most healthcare professionals need a set number of CE credits every year (or every few years) to renew their license or recertify in a particular specialty area. An accreditation process helps ensure consistent quality of NCPD or IPCE learning activities, holding accredited organizations to the highest standards in nursing and interprofessional education.

Write for Your Target Audience

Just like you would ask your traveling companions what they prefer to see and do before you go on your trip, you should know your target audience before you start writing. Who can benefit most from the information? Do they represent different professions? Are they new graduates or experienced clinicians? What are their educational backgrounds and current roles?

The answers to these questions will frame your learning activity. For example, if you want an article to reach a clinically diverse interprofessional audience, topics that pertain to multiple specialties, such as heart disease, might be a better option than topics specific to fewer specialties, such as shared governance. Likewise, an article geared to new graduates generally reads differently than one for experienced clinicians. You should write a learning activity that matches the educational background and clinical experience of the learner. When considering content for NCPD and IPCE activities, remember that the content needs to include more than just the basic recall of facts; the application of knowledge in the clinical setting as well as the importance of collaboration and communication, are cornerstones of CE courses (Howson, 2023).

Writing CE activities requires an understanding of adult learning principles (ALPs) because using these principles will increase the value and impact that the learning opportunity has on the learner (Howson, 2023). In addition to ALPs, authors must also consider other aspects of adult learning such as technology, brain maturity, memory/prior experience, cognition, and organizational perspectives when creating continuing education content (Merriam & Baumgartner, 2020).

Several resources can help you learn more about the demographics of your target audience. For *nurses*, look at results from the National Council of State Boards of Nursing (NCSBN) and the National Forum of State Nursing Workforce Centers' National Nursing Workforce Survey (NCSBN, 2022). This survey provides a summary of the number and characteristics of registered nurses in the United States, including age and educational background. For *physicians*, consider data from the Association of American Medical Colleges (AAMC), which includes demographics and practice patterns of physicians who graduated from MD-granting medical schools and trending data for select topics. For *pharmacists*, turn to the American Association of Colleges of Pharmacy (AACP) Pharmacy Workforce Center, which is a nonprofit corporation with the mission of serving the pharmacy profession and the public by actively researching, analyzing, and monitoring the size, demography, and activities of the pharmacy workforce.

Q *I keep hearing the term "interprofessional education," what does that really mean?*

A Interprofessional continuing education (IPCE) encourages students to learn together and broaden their knowledge and experiences to improve patient outcomes (ACCME, n.d.). IPCE may occur when members from two or more professions learn with, from, and about each other to promote effective collaboration and improve health outcomes (Joint Accreditation for Interprofessional Continuing Education, 2023).

When developing IPCE, the target audience is more diverse, and extra diligence is required to ensure the topic and discussion are relevant to all groups. IPCE differs from multidisciplinary education in that learners from the different professions learn from and together with each other, focusing on the importance of collaboration and communication. Conversely, multidisciplinary team education silos learning for each profession, so that health professionals learn about patient care in the context of their own professional role (Howson, 2023).

Joint Accreditation for Interprofessional Continuing Education, a collaboration of several associations, including the American Nurses Credentialing Center, Accreditation Council for Continuing Medical Education, and Accreditation Council for Pharmacy Education, offers organizations the opportunity to be simultaneously accredited to provide nursing, medical, and pharmacy continuing education through a single, unified application process and set of accreditation standards (Joint Accreditation for Interprofessional Continuing Education, 2023).

Review the author guidelines and read previously published content for the publication you are writing for to gain more insights into the target audience. The editors of the publication also can provide guidance, as needed.

Select a Topic/Identify a Gap in Knowledge

The following strategies can help you identify an NCPD or IPCE topic and provide support for a needs assessment, which you may be asked to provide:

- **Identify a clinical gap.** Focus on what would be of interest to your target audience. For example, is there a cutting-edge medication or treatment on the horizon or new discoveries about a particular disease or condition that clinicians need to know about? Or is there a state that has started requiring nurses to complete NCPD on a topic, such as human trafficking, as a condition for licensure? CE editors, like news editors, seek out the "wow effect," those topics that make readers clamor for more. But even a novel approach to a common topic might be of interest. In addition, you can conduct a literature review to identify holes in the literature—topics that haven't been covered by other publications. Identifying a gap in knowledge is the first step that authors must take in planning a learning activity. This gap assessment will help identify a gap in clinical performance, which will lead to the formation of the learning outcomes you want the learner to achieve.

- **Identify your target audience.** Knowing the demographics of your target audience will help you select an appropriate topic.

- **Identify the focus of the learning activity.** Will the activity expand a scope of practice or help clinicians to work more effectively with colleagues from other disciplines?

- **Conduct a literature review.** Collect a few sources to support the general need, along with evidence to support how this information applies to your target audience.

- **Develop a needs assessment.** Document how the evidence you collected supports your decision to plan this particular learning activity for the identified adult learners by considering the gap that exists between the current level of learner knowledge, skill, or practice and the desired level. Given the gap identified with this target audience, what outcome will tell you that the gap has been filled?

- **Start considering desired outcomes.** Based on your gap assessment, think down the road about measurable patient outcomes you would like your learners to achieve, and then develop your learning activity to enable learners to achieve these outcomes and improve patient safety. For example, if you are considering writing about how interprofessional members of your provider unit can collaborate to reduce central line-associated blood stream infections, you can examine the rate of infection among surgical patients at this time and then compare the infection rates three to six months from now to see if that number has decreased (the measurable outcome).

Once you have the topic, you're ready for the next step in your writing journey.

Q *How do I know at what level I should write my NCPD or IPCE article?*

A The content should go beyond the basic level of knowledge taught in undergraduate programs. For instance, an article on elementary assessment skills would not qualify as NCPD or IPCE for practicing clinicians, because they should already be knowledgeable about basic assessment skills. Application of knowledge is an important component of continuing education activities, as well as communication and collaboration.

Set Goals and Objectives

Before you start a journey, you have a destination in mind and know what you want to accomplish by the end of your trip. The same should be true with an NCPD or IPCE activity. Beginning with the end in mind will keep your educational activity on the right track.

Several frameworks can guide the planning phase of your learning activity, but one of the most widely used is Moore's Model of Outcomes Assessment. This model was initially developed in response to increased concern about medical errors and quality of care among physicians but was later revised to focus on all healthcare professionals (Sud et al., 2022). Moore's model is based on the fundamental belief that the design of a continuing professional education course must *begin* with the establishment of learner outcomes, so that these outcomes can be expected to happen (Moore et al., 2009). In applying this model, you first identify a gap in patient health status, which is then used to identify a gap in clinical performance or competency; this discovery leads you to the identification of the knowledge gap that you need to address in your learning activity. The goal and objectives are then designed around what you want the learning outcome to be.

The *goal* (or purpose) is a broad statement that helps you and the learner focus on the big picture. An example of a goal or purpose is:

> The goal of this program is to inform clinicians in the acute care setting about current prophylactic management strategies for the prevention of deep vein thrombosis (DVT).

Objectives, on the other hand, state what behavior is expected of the learner by the end of the activity. The use of instructional objectives as a measure of learning started with Benjamin Bloom, an American educational psychologist from the University of Chicago (Bloom et al., 1956).

Subsequent to Bloom's taxonomy, Robert F. Mager, PhD, a renowned instructional designer and developer, published his groundbreaking work, *Preparing Instructional Objectives*, in 1962. Mager's strategy for developing instructional objectives is widely used today. Mager (1997) identifies three characteristics of an instructional objective. Objectives should be:

1. Related to intended outcomes, not the process for achieving those outcomes
2. Specific and measurable, rather than broad or intangible
3. Focused on the learner, not the instructor

Mager further breaks instructional objectives into three main components:

1. **Performance:** what learners are expected to be able to do
2. **Conditions:** conditions under which the performance is expected to occur
3. **Criteria:** the level of competence that must be achieved

Bloom's Taxonomy of Learning

Bloom's taxonomy divides the *cognitive domain* (development of intellectual skills and knowledge) objectives into several categories of increasing complexity, which is a stair-step approach to thinking about levels of learning. The simple schematic, shown in Table 19.1, will help you understand the level of learning conveyed in the objectives and the verbs typically associated with each level.

Keep in mind that you can use the taxonomy when writing test questions, too.

The categories illustrate the increasing complexity of the types of learning, starting with knowledge (the most basic level) and progressing to evaluation (the most complex level).

TABLE 19.1 Summary of Bloom's Taxonomy

Level of Learning	Type of Learning	Verbs
Knowledge	Memorization and regurgitation	Define, identify, list, repeat, name, relate
Comprehension	Understanding and interpretation	Discuss, describe, report, explain, review, summarize
Application	Use of information in new situation	Translate, apply, interpret, demonstrate
Analysis	Breakup of the whole into parts	Distinguish, compare showing relationships, contrast, differentiate
Synthesis	Combination of elements, forming new structure	Formulate, prepare, design, assemble, plan
Evaluation	Situation assessment, based on criteria	Assess, compute, revise, measure, evaluate

Don't confuse learning objectives with competencies. *Learning objectives* describe a measurable learning goal that a learner will be able to accomplish by the end of the learning activity. This differs from a *competency*, which describes the knowledge, skills, and abilities that a learner needs to have to complete a task successfully and safely (Nabizadeh-Gharghozar et al., 2021).

Here are some tips for writing objectives:

- Keep objectives congruent with the goal, content, and teaching-learning strategies of the activity.
- Limit yourself to one behavior per objective.
- Keep the language simple.
- Use the performance, conditions, and criteria model whenever possible.
- Use verbs that describe actions that can be quantified; for example, "identify the signs and symptoms of heart disease" can easily be converted into a post-test question, but "enhance knowledge of heart disease" cannot.
- Describe learner outcomes.
- Write at the level of the learner, keeping in mind professional status, experience, and educational level.
- Focus on the learner, not the instructor (i.e., author).
- Make sure objectives are clearly stated.
- Make objectives realistic and measurable.

Take a closer look at some sample instructional objectives in Example 19.1.

Here are two more examples. Try to identify the characteristics that make them good objectives.

> State the two main components of extracellular fluid.

> Compare and contrast the clinical presentation of Alzheimer's disease and Lewy body dementia.

Understanding the basic characteristics of well-written objectives will help you write effective instructional objectives for your own learning activity.

Write Outcome Statements

Outcomes are starting to be used more often than objectives as a measure of learning. What's the difference? *Objectives* focus on the goal and process, with more emphasis on the instructor and learner, whereas an *outcome*, a desired end result, speaks to the goal with the focus on the learner, who must achieve a specific result or outcome. Outcome-based education is a learner-focused approach to curriculum design that focuses on the knowledge, skills, and abilities that help learners develop competency (Tan et al., 2018). As mentioned previously, Moore's Model of Outcomes assessment is a popular framework used in IPCE, but there are many other frameworks that can also be used, so it's wise to review the literature about them.

Writing outcome statements is similar to writing objectives. The *stem* (standard introductory text), for example, precedes the outcome statement as it does with the objective:

> After completing this program, the learner will be able to...

After you complete the program, you will be able to identify three reasons why neonates are more susceptible to cold stress than other patient populations.

- Objective is focused on the learner.
- Learners are alerted that they will learn what is expected of them after they complete the activity.
- "Identify" is a knowledge verb, a basic level. The verb "identify" is followed by "three reasons"—a specific quantity.
- The language is simple and expresses one idea.

EXAMPLE 19.1 A well-written instructional objective.

The goal of this wound care program is to prepare medical-surgical nurses to manage wounds in patients with burns. After completing this program, the learner will be able to:

Objective	Outcome Statement
State the four stages of wound healing.	Apply the four stages of wound management to your clinical setting.
Describe the aseptic technique that should be used for wound cultures.	Correctly obtain wound culture specimens without contamination.
Compare and contrast the benefits of hydrocolloid versus hydrogel dressings.	Correctly select the most appropriate wound dressing for a second-degree burn.

EXAMPLE 19.2 Comparison of objectives and outcome statements.

Changing from the use of objectives to outcomes encourages the educator to stay focused on the end result—the practice change expected from the learner upon completion of the activity and, ultimately, changes in patient outcomes.

Begin each statement with the highest-level verb (the more complex verb in the Bloom taxonomy) that relates to the content and is measurable. Use language that is familiar to learners and represents their actual practice. As with objectives, the language should be clear, concise, and pertinent, and the statement should speak to the core competencies. Using the SMART mnemonic (**S**pecific, **M**easurable, **A**ttainable, **R**elevant, and **T**imely) to develop learning objectives will ensure that the objectives are well-written, measurable, and include the knowledge, skills, and abilities that the learner can expect to gain from the educational activity (Andreev, 2023).

When writing outcome statements, consider what learners are expected to do after completing the course (Andreev, 2023). Is the expectation for a change in cognitive, affective, or psychomotor performance? Will learners need to demonstrate their knowledge or write about it?

Compare three traditional objectives with the outcome statements they have been converted to, shown in Example 19.2. Note that the verbs used in the objectives represent knowledge and comprehension, compared to the use of higher-level verbs, representing application and analysis, in the outcome statements. The outcome statements are more specific and performance-oriented, generally requiring learners to apply the information to their practice.

Write the Outline

With the goal and objectives or outcome statements completed, you can now write your outline, which many editors require before you start writing. An outline is like your trip's itinerary, showing the starting and ending points as well as where you will go between. A one-page outline is usually adequate for a single-contact-hour NCPD learning activity, but requirements vary with the publication. The editor needs to know how you plan to write the narrative to ensure it flows in a logical progression. You're not going to backtrack 100 miles on your road trip, and the same is true about a learning activity—the progression of the narrative should move the learner forward in a clear, coherent manner.

What should you include in an outline? Generally, an outline shows that your topic moves from broad to more specific information. It includes your goal statement; objectives; and, if you already know, the sentence or case study you plan to use to start the learning activity. Show the main topics within the narrative with some detail for each. Example 19.3 shows part of an outline for a single-contact-hour NCPD learning activity about disseminated intravascular coagulation (DIC).

> **When the Coagulation Cascade Goes Horribly Wrong**
>
> I. **Goal:** The goal of this program is to inform nurses of the pathophysiology, assessment, and treatment of disseminated intravascular coagulation (DIC).
>
> II. **Objectives:** After studying the information provided here, you will be able to:
>   A. Identify three factors that precipitate DIC.
>   B. Describe the assessment parameters and laboratory values associated with DIC.
>   C. Discuss four nursing interventions appropriate for care of patients who exhibit indications of DIC.
>
> III. **Introductory Case Study**
>
> IV. **Main Body**
>   A. DIC defined
>   B. Factors and diseases that contribute to DIC
>   1. Obstetric disorders
>   2. GI disorders
>   3. Tissue-damage factors
>   4. Infections
>   5. Hemolytic processes
>   6. Vascular disorders
>   C. Pathophysiology of DIC
>   1. Healthy clotting mechanisms outside DIC
>   2. Endovascular changes that contribute to DIC

EXAMPLE 19.3 Part of an outline for single-contact-hour NCPD learning activity.

After the editor accepts your goal statement, objectives, outline, and teaching-learning strategies, you're ready to start the trip.

Write the Narrative

Like any article, the CE activity has a beginning, a middle, and an end.

Off to a Good Start

What's going to make the learner want to jump on board with you? A topic of interest helps, but something else increases the chances even more: An enticing lead sentence (also known as a *lede*) or case study inspires the learner to begin the journey.

Check the journal's past CE articles to see what type of lede is preferred—an attention-grabbing lede, or one that is more traditional yet still engaging for the reader. To make your lede attention-grabbing, try using a compelling question, vivid metaphor, dramatic statistic, current event, or the mention of a well-known movie or book. Whatever the lede, you must relate it to your topic immediately with a transition sentence.

Here are examples of well-constructed, attention-grabbing ledes.

Gun Violence in the US

US gun violence has reached an all-time high. Data from the Gun Violence Archive in 2018 revealed that there is a mass shooting occurring, on average, every nine out of every 10 days (Morris & Guardian US Interactive Team, 2018). What do healthcare providers need to do to prepare for the increased incidence of multiple gunshot wounds (GSW) to the ED?

In the preceding example, the author uses a compelling statistic to grab the reader's attention. Try to identify what makes the following introductory paragraphs a good lede.

Facebook: Know the Policy Before Posting

Why are some nurses and other healthcare professionals losing their jobs because of Facebook postings? Celebrities use the popular social networking site, TV reporters use it, and chances are you and your friends use it, too. However, users can overlook the negative effects that social networking sites can have on their careers. In healthcare, Facebook postings can influence the hiring process, violate patient privacy, and result in termination of employment.

Food Gone Bad

What do peanut butter, chocolate, granola bars, cookie dough, ground beef, ground turkey, chicken, bacon, hot dogs, salami, sushi, cheese, eggs, spinach, green onions, lettuce, tomatoes, olives, alfalfa sprouts, clover sprouts, orange juice, apple juice, cantaloupes, raspberries, sesame, tahini, ice cream, hazelnuts, pine nuts, and strawberries have in common? The answer: contamination with foodborne pathogens.

Note how provocative questions are posed for readers. In the first example, we're reminded of the consequences of misusing social media. In the second example, we're drawn in because everyone has consumed one or more of the listed foods and has been potentially exposed to foodborne pathogens. In both cases, readers identify with the scenario, increasing their interest in the topic.

If the journal you are targeting prefers more matter-of-fact ledes, you might opt for a common technique of using an introductory case study. Case studies can

Teaching-Learning Strategies

You can use a variety of teaching-learning strategies in your NCPD or IPCE article:

- **Case studies:** As nurses, our primary interest is people. Case studies play off of that and allow readers to think about applying what they have learned in their own practice. Case studies also engage learners in *emotional learning*—achieving powerful emotional responses to a clinical scenario engages learners' cognitive flexibility, which helps with memory retention (Howson, 2023).

- **Illustrations:** Consider including illustrations, which play a key role in bolstering memory retention. For example, you could provide an illustration of the surgical technique for repairing a mitral valve for an article on nursing care of the patient undergoing mitral valve replacement.

- **Tables and charts:** Pull out key concepts into tables. Use charts to illustrate study results.

- **Study questions:** You can give the reader questions to consider before taking the post-test.

- **Exercises:** Allow the reader a chance to practice skills. For example, in an NCPD program on the interpretation of arterial blood gas results, give participants practice sets of results for them to interpret.

- **Self-assessments:** If you are writing a lengthy CE learning activity, periodically insert self-assessments so readers can test themselves on what they have learned so far.

- **Glossary and references:** Even simple tools, such as a glossary of terms and your list of references, are helpful teaching-learning strategies.

be used in multiple ways, including testing the learner midway or at the end of the activity. Although there is not a single definition of a case study (Heale & Twycross, 2018), it's usually a description of a situation, event, or story that is used to illustrate an intervention or outcome. Well-written, succinct case studies can also arouse the reader's curiosity. You want to choose a topic and scenario that fits your objectives and content.

You can choose a case study that highlights a clinical experience. Posing a question at the end of the case study (e.g., "What nursing care would be appropriate in this situation?") and then answering it at the end of the learning activity can be an effective way to draw in readers. Or providing readers with more details about the situation throughout the narrative can help move them along. Case studies are an example of experiential learning, in which the learner is immersed in a clinical scenario or learning event, has an opportunity to reflect on the best way to handle that situation, and then participates in formulating an appropriate response to the situation, often referred to as "knowing-in-action" (Howson, 2023).

Here's an example of an introductory case study:

Knife and Gun Club: The Biomechanics of Penetrating Trauma

An ear-splitting crack penetrates the silence of the night air. The smallest flash of orange pierces the darkness. Unseen to the human eye is a small metal object, cutting through the atmosphere at well over 1,500 feet per second.

The recipient feels nothing more than a sudden rush of air from his throat as the blast wave preceding the bullet strikes his chest. Less than a millisecond later, the bullet tears first through his shirt and then through his skin and intercostal muscles. As the leading edge of the bullet meets the resistance of the man's body, it deforms outward, creating a flat surface that crushes the lung tissue in its way. When the object strikes the anterior edge of the scapula, it shatters into numerous pieces, each carving a different path through the surrounding tissue. One piece tears through the nerve roots of the neighboring spinal column, severing it and causing the man's legs to crumple beneath him. Another piece projects upward into the man's neck, cutting through an artery. Within seconds, blood gushes into the tissue spaces around the structures of the airway, and the man's respirations become labored and noisy.

A race against time has begun. If the race is won, the gunshot victim will receive medical and surgical care quickly enough to save his life. If the race is lost, he will join the thousands who die every year around the world from penetrating trauma.

Note how the author sets the stage for the reader by describing the path of the bullet into the victim and its anatomical damage in detail.

Here is another example of an introductory case study. This one is slightly more formal in tone:

When the Coagulation Cascade Goes Horribly Wrong

The ambulance report seems routine: a patient transferring to the hospital from a nursing home for a possible urinary tract infection (UTI) caused by an indwelling catheter. But on arrival, it is apparent this 82-year-old patient does not have a routine UTI. Although the urine in the catheter bag does appear cloudy and tests positive for red and white blood cells, the patient is unusually confused and has a decreased level of consciousness. Clinicians observe petechiae all over the body.

Lab tests are drawn and sent as an IV line is initiated. The prescribing provider orders antibiotics for apparent sepsis before transfer to the med/surg unit. Within hours, the patient's condition declines. Lab tests demonstrate low platelet and fibrinogen levels and elevated prothrombin times. Bright red blood begins to ooze from the patient's rectum, and the venipuncture and IV sites begin to bleed. The patient is unresponsive. The physician diagnoses disseminated intravascular coagulation (DIC) and summons the family to determine whether aggressive treatment is warranted.

DIC refers to a complex disorder of the blood characterized by abnormal clotting, leading to consumption of clotting factors that ultimately results in abnormal bleeding.

This example relates to the content outline earlier in the chapter. It also illustrates the importance of defining the topic after you introduce it to ensure everyone starts from the same reference point.

> **Confidence Booster**
>
> Capturing readers' attention in the first paragraph is essential and can make the difference in their decision to read more or not. Writing lede sentences or introductory case studies can be fun and creative, but it takes time and practice. Try writing several different ledes, and then have your spouse, friends, and colleagues read them and tell you whether they're drawn into the narrative. Don't get discouraged if you don't achieve the wow effect at first; just keep trying and eventually you'll dazzle them.

In the Middle

You have already created an outline to follow. The narrative typically begins with more general information, introducing the main topics, and then subsequent paragraphs discuss them in detail, using headings to break up the text. Consider the example of writing about shingles. One logical way to discuss the topic is by etiology, risk factors, signs and symptoms, diagnosis, treatment options, and nursing interventions. Some publications may prefer a traditional approach to headings, such as "Signs and Symptoms," "Diagnosis," "Treatment," and "Nursing Interventions." Others may welcome a more creative use of words to give them pizzazz.

Adding meaningful clinical visual aids, such as tables, graphs, and diagrams, can illustrate information, enhance the narrative, and improve memory retention. The range of interactivity that can be built into online activities today has been revolutionized by ongoing technological advancements. Visual aids can also break up text-laden layouts, making the learning activity more reader friendly. (Learn more about these techniques in Chapter 7.) If you're writing the activity for an education company, you might ask if budget and resources make it possible for you to have short videos or interactive exercises (e.g., having the participant label a figure illustrating the coagulation cascade) within the activity to illustrate key points.

Writing for Different Specialties

Nursing specialties have a unique vocabulary, so you will need to simplify the language in a learning activity for nurses outside the specialty to increase readability and comprehension. For example, an oncology nurse writing about bone marrow transplantation for a general nursing population will need to define more terminology than if writing for peers.

> **Evidence-Based Practice**
>
> Evidence-based practice (EBP) is now an integral part of nursing. You already know that EBP combines clinical expertise with the best available evidence, as well as patient values and preferences, for improved outcomes. But now it's your job to find the strongest evidence to support the information in your CE. You can learn more about finding sources in Chapter 4.
>
> Once you find the evidence, evaluate it using appraisal tools such as those from the Johns Hopkins Nursing Evidence-Based Practice Model (https://browse.welch.jhmi.edu/nursing_resources/jhnebp) or those in the book *Evidence-Based Practice in Nursing & Healthcare: A Guide to Best Practice*, 5th Edition, by Melnyk and Fineout-Overholt (2023).

Often, a simple one- or two-word explanation helps to jolt the memory of your audience or explain technical jargon. Provide a brief but enlightening definition of a condition:

- *Bradykinesia*: Slow movement or slow reflexes, which is often an early sign of Parkinson's disease.
- *Costochondritis*: Pain in the chest caused by inflammation of the cartilage connecting the ribs to the sternum.

Developing IPCE presents additional challenges to ensure the appropriate wording is understandable to the healthcare disciplines targeted in the course. For example, consider this narrative from an IPCE activity for nurses and physical therapists:

> Functional electrical stimulation (FES) may reduce foot drop and improve obstacle avoidance when used on the peroneal nerve. Also called "neuromuscular stimulation," FES uses electrical current to stimulate nerves, innervating affected extremities.

In this case, a short definition is needed because although physical therapists will likely know FES, nurses may not be familiar with the term.

Conclude Your Learning Activity

At the end of your learning activity, include one or two summary paragraphs that highlight your main points and remind learners about the gist of the activity. You began with a broad approach, and now you finish with it.

Note how the author reiterates the key point in the following conclusion paragraph:

Traumatic Brain Injury (TBI)

TBI is a leading cause of trauma-related death. Nurses are critical in preventing or minimizing irreversible brain damage. The priorities center on proper oxygenation, ventilation, and adequate circulation. Preserving neurologic function and preventing secondary injury due to shock and hypoxia are also important. By becoming familiar with brain injuries and their care, nurses can better plan and provide the special care that a patient with TBI needs.

Depending on the style of the publication, it also may be appropriate to refer the learner to additional resources to further expand their knowledge on the topic to enhance patient care/outcomes. For example, if the activity includes information on aromatherapy, the National Center for Complementary and Integrative Health might be a good resource

You're on your way home, and it's time to look back and think about what you've experienced along the way. The next step is writing the post-test.

Test Knowledge

What level of knowledge do you want to test the learner on? Publications and organizations differ as to the requirements for questions and feedback designed to assess learning, based on the audience and accreditation types. For instance, some require authors to provide feedback as to why the right answer is correct, and why the distractors are wrong. You can learn about the requirements in the author guidelines.

Many educational activities today begin with a pre-test to establish baseline knowledge before the educational intervention starts. This score can be compared to the post-test results to demonstrate knowledge acquisition from the educational activity. In most cases, the questions in the pre- and post-tests are the same so that an effective comparison can be made between the two scores.

The size of the target audience also influences the type of exam. Fixed-choice questions that require learners to select the correct response from several choices or supply a word or short phrase to answer a question (e.g., multiple-choice questions and questions involving matching or completing phrases) are geared toward larger groups. Open-ended questions (e.g., short-answer essays, extended-response essays, or problem-solving quizzes) are better suited to smaller groups. Evaluations for interactive online learning activities might include short video clips of scenarios for learners to respond to.

Tests should cover all the objectives and desired outcomes. Mapping the questions to the objectives/outcomes helps. For example, if a single-contact-hour NCPD activity has four objectives/outcomes, and the publication standard is 12 test questions, you should have three questions that test the learner's ability to meet each of the objectives/outcomes.

Q *As the author, will I write the post-test?*

A The publication editors may write the post-test or ask you to. Check the journal's author guidelines to see what is required.

Remember Bloom's taxonomy, which is used to write objectives? You should also apply it to writing test questions by considering the cognitive levels described earlier in the chapter. The taxonomy reminds you about the types of thinking required to answer test questions.

Example 19.4 contains a summary of the taxonomy and an example of a question for each level.

Multiple-Choice Questions

Multiple-choice questions are the most widely used method to test learners' knowledge and comprehension. Typically, they have three parts:

- The stem (the question)
- The correct answer
- Multiple incorrect options (distractors)

Knowledge: Memorize and recall facts.

    Example: What is a major cause of respiratory depression?

Comprehension: Understand and interpret important information.

    Example: Hemorrhagic stroke is _____.

Application: Apply new concepts to another situation.

    Example: Which blood products would be used to improve tissue oxygenation if the complete blood count indicates a low hemoglobin and hematocrit?

Analysis: Break down new information into parts to differentiate between them.

    Example: What is the difference between a transfusion of packed red blood cells and whole blood?

Synthesis: Take various pieces of information and form a whole, creating a pattern where it didn't exist.

    Example: What nursing diagnosis can be formulated based on the patient's signs and symptoms, physical exam, and lab tests?

Evaluation: Assess and conclude the value of materials.

    Example: Of the two treatment options, which would be more efficacious for the patient's condition?

EXAMPLE 19.4 Taxonomy levels and sample questions.

It's best to write the correct answer before writing the distractors. This order helps you focus on the one clearly correct answer. It's also best to create distractors that are plausible to the less knowledgeable learner and are of similar length and complexity to the correct answer option (Minnesota State University, n.d.).

Multiple-choice questions are a highly structured, effective method to measure a learner's achievement and an easy, reliable format for scoring and performance comparison. Although multiple-choice questions offer several advantages, they have limitations, as well:

- Constructing the questions is time-consuming.
- Writing plausible distractors and testing higher levels of learning is difficult.

Here are a few tips for writing multiple-choice questions.

Strive to:

- Base the questions on the instructional objectives.
- Test for important information that affects clinical practice.
- Focus on a single problem or idea for each question.
- Provide plausible distractors. You might consider options that represent common practice mistakes.
- Test for higher-level thinking whenever possible.

Avoid:

- Providing cues from one question to another
- Being overly specific or including technical information
- Using verbatim phrasing
- Writing questions based on opinions
- Using absolute terms such as "always" or "never"

Tips for writing the stem include:

- Phrase it as clearly and succinctly as possible.
- Include the central idea in the stem.
- Include language in the stem that would have been repeated in each answer option.
- Use a question or completion form.
- Put a blank space at the end of completion questions.
- Avoid negative phrasing, such as "not" or "except"; if negative words must be used, highlight or capitalize them: for example, "NOT."

Writing answers can be just as challenging as writing the questions, particularly when it comes to developing distractors. Here are some tips you can use:

- Ensure there is only one correct answer.
- Keep the options about the same length, and parallel in grammatical structure.
- Limit the number of answers to three to five options.
- Use distractors that seem plausible but are incorrect.
- Avoid using phrases taken directly from the text.
- Use the following sparingly: all, always, never, usually, typically, all of the above, none of the above.
- Make options as similar as possible to increase the difficulty.
- Avoid offering trick answers.

Look at some examples of well-written multiple-choice questions. Try to identify what level of thinking the questions test the learner on and what makes them effective.

1. Which aneurysm is most common?
    a) Saccular
    b) Fusiform
    c) Mycotic
    d) Infectious

Note the clear central idea with only one correct answer and that the distractors are parallel in length.

2. In DIC, with low fibrinogen levels, the registered nurse can expect to administer _____.
    a) Vitamin K
    b) Cryoprecipitate
    c) Fresh frozen plasma
    d) Aminocaproic acid

Again, note the one central idea, a blank at the end of the question, and answers that are parallel in length and grammar.

1. a, 2. b

Multiple-Choice Questions and Case Studies

Using multiple-choice questions with case studies provides an opportunity to encourage critical thinking and test a higher level of thinking, such as the application level on Bloom's taxonomy scale. Case studies represent real-life clinical situations from which learners are challenged to apply the didactic information presented in the learning activity. They can range from short and simple to lengthy and complex.

Unlike the introductory case study leading into the CE learning activity, though, the case study with multiple-choice questions tests the learners' knowledge and comprehension of a topic. Sometimes used before starting the activity, this method pre-tests the learners' knowledge base.

Multiple-choice questions should require learners to apply the information gleaned from the activity to the case study. The rationale for correct and incorrect answers is often included for additional learning. This format works especially well online; after users answer a question, they can see the rationale or explanation, which reinforces learning.

Here is an example of a case study used to test learners' knowledge before and after the activity. What level of thinking does it test learners on? (Note that learners are told this is not a real patient. If you use a real patient, protect privacy by changing identifying information; state that the name of the patient and all identifying information have been changed.)

Cystic Fibrosis

Tim (not a real patient), a 32-year-old man with cystic fibrosis, arrived in the pulmonary clinic with a one-week history of increased cough, increased sputum production, intermittent fevers to 101 °F, and increased shortness of breath at rest. He had called the clinic three days earlier and spoke to the nurse practitioner, who started him on oral ciprofloxacin and inhaled tobramycin, with the understanding that if he didn't improve in one to two days, he should come in for evaluation and probable admission. Tim's symptoms continued to worsen. Vital signs upon arrival were temperature: 38.6 °F, respiratory rate: 28 breaths per minute, pulse: 110 beats per minute, blood pressure: 126/76 mm Hg, and oxygen saturation via pulse oximetry: 97% on room air. Tim reported a three-pound weight loss over the past week. Bloodwork revealed a blood sugar level of 200 mg/dL. Upon examination, he had significant crackles, mainly noted in the right upper lobe, was wheezing, and appeared very fatigued. Tim was admitted for IV antibiotics and aggressive pulmonary hygiene.

1. Upon Tim's arrival at the clinic, after obtaining the vital signs, the healthcare provider should:
    a) Place a nasal cannula to keep the patient's oxygen saturation above 95%
    b) Obtain a sputum culture
    c) Administer pancreatic enzymes
    d) Have the patient perform incentive spirometry

2. The most likely cause of Tim's elevated blood glucose level is:
    a) Physical stress
    b) Use of corticosteroids
    c) Dehydration
    d) Cystic fibrosis-related diabetes

3. To address Tim's weight loss during his exacerbation, the recommended diet should:
    a) Increase calories without restriction
    b) Decrease intake of dairy products
    c) Eliminate the intake of fats
    d) Limit calories to complex carbohydrates and protein

4. The provider prescribes albuterol for Tim's wheezing. The purpose of albuterol is to:
    a) Decrease viscosity of the mucus in the airway
    b) Open the airways and promote mucociliary clearance
    c) Decrease risk of pulmonary infection
    d) Decrease airway edema

1. b — Tim's three-day course of ciprofloxacin and tobramycin were ineffective. Sputum culture will determine the most effective antibiotic(s) for the infection.
2. d — Cystic fibrosis-related diabetes is the most common non-pulmonary complication in patients with cystic fibrosis.
3. a — Patients with cystic fibrosis should follow a diet without restrictions and add extra calories during a period of exacerbation.
4. b — Albuterol is a bronchodilator that is used to relax the smooth muscle surrounding the bronchi, to open the airways and help with mucociliary clearance.

Journey's End

Your journey has almost come to an end. You imparted new, important information that will affect the clinical practice of those who came along for the ride. You successfully developed your NCPD or IPCE activity by providing a broad, one-sentence goal statement; clear, succinct instructional objectives or outcome statements; an outline that shows the logical progression of the content; a well-written, researched narrative that reflects the outline; and a well-constructed exam and/or case study.

Whether nearby or in a distant land, clinicians who read your learning activity may change and improve their practice. As a final part of your journey, you can consider how you can measure the impact of your educational activity on patient outcomes. There are several ways to do this, including the use of post-activity evaluations, follow-up surveys at regular intervals, chart audits, and clinical observation of practice changes. Documenting the change in clinical practice and the subsequent improvements in patient outcomes is an important step that completes your journey and provides a meaningful destination or endpoint.

Write Now!

1. Describe the goal of an educational activity and form three learning objectives. Compare these with the sample objectives in this chapter.

2. Pick an NCPD article from a journal and develop one post-test question for it. Compare what you have written with the criteria in this chapter to evaluate the question.

References

Accreditation Council for Continuing Medical Education. (n.d.). *Defining interprofessional continuing education.* https://www.accme.org/resources/video-resources/cme-collaborations/defining-interprofessional-continuing-education

Andreev, I. (2023). Learning outcomes. *Valamis Learning Solutions.* https://www.valamis.com/hub/learning-outcomes

Bloom, B. S. (Ed.), Engelhart, M. D., Furst, E. J., Hill, W. H., & Krathwohl, D. R. (1956). *Taxonomy of educational objectives.* David McKay Company, Inc.

Heale, R., & Twycross, A. (2018). What is a case study? *Evidence-Based Nursing, 21*(1), 7–8. http://dx.doi.org/10.1136/eb-2017-102845

Howson, A. (2023). Practical strategies for creating CME/CE content: Insights from adult learning scholarship. *American Medical Writers Association Journal, 38*(2), 47–50. https://doi.org/10.55752/amwa.2023.192

Joint Accreditation for Interprofessional Continuing Education. (2023). *About us.* https://jointaccreditation.org/about-joint-accreditation/

Mager, R. F. (1997). *Preparing instructional objectives: A critical tool in development of effective instruction* (3rd ed.). Center for Effective Performance.

Melnyk, B. M., & Fineout-Overholt, E. (2023). *Evidence-based practice in nursing & healthcare: A guide to best practice* (5th ed.). Wolters Kluwer Health.

Merriam, S. B., & Baumgartner, L. M. (2020). *Learning in adulthood: A comprehensive guide* (4th ed.). Jossey-Bass.

Minnesota State University. (n.d.). *MNSU guide to writing good multiple choice quizzes and exams.* https://cornerstone.lib.mnsu.edu/cgi/viewcontent.cgi?article=1112&context=all

Moore, D. E., Jr., Green, J. S., & Gallis, H. A. (2009). Achieving desired results and improved outcomes: integrating planning and assessment throughout learning activities. *Journal of Continuing Education for Health Professionals, 29*(1), 1–15. https://doi.org/10.1002/chp.20001

Morris, S., & Guardian US Interactive Team. (2018, Feb. 15). Mass shootings in the US: There have been 1,624 in 1,870 days. *The Guardian.* Gun Violence Archive. https://www.theguardian.com/us-news/ng-interactive/2017/oct/02/america-mass-shootings-gun-violence

Nabizadeh-Gharghozar, Z., Masoudi Alavi, N., & Mirbagher Ajorpaz, N. (2021). Clinical competence in nursing: A hybrid concept analysis. *Nurse Education Today, 97.* https://doi.org/10.1016/j.nedt.2020.104728

National Council of State Boards of Nursing. (2022). *National nursing workforce study.* https://www.ncsbn.org/research/recent-research/workforce.page

Nayak, N. (2023, May 9). Artificial intelligence in healthcare: Transforming patient experience. *Classic Informatics.* https://www.classicinformatics.com/blog/artificial-intelligence-in-healthcare-transforming-patient-experience#:~:text=Providing%20Personalized%20Care%20To%20Improve%20Patient%20Condition&text=Using%20AI%20can%20help%20overcome,and%20asking%20patients%20relevant%20questions

Sud, A., Hodgson, K., Bloch, G. & Upshur, R. (2022). A conceptual framework for continuing medical education and population health. *Teaching and Learning in Medicine, 34*(5), 541–555. https://doi.org/10.1080/10401334.2021.1950540

Tan, K., Chong, M. C., Subramaniam, P., & Wong, L. P. (2018). The effectiveness of outcome-based education on the competencies of nursing students: A systematic review. *Nurse Education Today, 64,* 180–189. https://doi.org/10.1016/j.nedt.2017.12.030

Writing the Nursing Narrative

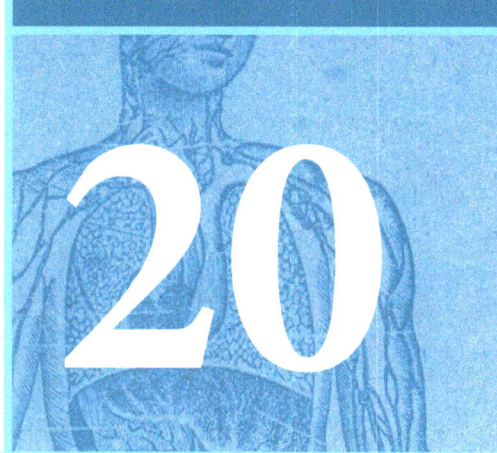

–Marianne Ditomassi, DNP, MBA, RN, NEA-BC, FAAN

WHAT YOU'LL LEARN IN THIS CHAPTER

- Nurses write narratives for personal reflection, professional advancement, and publication.
- Consider writing narratives about advocacy, error, interdisciplinary teamwork, reflection, resilience, and skill acquisition.
- When crafting the narrative, describe what you perceived with your senses; share your thoughts, reasoning processes, and feelings.

"We are all storytellers. We all live in a network of stories. There isn't a stronger connection between people than storytelling."
–Jimmy Neil Smith

Stories are authentic human experiences. Perhaps it's because storytelling is so woven into the human experience that we often minimize how central stories have been in shaping who we are, what we do, how we do it, and how we are perceived. This chapter demonstrates how the power of your stories of practice can not only expand your own understanding of your practice and opportunities for continued professional growth and development, but also influence the image of the nursing profession by making visible that which is often invisible—what nurses *do*.

Ask veteran nurses what they remember from student days, and they won't explain the flow of blood through the chambers of a normal heart or recite the stages of labor. They'll tell you a story about a patient they cared for and possibly the instructor or preceptor who guided them. Or watch how people in an audience raise their eyes from their cellphones and tablets when they hear the speaker say, "Let me tell you a story." People shift in their seats and lean forward in anticipation.

We use stories to drive home a point when we're teaching a student, a preceptee, or a patient. We also convey our feelings through stories, and we certainly juggle all kinds of feelings in our daily practice: awe, gratitude, weariness, sadness, joy, helplessness, anger, frustration, and satisfaction.

As readers or authors, some of us have already discovered the power of the written narrative to deepen our understanding of nursing and inspire our appreciation. This chapter will help you discover that power—and learn how to share it.

The author wishes to acknowledge the contributions of Mary Ellin Smith, who cowrote this chapter in previous editions.

The Nature of Narratives

The narrative differs from the types of writing described in other sections of this book. It's personal and subjective, and it's written in the first person. It flows from emotional experiences, sensory perceptions, and both intuitive and intellectual knowing. Narratives unearth golden nuggets of knowledge, sometimes hidden in clinical practice, and they enrich our understanding of our work. Just as important to the profession as clinical, research, and professional development articles, narrative writing educates, edifies, inspires, and clarifies; it may even serve as the springboard for a quality improvement (QI) project or formal research. Nursing and medical history tells us that specific observations in everyday practice have led to scientific discoveries and new theories.

In her classic 1984 book, *From Novice to Expert: Excellence and Power in Clinical Nursing Practice*, Patricia Benner opened the eyes of nurses and other healthcare providers around the world to the importance of the narrative. In the foreword to the 2000 commemorative edition of the book, Benner writes:

> In developing a narrative account of experiential learning, the storyteller learns from telling the story. Teaching reflection allows clinicians to identify concerns that organize the story; identify notions of good embedded in the story; identify relational, communicative, and collaborative skills; and articulate newly developing clinical knowledge. (Benner, 2000, pp. vii–viii)

Narratives allow clinicians to reflect on who the patient is and how that knowledge informs their care, their clinical decision-making, and their work with the members of the healthcare team. Narratives are also valuable for students (Benner et al., 2010). They can be used to articulate best practices in the classroom and in students' experience of integrating the theory they learned with the reality of the clinical setting. Using narratives with students is a way for them to learn about nursing and understand the complexity, nuance, the unique characteristics of each patient and family, and individual responses to illness, recovery, and loss (Benner et al., 1999). Nurse leaders also can benefit from writing narratives: Fitzpatrick and Kim (2023) reported that leaders who participated in a nursing narrative writing workshop for clinicians and leaders were able to share experiences and coping mechanisms that helped them navigate challenges and foster resilience.

Benefits of Narratives

Excellent nursing care is often invisible—patients leave the hospital without skin breakdown or infection; patients learn how to manage complex medication management and treatments; and, in situations of grief and trauma, patients receive support and compassion—but how does all this happen? Simply viewing the nurse in practice wouldn't fully answer the question. To know the complete answer, we need to hear nurses' stories that reveal what they were thinking and seeing, and perhaps how past experiences shaped their actions and reactions.

Through telling stories, we learn a great deal from one another—for example: how to prevent complications, recognize subtle changes in a patient's condition, approach patients with substance use disorders, communicate with team members, and teach and console family members. Anecdotes and stories can even serve as the basis of inquiry for evidence-based practice projects and research studies.

Many nurses dismiss the idea of writing and sharing narratives, believing that they were just doing their job and that anyone would know or do what they did. But it's this belief that has prevented the public, and even some nurses, from fully understanding the power, complexity, and influence that nurses have in healthcare. Sharing our stories through narratives is one way to enhance this understanding.

Narratives serve many other purposes too. Practicing in complex, rapidly changing environments can often prevent nurses from fully reflecting on what they are experiencing. We meet patients on their best days and on their worst; we bear witness to tragedy and injustice. For many of us, sharing those stories with friends and loved ones may not be possible because we know our stories can spark worry or distress in those outside the healthcare profession. But not expressing our reflections about events can lead to unhealthy rumination and difficulty learning from and moving on from the experience. Narratives have been thought to assist in avoiding these patterns (Newman, 2016; Sherman, 2018).

And even though nursing can exact an emotional toll on the most mature and well-adjusted person, narrative writing can serve as an antidote. In fact, researchers have found that storytelling is associated with beneficial effects in the form of decreased physical symptoms of disease and healing of emotional and mental trauma (DeSalvo, 2000; Gao, 2022; Newman, 2016; Smyth et al., 1999).

Types of Narratives

Benner's work has helped nurses understand the power of the personal narrative to teach, enlighten, reveal, and inspire. She provided guidelines for writing narratives and described many types of nursing situations that lend themselves to a narrative. Topics for narratives are as varied as the nurses who write them and include:

- Advocacy
- Error
- Interdisciplinary teamwork
- Reflection
- Resilience
- Skill acquisition

Here's a closer look at each of these.

Advocacy

Patient safety requires nurses to be a patient's advocate. Nurses use their position to support, protect, or speak out for the rights and interests of others, and have long claimed patient advocacy as fundamental to their practice. The American Nurses Association's *Code of Ethics for Nurses with Interpretive Statements* and *Scope and Standards of Nursing Practice* clearly identify nurses' ethical and professional responsibility for protecting the safety and rights of their patients (Zolnierek, 2012). The following excerpt from a narrative by Jenna Staid, RN, a clinical nurse on a general medical unit, demonstrates her advocacy for her patient. (Note: All names of patients in the "Types of Narratives" sections are fictitious, but the narratives are real.) Staid writes of caring for a patient with chronic obstructive pulmonary disease (COPD) whose anxiety is heightened during hospitalization:

> Mary arrived on the unit highly anxious and with elevated respirations to the high 30s with an oxygen saturation of 100% on 5 liters of oxygen via nasal cannula. She adamantly refused to allow her oxygen to be titrated down. At this point I felt safe taking the risk of having her oxygen level high because she had been living and had been compensating for her COPD; I knew the risk of Mary maintaining her oxygen levels at 100% was better than increasing her anxiety. I sat with her and helped her relax through conversation about her, her life, and her supports at home. Mary's breathing began to slow, I began a conversation with her about possibly starting to wean her respirations down slowly at her own pace today; I wanted to give Mary control of the process. Mary was hesitant at first but said "maybe later." I left the room knowing that she needed trust, time, and patience before she would agree to have her oxygen weaned.
>
> I consulted with the social worker, asking her to meet with Mary to better understand the reasons she was so anxious. After their visit, the social worker shared that Mary felt anxious about being in the hospital and hated going to the doctor. This reinforced my plan to make Mary an active participant in her care, including the schedule to wean down her oxygen. I huddled with the medical team before they entered her room and told them that while Mary remained anxious, we would work to decrease her oxygen level during the shift. They agreed with the plan and we entered her room.
>
> As the team introduced themselves, the intern walked to the head of the bed and decreased Mary's oxygen, which she immediately noticed. She became highly anxious, her oxygen level decreased, she called out for a nebulizer treatment, and she kicked everyone out of the room. While the intern had the best of intentions in wishing to decrease Mary's oxygen level, the patient was too fragile at that point; she felt betrayed that this would occur without warning.
>
> After the patient stabilized, I met with the intern. I told her that I knew she was trying to help Mary, but I also expressed how Mary felt about what was done—that her already fragile trust had been damaged. The intern recognized the impact of her actions and asked to apologize to Mary. Mary listened and accepted her apology. Mary asked that she be placed on 6 liters and the intern agreed; after that, her oxygen level returned to 100%.
>
> As Mary's anxiety decreased, I asked her if she was ready to begin to decrease her oxygen back to 5 liters and she agreed. I began to educate her about COPD and watched as she moved from looking puzzled to more engaged and asked for her oxygen to be lowered to 4 liters.

As I was preparing to leave at the end of my shift, I was called to Mary's room, I expected her to be anxious, but instead I was greeted by her request to have her oxygen lowered to 3 liters.

Notes on the Narrative

In this narrative, Staid uses both clinical knowledge and the ability to build a therapeutic relationship with Mary to advocate for her to control how many liters of oxygen she was comfortable with and to address the intern's actions. Staid recognizes the risk in maintaining Mary on such a high level of oxygen, but her advocacy allows the patient time to develop trust with the team; that trust is tested by the intern's actions. Staid quickly addresses the event and facilitates the intern's apology to Mary. Advocacy requires knowledge (of the patient and the clinical situation), skill, and, at times, clinically sound risk-taking. All these elements are present in Staid's narrative.

Another type of advocacy is writing a letter of recommendation for someone applying for school, a position, or an award. The use of a clinical narrative can help illustrate the traits you'd like to showcase for an applicant (Herrity, 2023). The following excerpt from a letter of recommendation by Stephanie Qualls, MSN, RN, ACCNS-AG, nurse director of a neuroscience ICU, for Kathryn Peters, RN, a clinical nurse pursuing her master's to become a family nurse practitioner in primary care, includes a clinical example demonstrating Peters's readiness to pursue an advanced degree.

> Please accept this letter of support for Kathryn Peters. She is a nurse who constantly demonstrates strong clinical knowledge, compassion, teamwork and patient and family relationships in her daily practice. Kathryn's critical thinking and collaborative nature are frequently highlighted as she is often assigned the most complex critically ill patients.
>
> Kathryn was caring for a gentleman in his forties who had bilateral ischemic strokes. His admission lasted six weeks and Kathryn cared for him most of his time on the unit and specifically on admission when he was extremely unstable and critically ill and on the day of transfer. During the initial admission period, the patient suffered from profound neurologic deficits due to the ischemia. He required mechanical ventilation due to decreased level of consciousness. The most concerning immediate complication was the amount of cerebral edema the patient had due to the ischemia. The edema was treated with two alternating hyperosmolar infusions which can cause profound metabolic disarray and carries a risk of acute kidney injury. Katheryn's excellent assessment skills were necessary to ensure there were no clinical signs or symptoms that the patient's cerebral edema was worsening. Her astute assessment found the patient to have a neurologic change. Quickly she alerted both the Neuro ICU responding clinician and the Neurosurgery resident who responded to the bedside. Kathryn knew the patient could not receive any further hyperosmolar therapy and her past experience allowed her to anticipate that the patient would likely be heading to surgery, so she notified the respiratory therapist and began preparing for transport for an emergent suboccipital craniectomy. Kathryn's preparedness allowed her to immediately start transporting the patient to the operating room, illustrating her ability to adapt and be flexible when managing unexpected clinical situations.
>
> While caring for this patient, Kathryn ensured she developed a strong rapport with the patient's wife who was constantly at his bedside. She recognized that family members often feel helpless in the early stages of their loved one's critical illness and encouraged her to share stories about the patient and to decorate the room with photos and some of the patient's favorite things. Later in the patient's admission, the time Kathryn devoted to developing the rapport with the patient's wife paid dividends. The patient had received a percutaneous gastrostomy and tracheostomy and it was time to start talking about what recovery might look like. The trust the patient's wife had in Kathryn allowed her to be vulnerable and express her fear about transferring to a different unit as Kathryn had become "her rock."

Notes on the Narrative

By including a narrative in her letter of reference, Qualls illustrates Peters's expert ability to manage complex critical care, family dynamics, and symptoms of her patient as one example of the holistic care she provides to her patient and families. Peters's nursing practice demonstrates excellent clinical knowledge, teamwork, communication, patient advocacy, and strong patient and family relationships. For these reasons, she's poised for success in the family nurse practitioner program.

Error

A narrative about an error is often the most challenging type for a nurse to write, yet the process of reflection through writing serves as a way for the nurse to recover from the error and to promote a just culture within an organization. Clinicians who have made an error are often described as "second victims," defined by Scott et al. (2009) as individuals who are "traumatized by the event…feel as though they have failed the patient and second guess their clinical skills and knowledge" (p. 326). They may fear loss of their position or standing with their patient and colleagues. But writing and, if desired, sharing the narrative not only helps clinicians heal but also identifies system issues that can be addressed to keep patients safe.

In a 2014 presentation at Massachusetts General Hospital, Barbara Mackoff said narratives of breakdown, error, and near misses can be "leveraged to create exemplary practice models and strategies for increased patient safety; they can create a safe environment to discuss a taboo but crucial topic by building trusting teams and a culture of trust; they can also evoke for the listener, their own stories." To do that, Mackoff recommends this framework for the end of the narrative:

- **Describe the impact:** How were you changed by what happened?

- **Describe your reflection:** What information could have helped avoid the situation? Are there alternatives you might have considered but did not? Were there small mistakes that led to a bigger mistake?

- **Give the story a different ending:** How could this situation have ended differently—without the event you described?

- **Revise the situation:** What are the relationships, systems, or choices that would lead to a different ending?

- **Describe your wisdom:** How would you behave differently if you were in the situation again? What new commitments and practices have resulted from what you learned?

The following excerpts of a narrative, written by Lisette Packer, RN, a clinical nurse on an oncology unit, tell the story of a medication error and demonstrate how writing about an error can identify a system issue and allow the nurse to reflect on what occurred. Packer's patient was admitted in a pain crisis and was started on high-concentration hydromorphone by patient-controlled analgesia (PCA), then switched to hydromorphone 0.5 mg/mL by continuous infusion at 3 mg/hr with clinician boluses as needed. Packer writes of returning to work the next day:

> I came back to work, and my nursing director told me an error had been made with Mrs. L.'s PCA pump that involved me and six other nurses. Mrs. L.'s PCA pump was set to administer high-concentration hydromorphone (10 mg/mL) rather than hydromorphone 0.5 mg/mL. We had the correct medication hanging, the PCA settings were correct, but the wrong concentration was programmed into the pump. This resulted in the patient receiving 0.15 mg/hr rather than the 3 mg/hr she was supposed to be receiving.

Here is how Packer applies Mackoff's framework to her narrative:

> **Describe the impact:** I was devastated to hear that I had made a mistake and that because I didn't catch the mistake, Mrs. L. was in significant pain for eight hours.
>
> **Describe your reflection:** If the PCA screen read differently, there would be less chance of this happening. The screen displays high concentration on one line and underneath it, it says hydromorphone. The concentration and drug should all be on the same line. Had I stopped to do the math, I would have realized that the bag would have needed to be changed. I also wonder if the team meant to change the order from high concentration to regular; she was receiving large amounts of hydromorphone, so a high-concentration order would make sense.
>
> **Give the story a different ending:** This patient should not have experienced the pain she did. Ideally, we should have started her on a PCA and titrated up as needed with comfort being the goal.

Revise the situation: Had the nurse who received the order to change the PCA to regular concentration from high concentration completely reset the pump and started as a new patient, this might not have happened. Had I stopped to do the math halfway through my shift, I would have realized the problem.

Describe your wisdom: Since this experience, I look at PCAs differently. I have shared this story with all the nurses on the unit, and I now triple check the PCA orders and medication concentration. One of the suggestions was having pharmacy highlight high-concentration medications to remind the nurse of the dose concentration.

Notes on the Narrative

Note how Packer states the facts of the event without interjecting her opinion, making excuses, or blaming others. Writing the narrative helped her move from blaming herself for the error to recognizing the various system issues that allowed the error, and then to problem-solving how this event could be avoided. Using Mackoff's framework, Packer is able to delve into what occurred and reflect on the personal impact of the event. The opportunity to write and share these narratives has an added benefit—they help organizations to move their safety culture in ways that build open and safe environments.

Interdisciplinary Teamwork

Teamwork and collaboration play an important role in quality and safety. While we often focus on interdisciplinary teamwork and collaboration when the team agrees, the strength of the team is most apparent when its members stay engaged to resolve conflict or disagreement. Jesse MacKinnon, RN, a clinical nurse on an oncology unit, writes about caring for a young patient with an end-stage cancer diagnosis. The patient returns to the hospital after a brief stay at home and makes the decision to stop treatment—a decision his physicians, still hoping for a better outcome, are unable to comprehend. Rather than walk away, MacKinnon engages with the team members so they can listen to and respect the patient's wishes. He writes:

> John was in severe pain, couldn't eat, and had no quality of life to speak of. He confided in me that he was ready to die. All he wanted was to be comfortable and no longer pursue treatment. But John wasn't dying of cancer, he was dying of an infection. Many of his doctors didn't want to give up. There was great disagreement among the team; some passionately wanted to try and save him, while some compassionately wanted to let him go.
>
> I reminded them that John no longer wanted treatment. I called a meeting so the team could hear it directly from John. I arranged for John to meet with a representative from patient advocacy. At a second meeting, with my support, John explained why he no longer wanted to live "this life." The team finally understood. Treatment was stopped, and John spent a comfortable final two days with his sister and his beloved dogs.

Notes on the Narrative

All of John's caregivers wanted the best for him; his physicians wanted to give him more time, and MacKinnon wanted John's wishes heard and followed. Similar situations play out every day, and too often end in a stalemate where roles and authority overtake communication and collaboration. MacKinnon's narrative shows us how we can create a space where clinicians can disagree respectfully and then work to come together in the best interest of the patient. It's also worth pointing out that small details can create connections between readers and those in the story. MacKinnon's introduction of John's sister and his "beloved" dogs helps us relate to him as a person.

Reflection

In "What Is Reflective Practice?" Joy Amulya writes that the key to reflection is

> learning how to take perspective on one's own actions and experience—in other words, to examine that experience rather than just living it. By developing the ability to explore and be curious about our own experience and actions, we suddenly open up the possibilities of purposeful learning—derived not from books or experts but from our work and our lives. This is the possibility of reflection: to allow the possibility of learning through experience…before, during or after it has occurred. (n.d., p. 1)

Writing your narrative allows you to bring the reader into your story to seek clarity on what you were thinking and experiencing, and the judgments you were making in the situation. By its very nature, the narrative raises questions not only for those who read it, but for the writer as well. The writing process brings writers back to the event, no matter how long ago it happened, as they reflect on what occurred and the impact it has had on them and their practice.

Consider a narrative from Jing Lee, RN, a clinical nurse on the cardiac surgical intensive care unit (CSICU). She reflects on how the care of her patient, Mrs. O., taught her to advocate for her patient and herself, and how to work with an interdisciplinary team. Mrs. O. was a young woman from a rural part of the state who was admitted with cardiomyopathy; she was intubated and required a ventricular assist device. Her only significant past medical history was for substance use disorder. Slowly Mrs. O. began to make the first steps toward recovery, and Lee asked for a meeting to update the family. She writes:

> Before caring for Mrs. O., I had never participated in a family meeting. I was nervous before it started. I thought to myself, "How should I approach this?" In the CSICU, it is a difficult balance between being overly optimistic and yet realistic given the clinical situation. Mrs. O.'s husband and I spoke daily about her progress and plan of care. The trust I felt they had in my ability and the information I reported to them every day felt simultaneously like a gift and a burden. The weight of my responsibility to my patient extended to caring for her family members as well. To help prepare for the family meeting, I consulted with our unit social worker on how to handle such a sensitive matter and how to update them regarding her clinical condition. I also met with the attending physician and asked that we go over our talking points for the meeting beforehand so that we would present a consistent and cohesive plan of care.

Reflecting on her care of Mrs. O., Lee writes:

> The month and a half I spent caring for Mrs. O. taught me so much about myself as a nurse. She challenged my critical thinking skills as well as my interpersonal communication skills with having to coordinate her care with the interdisciplinary team as well as ensuring that her family members were included in clinical conversations. The experience I gained through our interaction will continue to impact my practice for the better.

Notes on the Narrative

As you gain confidence and experience, it can be challenging to remember what brought you to that level. Lee's narrative opens the door to that memory and can serve as a teaching tool for less experienced nurses. Writing reflective narratives enables us to transform the present and shape the future by revisiting the past. Note that Lee uses the phrase "a gift and a burden" to describe how she felt about the trust the family had in her. She could have said that the trust made her feel "glad to be trusted, but uncomfortable too," but instead she chooses specific, contradictory words that immediate convey her feelings, making the effect much more powerful. She also clearly describes the steps (e.g., consulting with the social worker) she took to prepare for the meeting, giving the readers strategies they could apply in their own practice.

Resilience

Even for the relatively self-aware and emotionally adept, struggles can take us by surprise. But learning healthy ways to move through adversity can help you cope better, recover more quickly, or redirect yourself (Newman, 2016). Freshwater and colleagues define resiliency as "a positive adaptation to adverse situations combined with the ability to manage life-threatening situations successfully and courageously" (2023, p. 9). Rushton and colleagues (2015) write that resilience "involves the internal stability, awareness, and flexibility that enables a person to navigate high-stress situations in ways that reduce burnout and moral distress" (p. 418).

Newman (2016) points out that when something bad happens, we often relive the event over and over in our heads, rehashing the experience. This process is called *rumination*—a cognitive spinning of the wheels that doesn't promote healing or growth. The practice of expressive writing, writing about thoughts and feelings to help us cope with difficult situations, can move us forward by helping us gain new insights about the challenges in our lives (Lai et al., 2023; Newman, 2016). Sherman (2018) notes that researchers have found that negativity and rumination can become habits that need to be consciously managed and that reflective journaling can help break the habit.

Expressive writing starts with a "free write," where you write quickly and without judgment about an issue, exploring your deepest thoughts and feelings surrounding it. As Anne Lamott, author of the classic book *Bird by Bird: Some Instructions on Writing and Life*, advises, "Start by getting something—anything—down on paper" (1995, p. 25). Once this draft is completed, you can choose to contemplate some of the upsides of the situation, such as what you have learned. The more you can leverage challenges as opportunities to grow and evolve, the more resilient you are likely to be.

Elizabeth Hurton, RN, a nurse on general surgery, writes in her narrative:

> I try to remember the many patients who have helped me grow and develop as a clinician by writing a line or two about them in a notebook I keep in my locker at the end of the shift so that the lessons they have taught me are always forefront in my mind as I reread previous passages. As nurses, I find that we all have different ways to cope with the emotional toll our work can take. I know that by writing down these learning experiences from what may be an otherwise devastating patient can help me refocus my thinking and emotions.

Hurton notes how her care of a gender non-binary patient, Jade, made her reflect on issues of implicit bias: "Knowing that I grew up in a very traditional family setting and only meeting openly LGBTQ peers in college for the first time, I have worked toward making no assumptions about the relationships among the people in the room with the patient as well as the patient's relationship history. I know these steps will go a long way in making someone feel included and trusting of a healthcare setting."

Hurton describes her care of Jade, who was admitted for ostomy reversal, and how she worked to develop the nurse-patient relationship. While Jade initially recovered without incident, Hurton grew concerned as Jade complained of increasing pain and abdominal distention, all considered by the surgical team as not unusual given the surgery. However, Hurton knew Jade and recognized that this was unusual, though the surgical team focused on their assessment that Jade was following a slow but steady recovery trajectory. Hurton wasn't convinced and notified the nursing supervisor and the rapid response team. Jade was soon transferred to the ICU, where the source of the bleeding was identified; life support became necessary. As the patient's condition deteriorated, Jade's family made the difficult decision to withdraw care; Jade died surrounded by family and friends.

Notes on the Narrative

We imagine that for many nurses this narrative will sound familiar. There are occasions when you recognize subtle changes in your patient—so subtle that other members of the team who don't know the patient as well or don't have the same experience dismiss them, which can lead to delayed treatment. It's easy at these times to focus on what was not done and to become discouraged or disengaged. Hurton shows us that narratives provide the opportunity for the clinician to learn from the experience and to become more resilient. She writes:

> I think about Jade often, I hope that they knew just how much the nurses cared for them and were advocating for them. Though this particular experience will always stay with me as an instance I felt my concerns were not being addressed by the patient's responding team, I also feel it is an example of where my colleagues and I advocated for our patient. I will always be proud of that effort.

Skill Acquisition

Ives Erickson and colleagues (2015) note that narratives build skilled clinicians. Patricia Benner's classic book, *From Novice to Expert: Excellence and Power in Clinical Nursing Practice* (1984, 2000), uses narratives to articulate and describe nurses' changing clinical world as they transition along the continuum of novice to expert. Benner's work is built on the Dreyfus Model of Skill Acquisition (Dreyfus & Dreyfus, 1986). Together, the Dreyfus brothers' and Benner's research describes that skilled know-how comes not just from knowing what to do—the performance or a task, knowing the policy or attending a class—but how and when to do it, which occurs in the active engagement in clinical practice. Nurses at different levels of experience live in different clinical worlds, so their narratives reflect the world they are living in, what they are paying attention to, and how they make sense of the experience.

Many nursing departments require nurses to include at least one exemplar as part of a portfolio submitted for advancement or recognition. For recognition, your narrative should clearly portray a situation in which your level of expertise reflects the criteria for that level. Applications for designation as a Magnet facility by the American Nurses Credentialing Center (ANCC) include exemplars of practice, which help illustrate that nursing practice meets the ANCC's high standards.

The following excerpts are from narratives written by nurses at one of the four levels of skill acquisition (entry, clinician, advanced clinician, and clinical scholar) as defined by the MGH Clinical Recognition Program (Ives Erickson et al., 2008), which was based on the Dreyfus Model of Skill Acquisition and Benner's work. Clinicians at all levels are required to write a narrative in order to be recognized.

Entry level. Patrick Johnson, RN, then a new graduate, wrote about learning how a patient's wife processed information and how he needed to change his interactions with her to ensure she understood her husband's condition. He writes:

> Mrs. A. still panicked whenever Mr. A. did anything out of the ordinary, such as cough or sigh. I tried to think of something I could do to help her relax. Again, I offered her reassurance and explained our monitoring system. Even though I was repeating the same information I had told her earlier, this time it seemed to bring her relief. She said, "Thank you for explaining that to me." I realized that her elevated level of anxiety had prevented her from hearing or comprehending what I said the first time. I made a mental note that Mrs. A. would require ongoing reassurance and explanations.

Notes on the Narrative

Patients and families place tremendous trust in their caregivers. That trust is not conferred simply by being in a role or from the name of an institution, but rather from positive relationships. Patients and families are hypervigilant to the care, commitment, and skill of their care team as clinicians and support staff take the time to "know" them. As a new graduate, Johnson's focus is correctly attuned to the complexities inherent in caring for a patient as ill as Mr. A., but he shows in his narrative that he recognizes the anxiety Mr. A.'s wife is experiencing and seeks to decrease her anxiety and fear by recognizing her important role, not only as Mr. A's wife but as a caregiver.

Clinician level. At the clinician level, the nurse is comfortable in the clinical setting, and experience allows them to be flexible in managing rapidly changing situations. In her narrative, Riya Singh, RN, who practices in the operating room, reflects on her care of a pregnant patient undergoing a tracheal resection and reconstruction surgery. Given the complexity of the surgery, she asked the team leader to have the room double staffed with experienced scrub nurses in addition to a full delivery team. All her planning pays off as she describes the start of the case:

> Logistically, getting started was nearly overwhelming. Every team had its own set of needs, requiring me to move quickly around the operating table (even under it a couple of times) to accommodate everyone. Fortunately, we had an extra set of hands in the form of additional staffing for the day. Eventually, the case fell into the well-choreographed dance it always does.

Notes on the Narrative

Singh understood and anticipated the challenges related to her patient's complex surgery. That anticipation allowed surgery to progress smoothly and for resources and support to be available in case unanticipated events occurred. A point of interest in her narrative is the imagery she paints with the words "well-choreographed dance." Creating images in the reader's mind will drive home your points more effectively.

Advanced clinician level. Narratives from nurses at this level describe clinically sound risks in the care of the patient and in the development of clinical knowledge. In other words, they can anticipate what they need to do based on their experience and knowledge. Mirlande Dorsainvil, RN, a clinical nurse on a general medical unit, writes of caring for Mr. C., a 70-year-old man admitted with altered mental status and a history of end-stage renal disease for which he was receiving dialysis. His dialysis had to be ended early because of his agitation. On initial assessment, Mr. C is stable, but soon his systolic blood pressure drops to the 60s mm Hg range. Dorsainvil asks a colleague to notify the physician and begins preparing a bag of Lactated Ringers in anticipation of a fluid bolus. She writes:

The doctor ordered a bolus of 500 mL. I suggested that we start with 250 mL, given Mr. C.'s incomplete dialysis treatment and my concern for fluid overload, and the doctor agreed. Mr. C.'s blood pressure returned to baseline for a short time, but he soon began having a high volume of loose stools and his blood pressure dropped. Given his frequent hospital admissions, I was concerned that he had *C. difficile* infection, and the physician agreed with my recommendation to send a stool sample, blood cultures, and a new set of labs to check for infection. Despite Mr. C. being afebrile, I recognized that he might be septic, and a serum lactate was also checked. The results showed a high WBC and a serum lactate of 3. The physician and I agreed we would need to repeat over time to determine trending. I also anticipated the need for additional IV access and called the IV team. I started the ordered antibiotics and continued close monitoring of Mr. C.'s condition.

Notes on the Narrative

This narrative reflects Dorsainvil's comfort in a rapidly changing situation based on her past experience and expertise. She is able to tailor interventions, including the need to closely monitor Mr. C.'s fluid balance and the probability of sepsis even though he is afebrile. She also demonstrates her close partnership with her physician colleague as they work together to stabilize and understand the cause of Mr. C.'s deterioration.

Clinical scholar level. At this level, clinicians' practice is fluid and intuitive, they are leaders on the unit and in the organization, and they elevate the practice of others including members of other disciplines. Brenda Pignone, RN, a clinical nurse on a general surgical unit, writes about her care of a young woman, Mrs. A., who became paraplegic after a high-speed motor vehicle accident. At their first meeting, Mrs. A. has had a difficult night because of her nightmares of the accident. Pignone writes:

> Upon entering her room, I went to the head of the bed and leaned over so she could make eye contact with me. I immediately saw the fear and anxiety in her eyes. I introduced myself and told her I'd be her nurse for the next 12 hours. I spent time with Mrs. A. and her husband discussing her physical and emotional issues and helping staff manage the situation. Mrs. A. and her husband spoke about how important it was for her to be able to touch her surroundings and her caregivers—it helped remind her of where she was and reassured her she was safe. Mrs. A. shared that because she could no longer feel her legs, her sense of touch was vital to her sense of "who she was at that moment."
>
> Mrs. A. was a professional French horn player. She needed to feel that she could still use her arms, so she'd constantly move her arms, seeking things to touch. I quickly arranged a meeting with Mrs. A., her husband, the nurse practitioner, the social worker, and the psychiatric clinical nurse specialist. With this new information, I felt it was important for Mrs. A. to have a sitter (patient care associate), who could stay by her bed at night. When Mrs. A. reached out, the sitter could remind her that she was at MGH, that she'd had an accident, give her the date and time, and assure her that she was safe.

Notes on the Narrative

How do you rebuild a life? Slowly, and with a lot of guidance, support, and understanding. Pignone's expert knowledge and interventions allowed Mrs. A. and her family to be able to imagine and plan for the next chapter of their lives. It would have been easy to focus on Mrs. A's extensive physical injuries, but Lewis demonstrates how she gave equal attention to her mental and emotional needs.

Publishing Your Narrative

Every day, in all types of settings, nurses are writing narratives, such as those you have read, in the form of exemplars that are part of a recognition program. Unfortunately, many of these stories are read or heard by only a few people. If you tucked away an exemplar for promotion in a file drawer, dust it off and consider submitting it for publication. Narratives written for nursing journals and magazines can offer you more latitude to explore your experiences than exemplars written specifically for advancement.

> **Confidence Booster**
>
> You may think the world isn't interested in nurses' everyday practice, but consider nurse Theresa Brown. She submitted her personal essays about nursing to *The New York Times*, and they soon began to appear in that prestigious newspaper on a regular basis. Brown also published a book of nursing narratives (*Critical Care: A New Nurse Faces Death, Life, and Everything in Between*) in 2010. In one of the book's essays, titled "First Death," she writes, "Almost every job has its initiations and rites of passage. In nursing, especially in oncology nursing, the first death is a professional rite of passage" (Brown, 2010, p. 35).
>
> Brown continues to have articles published by *The New York Times* and other media outlets. She is the author of the books *The Shift: One Nurse, Twelve Hours, Four Patients' Lives* (2016) and *Healing: When a Nurse Becomes a Patient* (2022), where Brown, who worked as an oncology and hospice nurse, shares her personal experience with breast cancer.

As you saw in the earlier examples, narratives free you from the convention of the objective third-person voice, and you can simply tell a story from your own point of view. Whether you are writing about a meaningful relationship with a patient in the last days of her life, a highly technical assessment, or teaching an anxious mother how to nurse her newborn, you offer yourself to the reader in a way that is dramatically different from the presentation of information found in a research or clinical article.

Q *What other outlets are available for publishing narratives?*

A Hospital and nursing newsletters are a perfect starting point. In fact, for years, Massachusetts General Hospital in Boston has published clinical narratives describing practice in its nursing and patient care services newsletter *Caring Headlines*. You can read these narratives on the publication's website (www.mghpcs.org/caring/caring-previous.shtml). If your organization doesn't currently have a venue for publishing narratives, suggest it start one.

Seize opportunities to share your stories more widely. Flip to the final pages in a nursing magazine or journal, and you often find a personal narrative as a regular column. You can also share these narratives on blogs.

Short narratives in the form of vignettes can also enhance books and articles on professional development topics and help you become more comfortable with the format. In the book, *Fostering Nurse-Led Care: Professional Practice for the Bedside Leader from Massachusetts General Hospital* (2013), authors Ives Erickson, Jones, and Ditomassi use exemplars in each of the chapters—for example, on topics such as environmental care, healing spaces, intentional presencing, and mentoring the clinical nurse specialist.

Keeping a journal or diary might help you get started if you'd like to publish a personal narrative. Of course, although a narrative may spring from journal jottings, a published narrative is much more structured and polished and must be written as a complete story with a definite beginning, middle, and end. The conclusion or ending incorporates lessons learned, insights gained, truths discovered, or understandings about the essence of nursing realized—often an "Aha!" moment in your career.

How to Write a Narrative

Just the thought of putting fingers to keyboard or pen to paper might be intimidating, but it doesn't have to be. You now know some types of narratives you can consider, and you can review other narratives as examples for helping you write your own.

Q *I've looked over the types of narratives, but I'm still not sure what I should write about. Any suggestions?*

A Identifying a topic to write about can be challenging. Consider a situation in which you feel your intervention really made a difference in patient outcome, a situation that you commonly confront in your practice, a situation that was particularly demanding, or a situation that you think captures the essence of your discipline. These ideas should help get your creative juices flowing!

It helps to remember that your narrative is a first-person "story" about a clinical event or situation that holds some special meaning for you. Having a systematic approach will help you establish a clear purpose for your narrative (Sherwood et al., 2023). Whether you're writing the narrative for work or to be published, you'll want to include the following:

- Information about yourself: name, title, unit, and length of time in practice
- A detailed description of what happened
- Why this clinical situation is important to you
- What your concerns were at the time
- What you were thinking about as it was taking place
- What you were feeling during and after the situation
- What, if anything, stood out to you

Be sure to change the patient's name and any other identifying information to protect privacy and confidentiality. (See Chapter 11 for more information about protecting patients' privacy.)

Three Steps to Writing Your Narrative

One of today's communication phenomena has been the advent of TED talks—short (under 20 minutes), powerful presentations focused on presenting one idea, telling one story, and asking one question. You can apply the framework for TED talks to writing your narrative (Morgan, 2013):

1. Begin by choosing one idea. Select a clinical situation that has universal interest but where your specific experience and expertise can be showcased.

2. Next, pick one story to go with the one idea. Make it a story only you can tell. And make it a story with a point, or lesson.

3. Finally, ask one question. Use your story to engage others in learning from your experience.

You might want to tell your story into your mobile device or a tape recorder, then transcribe and edit the narrative, tightening it and filling in any needed details. As you edit, avoid vague summary statements or general phrases that do not communicate what actually occurred, such as:

"I analyzed the possible dangers to the patient and took action."

"I gave emotional support."

"The patient is improving."

More specific ways of stating what occurred are:

"The blood pressure was dropping, and the pulse rate was rising. I sensed the patient was going into shock, so I immediately called the intern."

"I sat and talked with the patient about how to tell his family about the diagnosis."

"The patient is able to sit independently, transfer out of bed with assistance, and is progressing with gait activities on the parallel bars and with a walker."

Be sure you have included your concerns or what you were anticipating when you took a particular action; this gives a window to your judgment. For example, "I thought the patient would be resistant, so I decided to..." (Ives Erickson et al., 2015, p. 174).

The Power of Storytelling

As nurses, we spend so much time in relationships: listening to our patients' stories and caring for people in crisis. Often, we are the only ones who experience life's momentous events with another human being. Sue Hagedorn, nurse storyteller, says, "We're the ones in a position to tell the story or help the patient tell the story and make some sense out of that story" (S. Hagedorn, personal communication, October 16, 2009).

Like anything worth doing, writing narrative accounts takes time and practice, but you have stories to tell and experiences to share—and now you have the tools to begin writing.

Write Now!

1. Visualize a patient you cared for or a situation that has stayed with you. Recall what you saw, heard, smelled, and felt. Write the experience as you remember it. Include dialogue and the thoughts and feelings you had at the time.

2. Use a mobile device or a tape recorder to tell a story to yourself or speak to a trusted colleague about a patient you cared for. Tell it quickly, without judgment or editing yourself. Then listen to the story for key points you might include in a narrative.

References

Amulya, J. (n.d.). *What is reflective practice?* http://itslifejimbutnotasweknowit.org.uk/files/whatisreflectivepractice.pdf

Benner, P. (1984, 2000). *From novice to expert: Excellence and power in clinical practice*. Addison-Wesley Publishing Company.

Benner, P., Hooper-Kyriakidis, P., & Stannard, D. (1999). *Clinical wisdom and interventions in critical care: A thinking-in-action approach*. W. B. Saunders.

Benner, P., Sutphen, M., Leonard, V., & Day, L. (2010). *Educating nurses: A call for radical transformation*. The Carnegie Foundation for the Advancement of Teaching. Jossey-Bass.

Brown, T. (2010). *Critical care: A new nurse faces death, life and everything in between*. HarperCollins Publishers.

Brown, T. (2016). *The shift: One nurse, twelve hours, four patients' lives*. Algonquin Books.

Brown, T. (2022). *Healing: When a nurse becomes a patient*. Algonquin Books.

DeSalvo, L. (2000). *Writing as a way of healing: How telling our stories transforms our lives*. Beacon Press.

Dreyfus, H. L., & Dreyfus, E. E. (with Athanasiou, T.). (1986). *Mind over machine*. Free Press.

Fitzpatrick, J. J., & Kim, M. (2023, Dec. 12). Narrative nursing. *Nurse Leader*. In press. https://doi.org/10.1016/j.mnl.2023.11.007

Freshwater, D., Horton-Deutsch, S., & Sherwood, G. (2023). Reimagining ourselves: The role of reflection on critical Caritas consciousness and knowledge development. In S. Horton-Deutsch & G. D. Sherwood, *Reflective practice: Reimagining ourselves, reimagining nursing* (pp. 3–18). Sigma Theta Tau International.

Gao, X. (2022). Research on expressive writing in psychology: A forty-year bibliometric analysis and visualization of current status and research trends. *Frontiers in Psychology, 13*, 825626. https://doi.org/10.3389/fpsyg.2022.825626

Herrity, J. (2023, Sept. 27). How to write a letter of recommendation with example. *Indeed*. https://www.indeed.com/career-advice/career-development/how-to-write-a-letter-of-recommendation-with-examples

Ives Erickson, J., Daniels, A. A., Smith, M. E., & Vega-Barachowitz, C. D. (2008). Recognizing clinical excellence at all levels of practice. *Journal of Nursing Administration, 38*(2), 68–75. https://doi.org/10.1097/01.NNA.0000310716.15474.be

Ives Erickson, J, Ditomassi, M., Sabia, S., & Smith, M. E. (2015). *Fostering clinical success: Using narratives for interprofessional team partnerships from Massachusetts General Hospital*. Sigma Theta Tau International.

Ives Erickson, J., Jones, D. A., & Ditomassi, M. (2013). *Fostering nurse-led care: Professional practice for the bedside leader from Massachusetts General Hospital*. Sigma Theta Tau International.

Lai, J., Song, H., Wang, Y., Ren, Y., Li, S. Xiao, F., Liao, S., Xie, T., & Zhuang, W. (2023). Efficacy of expressive writing versus positive writing in different populations: Systemic review and meta-analysis. *Nursing Open, 10*(9), 5961–5974. https://doi.org/10.1002/nop2.1897

Lamott, A. (1995). *Bird by bird: Some instructions on writing and life*. Anchor.

Mackoff, B. (2014, Oct. 27). *The wisdom of experience: How stories become strategies*. Presentation at Massachusetts General Hospital.

Morgan, N. (2013, April 30). How to prepare a 20-minute TED-like talk. *Public Words*. http://www.publicwords.com/2013/04/30/how-to-prepare-a-20-minute-ted-like-talk

Newman, K. M. (2016, Nov. 9). Five science-backed strategies to build resilience. *Greater Good*. https://greatergood.berkeley.edu/article/item/five_science_backed_strategies_to_build_resilience

Rushton, C. H., Batcheller, J., Schroeder, K., & Donohue, P. (2015). Burnout and resilience among nurses practicing in high-intensity settings. *American Journal of Critical Care, 24*(5), 412–420. http://dx.doi.org/10.4037/ajcc2015291

Scott, S. D., Hirschinger, L. E., Cox, K. R., McCoig, M., Brandt, J., & Hall, L. W. (2009). The natural history of recovery for the "healthcare provider second victim" after adverse patient events. *Quality and Safety in Health Care Journal, 18*(5), 325–330. https://doi.org/10.1136/qshc.2009.032870

Sherman, R. O. (2018). Building your resiliency. *American Nurse Journal, 13*(9), 26–28. https://www.myamericannurse.com/wp-content/uploads/2018/09/ant9-Resiliency-831.pdf

Sherwood, G., Moorman, M., & Morales, C. (2023). Deepening our foundations: Reimagining ourselves, reimagining nursing identity. In S. Horton-Deutsch & G. D. Sherwood, *Reflective practice: Reimagining ourselves, reimagining nursing* (pp. 89–113). Sigma Theta Tau International.

Smyth, J. M., Stone, A. A., Hurewitz, A., & Kaell, A. (1999). Effects of writing about stressful experiences on symptom reduction in patients with asthma or rheumatoid arthritis: A randomized trial. *Journal of the American Medical Association, 281*(14), 1304–1309. https://doi.org/10.1001/jama.281.14.1304

Zolnierek, C. (2012). Speak to be heard: Effective nurse advocacy. *American Nurse Journal, 7*(10). https://www.americannursetoday.com/speak-to-be-heard-effective-nurse-advocacy

Think Outside the Journal: Alternative Publication Options

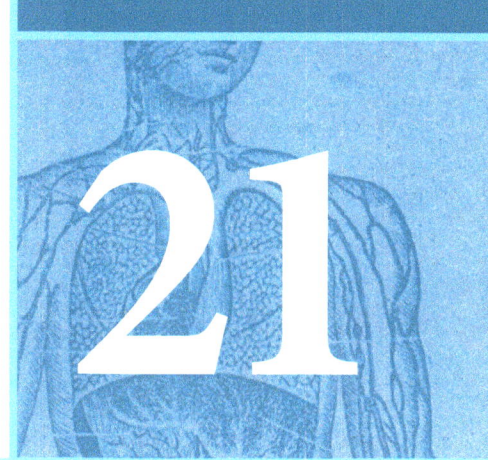

–Demetrius J. Porche, DNS, PhD, PCC, ANEF, FACHE, FAANP, FAAN

> *"The idea is to write it so that people hear it and it slides through the brain and goes straight to the heart."*
> –Maya Angelou

WHAT YOU'LL LEARN IN THIS CHAPTER

- Alternative publication options, which include letters to the editor, editorials, columns, book reviews, newsletters, and blogs, can help you gain confidence as a writer and provide another way to disseminate key information.

- Writing letters to the editor or guest editorials allows you to share your thoughts, present information, and possibly call for specific actions.

- You can help keep people engaged with an organization by contributing to a newsletter.

- Professional blogs provide a forum for engaging both professionals and the lay community.

Although nurses engage in communication every day using the spoken and written word, writing for publication can be an intimidating process. Fortunately, if you're a novice nurse author, you have a variety of writing options beyond the traditional journal article or book chapter to begin your writing career. Publishing through these alternative options helps you develop your writing skills, build confidence, and establish yourself as a knowledgeable content expert. These small writing projects may seem more achievable, since many of the options are shorter pieces, such as book reviews or professional blogs.

If you're an experienced nurse author, you might be comfortable with publishing a journal article, but now you're looking for a way to disseminate your opinion (editorial), share your expertise on a regular basis (column or professional blog), or simply communicate with an audience through your writing.

Alternative publication options allow you to document your knowledge and experience in a defined area, state an opinion regarding an issue, make a call for action, or just serve as an outlet to communicate with a professional group of like-minded nurses or with the general public. These other publication options include letters to the editor, editorials, columns, book reviews, newsletters, and professional blogs.

Letters to the Editor

A letter to the editor is generally written in response to something the editor has written in previous editorials or in response to a published article. In professional nursing society or organization publications, the letter to the editor may be a statement about a position, issue, or current situation within the respective nursing organization. Like an editorial, letters to the editor are one of the most frequently read components of a publication; they are a great strategy for focusing attention on an issue and influencing others by sharing your opinion.

When to Write a Letter to the Editor

Consider a letter to the editor when you want to:

- Suggest an idea, solution, different perspective, or position on an issue
- Influence the opinion of a political leader or that of the public
- Educate the general public or readership on an issue
- Provide corrective or supplemental data and information on an issue
- Publicize your scholarly work in an area related to an issue
- Praise an article, editorial, or opinion
- Use the letter to illustrate your authority or experience
- Attract attention to your professional group

Q *I've decided to write a letter to the editor. How do I get started?*

A First, review the mission and purpose of the publication to which you plan to write a letter to the editor. Find the editor's name, title, credentials, and email address. Read a few previously written letters to the editor in the publication. Although "letter" remains in the name of the communication, you should send an email or use the designated section on the journal's website, rather than send a hard copy through the mail. You may also find submission information in the author guidelines. Keep in mind that you must respond to an article quickly or your letter will have less chance of being published. Ensure that the letter has a clearly defined purpose, intent, message, and tone, both for the editor and for the publication's readers.

Writing the Letter to the Editor

Letters to the editor can be influential if grounded in a conversation about an issue from a larger community, organizational, or disciplinary perspective. A general rule is to open the letter with a simple sentence that is important, dramatic, and grabs the reader's attention. Consider the following examples:

> Dear Editor,
> In a recent article, Walsh and Stephenson (2021) noted that sexual minorities, particularly gay, bisexual, and other men who have sex with men (GBMSM), have increased mental and emotional stress during the pandemic because a majority of them have lingering morbidities and underlying conditions that make them highly vulnerable to grave illnesses and death from the COVID-19 virus. I would argue that social inequality and exclusionary tendencies against the LGBTQI+ community, in general, have been more evident within the pandemic and that further impinged upon their conditions and health. (Macaraan, 2022, para. 1)

> Dear Editor,
> It is commendable that in a recent article [letter to the editor] published in the *American Journal of Men's Health*, Macaraan (2022) pointed out the 'social inequalities and exclusionary tendencies' toward lesbians, gays, bisexuals, transgenders, queers, intersex, asexuals and other individuals with diverse sexualities and genders (LGBTQIA+) community have been more exacerbated by the COVID-19 pandemic. I would like to add an important consideration for policymakers and for the global audience that one needs to reexamine the root causes of the stigmatization, discrimination, and criminalization of LGBTQIA+. The deeply embedded homophobic and transphobic attitudes expose many LGBTQIA+ people of all ages and in all regions of the world to a blatant violations of their human rights. In line with the proposal of Macaraan (2022), the value of openness, hospitality, and acceptance through equitable laws and education are important factors to move forward toward inclusive praxis. (Corpuz, 2023, para. 1)

Before or immediately after your opening statement, include the name of the article (whether in print or online) and when it was published. Next, explain why you are writing the letter—state the problem or issue to which your concerns are directed. Clearly articulate how the issue or concern affects you, others, and especially the publication's readership. At this point, it would be beneficial to provide some strong statistical or epidemiological data to substantiate your opinion or concerns. Finally, communicate your proposed *call to action* (if you think one is needed) in response to the issue.

It's good practice to link an issue of concern to an influential person. For example, if the course of action you are proposing is in line with the current position, or a strategy supported by a professional association or leader, state that your position supports or is consistent with the respective organization or person's stance.

As you write, remember the "five Bs" of writing a letter to the editor. It should:

- Be easy to read
- Be brief
- Be concise
- Be factual
- Be stimulating

Before concluding the letter to the editor, ensure that you have clearly communicated your recommendation, call to action, and expected action. Date the letter and sign with your name, title, credentials, email address, city, state, and preferred method of contact (phone or email). If you decide to mail your letter (which is not advised because of lag time), address the envelope to the attention of the editor.

Example 21.1 shows an effective letter to the editor.

Common errors with writing a letter to the editor include wordiness, addressing too many issues in one letter, taking several positions or presenting multiple opinions on the issue (which leads to an unfocused letter), using slang or having a tone that is either too informal or too aggressive, factual inaccuracies or a lack of facts to support your statement, and not being original in your information or presentation of your opinion.

The publication's editorial staff will decide whether to publish the letter. They consider factors such as timeliness, grammar, purpose and clarity of content, and how well assertions are supported (Owens, 2020). Letters may be edited for length, grammar, and the publication's style. In some cases, you will receive a proof of the letter to review before publication.

I was pleased to read about the Rhode Island Nurses Institute (RINI) Middle College Charter School ("Starting Nursing Careers in High School," *In the News*, September 2019). An alternative public school focused on recruiting urban youth from low-income and underrepresented backgrounds is an amazing concept. As an African American male from a similar target demographic, I was fortunate to be introduced to nursing as a high school student.

I believe diversity in nursing is an important issue, as minorities, which made up 38% of the US population in 2014, are expected to become the majority by 2044. Despite these historic demographic shifts, the US RN workforce is failing to reflect the population changes. I work as an ICU nurse in a community that is 48.6% Hispanic or Latino. Although my facility has many interpreting options available to staff, I believe having an intimate understanding of a community's culture is necessary to the delivery of culturally competent care. To accomplish this, more efforts should be concentrated on initiating programs like the RINI Middle College Charter School in districts around the United States.

Aron King, BSN, RN
Sacramento, CA

American Journal of Nursing, 2020, p. 13

EXAMPLE 21.1 A persuasive letter to the editor.

Tips for Getting Your Letter to the Editor Accepted

Here are several tips for getting your letter to the editor accepted:

- Write a provocative, catchy, and stimulating opening statement; make a dramatic point with statistics or epidemiological data.
- Keep the letter shorter than 300 words.
- Depending on the nature of the publication, aim for a 5th-grade reading level.
- Make the letter relevant to the editor and readership by connecting the letter to recent publications, current events, or new information.
- Connect the letter to your readership through personal experiences.
- Use statistics that are relevant to the readership.
- Use easily validated information to make your points.
- Illustrate your points with personal stories.
- Conclude the letter with your name, title, and credentials.
- Proofread, proofread, and proofread again.

Q *I want to write a letter to the editor, but I don't want to use my name. Can letters to the editor be published anonymously?*

A If you do not want your name used (e.g., if you want to share your personal experience with intimate partner violence but don't want to be identified), you may say so when you write the editor and provide a brief rationale. An effective way to ask is to end your letter with a simple line like, "I would prefer to have my name withheld if the letter is published." Make sure, though, to include your contact information, because typically editors won't publish letters that they can't verify. The letter will most often be published with the signature, "Name withheld by request." Even if you decide to withhold your name, consider publishing your professional credentials or discipline.

Confidence Booster

"I read an article about buying pedigree dogs in an inflight magazine. As a volunteer at an animal shelter, I was appalled that adoption wasn't even mentioned as an option. I felt so passionate about this issue that I wrote my first letter to the editor—and it was published!" This story from a nurse illustrates a key point about writing letters to the editor. Try to relate your topic to a passion you have; of course, remember to harness that passion so that your letter is objective.

Letters to the editor are frequently missed opportunities to communicate evidence-based information. Seize the opportunity by ensuring that your letter to the editor contains data and other evidence to support your opinion. This simple letter begins to document in writing your knowledge of the topic under discussion.

Editorials

An *editorial* is an opinion, a factual point of information or clarification, an argumentative stance, or a thought-provoking substantive narrative. Editorials are composed by editors, associate or assistant editors, or guest editors. The editorial, one of the most widely read features of a newspaper, newsletter, or journal, is a communication channel through which a nurse can disseminate information to a large audience in a short narrative, while establishing a position and knowledge base on a specific topic. Publicly elected officials are known to have daily briefings on editorials written about current events and political affairs, especially through newspapers. The four basic types of editorials are (Nundy et al., 2021):

1. Explaining or interpreting a stance, topic, or subject area
2. Criticizing actions or decisions
3. Persuading readers to take a specific action or opinion on a topic
4. Praising to demonstrate support

An editorial communicates an opinion but should be positive, negative, or informative in tone. Regardless of tone, the editorial should always be factual and professional in word selection and presentation. The tone of an editorial can be emotional, but it should always be objective in nature.

Consider the start of an editorial on interprofessional men's health practice (Porche, 2016):

> As health care professionals continue to focus on quality, safety, and access to affordable health care, interprofessional practice seems to be the imperative practice linkage. The current health care arena presents a complex environment plagued with communication breakdowns that lead to errors in care and errors of omission in health care. (p. 89)

Note that the author enters an emotional and controversial topic by starting with a simple declarative statement, but then backs up the statement with information to support the primary statement.

The best editorials are simple, easy to read, and short. Editorials are generally about 250 to 750 words; check if the publication's author guidelines specify a range (Nundy et al., 2021; Porche, 2011).

Some simple guidelines for constructing an editorial are (Porche, 2017):

- The opening paragraph should include an outline of the issue or problem; a statement challenging an opinion, agreeing with an opinion, or presenting a new perspective on an issue; and factual and dramatic information.
- The second paragraph should present your position and clearly communicate your rationale for your position.
- The third paragraph acknowledges opposing thoughts or opinions and presents a counterargument, thought, or opinion from your perspective on each of the thoughts and opinions presented.
- The last paragraph concludes with a call to action. A call to action is typically behaviorally focused and states the action you expect someone to take or the action-oriented challenge you are putting forth to the readers. The call to action should be specific and not a laundry list of potential options.
- Conclude editorials with your name, title (if permitted by employer), credentials, affiliation, city, and state.

Tips for Getting Your Editorial Accepted

Here are several tips for getting your editorial accepted:

- Be sure the topic or issue is relevant and timely.
- Make the editorial informative by including new information.
- Make the editorial specific to a recently published article or national issue.
- Build on a previous editorial or present a contradictory or different paradigm of a previous editorial.
- Write in the active voice. (You can read more about using active voice in Chapter 6.)

Here are additional tips for editorial writing:

- Select an influential interesting topic.
- Make an outline.
- Start writing.
- Ensure all your facts are correct.
- Keep the tone friendly.
- Begin with a dramatic thesis statement.
- Present the opposing argument first.
- Provide evidence that refutes the opposing argument.
- Present your argument.
- Conclude with an editorial punch or striking remark.

Here is an example of a call to action from an editorial on developing a specialty men's health clinic (Porche, 2015):

> Men's health care providers may want to consider developing a specialty clinic within their men's health practice. This specialty 'Gender Identity Clinic' would consist of an interprofessional integrated clinic that focuses on gender identity disorder/dysphoria. In addition, it is suggested that the clinic should consider a life span approach that integrates both pediatric,

adult, and geriatric care services for patients at different points in the gender identity disorder—gender reassignment and life after reassignment… (p. 261)

The call to action is quite clear as to who should do what. The editorial also progresses the concept as it moves forward.

Columns

Columns are brief articles or features written for newspapers, newsletters, magazines, or professional journals. In professional journals, columns are sometimes referred to as *departments*. A column can be in every issue of a publication or scheduled periodically. Columns are generally short—about 700 to 1,500 words—and may focus on a specific content area or theme, such as research methods, policy updates, research briefs, or new pharmacology information. An associate editor, rather than the editor, may be responsible for columns.

Tips for writing a column include:

- Identify an informational need. Is there an information gap in the literature? Is there a new technique? Do you have a new model or strategy to share? Do you have new data or research findings?

- Determine your target audience. What component of the journal's readership are you targeting (e.g., clinicians, administrators, or the general audience)?

- Determine the column's purpose. Is the column to inform the readers? Present information in a new manner? Influence best practices?

- Review the author guidelines for the expected column format and comply with that format. Read and review the general structure of previously published columns in the publication.

- Obtain factual information by conducting a review of the literature. Ensure that you have the most current and relevant information and statistics.

- Synthesize the information. Because a column is short, the information needs to be presented in a concise manner with a logical flow. For example, if you are writing a column on a new intervention for an existing health problem, the flow of the column might be incidence, etiology, pathophysiology, signs/symptoms, diagnostic criteria, clinical management (this would represent the bulk of the column since this column would be focusing on a new intervention), expected clinical outcomes, conclusion, and references.

- Outline the column.

- Write the column by inserting narrative content into the column outline.

- Proofread, edit, proofread, edit, then have a colleague do the same. Do not read or think about the column for a few days, then read it again, and edit and proofread a final time.

- Submit the column to the correct editor, as instructed by the author guidelines.

Generally, some level of peer review is conducted for column articles regarding the scientific merit (if appropriate) and accuracy of the information presented. For most professional journals, a column is peer reviewed by the editor, associate editor, or an editorial board member, so the peer-review process usually doesn't require as much time. Some columns have a designated member of the editorial board to serve as the column editor. This makes journal columns a great feature through which to rapidly disseminate your scholarly work or research. Keep in mind, however, that more clinically oriented articles will undergo a more detailed peer-review process.

Book Reviews

Nurses face a time barrier when trying to keep up to date with the latest evidence-based practice while continuing to practice nursing full time. A strategy to help nurses decide what to read—and what not to read—is the book review. Book reviews help nurses focus their reading time on the most beneficial information source (Davis, 2020).

Book reviews are published by some journals and other publications, and generally appear in the beginning or ending of the journal among the non-peer-reviewed material. It is always a good idea to send a query to the editor before submitting a book review. Editors frequently receive complimentary copies of books, from either the author or the author's marketing team, that align with the journal's mission—so check with the editor first.

A book review is more than a description of the published book; it's a critical appraisal and evaluation of the quality and significance of the book to nursing practice. The review generally concludes with the reviewer's overall impression of the book and a recommendation on the utility of the book for nursing practice. The length of a book review varies, anywhere from about 50 to 1,500 words (Davis, 2020; Nickerson, 2016).

Before writing a book review, read the entire book, highlight any key sections (use the highlighting feature if you are reading it in an ebook format), and take notes that summarize the major points. Generally, the first two-thirds of the book review should cover background information and summarize the book; the reviewer's critical appraisal and evaluation of the book should represent at least one-third of the book review's content.

Here is an example from the beginning of a review of the book *Appreciative Leadership: Focus on What Works to Drive Winning Performance and Build a Thriving Organization*:

> The author's research into appreciative inquiry is used to develop a map of leadership strategies and practices that inspires high levels of contribution, engagement, and performance. They use straightforward language and compelling stories to demonstrate how to get results with "positive power." (Sakallaris, 2020, p. 18)

The components of a book review, in order, are:

- A *bibliographic notation* on the book that includes the title, author, copyright date, place of publication, publisher, number of pages, type of book or genre, general content or focus of the book, special book features, price, and ISBN number.

- The *background information*, which consists of the author's purpose for writing the book, intended audience, book theme or subject matter, author's primary thesis about the book's subject matter, and prior publications by the author.

- A *summary of the book's content*. The book content summary reviews the overall structure of the book, organization and flow of the book content, a short review of the book's table of contents, and information on the substantive content covered throughout the book's chapters.

- The reviewer's *critical appraisal and evaluation of the book*, which should consist of the extent to which the book achieved its stated purpose, comparison of the book to other books on the same or similar topic, content omitted or unique content presented in the book, persuasiveness of the content, placement or position of the book within the existing books on the same or similar topic, extent to which the book meets the intended audience's needs, and the content's accuracy, objectivity, and thoroughness.

- A *concluding recommendation* about the usefulness of the book, and the extent to which the reviewer recommends the book to other nurses. The concluding recommendation is an honest explanation regarding the reviewer's opinion about the book's utility, significance, and contribution to the nursing literature.

Q *I have never written a book review. Do you have any more tips?*

A It seems obvious, but still worth stating again, that you should read the entire book first. Start with the book's preface (or introduction), which outlines the book's intended purpose and structure. Reading the preface will help you understand the organization of the book's content. Check if the preface identifies the intended audience. After reading the book, ask yourself, "Do I agree that the book was focused on the intended audience? How does this book fit within the context of other books on the same topic?" Reflect on the book to generate a critical appraisal and evaluation. Finally, write your opinion about the book's value. Be clear with your analysis, but never disparage the author if you didn't find the book to be of much value; rather, keep your tone neutral and focus on the content.

Newsletters

Newsletters are a communication tool for professional associations, organizations, and institutions. Some boards of directors consider newsletters to be the communication glue that holds the organization together and keeps members engaged with the professional association. Generally, the newsletter is a document to inform, announce, remind, advise, educate, advertise, or communicate with a large audience in a short publication. Professional association and institutional newsletters frequently have an open call for submissions.

An organization's newsletter, whether disseminated in print or electronically (e-newsletter), is a critical element to the strategic success of an organization. As a critical communication tool, the newsletter is used to disseminate information to the membership or constituents of an organization or institution in a timely manner. The key to a successful newsletter is in its name—*NEW*sletter. The information must be "new."

Regular newsletter readers tend to focus on three things in the newsletter:

- Who they know and what they are doing
- New events or announcements
- Recent activities of the association or organization that directly affect them

All these areas make good ideas for potential newsletter articles.

Newsletters have an editor who compiles all the features, solicits and edits information, and ensures that the newsletter is disseminated on schedule. Some newsletters are indexed in various literature databases.

The ease in getting published in a newsletter varies according to the source. For example, getting published in your hospital's newsletter is easier than getting published in a more scholarly newsletter that is indexed in a database. As with other types of articles, first contact the editor with your idea and access any author guidelines that are available.

Some tips for writing a newsletter article include (Buck, 2017):

- When developing a title, remember that readers scan for keywords and that newsletter titles are typically short in length.
- Start with a catchy opening statement that states the purpose of the article: who, what, where, when, why, and how.
- Include new content. Remember the "new" in newsletter.
- Keep messages short and concise, and focus on one topic at a time.
- Keep sentence structure simple; sentences should be no more than 15 to 20 words long.
- Keep paragraphs simple, with a length of no more than five sentences.
- Write in a conversational tone.
- Use bulleted and numbered lists to facilitate reading.
- Integrate pictures and figures to attract the readers' attention.

Remember, newsletters are an excellent way to get started in writing for publication.

Professional Blog

A professional blogger is not the same as a professional blog, even though a professional blogger can write a professional blog. A *professional blogger* is someone who blogs as a career choice. A *professional blog* is a blog that focuses on a specific topical area with the intent of providing information and knowledge specific to a profession or discipline. Nurses can use a professional blog as a channel for communicating research findings, evidence-based knowledge, and ideas in an informal, conversational tone. A regular blog also can help improve your writing and obtain feedback for your ideas (Chinn, 2023). Blogs have grown in popularity and impact and are being recognized as a form of scholarly communication (Chinn, 2023).

Some important tips for creating professional blogs are (Goodman, 2018):

- Determine the mission and purpose of your blog.
- Register your blog with searchable keywords aligned to topic.
- Establish your voice and credibility on the professional topic.
- Use searchable terms or create topic tags.
- Write short, attention-grabbing titles.
- Create white space and use images and illustrations (obtain permission first).
- Write in a conversational tone.
- Include anecdotes and case studies to illustrate points.

- Use adjectives and adverbs sparingly.
- Choose calls to action and phrases that can be easily remembered and repeated.
- Cite authoritative sources.
- Keep entries short, no more than 1,000 words—shorter is better (Chinn, 2023)
- Post or reference your blog through various social media outlets.
- Keep the content current.
- Develop an editorial calendar of your blogs.
- Plan and time your blog post to coincide with professional events, such as blogs on breast cancer during October.
- Keep archives of your blog for legal purposes.

Be sure to write an attention-getting headline that will draw readers in and result in optimal search engine results. You can use free online tools such as Capitalize My Title (https://capitalizemytitle.com/headline-analyzer) and the tools from Sharethrough (https://headlines.sharethrough.com) and MonsterInsights (https://www.monsterinsights.com/headline-analyzer) to determine the effectiveness of your headline.

You can choose to submit guest blogs to websites for organizations or other bloggers, or you can create a simple website where you publish them (Chinn, 2023). Check websites for professional associations and nursing journals to see if they accept guest blogs (you may need to be a member to contribute). Some sites, such as Nursology.net, have specific guidelines for submitting blogs and provide tips (Nursology.net, n.d.). A resource for creating your own website is WebsiteSetup (https://websitesetup.org).

You'll want to analyze blog metrics such as number of readers, subscribers, number of page views per post, number of conversations, number of back links, number of referrals, and overall traffic to and from the blog.

Expand Your Writing Potential

Expand your writing potential by using other avenues for publishing, such as letters to the editor, editorials, columns, book reviews, newsletters, and professional blogs. These other avenues help you develop your writing skills and build your confidence, while engaging in a less laborious and lengthy publication process. These publications also build your documented level of knowledge and expertise in a nursing area.

Write Now!

1. Write a letter to the editor and submit it. You might first try your local newspaper.
2. Select a journal you read routinely. Does the journal publish columns? If so, read the author guidelines for writing a column. Review the last three years of the journal for relevant and "hot" topics not covered. Contact the editor to see if there is interest in your topic.
3. Review your professional association's newsletter. Identify the three main areas that are the focus. What can you contribute as an article in one of these areas?
4. Write a blog on a nursing topic you feel passionate about.

References

Buck, S. (2017). *The ultimate guide to newsletters: Your secret weapon for doubling referrals and tripling retention* (Kindle edition). Amazon.com Services LLC.

Chinn, P. (2023). On blogging. *Nurse Author & Editor, 33*(1-2), 10–12. https://doi.org/1111.nae2.12052

Corpuz, J. C. G. (2023). Beyond tolerance: An urgent call for LGBTQIA+ inclusive praxis. *American Journal of Men's Health, 17*(3). https://doi.org/10.1177/15579883231177635

Davis, S. S. (2020). *How to write a book review: A template for reviewing books.* Broke by Books Press.

Goodman, T. (2018). *Building a professional blog* (Kindle edition). Amazon.com Services LLC.

King, A. (2020). Diversity in nursing. *American Journal of Nursing, 120*(4), 13. https://doi.org/10.1097/01.NAJ.0000659940.41237.ac

Macaraan, W. E. R. (2022). The state and the LGBTQI+ people: Toward an inclusive COVID-19 humanitarian response. *American Journal of Men's Health, 16*(6). https://doi.org/10.1177/15579883221144376

Nickerson, L. A. (2016). *How to write a book review in 10 easy steps* (Kindle edition). Amazon.com Services LLC.

Nundy, S., Kakar, A., & Bhutta Z. A. (2021), How to write an editorial? In S. Nundy, A. Kakar, Z. A. Bhutta. *How to practice academic medicine and publish from developing countries? A practical guide* (pp. 263–266). Springer.

Nursology.net. (n.d.). *Contribute to the Nursology.net blog!* https://nursology.net/about/contribute-to-the-nursology-net-blog/

Owens, J. K. (2020). Writing a letter to the editor: Tips for success. *Nurse Author & Editor, 30*(3), 15–17. https://doi.org/10.1111/nae2.5

Porche, D. (2011). *Health policy: Application for nurses and other health care professionals.* Jones & Bartlett Learning.

Porche, D. (2015). Evolution of men's health issues: Impact of gender identity and reassignment on the clinical area. *American Journal of Men's Health, 9*(4), 261. https://doi.org/10.1177/1557988315589628

Porche, D. (2016). Interprofessional men's health practice. *American Journal of Men's Health, 10*(2), 89. https://doi.org/10.1177/1557988315626263

Porche, D. (2017). *Health policy: Application for nurses and other health care professionals* (2nd ed.). Jones & Bartlett Learning.

Sakallaris, B. R. (2020). LeaderRead: Appreciative leadership: Focus on what works to drive winning performance and build a thriving organization. [Book review]. *Voice of Nursing Leadership, 18*(1), 18. https://www.aonl.org/system/files/media/file/2020/01/voice-jan-2020.pdf

Walsh A. R., & Stephenson R. (2021). Positive and negative impacts of the COVID-19 pandemic on relationship satisfaction in male couples. *American Journal of Men's Health, 15*(3). https://doi.org/10.1177/15579883211022180

Writing a Book or Book Chapter

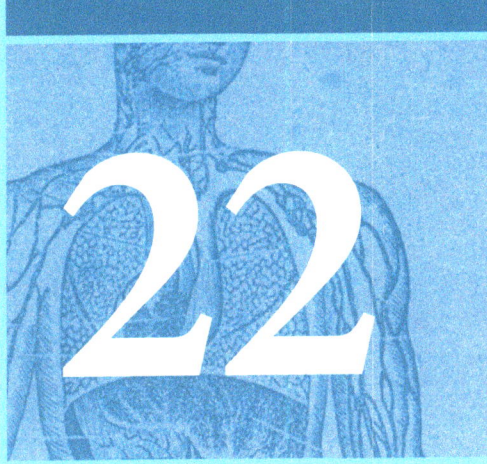

–Sandra M. Nettina, MSN, ANP-BC

"The power of a book lies in its power to turn a solitary act into a shared vision."
—Laura Bush

WHAT YOU'LL LEARN IN THIS CHAPTER

- To prepare a book proposal, articulate your idea and consult publisher websites.
- Develop a table of contents, templates, and a sample chapter to organize content and avoid overlap.
- Choose contributors carefully and outline their responsibilities in a letter of intent.
- Manage the project according to a plan and timeline with plenty of communication and focus on the goal.

Have you ever read a book and thought, "I could have written that"? Or maybe you simply have a secret desire to write a book of your own but are afraid to try. Writing a book (or even a chapter in a book) can seem overwhelming. Some nurses have taken on the task and have found themselves in a nightmare of disorganization, miscommunication, and missed deadlines. Others have encountered challenges but ultimately achieved a highly satisfying outcome. Although writing a book or book chapter isn't for the faint of heart, a systematic approach will help you achieve positive outcomes.

This chapter takes you through the steps of that approach. Much like other writing projects, the process starts with a rough idea that is further elucidated; in the case of a book, this means developing a table of contents. A major difference, however, is the organization, time frame, and flow of a multistep or multilayered project: You need to be a good project manager to produce a book with multiple chapters. And you might need to recruit, supervise, and coordinate the efforts of multiple contributors and reviewers.

Whether you are a single author or working with contributors, all books start with an idea.

Idea to Proposal

A good book begins with an idea, often in the form of a passion or a burning question. If an idea isn't articulated and explored, however, it may languish in the recesses of your mind or be forgotten. If an idea sticks, why not nurture it until it blossoms into content with a specific purpose for a specific audience?

Q *How do I know if I have enough material for a book?*

A You might debate whether you have enough material for a book—or whether your idea is best portrayed in an article. Writing an article is certainly easier, but it's limiting. A two- or three-part series of articles might be appropriate for a topic that can clearly be broken down into parts that could stand alone. Comparatively, you might have enough content for a book if your idea is multifaceted, covers many different aspects of the general theme, is a collection of topics, or contains so much detail that it encompasses multiple chapters.

When you create a book, you must have an overall theme and construct it in a way that provides a broader service to the reader than a single article or series of articles could do. If your book focuses on research, tease out the important strands from other studies and pull them together into a theme. Writing in a way that balances the complexity of the information with accessibility to keep the reader engaged may set you apart (*Nature Cancer*, 2023). The longer length of a book allows a thorough systematic review of the theme, with both historical review and application to practice included.

Targeting the Right Publisher

Your proposal will more likely be accepted if you target a publisher who has released books in line with your idea. Your idea should not be in direct competition with a publisher's books, but it should be relevant to a similar audience. For instance, you wouldn't pitch an idea for a memoir of hospice nurses to a publisher who prepares only study guides for nursing certification exams. Nor would you pitch your idea for a scholarly review of research studies on cardiovascular risk reduction to a publisher of exclusively consumer health books.

Check several publisher websites to learn about the types of books they publish before submitting a proposal. Look for publishers marketing books of similar topics to yours. You would not want to pitch the same idea, but if your book can be complementary to what the publisher already has in print, it may be a great fit. For example, a publisher might have a strong emphasis on end-of-life care but doesn't have a book on end-of-life care for pediatric patients, giving you an opening for your idea in this area.

After you have a publisher in mind, you're ready to tackle the proposal.

Crafting a Successful Proposal

Submit a proposal in the requested format, which is usually found on the publisher's website in the section for prospective authors. Although publishers' formats vary, they generally want to see the same key items: your plan and vision for the book, along with a *prospectus* (document that provides specific information about your offering), table of contents, and sample chapter. For example, here is information that Sigma Theta Tau International requests for book proposals (Sigma Theta Tau International, 2023):

Working title: Include any descriptors, subtitle, or positioning statement to reflect the content and purpose of the book. The publisher may change the title during the process, but you should still create one.

Names of authors, editors, and contributors already identified: Include brief biographies including credentials and affiliations and what chapters contributors will be creating.

Description of topic and how the book uniquely addresses a need in the market: Why is this book needed? How will this book meet a current need?

Primary audience: Who are the main readers you are targeting? Will it be a clinical text or a reference for professionals? Be as specific as possible and include what organizations or groups could be effectively marketed.

Number of chapters and length: What is the general length and number of chapters that will form the book?

Special features: Will there be stories from the field? Will it include tips, checklists, and resources?

Images: About how many photos, illustrations, tables, or figures will be in each chapter or within the book?

Projected word count: (Perhaps the most difficult for you to envision, but very important information for the publisher; review other books to estimate.)

Time frame: How long will it take to prepare the manuscript to submit to the publisher?

Goals for writing this book: Will it inform, expand, or influence current thinking?

Competitive works: List books that will compete with your planned book. Include publishers, authors, titles, and prices. Then explain how your book differs from these.

Table of contents: List what you plan to cover in the book and breakdown of content by chapter, including subheads for each chapter or a detailed description of what will be covered in each chapter.

Sample chapter: Create a chapter that shows the style of writing, depth of content, and variety of features that you plan for the book.

Don't submit your proposal to more than one publisher at a time unless you're working with a literary agent. (Agents aren't necessary for most nursing books.) Most proposals are submitted electronically via forms on publisher websites or emailed directly to an acquisitions editor, who will review them.

Q *I thought I had a one-of-a-kind idea. However, the publisher I submitted it to said that it already had a book just like it in the works. What keeps them from stealing my idea?*

A Ethical issues prevent publishers from stealing ideas. However, know that publishers might receive the same idea from multiple writers; it's the writer who first develops the most effective proposal and is the best fit for the book who will likely be approached as an author.

Waiting for a Reply

Usually, a review of your proposal takes about six to ten weeks but might take longer, based on the publisher's use of external reviewers and in-house schedule. Faculty, practicing nurses, and students may serve as reviewers. You may be contacted for more information during the process. After a proposal has been favorably reviewed, cost and sales forecasts are made, a development and marketing plan often are designed, and the project is presented to the in-house publishing committee for final approval.

If you don't receive confirmation after submitting, follow up by email or telephone to make sure your submission was received by the appropriate contact person and that no other information is needed. If you hear no news eight weeks after you have confirmed receipt, follow up again. Your contact might ask for more information or for revisions based on internal or external review of your proposal.

Q *Is writing or editing a book worth the effort?*

A This question can't be easily answered. Each authorship experience is unique. It is seldom financially lucrative, but there are other benefits, such as pride in accomplishment, gaining a deeper understanding of the topic, and building your reputation, which can result in professional advancement (Haberman & Wilson, 2023). As one nurse-author describes, the craft or art of writing is similar to the art of nursing, eliciting skill, practice, dedication, aesthetics, resilience, and joy. Just as relationship with those in our care is fundamental to the art of nursing, writing can be relational as well. We must form a connection with our intended audience that prompts us to write in a way that our readers will understand. To create something aesthetically pleasing that reaches one nurse, one patient, one family, or one community that gains comfort or insight can bring joy (Kagan, 2023).

Developing a Table of Contents

Most publishers will ask for a table of contents as part of your proposal. A *table of contents*—an outline or blueprint of your book project—is the most complete way to show publishers exactly what you intend to cover. Not only will this outline help guide you while you complete the project, it will also be used in the final product to lead readers to specific information. Detailed tables of contents are especially helpful for large projects that include multiple writers or contributors to ensure that all topic areas are covered without overlap.

A table of contents is organizational and topical. It should flow in a logical and predictable pattern. For example, for a physical assessment book, a head-to-toe format is logical, as is an organ system that begins with more critical (heart, lungs) and moves to less critical (skin).

To decide how to break down content into chapters or sections, start with major topic areas of your subject. Decide whether any major area is so broad that it needs to be divided: for example, *genitourinary* into *urologic*, *gynecologic*, and *male reproductive*; or *endocrine* into *diabetes mellitus*, *pituitary disorders*, and *disorders of the thyroid and parathyroid glands*. Likewise, determine whether any major area is shorter than the rest and could naturally be combined, such as *eye, ear, nose, and throat disorders*.

After you document in a logical format all the major areas you want to cover, determine what subheadings of information need to be addressed. List these in bullet points or write a paragraph under each major topic area. Include estimated page or word counts for each section of your table of contents.

While you're preparing the table of contents, keep in mind your target audience and purpose of the book or chapter. Is it a nursing textbook that might include ancillary materials, or a general nursing book that might be used for reference or inspiration? If you have not gathered enough information about the topic(s) you are going to write about, do an extensive but general review before you finalize your table of contents. Have your table of contents reviewed by several people in the field and then reorganize, rework, or supplement as indicated. Keep in mind that you want your book to be relevant for three to five years, not just the day it is published (Haberman & Wilson, 2023).

Using a Template

Most clinical books, as well as some nonclinical books, are composed of chapters and entries within chapters that follow a consistent format. If you find that "Clinical Manifestations" is the third subheading in the first chapter or entry, it could well end up being the third subheading in subsequent chapters or entries.

Just like an outline helps you write an article without leaving out any critical content areas, you can use a template to help organize your writing and ensure that everything has a place in the book or chapter. For example, for nursing books about the care of patients with certain diseases and disorders, the reader consistently wants to know about the pathophysiology, clinical manifestations, diagnostic test findings, and treatments and nursing interventions to provide. Use these guideposts for each chapter.

One template does not always fit all topic areas, however. Variations on the template might be necessary.

Within the template, identify the level of headings and subheadings that best portray the information.

Estimating Page Counts

Assigning page or word counts to the table of contents is important for your own writing schedule as well as for a publisher to assess the proposal as a business proposition. Estimating page count depends on the trim size of the book, font size, spacing, number and size of illustrations and tables, and additional elements such as table of contents and index. You can query the publisher for standard book trim sizes and page conversions. For a standard size 8.5" × 11", use three to four double-spaced manuscript pages in a 12-point font to one printed book page. Use roughly two manuscript pages to one print page for smaller trim-size books. Setting page limits will also help keep multiple contributors to similar levels of detail. Here are some tips to keep in mind:

- Determine page counts by evaluating other available literature on the topic areas, dividing the sum by the number of parts, and weighing the importance of each content area so that more important or complicated topics are allocated more pages.

- In most cases, per-chapter page counts are flexible as long as you stay within the total for the entire book.

- Have some optional content in mind to add if your project falls short. Also put some thought into what you could cut if the project runs long.

- You can refer the reader to internet resources for additional information, and cross-reference to previous sections of the book to save space. Books that will be offered in electronic formats can add digital content, and even print books can be enhanced by their own web pages for additional content.

For example, the highest level of heading after the title of the chapter could be the name of a disease or disorder. The second level of heading could be "Pathophysiology" or "Diagnostic Test Findings." To organize information further, a third level of heading such as "Laboratory," "Imaging," or "Physiologic Tests" might be used.

You can set up templates in most word-processing systems, including formatting for headings and other key sections. Consider using a template or the level headings feature in your word-processing program. However, be aware that some publishers may request specific formatting or require that formatting be removed before final submission of the manuscript. It's best to ask the editor you work with if the publisher has any word processing templates that should be used. You can then share them with your contributors. Setting up correctly from the beginning can save time before submission.

If you're working with other authors, you might consider inserting instructions into the various sections, which can then be deleted by the contributor. Here is an example of a template for a book on nursing management of chronic diseases.

Chapter 7 Inflammatory Bowel Disease

Overview *(introduction explaining how common the condition is, types and stages of the condition, how the condition can affect the patient, and the main goals of care; 2–4 paragraphs)*

Pathophysiology *(include cause, anatomic and physiologic changes, and complications; 4–8 paragraphs—do not use subheads but present each category in this order.)*

Clinical Findings *(include assessment findings, laboratory tests, and imaging results associated with the condition)*

    Signs and Symptoms *(4–6 paragraphs)*

    Diagnostic Test Results *(4–6 paragraphs)*

Treatment *(describe treatment modalities for this condition, including their indication, pharmacologic information, and expected results)*

    Pharmacologic Treatment *(1 paragraph for each drug or drug class)*

    Surgical Treatment *(2–4 paragraphs)*

    Supportive Treatment *(2–4 paragraphs to include hydration, nutrition, and other supportive measures)*

    Other Treatments *(e.g., physical therapy, alternative treatments, and investigational treatment)*

Nursing Management *(describe nursing interventions in detail, grouped by patient problem/nursing care focus; Note: refer to previous entries in the chapter to avoid repetition)*

    Acute Care Interventions *(8–12 paragraphs)*

    Chronic Care Management *(8–12 paragraphs)*

    Patient Education *(4–6 paragraphs)*

    Palliative Care Considerations *(1–2 paragraphs)*

References *(12–24 evidence-based primary resources in APA format)*

Creating a Sample Chapter or Entry

At the start of a project, writing a sample chapter or entry within a chapter is often helpful, especially if you're leading a team of contributors. A sample is also usually required in a proposal. Pick an area that you are most familiar with or that will fit the template best. By putting the information into the template format, you will see what doesn't work and make revisions accordingly. You can identify areas that fall outside the template and consider how to handle them differently.

Within the sample, try to include recurring or suggested features, such as tables, boxes, tips, case studies, key points, online resources, or questions and answers. Show their placement within the sample. Highlight the type of information to include in these features as well as the format to use. Identifying features early helps ensure that a good number of these will be included in the finished project and also that they will be consistent and appropriate. Lori Dambaugh (DNP, CNS, RN, ACCN-AG, Associate Professor and Associate Dean of Undergraduate Affairs, Wegmans School of Nursing, St. John Fisher College in Rochester, New York) advises, "While constructing a table in a chapter, focus on incorporating significant information that adds value to the subject matter. Consider including data, statistics, or insights that have not been discussed elsewhere. Specific features such as tables and figures contribute to the originality of the chapter and help provide depth to the material" (personal communication, October 23, 2023).

Writing style should also be highlighted in a sample. You will likely have writing guidelines, but use your sample to show thoughtful and deliberate implementation of the guidelines. The sample will also set the tone of the writing style, depth of information, and frequency and format of references.

Contributors and Coauthors

Just like the actors in a movie can make or break its success, having the right contributors, who understand and are committed to the project, can ease your workload and improve the outcome. A book might have one main author, who writes some parts of the book but also acts as an editor who coordinates a team of contributors, or several coauthors who divide sections or topics within the book. The more contributors you have, the less writing for everyone, which can speed the process. However, the more contributors, the more coordination and time you will spend orienting them to the project and editing for uniform style, repetition, and flow between sections or chapters. Table 22.1 compares single author and multiple contributors.

Finding Contributors

Matching content area with expertise to assign sections of the project can take several weeks to even months. Start by using your network of dependable experts. Look for potential contributors who have prior experience, interest and passion, and understanding of the responsibility and deadline of the project (Indeed Editorial Team, 2022). Perhaps you can find colleagues who are willing to do more than one section or chapter. Some colleagues may not want to commit to a whole chapter, but would be willing to split a chapter with someone they are used to working with.

After you exhaust your own network for contributors, look further. Ideas for finding good writers in fields out of your area of expertise include the following:

- Check recent journals for authors of articles on the general topic, or check specialty journals for their editorial board.

- Contact specialty organizations to see whether they can put out a call for authors to their members.

- Network wherever you go—professional meetings, alumni gatherings, community events, and even social engagements.

TABLE 22.1 Comparison of Single Author and Multiple Contributors

	Single Author	**Multiple Contributors**
Writing style	Consistent writing style	Variable writing styles
Format	Consistent format	Potential for more variability
Deadline	More difficult to meet deadline with large amount of content, but only one person is accountable to that deadline	Deadline may be easier to reach with less content per person, but everyone needs to be accountable to deadline
Administrative duties	Less time spent in organization and supervision of others	More time spent planning, organizing, and collaborating
Compensation	Royalties do not need to be split	Need to split royalties or pay contributors out of author royalties
Development	No overlap, consistent depth through chapters	Inconsistent depth and possible overlap among chapters
Content	Limited to one person's expertise and perspective	Expertise and perspective of multiple authors may provide richer content

- Use social media as outreach and conduct online searches to check conference programs or proceedings to see who has spoken on the topic.
- Partner with a school of nursing or hospital department of continuing education to find contributors who are being encouraged by their institution to write for publication.
- Consult with your initial contact—usually the acquisitions editor—at the publisher. There may be a list of experts on file.

Some (but not all) book projects and some chapter projects have an author allowance budgeted; depending on the contract, this might be an advance on royalties or a grant for the creation of the book. You might need to use some of this money to help find or incentivize those hard-to-find contributors. Give potential contributors complete information—a synopsis of the project, the breadth and depth of the topic you want covered, page count, deadlines, additional duties such as reviewing page proofs, and any honorarium or incentive—to help them determine whether the work is a good fit. The last thing you need is a contributor who says yes but fails to deliver.

Q *I've been asked to write a book chapter, but I'm not sure if I should do it. What should I consider?*

A If you have been asked to write or revise a chapter for a book, you can feel honored but should not feel obligated to accept. You may consider many aspects of the offer, but your main consideration should be the time commitment (Oermann, 2022). If you don't have adequate time to successfully complete the project, you will be a hindrance rather than a help to the project. To estimate the time commitment, find out as much about the project as you can, and speak to others in your field who may have done similar work. In the end, only you can decide how much free time your schedule allows, and how you would like to spend it.

Collecting Contributor Forms

Even if you're using a network of friends and trusted colleagues to help you with your project, don't neglect to have a contributor agreement and all official documents in place, including the letter of intent, biography form, and contributor agreement. Your contract with your publisher will require it, and the publisher may have company forms or electronic filing for this information. To help with organization of documents and working toward the deadline, keep a spreadsheet listing the following for each chapter: title, contributor, contact information (including phone numbers, email addresses, work and home addresses, fax number), number of pages, honorarium (include space for check number if you will be paying the honorarium), deadlines, when forms were sent out and when they were returned, and any special notes such as the best time to call.

Q *I asked a friend to contribute to my book. I didn't think I'd need a contributor agreement because we're so close, but now she's late on her deadline, and my publisher is unhappy with us. What can I do to avoid losing a contributor—and a friend?*

A You might need to consider replacing her with another author because ultimately, your professional career is your priority. Be open and honest about a missed deadline before your whole project is in jeopardy. By suggesting a replacement, you may be giving your friend a graceful "out." For the future, remember that it's hard to do business with friends. A contributor agreement is a business agreement; it's a simple transaction to protect you both.

Letter of intent. One of the first forms you should provide for the contributor is a *letter of intent* or *project letter*. This should describe the project and identify the contributor's role, including topic area, length, due dates, publishing date, and honorarium. The letter, which summarizes what you described to the contributor verbally or via email, serves as a document that the contributor can refer to during the project for basic information. Some authors have contributors sign this letter as an agreement, but it is not the same as the contributor agreement. Example 22.1 shows elements of a contributor letter of intent.

Contributor agreement. An essential form is the contributor agreement for the publisher. The publisher might offer a standard form that identifies the responsibilities of the contributor to the main author(s) and publisher, verifies that the work has not been published previously, and assigns copyright to the publisher. Both the contributor and the publisher

Carol Stevens, MSN, RN
University Hospital
Address
City/State/Zip

Dear Ms. Stevens:

Thank you for agreeing to contribute to *Chronic Disease Management for Nurses: From Acute Care to Palliative Care*. Sigma Theta Tau International will publish this reference book next year. This book will be used as a field guide and quick reference book for nurses working in a variety of settings with patients with chronic diseases. I would like it to reflect best practices and research in the areas of chronic disease management and care across the time and severity continuum, from acute care to palliative care. ←—— *Title of book, publisher, and planned publication date / Purpose of the book*

Your chapter is Chapter 7, "Chronic Obstructive Pulmonary Disease," which has been allocated 11 pages. I will send you an electronic template that explicitly outlines the headings and flow of information. ←—— *Chapter topic and page allotment*

I need your completed manuscript by February 15, 2026, to allow for editing and production time. Approximately six weeks after submission of your manuscript, you will receive an edited copy with questions for your review. Later in the process, you will be asked to read page proofs of the chapter to ensure its accuracy and possibly add any last-minute changes. ←—— *Deadline and editing process*

Please keep a copy of your manuscript, revisions along the way, and the reference materials you used in case I have any questions during the process. When the entire book is complete, you will be sent an honorarium of $200 and a copy of the book. Your name will be listed in the front of the book as a contributor. ←—— *Honorarium*

Because this is both a practice manual guide and reference book, the material should be written in a practical manner, but please supply authoritative references within the chapter, such as those that come from published clinical trials, meta-analyses, approved guidelines, and position papers, using American Psychological Association (APA) format. The majority of references should be no more than three years old at the time of publication. ←—— *Writing and referencing style*

Special features in this book are three to six learning objectives for each chapter, tables that outline the most common drugs and their actions, a list of community resources for each topic area, and patient education alerts. You will see examples of these in the electronic template that I will send to you. ←—— *Special features of the book*

Please contact me when you have reviewed all the material and would like to discuss the details further. You can reach me by email or cellphone at any time during the process. Thank you again for your participation. ←—— *How to contact you with any questions*

Sincerely,
(your name and credentials)

EXAMPLE 22.1 Components of a contributor letter of intent.

sign the form. This is a legal agreement. In some cases (e.g., if the author will retain copyright of the book), the contributor agreement is between the author and contributor, rather than the publisher and contributor; in this situation, the publisher requires the author to ensure agreements are signed and kept on file.

Biography form. A biography form is another important form to have completed early in the process. You need each contributor's correct spelling of name and their credentials, professional title and affiliations, preferred address, email address, and contact numbers (work, cell, home, and fax). Collecting this information early will ensure that you can reach your contributors with questions and comments as deadlines approach. You can also use this information when compiling a list of contributors in the book, or for finding expertise if you need additional help in certain areas. Ask each contributor to provide a short narrative bio (100 to 150 words) that describes their expertise in relation to the book, including education, clinical practice, academic appointment, and other professional accomplishments. In addition, a social security number may be required if an honorarium will be paid.

Q *Can an author or contributor retain copyright for their work?*

A The answer is yes and no. Copyright law is meant to protect the format or expression of a work, not the ideas or facts that the work is based on. The publisher is investing significant time and money into the development of the publication and wants to protect their investment. Read the wording of the agreement. Some publishers may allow their authors and contributors the right to use up to 10% of content for scholarly purposes without seeking permission, providing the work is appropriately cited. For more information about copyright, see Chapter 11.

Contract

After the publisher accepts your proposal, a contract is drawn up and signed between the author and the publisher. Publishers usually have a template contract that includes items such as payment of author royalties, copyright ownership, number of copies to be published, publication date, and general responsibilities of the author and publisher. The author is generally responsible for preparing an original manuscript and submitting it according to deadline, then reviewing proofs and making corrections. The publisher is responsible for producing the book (copyediting, design, printing), marketing the book, and paying royalties or honoraria according to negotiated terms. There may be additional provisions about revised editions, derivative works, permission and licensing fees, use of the author's name, and "force majeure" (delay due to unforeseen circumstances such as war, terrorism, or "acts of God" [e.g., natural disasters]). As with any contract, read carefully before signing and consult an attorney as needed.

Q *How can I be sure to meet the deadline in my contact?*

A Through no fault of your own, you might find yourself slipping behind because of too many commitments, family emergencies, regional disasters, or the need to revise what you have written because of newly released information. At the start of the project, have a backup plan to handle situations that may threaten your deadline. You need to be proactive to keep a project on track. One young entrepreneur, Andrew Howlett, suggests doing a pre-mortem at the beginning of any project—identify ways the project may go wrong and ways to avoid that, such as reviewing everyone's vacation schedule and planning for holidays (Forbes Young Entrepreneur Council, 2022). You may need to line up a potential second editor who could step in if needed, and identify times you can "burn the midnight oil" in order to catch up. Good communication is always helpful. Check in with contributors regularly to check their progress and offer objective feedback, suggests Andrew Schrage. And frequently remind yourself why you got started on the project in the first place, offers Nick Venditti, to help you and your team stay motivated (Forbes Young Entrepreneur Council, 2022).

Setting a Schedule

The publisher has accepted your proposal with projected manuscript transmittal and publication dates. Whether you're writing your project alone or working with a team of 50 people, you need a schedule. You now need to work backward to establish a timeline. Front-end planning time is needed to ensure that content can be reviewed, edited, and revised as needed before submission to the publisher.

Q *Why does it take so long to produce a book?*

A The larger and more complex the project is (e.g., if it has many contributors), the longer the preparation time. Time is needed for the initial preparation of the manuscript by the main author(s). Then it is sent to the publisher, where more editing and copyediting are done. After that, you need to answer editors' questions and make revisions as needed. A production staff takes over, you review page proofs, the work goes out to a printer, and (finally) it arrives in a distribution center for sale. That whole process can take from eight months to two years. Electronic publications are on the shorter side, but still take considerable planning and production time. Fortunately, you—as the author—are concerned only about the preparation of the manuscript and reviewing the edited pages and page proofs.

Naturally, your schedule becomes a bit more complex if you're using contributors or coauthors. Because you will be providing outlines, templates, and a sample chapter to the contributors, you might not need to see rough drafts or expanded outlines from them. You should give enough time, however, for you to send their contributions for peer review and to edit them, then return to the contributors for revisions. Add in extra time for revisions in case the chapter or section does not come in as you intended. Some authors give a monetary bonus to contributors who get in their material ahead of the deadline. Despite incentives, frequent communication, and helpful support, expect that some contributors will be late. As an author, you must balance the schedule with enough time for contributors to produce their manuscript, adding your time spent editing all sections and melding them into one cohesive work. If possible, work on one chapter at a time. It takes more time to start multiple chapters than to concentrate on one chapter and getting it completed (Oermann, 2022).

One tip for managing a schedule and encouraging on-time submissions by contributors is to have virtual office hours at least once a week at a time that will be convenient to many. You can let your team know you are available for questions and communication by phone or electronic means. You also can pass information back and forth through various programs such as the publisher's editorial site, Google Docs, or even your Facebook page (limit who can view the page). It's helpful to send out reminders, words of encouragement, tips, and examples of best practices. Be aware that you will need to be available 24/7 for those who work best during off hours.

Although you'll want to keep the documents private, you might want to use blogs or social media such as Facebook, Instagram, and X to give people a taste of what is coming in your book to build anticipation—and sales. Writing blogs and holding workshops based on your planned material can be helpful to test your assumptions about what your target audience wants and needs to know (Haberman & Wilson, 2023).

> **Confidence Booster**
>
> Even though you may have had a negative experience with writing or publishing in the past, don't give up on your dream project! With enough organization, support, commitment, and guts, you can succeed.

Following Guidelines

Each publisher has *author guidelines*, also called *submission guidelines* or *publisher's guidelines*, which give you information on each step of the process, such as how to prepare your manuscript, how to obtain permission for copyrighted material, and how to submit your manuscript. Guidelines also cover any of the publisher's *house style* issues, such as how to handle titles or credentials or how to spell certain words (e.g., *health care* versus *healthcare*), and which stylebook you should use as a reference. Base your instructions to any contributors on these guidelines, and check them again during the editing and final preparation of your manuscript. Be sure that you have all parts of the book covered.

You'll also likely need to submit a list of figures. It's easiest to set this up as a spreadsheet, with the figure number, short title, and permission information (whether permission is needed; if so, whether it was obtained and how the copyright holder needs to be listed in the book) for each chapter. You may also be required to submit evidence documenting that permission has been obtained.

The author's guidelines detail how to set up paragraphs, pages, tables, illustrations, footnotes or endnotes, references, and other aspects of the manuscript.

As the author, this is your responsibility, but you will save time and effort by highlighting these guidelines for your contributors. An important aspect of guidelines is how to submit illustrations. Many contributors do not know how to obtain illustrations or obtain permission for published illustrations. In most cases, you can submit photos or illustrations in the form of electronic files. You must obtain permission from the copyright holder of anything that has been published and from people who are identified in photographs.

Submission guidelines explain this process. (You can learn more about permissions in Chapter 11.)

The electronic format in which you transmit the manuscript depends on the author guidelines. Typically, each chapter and other parts of the manuscript, such as the appendices, should be in separate files and identified by author last name and chapter number. Once you submit your manuscript, any changes you feel are necessary should be held for the review stage.

Parts of a Book

Here are typical parts of a book that you'll need to submit to the publisher:

Front matter
- **Title page:** This includes the book title and author names with credentials.
- **Dedication:** A dedication is a personal thank-you, usually to a family member, friend, or special colleague. It should be short and to the point.
- **Acknowledgments:** This section recognizes those who have helped with the book content—for example, a librarian who conducted extra research for you, or the person who designed the cover. It's longer than the dedication.
- **Author and contributors:** List names, credentials, and a short bio. The lead author is listed first, with contributors in alphabetical order. Try to keep contributor bios similar in length (about 100 to 150 words), with the focus on what qualifies each person to write the chapter.
- **Table of contents:** Be sure to include any appendices.
- **Foreword:** This is written by an expert and explains why the book is important. Try to choose a foreword author who is well known in the book's content area, but don't use one of the contributors.
- **Introduction or preface:** This is where you get to set the stage for readers. Give them an overview of the purpose of the book, any special features such as checklists, and what they can expect to gain from the content.

Chapters
- Identify each chapter with the number, short title, and, if applicable, contributor name.

Back matter
Not all of these elements will be included in every book.

- **Appendices:** These provide the opportunity to give readers supplemental information that would be too long to include in a chapter, relates to multiple chapters, or is helpful but not essential to include in the main book. For example, Appendix C in this book is on publishing terminology, which is helpful for authors to know. Appendices are usually labeled by letter: Appendix A, Appendix B, and so on.
- **Glossary:** If your book is highly technical and uses terms that readers might struggle with, a glossary can be helpful.
- **Bibliography:** Sometimes readers can benefit from a list of references and resources that aren't cited in the chapters but might be helpful.
- **Index:** Usually the publisher, not the author, prepares the index. If you are required to do so by your contract, it's best to hire a professional indexer to do this work.

The order of front and back matter may vary slightly.

Q *Who picks the title and creates the book cover?*

A Although your ideas on title and cover design are usually welcome, the publisher makes the final decision on these items. Both title and design depend on several marketing considerations, such as other book titles in your content area; whether the book is positioned as a textbook, continuing education product, reference manual, or another type; and what will work well on the planned cover size.

Yes, You Can

Potential book authors usually ask themselves, "Can I do this?" If you believe you can't, you won't. However, if you reject negative thoughts and negative self-talk, and focus on positive affirmations about your ability to write a book, your outlook and outcome will be different. Enlist help from colleagues, family, and friends as a network of support. Set goals and timelines and start writing. Through upfront planning and careful project management, you *can* produce a finished book.

Write Now!

1. Think of an idea for a book or book chapter. Using the Sigma Theta Tau proposal format in this chapter, make notes on how you would accomplish each step.

2. Compare the table of contents from three different books to identify different formats. Analyze how well the table of contents reflects the book's stated purpose and title.

References

Forbes Young Entrepreneur Council. (2022, April 20). Nine effective tips to keep a long-term project on track. *Forbes.* https://www.forbes.com/sites/theyec/2022/04/20/nine-effective-tips-to-keep-a-long-term-project-on-track/?sh=1374f6b83759

Haberman, J., & Wilson, G. (2023). Ten simple rules for writing a technical book. *PLoS Computational Biology, 19*(8), e1011305. https://doi.org/10.1371/journal.pcbi.1011305

Indeed Editorial Team. (2022, June 24). *11 tips for managing large projects.* https://www.indeed.com/career-advice/career-development/managing-large-projects

Kagan, S. H. (2023). The art of nursing, the craft of writing [Editorial]. *International Journal of Older People Nursing, 18*(2), e12531. https://doi.org/10.1111/opn.12531

Nature Cancer. (2023). The craft (and art) of scientific writing [Editorial]. *Nature Cancer, 4,* 583–584. https://doi.org/10.1038/s43018-023-00579-y

Oermann, M. H. (2022). Writing a book: Strategies for your success. *Nurse Author & Editor, 32*(2), 38–41. https://doi.org/10.1111/nae2.12041

Sigma Theta Tau International. (2023). *Becoming a book author.* https://www.sigmanursing.org/learn-grow/publications/book-proposal-guidelines

Writing for a General Audience

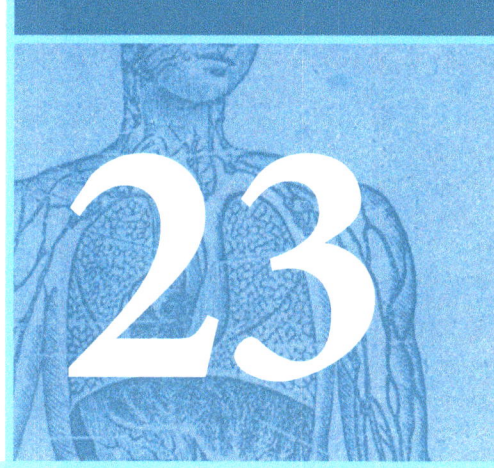

23

–Pamela J. Haylock, PhD, RN, FAAN

> *"The point of writing is not just to exist; it's to be read."*
> –Nicholas Kristof

WHAT YOU'LL LEARN IN THIS CHAPTER

- Nurse writers use curiosity, interests, knowledge, expertise, and scientific writing experience to craft effective health communications for general audiences.

- Crucial elements of any writing project include the author's attention to general literacy, reading level, and cultural awareness as they apply to targeted readers.

- Plain language, readability assessment, and other tools can help improve comprehension of material.

Have you noticed? Changes in learning needs and information sources are ongoing and constant within an environment of health literacy differences among populations and demographic groups. The COVID-19 pandemic continues to affect many aspects of healthcare, including health communications. For example, misinformation and mistrust are troubling in the fast-changing worlds of science and healthcare (Grace, 2021).

Readily available sources of health-related information and advice include professional journals, magazines, newspapers, self-help books, community-based lectures and presentations, the internet, social media platforms, podcasts, and yes, supermarket tabloids. Not all sources are reliable, nor are all reliable sources available or readable by people who need and want information.

That's where nurses come in. In addition to writing for scientific and professional literature, nurses can provide high-quality health information for the general public to motivate behavior changes among individuals, families, communities, and populations. Given the complex nature of healthcare and the public's ready access to misinformation, credible and clear health communications must be available to guide decision-making and self-care, influence public policy, address population-specific and environmental challenges, and teach effective family and community caregiving skills (Klein et al., 2023; Office of the Surgeon General, 2021). Using strategies in this chapter, you can provide that communication by writing for the general public.

What to Write

Potential health-related topics present themselves everywhere we look—subject matter about which nurses have informed perspectives. Journal articles; local, state, and federal health-related measures; organizations' position papers; and treatment guidelines will surely spark ideas for topics of interest to the public, neighbors, and colleagues. Current events and related issues that are unlikely to vanish anytime soon and about which nurses' observations, opinions, and suggestions are relevant include COVID-19 and other infectious disease outbreaks, health effects related to climate change, nurse staffing, health misinformation, and artificial intelligence. Pick a topic you find interesting and about which you are knowledgeable and passionate.

Before You Write

Before jumping into writing an article, book chapter, or other form of publication, take time to plan your project, including setting goals and creating a timeline. Too often authors skip this step, but planning is essential for successful completion. (See Chapter 1 for more information about planning your project.) To plan effectively, you need to understand how literacy, reading level, and cultural and linguistic factors can affect comprehension of material for a general audience.

Literacy

Literacy and, specifically, health literacy are recognized as social determinants of health (Coughlin et al., 2020; Nutbeam & Lloyd, 2021). A person's health and ability to access healthcare services depend on success in seeking, using, and understanding health information. Barriers in speaking, reading, and writing can lead to significant health challenges for individuals and disparities in outcomes.

Literacy. The National Center for Education Statistics (NCES) Program for the International Assessment of Adult Competencies (PIAAC) defines literacy as "understanding, evaluating, using and engaging with written text to participate in the society, to achieve one's goals and to develop one's knowledge and potential" (2019, para. 2).

Several agencies report national and international literacy data. PIACC survey findings indicate that 79% (four in five) of adults in the United States can complete tasks that allow them to compare and contrast information, paraphrase, and make low-level inferences—in essence, literacy skills at level 2 or above (Mamedova & Pawloski, 2019). The remaining one in five adults (21%, or 43 million adults) find these tasks difficult to complete. Adults below level 1 literacy may be considered "functionally illiterate" in English. US-born adults comprise the majority (66%) of adults with low English literacy skills, but adults not born in the US are over-represented in this category—they comprise 34% of the population with low literacy skills compared to 15% of the total population (Mamedova & Pawloski, 2019).

Crucial variations in literacy rates in individual states are often overlooked, particularly in publications and other media aimed at entire populations. ThinkImpact, a project that provides research and trends in education and business (https://www.thinkimpact.com), reports literacy rates by state.

Health literacy. The Healthy People Initiative, established by the US Department of Health and Human Services (HHS) in 1979, seeks to improve the health and well-being of Americans (Ochiai et al., 2021). The fifth iteration of the initiative, Healthy People 2030,

> ### Confidence Booster
>
> As nurses and advocates, we share knowledge and experience. For example, a friend risked life and limb—literally—as she fought an infection that started with edema and painful skin breakdown on both legs. After several days of activity-limiting pain, she was hospitalized for four days and treated with bed rest, intravenous antibiotics, pain management, and applications of compression dressings twice-daily. She didn't know the sores and edema were symptoms of lymphedema, most likely secondary to surgery and radiation therapy in treatment for uterine cancer more than 10 years ago.
>
> In another situation, a young woman (I'll call her Ava) talked with her obstetrician about planning for a second baby. Ava said she was "a little nervous" about a lump in her breast. The physician dismissed Ava's concern, saying, "Don't worry—you're too young to have breast cancer." Just months later, Ava learned the doctor was wrong; she is not too young. Ava had late-stage breast cancer at diagnosis, started traditional chemotherapy, and then moved on to clinical trials using medications not yet approved for use in the United States.
>
> We have all heard too many similar stories. It is among nurses' duties and responsibilities to learn and to teach. Sharing what we know, and seeing people benefit from our knowledge, is one of the great joys of being a nurse.

focuses on national health objectives and improvement of health and well-being. This iteration includes health literacy as a foundational principle of promoting health equity and reducing disparities in social determinants of health (Ochiai et al., 2021; Santana et al., 2021). Healthy People 2030 clarifies individual and organizational roles in health literacy with these definitions:

- *Personal health literacy* is the degree to which individuals have the ability to find, understand, and use information and services to inform health-related decisions and actions for themselves and others.

- *Organizational health literacy* is the degree to which organizations equitably enable individuals to find, understand, and use information and services to inform health-related decisions and actions for themselves and others.

Low health literacy is a barrier to effective communication between patients, families, and healthcare providers and affects people's health outcomes. Evidence indicates links between limited health literacy and fewer health promotion and early detection activities, lower abilities to manage chronic illnesses, increased hospitalization and re-hospitalization, and higher morbidity and mortality (Navarro-Rubio et al., 2016; Rudd et al., 2013). In a scoping review examining connections between health literacy and cancer-related outcomes, Samoil and colleagues (2021) found that inadequate health literacy was associated with several negative effects, including less engagement in preventative behaviors and a longer lag time between symptom identification and seeking medical treatment.

People with low health literacy are unable to absorb complicated concepts related to health, so explanations for these populations must be clear and concise. The Plain Writing Act of 2010 requires federal agencies to use clear communication that the public can understand (PlainLanguage.gov, 2011). You also should use plain language to improve readability and facilitate understanding when writing for a general audience.

Reading Level

Using plain language and writing at an appropriate reading level pay off in effective communication. Consider the classic study of parents' grasp of two polio vaccine information pamphlets (Davis et al., 1996). Researchers used two versions of a pamphlet on the vaccine. One version was developed by the Centers for Disease Control and Prevention (CDC); the second was a simplified version that maintained the essential information. Parents were more likely to read the revised pamphlet, and their comprehension and reading time improved.

Unfortunately, information for the public is often not written in plain language. That includes patient education materials. For example, a 20-year analysis of patient education materials from "high-impact medical journals" found readability grade levels ranging from grades 11.2 to 13.8 (Rooney et al., 2021). In addition, a study of patient education materials used in Canadian provincial cancer agencies found that of the nearly 800 patient education materials analyzed, the average grade level was 9.3 ± 2.1 (van Ballegooie et al., 2023).

The problem extends to online material as well. Of 18 websites, online health information about COVID-19 exceeded reading levels of grades 6 through 8. State-generated materials were written above 8th grade levels for every state and used more difficult terms. Of 10 states with high illiteracy rates, 9 had information written above grade 10 level (Mishra & Dexter, 2020).

Q *What resources are available if I want to become more skilled in writing health information materials for the public?*

A Take every opportunity that comes your way to hone your writing skills and improve your ability to share health-related information. Peruse the local library and bookstores for how-to books that seem to match your interest areas. Look for writing interest groups in your community and local or university-sponsored writing workshops.

Online and in-person continuing education courses offered by academic institutions and writers' associations are also options. The American Medical Writers Association (www.amwa.org), the Association of Health Care Journalists (www.healthjournalism.org), and the European Medical Writers Association (www.emwa.org) are three member associations that support writers who focus on medical communications, including writing for a general audience. These organizations' websites provide resources for writers of any level, and some resources are available to nonmembers at no cost.

What reading level should you target for your written material? Recommendations vary and are frustratingly inconsistent. The American Medical Association (AMA) and the National Institutes of Health (NIH) agree that health information directed toward patients should be written at 6th- to 7th-grade reading levels (Abu-Heija et al., 2019). Hill-Briggs and Fitzpatrick (2023) and Hill-Briggs et al. (2012) suggest 5th-grade reading levels for low-literacy populations. Consider your target audience and reading levels of materials offered by publication outlets you'll target.

Cultural and Linguistic Considerations

Under-studied aspects of health education include cultural sensitivity and cultural appropriateness (Kirmayer, 2012; Knoerl et al., 2011; Williamson & Harrison, 2010). Kirmayer (2012) writes that evidence-based practices (EBP) demanded in today's healthcare settings are culturally determined, possibly biased, and inappropriate. He suggests that culturally diverse communities have "ways of knowing" that don't rely on the methods that characterize EBP. In addition, cultural beliefs, norms, and perspectives may impact how health information is interpreted.

Linguistic issues are also important to consider when writing for the general public. According to 2019 Census Bureau data, 68 million residents in the United States speak a language other than English at home (Dietrich & Hernandez, 2022). Many of these residents have limited English proficiency, possibly making it difficult for them to communicate with healthcare providers and other healthcare personnel, resulting in suboptimal care.

The National Standards for Competency and Linguistically Appropriate Services (CLAS) in Health and Health Care, published by the US Department of Health and Human Services Office of Minority Health (n.d.), are intended to help organizations take steps to reduce health disparities by addressing linguistic needs. The standards take into account health literacy and state the need to provide information, including printed material, in languages commonly used in the population the organization serves.

Be sensitive to linguistic and cultural issues when writing so readers can understand and apply the information you offer. You'll want to use bias-free language, particularly in sensitive areas such as age, religion, racial or ethnic identity, sexual orientation, socioeconomic status, and immigration status (American Psychological Association, 2020). See Chapter 6 for more information about bias-free language.

Crafting Your Work

Now that you understand how literacy, reading level, and cultural and linguistic factors can affect reader comprehension, and you have your goals and timeline in place, you're ready to start writing. Writing your article, letter, or another type of work will be easier if you follow some basic tips.

Culturally Sensitive Materials

Creation and use of culturally appropriate materials come with complex and often related challenges. Overcoming these challenges depends on cultural understanding. Consider pain-related materials for American Indians (AI) and Alaska Natives (AN) as examples. Relevant cultural beliefs include (Haozous et al., 2010; Hendrix, 2001):

- Enduring pain is looked upon as a survival skill.
- Verbal and nonverbal expressions of pain are unacceptable in many AI cultures.
- People who violate the social norm by admitting to pain experience a high degree of social isolation and guilt.
- Older AI/AN have difficulties describing pain, and as a result may be less likely to ask for pain medication and more likely to use internal resources to manage pain.

Tribal culture and socioeconomic variations are important cultural sensitivity, health literacy, and readability considerations—vital to preparing written materials. As exemplars, suggestions for writing effective pain educational material for AI/AN patients include (Haozous & Knobf, 2013; Jimenez et al., 2011):

- Consider the multidimensional nature of AI's perceptions of pain.
- Use metaphors and storytelling traditions.
- Use appropriate quality-of-life measures and terms.
- Include culturally based traditional treatments for pain management.
- Know that a numeric pain scale is often not appropriate for assessment.

Know Your Audience

Knowing your intended audience helps you organize and present your topic in ways that encourage someone to read, take note of, and possibly even act on what you write. Background information and answering certain questions can clarify your intended audience. Consider the scenario of preparing to write a new CDC pamphlet to encourage adults to adhere to the current recommended vaccination schedule. You learn that adult vaccination rates in the United States are extremely low. According to the CDC, thousands of adults become ill, are hospitalized, and die from vaccine-preventable diseases (CDC, 2023). Unfortunately, most adults don't know they need lifelong vaccinations.

Armed with this information, you ask yourself these questions: Is this work intended for younger or older adults? What do people already know about vaccines, what do they want to know, and what do they need to know? What are their views on vaccination in general? The answers will help you develop a concise message. You may want to hold focus groups for members of your potential target audience to gain more insights and validate that your planned content is on track.

Know Your Message

Your message should be one that helps you achieve your desired outcome. For example, in the vaccine scenario, you want people to follow the recommended schedule. You should have one main message. Craft that message before writing a first draft; consider the diversity in the population you are writing for, including variations in health-seeking behaviors. Translate that message into a clear and compelling statement. Every sentence in the final work should support the message. Keep in mind a quotation attributed to Einstein:

> If you can't explain something simply, you don't understand it well. Most of the fundamental ideas of science are essentially simple, and may, as a rule, be expressed in a language comprehensible to everyone. Everything should be as simple as it can be, yet no simpler. (PlainLanguage.gov, n.d., para. 5)

Follow a Process

Once you know the intended audience and have a message, you're ready to begin writing. As you write, use language your intended readers know. You can determine this by reading other materials that the publisher provides its readers.

Start by writing an initial draft, a first quick effort to get your thoughts down. Consider what format will work best to deliver your message. Examples include article, tip sheet, quiz, and infographic (CDC and Prevention Agency for Toxic Substances and Disease Registry, n.d.). If you're writing for national government entities, you'll need to adhere to the Federal Plain Language Guidelines mentioned earlier in this chapter. You should also apply these guidelines in items you write for the general public.

Consider these suggestions (CDC and Prevention Agency for Toxic Substances and Disease Registry, n.d.; Center for Health Care Strategies, Inc., 2013):

- Use simple illustrations and pictures along with text to help readers focus on what is important. Consider diversity in images and avoid ones that look staged.
- Use clear headings and bullets instead of paragraphs.
- Use short sentences, active voice, and conversational language.
- Use clear and inclusive language.
- Avoid jargon and define any medical terms you need to include in plain language.
- Make any advice easy to act on by providing clear action steps that are doable.
- Strive to deliver a clear and persuasive message.

Experienced writers suggest putting your first draft aside for a time. Then come back to it, read it, and consider changes to clarify the content. Pay particular attention to the beginning of your work. People choose to read, and they can choose not to read. Capture readers' interests in the topic as early as possible—in the first sentence or at least in the first few sentences. You might begin with a startling fact or dramatic example of how the topic affects members of the population for whom you are writing.

Consider these questions as you form those all-important first sentences:

- Why is this information important to the reader?
- What difference will this information make?
- How will the information be helpful?

After you've reworked the draft, ask a colleague to review it and provide feedback. If possible, you also should seek feedback from a person representative of your target readers. Consider this feedback, along with your own insights, as you revise the work.

After revision it's time to edit, which includes conducting a careful review of the basic elements of your writing for correctness and clarity (grammar, punctuation, spelling, sentence structure). Proofreading is the final check and provides opportunities to catch errors before submitting your work to an editor or publisher. (You can access editing and proofing checklists in Appendices A and B.)

During this process, you'll want to be sure you assess your work for readability.

Q *Are there other resources I could access to improve my writing for the public (and my professional writing too)?*

A Here are a few additional resources:

- Clear Writing Hub (https://www.cdc.gov/nceh/clearwriting/index.html), part of the CDC website, contains many free resources, including the *Clear Writing Guide*.

- Coursera lists universities that offer free online writing courses for many genres (www.coursera.org).

- The Purdue OWL (https://owl.purdue.edu/owl/purdue_owl.html) has a variety of free writing resources.

Writing workshops can be particularly helpful. The combination of fascinating and inspiring environs, accomplished mentors, and willing fellow students can motivate participants to adopt the habit of writing—and with each effort, write better. Shaw Guides' Guide to Writers Conferences & Writing Workshops (http://writing.shawguides.com) is a source for these.

Assess Readability

After your initial draft is finished, but before you consider it ready to submit, check readability using an established tool to obtain a readability score. (*Readability scores* are computer-calculated indices that reveal the level of education someone is likely to need to read a piece of text with ease.) Such tools are most often based on two central features that translate to easier readability (lower grade levels):

- Minimize the number of words with three or more syllables.

- Minimize average sentence length.

You can use online resources and tools in software programs to easily calculate readability. An online example is the **Readability Calculator** (www.wordcalc.com/readability), which provides a score for eight readability metrics. Although for the most part calculations are automated, it's still helpful to understand what's behind common readability tools.

SMOG (Simplified Measure of Gobbledygook) Readability Formula. The SMOG formula is based on the number of polysyllabic words in the text. It's a quick and simple way to grade readability and is especially useful for materials that are short in length, such as an information pamphlet or consent form. The SMOG reading level (whether you complete this manually or use a third-party resource) is calculated by using these steps (Arian et al., 2016):

1. Count off 10 consecutive sentences near the beginning, middle, and end of the text. For materials with fewer than 30 sentences, use the entire text.

2. Count the number of words with three or more syllables, including repetitions of the same word.

3. Use the SMOG conversion table (see Table 23.1) to determine the approximate grade level.

TABLE 23.1 SMOG Conversion Table

Total Polysyllabic Word Count	Approximate Grade Level
1–6	5
7–12	6
13–20	7
21–30	8
31–42	9
43–56	10
57–72	11
73–90	12

Note: The SMOG conversion table, developed by Harold C. McGraw, Office of Educational Research, Baltimore Co. Public Schools, Towson, MD. The actual table extends through Grade Level 18.

Making the Conversion

Converting professional or scholarly information to information for consumers is common. Hill-Briggs et al. (2012) devised a method for evaluating and adapting print materials to meet a "less than fifth grade readability" criterion. Three low-literacy criteria are useful to assess and modify text:

- Sentence length less than 15 words
- Writing in active voice (You can learn more about active voice in Chapter 6.)
- Use of common words (use of multisyllabic words—words more than two to three syllables long—is minimized or avoided)

Here, an example shows commonly used medical information translated to material useful to consumers. At the end is an estimate of the reading level based on the Flesh-Kincaid tool.

Healthcare professionals: Early assessment of current and potential vascular access needs (preferably at admission) in all patient settings promotes timely and appropriate vascular access insertion, reduces vascular access-associated complications, and promotes vessel health and preservation. A consultation between the vascular access specialist and the patient and family is critical in achieving the optimal outcome of selecting the right device, placing it in the right location, at the right time.

(Readability Statistics: Passive sentences–0; Words per sentence–34.5; Flesch-Kincaid Grade Level–21.4)

General public: You will meet with the vascular access nurse soon after you arrive. This nurse helps us plan for the treatment you will have. This allows us to plan to meet your needs. This helps reduce your chances of problems while you are here and when you are at home. You will get the best outcome from your treatment when we:

- Use the right kind of device
- Put the device in the right place
- Use the device at the right time
- Remove the device when it is no longer needed

(Readability Statistics: Passive sentences–0; Words per sentence–12.6; Flesch-Kincaid Grade Level–3.7)

This example shows how you can convert language that healthcare professionals commonly use to communicate with each other to language that conveys the same information to lay readers. Notice how the second example strips away medical jargon, replacing it with simple words to make the point. Shorter sentences and, with a few exceptions, sticking to words with fewer than three syllables lower reading grade levels.

The website Plainlanguage.gov provides an online link to the Plain Language Thesaurus for Health Communications—a list of common medical terms with suggested alternate words and phrases aimed at creating patient education and consent materials at 5th-grade levels.

Flesch-Kincaid Grade Level/Flesch Reading Ease Tests. These tests compute readability based on the average number of syllables per word and the average number of words per sentence. Both can be equated to a grade level (Arian et al., 2016; Readable, n.d.). The past several Microsoft Word versions include these features. With the Windows version, go to File, then Options, then Proofing and select "Show readability statistics." With the Mac version, select the Editor feature, then click on Insights (Document stats). (The process may be different depending on which software version you have.)

SAM (Suitability Assessment of Materials). SAM can guide development of your material and assess suitability in six areas: content, literacy demand, graphics, layout and typography, learning stimulation and motivation, and cultural appropriateness. The SAM assessment process provides a score that falls in one of three categories: superior, adequate, or not suitable (Doak et al., 1996).

REALM (Rapid Estimate of Adult Literacy in Medicine) Tool. The REALM assessment tool uses medical word recognition and pronunciation tests to screen patient's reading ability in medical settings (Zulick et al., 2009). Like other readability assessment tools, REALM uses the number of syllables, along with pronunciation difficulty. Scores are translated into four reading levels based on grades: grade 0–3, 4–6, 7–8, and grade 9 and above. The REALM scale is available in English and Spanish (Agency for Healthcare Research and Quality, 2022)

Publishing Opportunities

Now that you understand the process of writing for the general public, consider where you would like to publish your work. Magazines featuring health articles are an especially important but underused outlet for nurses to reach the public. News, parenting, fitness, and beauty magazines all publish health-related articles. Newspaper and magazine journalists who write health-related stories often get information from nurses. Why shouldn't nurses do the writing and get the credit (and maybe even be paid) for what they know?

The simplest place to look for publishing opportunities may be your local public library. Bookstore shelves and magazine racks offer resources to consider—compare and contrast consumer-directed publications to determine the best fit for your idea. *Writer's Digest* magazine and website (www.writersdigest.com) cover nearly every genre you could consider. The *Writer's Market* book series is another source for identifying publication outlets. Many publications have websites and blogs, or are entirely online, offering venues for essays, stories, and practical advice for nurse writers.

Reader Feedback

Providing feedback on what has been published is an easy way to start writing for the public. The most common form of reader feedback is the "letter to the editor," most often submitted digitally.

Letter to the Editor

Letters to the editor in newspapers, magazines, and digital publications allow readers, including nurses, to respond to articles and contribute ideas to local, national, and international issues. These letters are useful ways for nurses to advocate for health-related topics and causes with prominent placement in publications and visibility through public forums such as websites.

Letters must adhere to guidelines usually listed on a publication's editorial page or on its website. In general, these letters should be short and concise, and support, rebut, or give an opinion on an article published within a given time frame.

Tips for writing a letter to the editor include:

- Construct your letter deliberately, with a beginning, a middle, and an end.
- Start by stating why you are writing (grab the editor's attention immediately).
- Cover only one main point so your idea is focused.
- Do not attack a person or use a letter to vent anger; instead, be objective and use facts to support your opinion.
- Use expert opinions to strengthen your position, as appropriate.

Example 23.1 shows a letter to the editor of a fictitious magazine.

Editors appreciate receiving letters from readers, and you might be surprised at how often your letters are published if you follow the guidelines. For more about letters to the editor and editorials, see Chapter 21.

Other forms of feedback, including commenting on an online article, blog entry, or social media post, should follow the same principles as letters to the editor.

Editorials

Editorials are another way you can provide reader feedback and reach a general audience by sharing your opinion about an issue. Editorials written by those not on a publication's staff are sometimes referred to as op-eds (short for "opposite editorial" because in print publications, they typically appear on the opposite page of staff-written editorials). Another term you may see is "guest essay" (Kingsbury, 2021).

One resource for learning how to write editorials is the nonprofit OpEd Project (theopedproject.org), which partners with organizations to offer mentoring, coaching, fellowships, webinars, and other

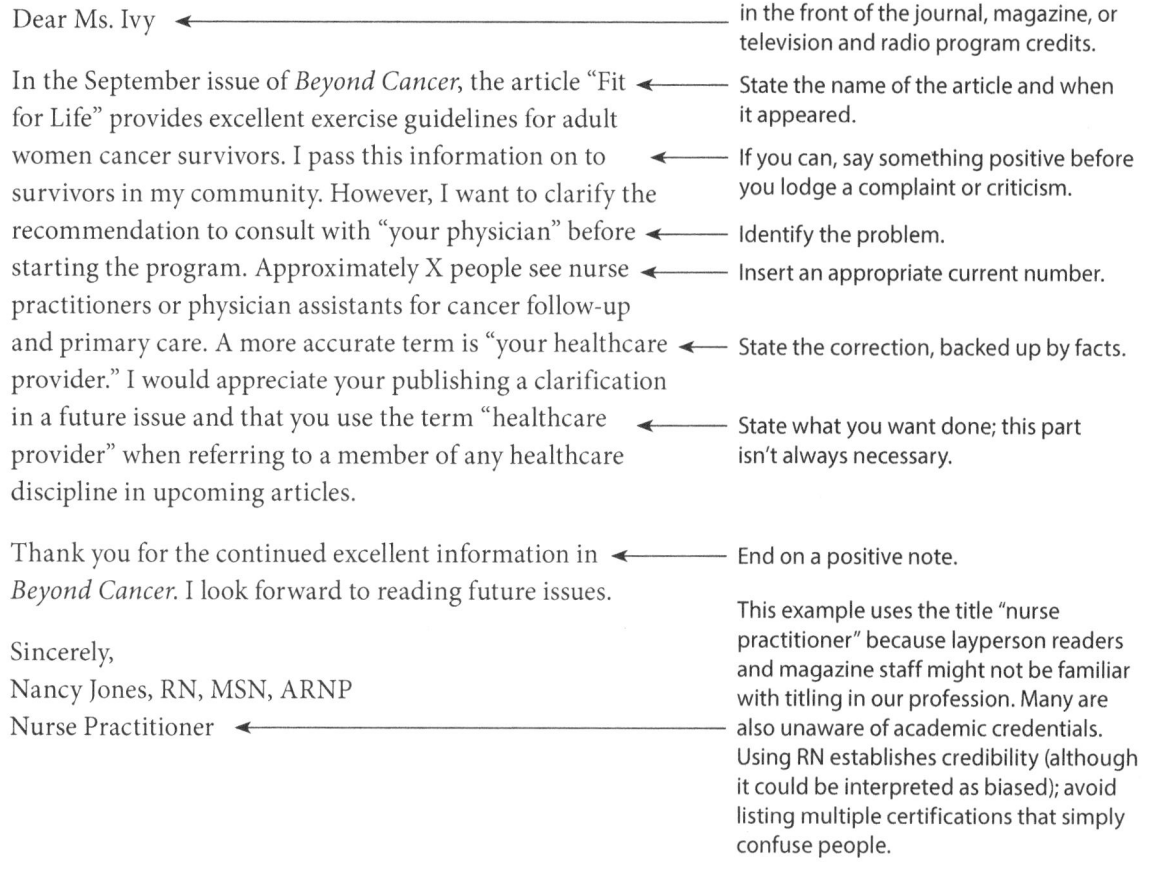

EXAMPLE 23.1 Sample letter to the editor of a fictitious magazine.

resources that support its mission ("to change who writes history") by encouraging those from all backgrounds to make their voices heard. Project participants are encouraged to ask big questions: "What do you know, Why does it matter, and How can you use it to change the world?" In short, the underpinning theme is "What could we accomplish if together we invested in all of our brain power?" (OpEd Project, n.d., para. 3 and 4).

Nicholas Kristof, an opinion columnist for *The New York Times*, provides these tips for writing editorials (Kristof, n.d.):

1. Start out with a very clear idea in your own mind about what point you want to make.
2. Don't choose a topic, choose an argument.
3. Start with a bang.
4. Personal stories are often very powerful to make a point.
5. If the platform allows it, use photos or video or music or whatever.
6. Don't feel the need to be formal or stodgy.
7. Acknowledge shortcomings in your arguments.
8. It's often useful to cite an example of what you're criticizing, or a quote from an antagonist.
9. If you're really trying to persuade people who are on the fence, remember their way of thinking may not be yours.
10. When your work is published, spread the word through social media or e-mails or any other avenue you can think of.

You can read an annotated version of one of Kristof's columns to gain insights into the writing process (Kristof, 2020).

Make the Leap

Nurse authors today enjoy limitless opportunities to provide accurate information to patients, families, and the public through writing. As nurses, we also are best positioned to write about what we do, an important task for influencing policy and inspiring potential new nurses.

We often begin our writing experience by creating patient education tools that meet specific informational needs in clinical practice settings. From there, it's a short leap to submitting work to newspapers, newsletters, magazines, social media, and journals. By following a few basics of writing for a general audience, you can open doors that widen your sphere of influence and experience professional satisfaction by contributing meaningful information to the public.

Write Now!

1. Write a letter to the editor of your local newspaper or a national magazine.
2. Write a paragraph designed for the public, and then test its readability level, using one of the tools discussed in this chapter.

References

Abu-Heija, A. A., Shatta, M., Ajam, M., Abu-Heija, U., Imran, N., & Levine, D. (2019). Quantitative readability assessment of the internal medicine content online patient information on Annals.org. *Cureus, 11*(3), e4184. https://doi.org/10.7759/cureus.4184

Agency for Healthcare Research and Quality. (2022). *Personal health literacy measurement tools.* https://www.ahrq.gov/health-literacy/research/tools/index.html

American Psychological Association. (2020). *Publication manual of the American Psychological Association* (7th ed.). https://doi.org/10.1037/0000165-000

Arian, M., Ramezani, M., Tabatabaeichehr, M., & Kamali, A. (2016). Designing and evaluating patient education pamphlets based on readability indexes and comparison with literacy levels of society. *Evidence Based Care Journal, 6*(2), 19–28. https://doi.org/10.22038/ebcj.2016.7304

Center for Health Care Strategies, Inc. (2013). *Improving print communication to promote health literacy.* https://www.chcs.org/media/CHCS_Health_Literacy_Fact_Sheets_2013_1.pdf

Centers for Disease Control and Prevention. (2023, July 19). *Vaccination coverage among adults in the United States, National Health Interview Survey, 2021.* https://www.cdc.gov/vaccines/imz-managers/coverage/adultvaxview/pubs-resources/vaccination-coverage-adults-2021.html

Centers for Disease Control and Prevention Agency for Toxic Substances and Disease Registry. (n.d.). *Your guide to clear writing.* https://www.cdc.gov/nceh/clearwriting/docs/clear-writing-guide-508.pdf

Coughlin, S. S., Vernon, M., Hatzigeorgiou, C., & George, V. (2020). Health literacy, social determinants of health, and disease prevention and control. *Journal of the Environment and Health Sciences, 6*(1), 3061.

Davis, T. C., Bocchini, J. A., Jr., Fredrickson, D., Arnold, C., Mayeaux, E. J., Murphy P. W., Jackson, R. H., Hanna, N., & Paterson, M. (1996). Parent comprehension of polio vaccine information pamphlets. *Pediatrics, 97*(6), 804–810. https://doi.org/10.1542/peds.97.6.804

Dietrich, S., & Hernandez, E. (2022, Dec. 6). *Nearly 68 million people spoke a language other than English at home in 2019.* US Census Bureau. https://www.census.gov/library/stories/2022/12/languages-we-speak-in-united-states.html

Doak, C., Doak, L., & Root, J. (1996). *Teaching patients with low literacy skills* (2nd ed.). Lippincott Williams & Wilkins.

Grace, P. J. (2021). Nurses spreading misinformation. *American Journal of Nursing, 121*(12), 49–53. https://doi.org/10.1097/01.NAJ.0000803200.65113.fd

Haozous, E. A., & Knobf, M. T. (2013). "All my tears were gone": Suffering and cancer pain in Southwest American Indians. *Journal of Pain and Symptom Management, 45*(6), 1050–1060. https://doi.org/10.1016/j.jpainsymman.2012.06.001

Haozous, E. A., Knobf, M. T., & Brant, J. M. (2010). Understanding the cancer pain experience in American Indians of the Northern Plains. *Psycho-Oncology, 20*(4), 404–410. https://doi.org/10.1002/pon.1741

Hendrix, L. R. (2001). *Health and health care of American Indians and Alaska Native Elders.* Stanford Geriatric Education Center.

Hill-Briggs, F., & Fitzpatrick, S. L. (2023). Overview of social determinants of health in the development of diabetes. *Diabetes Care, 46*(9), 1590–1598. https://doi.org/10.2337/dci23-0001

Hill-Briggs, F., Schumann, K. P., & Dike, O. (2012). Five-step methodology for evaluation and adaptation of print patient health information to meet the <5th grade readability criterion. *Medical Care, 50*(4), 294–301. https://doi.org/10.1097/MLR.0b013e318249d6c8

Jimenez, N., Garroutte, E., Kundu, A., Morales, L, & Buchwald, D. (2011). A review of the experience, epidemiology, and management of pain among American Indian, Alaska Native, and Aboriginal Canadian peoples. *Journal of Pain, 12*(5), 511–522. https://doi.org/10.1016/j.jpain.2010.12.002

Kingsbury, K. (2021, April 26). Why The New York Times is retiring the term 'op-ed' [Opinion]. *The New York Times*. https://www.nytimes.com/2021/04/26/opinion/nyt-opinion-oped-redesign.html

Kirmayer, L. J. (2012). Cultural competence and evidence-based practice in mental health: Epistemic communities and the politics of pluralism. *Social Science & Medicine, 75*(2), 249–256. https://doi.org/10.1016/j.socscimed.2012.03.018

Klein, W. M. P., Chou, W. S., & Vanderpool, R. C. (2023). Health information in 2023 (and beyond): Confronting emergent realities with health communication science [Viewpoint]. *JAMA, 330*(12), 1131–1132. https://doi.org/10.1001/jama.2023.15817

Knoerl, A. M., Esper, K. W., & Hasenau, S. M. (2011). Cultural sensitivity in patient health education. *Nursing Clinics of North America, 46*(3), 335–340. https://doi.org/10.1016/j.cnur.2011.05.008

Kristof, N. (n.d). *How to write op-eds*. https://www.hks.harvard.edu/sites/default/files/Academic%20Dean's%20Office/communications_program/workshop-materials/ho_kristof_oped_10_16_17.pdf

Kristof, N. (2020, Feb. 12). Annotated by the author: 'She helped a customer in need. Then U.S. bank fired her.' *The New York Times*. https://www.nytimes.com/2020/02/12/learning/annotated-by-the-author-she-helped-a-customer-in-need-then-us-bank-fired-her.html

Mamedova, S., & Pawlowski, E. (2019). Adult literacy in the United States. *Data Point*. https://nces.ed.gov/pubs2019/2019179/index.asp

Mishra, V., & Dexter, J. P. (2020). Comparison of readability of official public health information about COVID-19 on websites of international agencies and the governments of 15 countries [Letter]. *JAMA Network Open, 3*(8), e2018033. https://doi.org/10.1001/jamanetworkopen.2020.18033

National Center for Education Statistics. (2019). *Program for International Assessment of Adult Competencies (PIAAC): Literacy domain*. https://nces.ed.gov/surveys/piaac/literacy.asp

Navarro-Rubio, M. D., Rudd, R., Rosenfeld, L., & Arrighi, E. (2016). Alfabetización en salud: Implicación en el sistema sanitario [Health literacy: Implications for the health system]. *Medicina Clínica, 147*(4), 171–175. https://doi.org/10.1016/j.medcli.2016.02.010

Nutbeam, D., & Lloyd, J. E. (2021). Understanding and responding to health literacy as a social determinant of health. *Annual Review of Public Health, 42*(1), 159–173. https://doi.org/10.1146/annurev-publhealth-090419-102529

Ochiai, E., Blakey, C., McGowan, A., & Lin, Y. (2021). The evolution of the Healthy People Initiative: A look through the decades. *Journal of Public Health Management & Practice, 27*(Suppl 6), S225–S234. https://doi.org/10.1097/PHH.0000000000001377

Office of the Surgeon General. (2021). *Confronting health misinformation: The U.S. Surgeon General's advisory on building a healthy information environment*. https://www.hhs.gov/sites/default/files/surgeon-general-misinformation-advisory.pdf

OpEd Project. (n.d.). *What we care about*. https://www.theopedproject.org/mission

PlainLanguage.gov. (n.d.). *Science and industry quotes*. https://www.plainlanguage.gov/resources/quotes/science-and-industry-quotes/

PlainLanguage.gov. (2011). *Federal plain language guidelines*. https://www.plainlanguage.gov/media/FederalPLGuidelines.pdf

Readable. (n.d.). *Flesch reading ease and the Flesch Kincaid grade level*. https://readable.com/readability/flesch-reading-ease-flesch-kincaid-grade-level/

Rooney, M. K., Santiago, G., Perni, S., Horowitz, D. P., McCall, A. R., Einstein, A. J., Jagsi, R., & Golden, D. W. (2021). Readability of patient education materials from high-impact medical journals: A 20-year analysis. *Journal of Patient Experience, 8*. https://doi.org/10.1177/2374373521998847

Rudd, R. E., Groene, O. R., & Navarro-Rubio, M. D. (2013). Sobre alfabetismo y resultados en salud: Antecedentes, impacto y tendencias [On health literacy and health outcomes: Background, impact, and future directions]. *Revista de Calidad Asistencial, 28*(3), 188–192. https://doi.org/10.1016/j.cali.2013.03.003

Samoil, D., Kim, J., Fox, C., & Papadakos, J. K. (2021). The importance of health literacy on clinical cancer outcomes: A scoping review. *Annals of Cancer Epidemiology, 5*. https://doi.org/10.21037/ace-20-30

Santana, S., Brach, C., Harris, L., Ochiai, E., Blakey, C., Bevington, F., Kleinman, D., & Pronk, N. (2021). Updating health literacy for Healthy People 2030: Defining its importance for a new decade in public health. *Journal of Public Health Management & Practice, 27*(Suppl 6), S258–S264. https://doi.org/10.1097/PHH.0000000000001324

US Department of Health and Human Services Office of Minority Health. (n.d.). *National standards for culturally and linguistically appropriate services (CLAS) in health and health care*. https://thinkculturalhealth.hhs.gov/clas/standards

van Ballegooie, C., Heroux, D., Hoang, P., & Garg, S. (2023). Assessing the functional accessibility, actionability, and quality of patient education materials from Canadian cancer agencies. *Current Oncology, 30*(2), 1439–1449. https://doi.org/10.3390/curroncol30020110

Williamson, M., & Harrison, L. (2010). Providing culturally appropriate care: A literature review. *International Journal of Nursing Studies, 47*(6), 761–769. https://doi.org/10.1016/j.ijnurstu.2009.12.012

Zulick, K. M., Zulick, P. A., & Rothrock, J. C. (2009). Patient education and health literacy. *Perioperative Nursing Clinics, 4*(2), 131–139. https://doi.org/10.1016/j.cpen.2009.02.001

Part III
Appendices

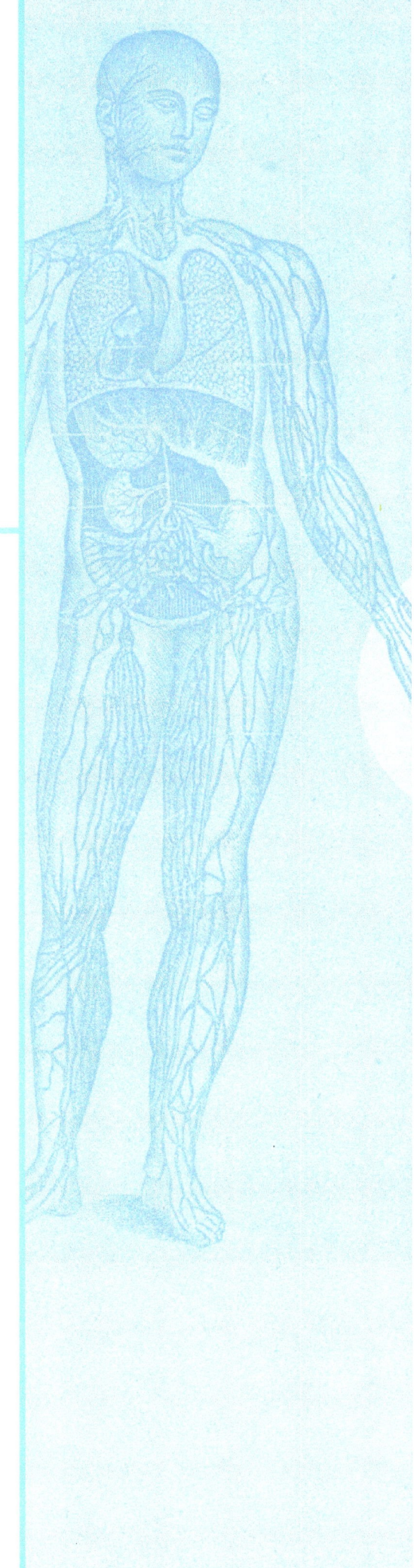

A	Tips for Editing Checklist	333
B	Proofing Checklist	335
C	Publishing Terminology	337
D	Guidelines for Reporting Results	341
E	Statistical Abbreviations	345
F	What Editors and Writers Want	347
G	Publishing Advice From Editors	349

Tips for Editing Checklist

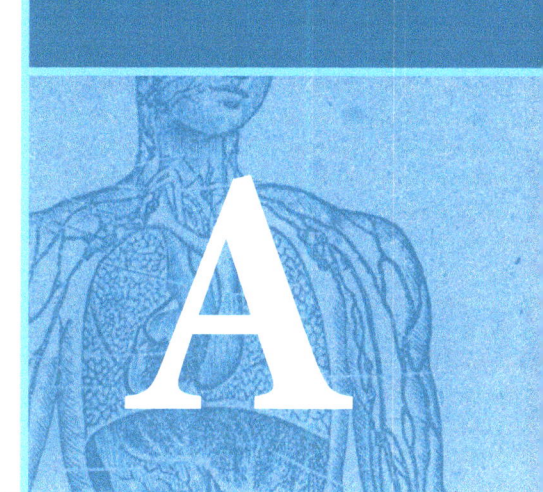

Here are some questions to ask yourself when editing your article.

Yes	No	
Overall		
☐	☐	Do the title and abstract accurately reflect the content?
☐	☐	Is the tone appropriate for the readership?
☐	☐	Is the text bias-free and respectful to patients (e.g., "patient with diabetes" instead of "diabetic")?
☐	☐	Is the organization of the article logical? Are there any information gaps?
☐	☐	Is the voice consistent? For example, check for switching back and forth from first person (I, we) to third person (he, she, they).
☐	☐	Does the opening make the reader want to read more and set up what is to come?
☐	☐	Are transitions used to move from one point to another and from one paragraph to another?
☐	☐	Are citations and references noted where appropriate but not overused?
☐	☐	Is there a take-home message for the reader? Will the article hold the reader's interest?
Details		
☐	☐	Are the lengths of sentences and paragraphs appropriate?
☐	☐	Have I used active voice when possible and appropriate?
☐	☐	Have I eliminated unnecessary words?
☐	☐	Have I eliminated unnecessary qualifiers such as "might" or "perhaps"?
☐	☐	Are verb tenses (past, present, and future) used correctly, and do subjects agree with verbs?
☐	☐	Do tables, figures, and illustrations support (rather than repeat) the content? Do they have labels, and are they referred to in the text?
☐	☐	Are grammar, punctuation, and spelling correct? Remember to run a final spelling and grammar check.
☐	☐	Are citations and references in the format requested by the publication?

Copyright 2024. Cynthia Saver.

Proofing Checklist

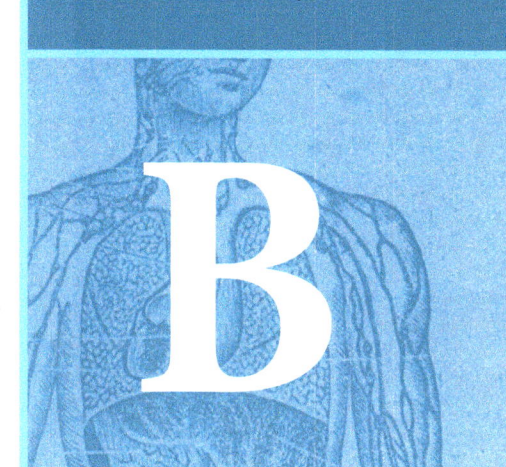

Immediately before submission, do a final proof, checking for the following:

Yes	No	
☐	☐	Are titles and subheads spelled correctly?
☐	☐	Are all organization names spelled correctly?
☐	☐	Are all names of people spelled correctly? Is my biography correct?
☐	☐	Is the sequence of tables, figures, and other graphics correct, and are they called out in the text?
☐	☐	Is each graphic referenced in the text (per author guidelines)?
☐	☐	Are photo and illustration captions accurate, and are people in photos identified correctly?
☐	☐	Are credits for graphics included where needed?
☐	☐	Are tables aligned properly?
☐	☐	Is the math correct in all calculations, and are all numbers correct? (If numbers won't add up to 100%, be sure the reason is stated—e.g., survey results have been rounded.)
☐	☐	Are acronyms spelled out the first time they appear in text?
☐	☐	Are terms consistent? (For example, *healthcare* and *health care* are both acceptable, but pick one and use it consistently. Before picking one, check the publication's style guide for preference.)
☐	☐	If a source is cited within the text, is the complete reference to the work also provided (per style guidelines)?
☐	☐	Are the references formatted correctly, per the publication's guidelines?

If your article is accepted for publication, you may receive a PDF of the layed out article, which shows how it will look when published. If so, be sure to check the above and the following:

Yes	No	
☐	☐	Are pages numbered sequentially?
☐	☐	Is the information in the footer (bottom of page) correct? (The footer typically contains the journal title, volume, and issue date.)
☐	☐	If the reader is referred to another page, is the page number correct?
☐	☐	Are the fonts consistent?
☐	☐	Are headings of different sections the right size, and are sizes consistent? (During the layout process, what should be a subheading may inadvertently be switched to a main head and vice versa.)
☐	☐	Are special characters such as an alpha or beta symbol formatted correctly? (Occasionally these characters don't display correctly.)
☐	☐	Are figure and other captions complete? (Sometimes they can get cut off when imported into the layout program.)
☐	☐	Are online links in the article correct?
☐	☐	Are titles in references italicized per the journal's style? (Sometimes italics are "lost" when going from document to layout.)

If you are proofing a computer-based program, also check the following:

Yes	No	
☐	☐	Can you navigate in the file (e.g., go back a page, return to home, return to the table of contents)?
☐	☐	Are the links active, and do they take you to the correct page?
☐	☐	Do pages contain too much text?
☐	☐	Are all levels of headings consistent in size, color, and font?
☐	☐	Do graphics load onto the page at an acceptable speed?
☐	☐	Can you access help files?

Copyright 2024. Cynthia Saver.

Publishing Terminology

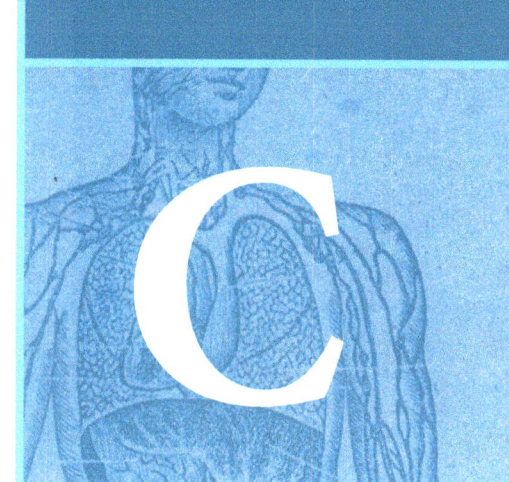

Editors and publishers use jargon that can be just as confusing as medical jargon is to a layperson. This appendix explains some of the terms you might hear.

acknowledgment A statement in the front of a book or at the end of a journal article that expresses the author's gratitude for help with the content.

Adobe Acrobat A software program used to create a portable document file (PDF), which allows files to be easily shared. The program used to access these files is free. PDF files are typically used for proofing (and indicating any corrections in) the final version of the article.

appendix Supplemental information to text in a book, placed in the back of the book.

art (artwork) A general term for tables, figures, graphs, photographs, and illustrations.

axis Reference line in a graph: The x-axis is the horizontal line that represents the independent variable, and the y-axis is the vertical line that represents the dependent variable.

back matter The material that follows the main body of a book, such as the index or appendices.

bad break Occurs when a word or line breaks at the right margin of a page in a way that results in too much space; also occurs when a word is hyphenated incorrectly.

bibliography A list of articles, books, and other references that are not cited in the text.

bleed A printed image that runs off the page.

blog An online entry that shares insights and viewpoints.

byline The name of the author, which appears at the start or the end of an article.

callout A short string of text connected by a line, arrow, or similar graphic to a feature of an illustration or technical drawing; the text provides information about that feature.

caption The text that explains a photo or illustration; also called a legend.

citation Information in the text that directs readers to a corresponding reference at the end of the article; it consists of the author and year in parentheses or in text, or a superscript number. (Note: Databases tend to use the term to refer to the complete information for a reference, including criteria such as author, journal, volume, issue number, and page numbers.)

CMYK Refers to the four colors used in printing color materials: cyan, magenta, yellow, and black.

content management system (CMS) A program that multiple people use to manage content for print or online. For example, photos or videos can be linked to text for posting online, or peer reviewers can access a manuscript, make comments, and return.

copyedit Editing the manuscript for details such as proper use of grammar and punctuation.

copyright The exclusive legal right, given to an original author or an assignee to print, publish, perform, film, or record literary, artistic, or musical material, and to others to do the same.

credit (credit line) The text that credits the source of an image or text that has been reproduced with permission; it usually appears under the reproduced material.

drop marks Define the edge of a photo or printed page. In photography, used to indicate where the image should be trimmed.

dash Two types of dashes are commonly used. An *en* dash is slightly longer than a hyphen and is about the width of the letter "n." En dashes imply "through." For example, you would write the January–March issue of a magazine instead of January-March because there is another month in between. An *em* dash is the widest dash and is the width of the letter "m." Em dashes are used to set off part of a sentence that the writer wants to emphasize—like this.

deck Refers to some additional information about the article that falls after the headline but before the byline and main text.

dedication An inscription in the front of a book dedicating it to a person; dedications are personal in nature, as opposed to acknowledgments.

DOI Stands for Digital Object Identifier, a unique code assigned to an article on publication (whether in print or online) that enables someone to retrieve the article using the DOI as a search term.

drop cap Refers to when the initial letter of the first word in a paragraph is larger and drops down into the paragraph (and sometimes is a different color than the rest of the text) starting an article.

ellipsis Three dots that indicate an intentional omission of a word or group of words.

em dash The widest dash, an em dash is the width of the letter "m." Often used to indicate a change in thought.

en dash A dash character that is slightly longer than a hyphen and is about the width of the letter "n." Often used to connect numbers, as in 50–60.

endnote Note or reference at the end of a portion of a text.

erratum Note of correction for previously published information.

figure A general term for charts, graphs, photographs, and illustrations.

flush Used in combination with left or right, such as "flush left," which means the text is aligned with the left margin, or "flush right," which means the text is aligned with the right margin. Text also may be flush on both sides, which is referred to as "justified."

folio The text that appears at the bottom of each page of a magazine or journal. It includes the page number and may also include the name of the publication, website, and year, volume, and issue number.

font A typeface.

footnote Information placed at the bottom of the page in a book, article, or other document.

foreword A short introduction to a book by someone other than the author.

front matter The pages before the main text of the book; typically includes the title page, table of contents, foreword, and preface.

four color Refers to a full-color publication that is printed using cyan, magenta, yellow, and black (CMYK).

galley A term for a prepublication version of an article or book. In the case of books, it's used to obtain prepublication endorsements from experts. Most publishers provide an electronic PDF proof for prepublication rather than paper galleys, which were used in the past.

gif Stands for *graphics interchange format*, a type of graphics file.

graph A figure that shows comparisons, trends, and amounts of data.

HEX (Hexadecimal) Code Code numbers used to identify specific RGB colors on a computer screen.

illustration A figure that is drawn or needs to be drawn; can include graphs and flowcharts, as well as pictures.

infographic Refers to presenting information visually with minimum text.

ISBN A product identifier used by publishers, booksellers, libraries, internet retailers, and others for ordering and archiving.

jpg (jpeg) Stands for *joint photographic experts group*, a type of graphics file.

kerning The space between the letters of a word. Kerning is sometimes adjusted for a better "look" to the text.

layout Refers to the composition or graphic design of a page or article. In essence, it is how the final publication will look. Usually, authors review the layout in a portable document file (PDF).

lead or **lede** The start of an article, designed to draw the reader in.

leading The space between lines of type, typically measured in *points*. Leading is sometimes adjusted for a better "look" to the text.

legend The caption for a figure, photograph, or illustration.

lorem epsum Dummy text made up of random letters, used as a placeholder for text to come and to estimate text length needed in a layout. Sometimes called "placeholder text."

marginalia Another term for sidebars, mainly used with books.

mov Represents a QuickTime video file.

MP4 A digital multimedia format commonly used to store video and audio data as well as other types of data.

mpg (mpeg) Stands for *motion picture experts group*; these files are used for computer video.

orphan A word or a few words that appear alone at the top of a column or page. Adjustments are usually made to avoid this. Definitions of widow and orphan vary; the point is that a word or line of text is separated from the rest of the text by too much distance.

page proof Shows how the final publication will look. Usually authors review the layout in a portable document file (PDF).

PDF Stands for *portable document file*; it shows how an article will look when it is published, and typically is the final published product in digital publishing.

permissions An official document giving authorization to reproduce copyright material.

photograph A photograph can be a black-and-white or color figure, but keep in mind that color photographs that need to be converted to black and white may not convert well and appear washed out in the final product.

PMS (Pantone Color Matching System) A numbered set of standard defined colors that can be printed as a single ink or converted into CMYK or RGB.

png Stands for *portable network graphic*, a type of graphics file.

preface The introduction to a book written by the author; it states the purpose of the book and its scope.

pull quote Pull quotes are made up of text that is pulled from the text—that is, duplicated—and presented on the page as an attention-grabbing visual element.

raster An image made up of pixels, which are resolution dependent. A raster loses quality when it is sized larger. Rasters are commonly jpg, psd, gif, tif, and png file types.

reference list A list of all references (with complete information) that are cited in the article.

resolution A number identifying the quality of an image. Screen resolution is typically 72 dpi (low resolution). Print resolution is typically 275 to 300 dpi (high resolution).

RGB Refers to the three colors used to achieve online color: red, green, and blue.

running header or footer Copy that appears at the top (header) or bottom (footer) of each page of a book or journal.

sans serif A typeface without serifs. Sometimes referred to as "block" lettering.

script A typeface that is tilted and flowing, like cursive handwriting or calligraphy.

serif A typeface with extra strokes or curves at the ends of letters.

sidebar A box of text with or without visuals that is set off from the main text. Sidebars are also referred to as marginalia.

spread Refers to two facing pages of a magazine or journal.

stet Proofreading or editorial mark that means to ignore a previously indicated change.

style guide A set of standards for editors or designers to follow so that information is presented consistently. In addition to general guides such as those from the American Psychological Association and the American Medical Association, publications usually also have a "house" style guide that addresses issues such as whether healthcare will be one word or two words (both are considered correct) and may pull from elements of general style guides.

subhead These are smaller in size than (and subordinate to) the main headings and are used to break up text. Subheads are typically bold and are sized a couple of points larger than body text.

subscript Letter, word, symbol, or number written or printed (in a smaller size) slightly below a line of text.

substantive edit During this edit, the focus is on the big picture of the work, such as organization and flow. Sometimes referred to as the developmental edit.

superscript Letter, word, symbol, or number written or printed (in a smaller size) slightly above a line of text.

supplement A special section to a journal or magazine that is separate from the publication but distributed with a particular issue.

table Presentation of numeric information or short bullet points set aside from the text in a column format. Typically contains at least two columns to be called a table as opposed to a box. Note that having more than four columns can create a design problem and should be avoided if possible.

thumbnail A small or concise description, sketch, representation, or summary.

tiff or tif Stands for *tagged image file format*, a type of graphics file. This is the preferred format for images such as photographs.

TOC Stands for Table of Contents, the section in the front of the publication that lists what is contained within.

two color Printing in which the final product is black and one other color (typically a PMS [Pantone Matching System] color).

typeface A type font that has a name, such as Times New Roman.

upload Refers to the transfer of files from a person's computer to a website.

URL Stands for Uniform Resource Locator. This is the online "address" for a specific piece of content, such as an article, web page, or photo.

vector An image made up of geometric shapes and patterns. Vector images do not lose quality when they are sized larger. Vectors are commonly an eps file type.

white space The area of a page that does not have any text or graphics. Sufficient white space makes pages easier to read.

widow A word or a few words that appear alone at the bottom of a page under a paragraph. Adjustments are usually made to avoid this. Definitions of widow and orphan vary; the point is that a word or line of text is separated from the rest of the text by too much distance.

wrap text Refers to moving sentences or words so that they wrap around a shape or graphic.

XML Stands for *extensible markup language*, used in formatting text and graphics that will appear online.

zip file A type of file that is compressed so that it can contain more files while not using too much computer space.

Copyright 2024. Cynthia Saver, with input from David Beverage and Patricia Dwyer Schull.

Guidelines for Reporting Results

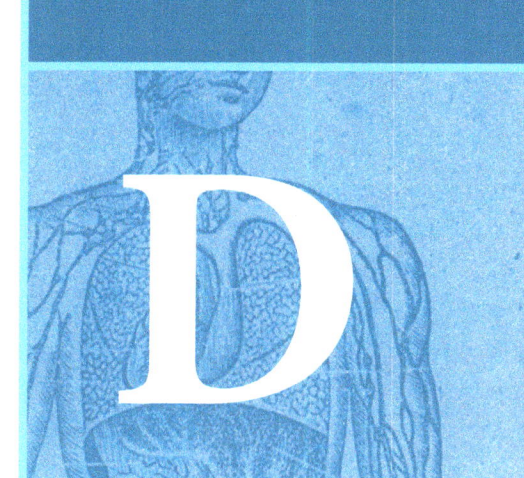

The following guidelines are tools that can help you craft your article. They also help ensure information is presented in a way that facilitates readers' ability to understand your work and evaluate how it fits with their practice. Many of these guidelines, often available in multiple languages, contain a checklist for assessing different sections of the manuscript.

Check the author guidelines to see if a publication requires you to use a specific guideline for reporting your work, then go to the corresponding website and download what you need. Keep in mind that even if a publication doesn't require you to follow certain guidelines, you can use them to organize and evaluate your manuscript before submission, which may improve your likelihood of acceptance.

If you're not sure which guidelines are best for your project, visit the website for EQUATOR (Enhancing the QUAlity and Transparency Of health Research) Network (http://www.equator-network.org), which includes a searchable database of reporting guidelines as well as a flowchart and online wizard for determining which are the most appropriate for your article. EQUATOR also includes information about additional guidelines not cited here.

The following table is a directory of guideline sources. (Preceding it is a brief bullet list—categorized based on type of study or project—to help you navigate the table.)

- Case reports: CARE
- Clinical practice guidelines: AGREE II, RIGHT
- Economic evaluations of healthcare: CHEERS
- Evidence-based practice: Evidence-Based Practice Dissemination Guide
- Implementation studies: StaRI
- Nonrandomized studies of behavioral and public health interventions: TREND
- Observational studies in epidemiology: STROBE
- Qualitative research: COREQ, eMERGe, ENTREQ, SRQR
- Quality improvement projects: SQUIRE 2.0, SQUIRE-EDU
- Randomized clinical trials: CONSORT
- Reviews: PRISMA

Title	Ideal for Reporting...	Comments
AGREE II (**A**ppraisal of **G**uidelines for **RE**search & **E**valuation) http://www.agreetrust.org/resource-centre/agree-reporting-checklist	Clinical practice guidelines	Checklist available as fillable PDF and Microsoft Word documents
CARE (**CA**se **RE**port Reporting Guidelines) http://www.care-statement.org	Case reports	Website includes a writing template that helps authors follow the guidelines

continues

Title	Ideal for Reporting...	Comments
CHEERS (**C**onsolidated **H**ealth **E**conomic **E**valuation **R**eporting **S**tandards) https://www.ispor.org/heor-resources/good-practices/cheers	Economic evaluations of healthcare	Website includes checklist and video resources
CONSORT (**CON**solidated **S**tandards **O**f **R**eporting **T**rials) http://www.consort-statement.org	Randomized clinical trials	Website includes checklist, flow diagram, and examples
COREQ (**CO**nsolidated criteria for **RE**porting **Q**ualitative research) https://academic.oup.com/intqhc/article/19/6/349/1791966/Consolidated-criteria-for-reporting-qualitative	Qualitative research that includes in-depth interviews and focus groups	Covers three domains: research team and reflexivity, study design, and analysis and findings
eMERGe Guideline https://emergeproject.org/	Meta-ethnography: synthesis of qualitative studies	Website includes video resources
ENTREQ (**En**hancing **T**ransparency in **RE**porting the Synthesis of **Q**ualitative Research) https://bmcmedresmethodol.biomedcentral.com/articles/10.1186/1471-2288-12-181	Synthesis of multiple qualitative studies	Includes 21 items grouped into five domains: introduction, methods and methodology, literature search and selection, appraisal, and synthesis of findings
Evidence-Based Practice Dissemination Guide Dean, J., & Gallagher-Ford, L. (2021) Evidence-based practice: A new dissemination guide. *Worldviews on Evidence-Based Nursing*, 18(1), 4–7. https://doi.org/10.1111/wvn.12489	Evidence-based practice projects	Includes seven steps of evidence-based practice
PRISMA (**P**referred **R**eporting **I**tems for **S**ystematic reviews and **M**eta-**A**nalyses) http://www.prisma-statement.org	Systematic reviews and meta-analyses	Website has checklist and helpful flow diagrams
RIGHT (Essential **R**eporting **I**tems for Practice **G**uidelines in **H**ealt**h**care) http://www.right-statement.org	Clinical practice guidelines	Website includes extensions, a checklist, and multiple translations
SQUIRE 2.0 (Revised **S**tandards for **QU**ality **I**mprovement **R**eporting **E**xcellence) http://www.squire-statement.org/index.cfm?fuseaction=Page.ViewPage&pageId=471	Quality improvement projects	Website includes examples of well-written items
SQUIRE-EDU (**S**tandards for **QU**ality **I**mprovement **R**eporting **E**xcellence for **E**ducation) https://www.squire-statement.org/index.cfm?fuseaction=Page.ViewPage&pageId=515	Quality improvement projects related to education	Website includes examples of well-written items

Appendix D Guidelines for Reporting Results

Title	Ideal for Reporting...	Comments
SRQR (**S**tandards for **R**eporting **Q**ualitative **R**esearch) https://journals.lww.com/academicmedicine/fulltext/2014/09000/Standards_for_Reporting_Qualitative_Research__A.21.aspx	Qualitative research	Consists of 21 points to address
StaRI (**Sta**ndards for **R**eporting **I**mplementation Studies) https://www.bmj.com/content/356/bmj.i6795	Implementation studies	Includes a 27-item checklist
STROBE (**S**trengthening the **R**eporting of **OB**servational Studies in **E**pidemiology) https://www.strobe-statement.org/index.php?id=strobe-home	Observational (cohort, case-control, and cross-sectional)	Multiple checklists and translations available
TREND (**T**ransparent **R**eporting of **E**valuations with **N**onrandomized **D**esigns) https://www.cdc.gov/trendstatement	Nonrandomized studies of behavioral and public health interventions	Has 22-item checklist

Statistical Abbreviations

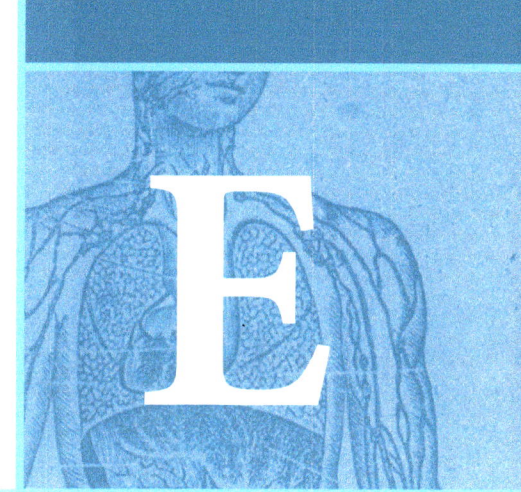

You might find this list of common statistical abbreviations helpful in writing and reviewing articles. Refer to the appropriate style guide and author guidelines for information about how to report statistics.

α—Alpha (level of significance, the probability of rejecting the null hypothesis when the null hypothesis is true)

ANCOVA—Analysis of covariance

ANOVA—Analysis of variance

AR—Absolute risk

CI—Confidence interval

df—Degrees of freedom

F—F ratio

f—Frequency

M or $\overline{X}$—Mean

MANCOVA—Multivariate analysis of covariance

MANOVA—Multivariate analysis of variance

Mdn—median

N—Total sample size

n—Subsample size

ns—Not statistically significant

OR—Odds ratio

p—Probability

r—Pearson's correlation

r_s—Spearman rank order correlation

RR—Relative risk

SD—Standard deviation

SE—Standard error

SEM—Standard error of the mean

σ—Sigma, designating the population standard deviation

SS—Sum of squares

T—Wilcoxon signed-rank test value

t—Student's t distribution

U or MWU—Mann–Whitney U test; also called the Mann-Whitney-Wilcoxon (MWW) test

x^2—Chi-square distributions

References

American Psychological Association. (2020). *Publication manual of the American Psychological Association* (7th ed.). https://doi.org/10.1037/0000165-000

JAMA Network Editors. (2020). *AMA manual of style: A guide for authors and editors* (11th ed.). Oxford University Press.

Tabachnick, B. G., & Fidell, L. S. (2019). *Using multivariate statistics* (7th ed.). Pearson.

Reviewed by Scott Emory Moore, PhD, MSN, RN, AGPCNP-BC, FAAN

What Editors and Writers Want

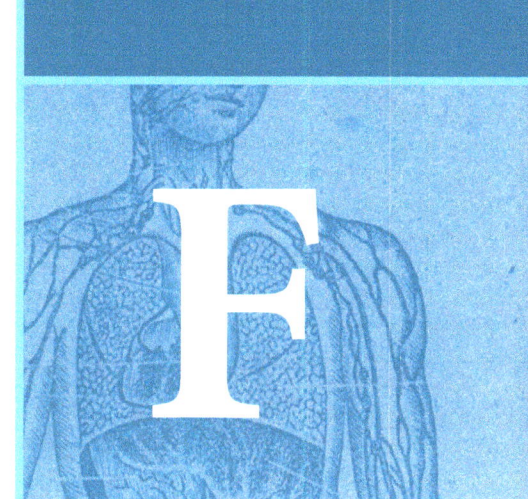

What Editors Want

Here's what editors would like you to do as an author:

- Follow our publication's author guidelines carefully.
- Use your last name, title of article, and name of publication (and assigned manuscript number if applicable) when corresponding by email.
- In a query letter, give us two or three sentences on why our readers would be interested in your topic and why you should be the one to write the article.
- Carefully read your manuscript before submitting it to catch errors.
- Meet your deadline. If you can't, let us know as soon as possible, and be honest about whether you can meet a later deadline.
- Stay calm if your manuscript is rejected because of peer-review comments; ask to see the reviewers' comments if they aren't included, but know that not all journals will share them.
- Respond to peer-review comments when you revise. If you choose not to make a suggested revision, briefly tell us why so we know you didn't overlook it.
- Understand that it can take more than a year for your article to be published if it is accepted for publication. If you haven't heard anything for four or five months, it's fine to email us for an update.
- Understand that each publication has a unique style. Our editors know how to edit for our readership. We ask that you respect their expertise in this area, just as we respect your expertise in the subject matter.
- Know that English is a living language. Rules you learned in high school may no longer apply.
- Realize that we know it's frustrating when we have your article for a year and then ask you to turn around your review of the edited manuscript in five days. Unfortunately, that sometimes occurs with the publishing cycle.
- Write for us more than once and tell others that you enjoyed the experience of working with us.
- Follow our author guidelines carefully. (Yes, this is a repeat!)

Cynthia Saver, MS, RN, with input from multiple journal editors. Copyright 2024.

What Writers Want

Writers appreciate it when editors:

- Make the author guidelines readable and as succinct as possible.
- Explain publishing terms we might not understand.
- Provide a realistic idea as to time frames. If we know it takes eight weeks for peer review, we won't bother you about the status of the manuscript after four weeks.
- Choose peer reviewers who are experts and provide feedback that is specific and considerate.
- Respect our input. We know you have an editorial style for you publication, but please don't change our words just for the sake of changing them.

- Double- and triple-check the spelling of our names, credentials, and affiliations.
- Keep us informed of the status of the submitted manuscript. It's hard to wait to hear whether an article has been accepted, and, if it's been accepted, when it's going to be published.
- Understand that writing is just one component of our busy world.
- Send us at least one copy (hopefully more) of the published article and the link to where it is online.
- Let us know if you have received feedback (positive and negative) about our articles after publication.
- Give us encouragement along the way.
- Thank us for taking the time to write the article.

Copyright 2024 by Cynthia Saver, with input from Susan Stallard, MSN, APRN-CNS, CCNS

Publishing Advice From Editors

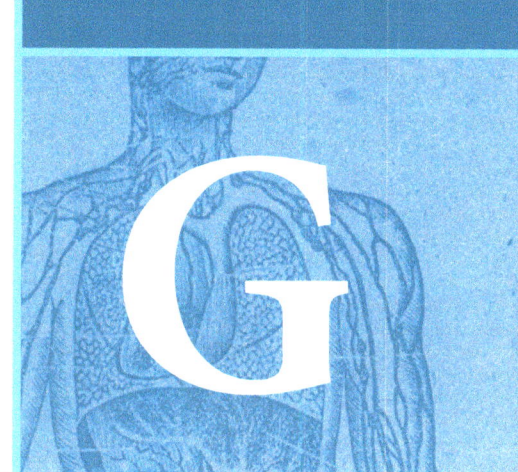

When working on an earlier edition of this book, I (Cynthia Saver) reached out to my editorial colleagues to solicit their advice related to nursing publishing. These nurse editors have also walked in the shoes of writers, peer reviewers, and editorial advisory board members. They provide straight talk in several areas that you can use to enhance your own publishing experience.

Getting Published

1. **Following the author guidelines increases your chance of getting published.** The guidelines contain all you need to know: the types of articles we want, length, writing style, what style guide to use, how to submit tables and figures, and other important information. The most common complaint among editors is that authors don't follow the guidelines. For example, American Psychological Association (APA) style for citations means APA style and not American Medical Association (AMA) style. When you don't follow the guidelines, we're already put off by your manuscript.

2. **We sometimes desperately need articles for a particular topic, especially if it's a special issue.** If your manuscript arrives during one of those times, you're more likely to be published quickly, and we'll be more willing to work extensively with you. Check the journal's website for notices of upcoming focus or themed issues.

3. **Regular journal departments are sometimes the hardest for us to fill.** That means we'll be more receptive to a topic that could be used there.

4. **The publication process takes time.** Sometimes articles are published quickly (within one to three months), but it also can take nearly two years from initial submission to final publication. If you need publications for your scholarly portfolio, plan accordingly.

5. **Keep track of documents and be organized.** If you are a faculty member on tenure track, keep a copy of your acceptance letter. We may not be able to produce a copy for you two to five years later. Similarly, add the publication citation to your resume, and make sure it's accurate, with the correct date, journal name, year, volume, issue, page numbers, and Digital Object Identifier (DOI).

Cover Letters

1. **Your cover letter praising the journal won't influence the decision to accept or decline your manuscript.** Keep the letter brief and stick with the facts of your submission: title, author names, and author affiliations.

2. **If you send us a cover letter addressed to another editor or with the name of another journal or editor, we'll be concerned about your attention to detail.** All editors know we get manuscripts that have been submitted to other journals because sometimes it takes a couple of tries to find the right home for a manuscript. But please get the name of the journal and editor correct. (And don't submit your manuscript to more than one journal at a time.)

Writing

1. **More words doesn't mean you've said anything more important or more clearly.** It's rare that a manuscript warrants more words than the stated limit. If you feel it does, you likely need to narrow the topic. The editor can sometimes help you with this.

2. **We appreciate authors who write in a simple and direct manner.** Poor grammar, misplaced phrases, and multisyllabic words when a simpler one would do are off-putting. Don't make your sentences overly complex and strip them of jargon. Remember that a paragraph typically consists of four to five sentences related to a single idea.

3. **Make sure your references are current.** If time has passed since you first drafted the manuscript (perhaps since you submitted somewhere else and received a rejection letter) your references might not be current. Reviewers and editors notice the years on your reference list. Older references may be appropriate for some types of articles (such as review articles), but in general, you want up-to-date citations so readers have current information.

4. **Make it easy for the reader to read your article.** Use headings and subheadings to organize your thoughts and develop ideas in a logical manner. Write so that the reader should not have to ask a single question, and write with an image of your target audience in mind. The goal is to communicate the information quickly—readers have many other tasks on their radar.

5. **Think about citations and use them wisely.** When you write, "Studies have shown…," you need to include citations to the studies that document your statement. On the other hand, when citing a statistic, such as, "One in eight women will be diagnosed with breast cancer in her lifetime," then you only need one citation—not four or five. And some statements, such as, "Pain in patients with cancer is a nearly universal experience," probably don't need a citation at all.

6. **Make sure your manuscript is formatted correctly.** Don't use the space bar to indent paragraphs—use the tab key. Don't press enter at the end of every line, and use one space (not two) between sentences. Check the author guidelines for formatting instructions.

Civility

1. **The publishing process will be smoother and more positive if you're professional when communicating with the editor.** For example, "Seriously?!" or, "You've got to be kidding!" are not the best responses to requests from the editor to revise your manuscript. When you first contact the editor about interest in your topic, use a formal address such as, "Dear Ms. Smith," as opposed to, "Hi, Mary!"

2. **We'll be pleasant when you try to rewrite our professional edit, but we are less likely to accept another manuscript from you.** Authors are experts on content, and editors are experts on editing. Both deserve equal respect for what they do.

Peer Review

1. **You don't have to take every suggestion from peer reviewers.** Peer reviewers are experts, but sometimes there is a legitimate disagreement between what is requested and what you feel is correct. When you return the manuscript, note why you did not make a revision so that we know you didn't overlook it and can understand your rationale for not making the change. However, know that if you ignore most of the reviewers' suggestions, your manuscript will be rejected.

2. **A letter saying "revise and resubmit" means we are interested in your article.** Please don't withdraw your manuscript and submit to another journal. Also, don't give up on getting published! Being asked to revise is a sign that we're still interested in your work.

Editing

1. **We respect that your name is on the article.** We take our responsibility to you seriously and will do everything in our power to ensure you publish a high-quality article.

2. **Don't send your rough draft for me to review before you submit (unless I've agreed to it in advance).** You are responsible for your manuscript. That's not to say, however, that in some cases where the topic is complex, we won't take a quick look. Ask ahead of time, and understand that although we might like the manuscript, that doesn't mean it will be accepted—that depends on peer review.

3. **We wonder about the accuracy of your content when it's clear you didn't make a final check of the manuscript before submitting.** When we can see that you didn't run spell-check, or we find that your percentages don't add up to 100 (without an explanation), it makes us wonder about the amount of care you took in presenting the information.

4. **Multiple editors and reviewers will evaluate your article.** Some editors are looking at the big picture, such as organization, while others are more focused on the details, such as grammar. All of us are part of your publishing team.

Student Papers

1. **Writing a paper for a school assignment isn't the same as writing an article for a journal.** School assignments can be a great starting point for a manuscript, but they must be revised to fit the journal's audience, aims, and format.

2. **We don't care that your teacher thought your manuscript was great.** Please don't tell us that when you ask to submit it.

3. **Please don't "cut and paste" a dissertation or capstone paper into a manuscript for a journal.** You'll never be successful, and the resulting manuscript will be unorganized and probably too long. Do not try to write a manuscript "from" your dissertation. Instead, go back to the study and write a report of the findings in a format that is appropriate for your selected journal.

Reporting Research

1. **If you used human subjects, your study must have been reviewed and approved by an Institutional Review Board (IRB).** All published research must include a statement about ethical review and approval. In the US, this is done by an IRB. If you are from another country, include the name of the reviewing committee and make clear to us what is in their scope of review. Without a statement of review by an IRB (or equivalent), your study won't be published.

2. **Statistical reporting is picky and detailed, and we are too.** Look at articles in the journal to see if p (probability) should be in capitals or italics or both. Same for N (for population) and n (for sample). Note if there are spaces around equal (=) and less than (<) signs, and format your manuscript accordingly.

Ethics

1. **Please don't tell me that there are no copyrighted items in your article and then include four figures with attributions to previously published works, all without written permission.** The rule is that if you found it in a publication (in print or online), it's copyrighted, and you must ask permission to use it. Most publications will willingly grant permission. If there is a fee, note in your submission that you will obtain permission and pay the fee if the article is accepted for publication.

2. **Just because someone participated in a project doesn't mean they deserve authorship credit.** Authorship represents a significant contribution to the manuscript. Listing 15 authors for a 1,200-word manuscript simply because they were involved in the project isn't appropriate. Only those who wrote (not reviewed) the article should be listed.

Rejection

1. **Often, it's hard for us to reject your article.** Many of us are writers ourselves, so we feel bad about having to disappoint you. However, our first duty is to our readers, who expect high-quality content.

2. **If you receive a rejection notice, don't write the editor incredulous that this happened because you had two people with PhDs and a physician on your research committee.** We rely on our peer reviewers. Consider that sometimes people are too close to the manuscript to give it a useful review.

Editors

1. **We suffer from short staffing just like you do.** The number of people who make up the editorial staff for a publication has shrunk over the years. That's why we might send your manuscript back for you to fix the reference list instead of doing it ourselves. Many editors of nursing journals have additional full-time jobs.

2. **We're happy to answer questions.** Part of our job is to support authors. Don't be afraid to ask us a question.

3. **We know resources that can help you.** Many nurses aren't familiar with resources such as the publication *Nurse Author & Editor.*

4. **We love what we do!** We are committed to publishing great articles with information that nurses can use in their practice. Give publishing a whirl!

Thank you to the following editors who contributed their advice: Maureen Anthony, Lucy Bradley-Springer, Marion Broome, Jan Fulton, Elizabeth Heavey, Anne Katz, Francie Likis, Tina Marrelli, Leslie Nicoll, Marilyn Oermann, Carol Patton, Geri Pearson, Susan Shropshire, Kathleen Simpson, and Sally Thorne.

Adapted from *40 Things Editors Won't Tell You (But You Need to Know)*, by C. Saver, 2016, *Nurse Author & Editor,* 26, p. 6. Copyright 2016 by Cynthia Saver. Reprinted with permission. http://naepub.com/publishing/2016-26-1-6

Index

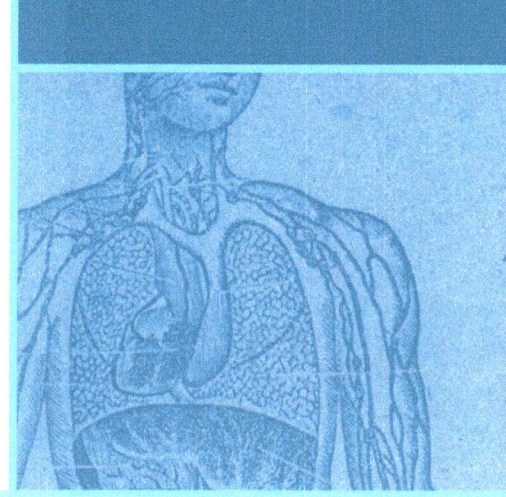

NOTE: Page references noted with an *f* are figures; page references noted with a *t* are tables.

A

abbreviations
    statistical, 345
    use of, 94–95
abstracts
    audience, 244
    call for, 242, 243, 244
    case examples, 246–248
    creating impressions, 244–245
    designing, 78
    evidence-based practice (EBP) articles, 234
    formatting, 77
    graphical abstracts (GAs), 77–79, 173
    guidelines, 245
    presentations, 241–244, 248–251, 252
    quality-improvement (QI) articles, 234
    quantitative articles, 200–201
    reviewing, 245–246
    scoping reviews, 224
    submitting, 245
    systematic reviews, 221
    video, 173–174
    writing, 201
academic social media sites, 175*t*–176*t*
acceptances, 128. *See also* submitting
    letters to the editor, 300
access
    closed, 39
    paying for article sources, 68
    selecting journals, 39–44
accountability partners, 12
accreditation, 268
Accreditation Council for Continuing Medical Education (ACCME), 268
acknowledgments, 317
active learning strategies (ALSs), 257
active voice, 90, 91, 193–195, 195*f*
adaptive publication, 166
adjectives, 90
adult learning principles (ALPs), 269
adverbs, 90
advocacy narrative, 285–287
agreements, contributor, 313–315
Alaska Natives (AN), 322
alternative publishing options, 297
    blogs, 304–305
    book reviews, 302–303
    columns, 302
    editorials, 300–302
    letters to the editor, 297–300
    newsletters, 303–304
altmetrics, 47
AMA Manual of Style: A Guide for Authors and Editors, 29, 60, 62, 69
American Association of Colleges of Pharmacy (AACP) Pharmacy Workforce Center, 269
American Indians (AI), 322
American Nurse Journal, 6, 29, 257
American Nurses Association (ANA), 4, 285. *See also* ethics
American Nurses Credentialing Center (ANCC), 268
analysis
    data analyses, 205, 226
    meta-analysis, 216
    of scientific data, 81
    scoping reviews, 225
anecdotes, adding, 7
APA (Publication Manual of the American Psychological Association), 60, 62, 69
appendices, 317
applicability, scope of (topics), 31
appraisal of evidence, 81
approval of manuscripts, 18–19
article processing charges (APCs), 41
articles. *See also* blog posts; writing
    audience for, 27
    case studies, 84–85
    clinical, 83, 187 (*see also* clinical articles)
    conference presentation, 251–253
    describing, 50–51
    editing, 8–9
    evidence-based practice (EBP), 81–82, 231 (*see also* evidence-based practice [EBP] articles)
    exemplars, 85
    flow of, 5
    formatting, 74–79
    how-to, 192
    information in, 7–8
    literature reviews, 83
    nursing narratives, 85
    organizing, 73 (*see also* organizing)
    outlines, 5–7
    publishing process, 16–19 (*see also* publishing)
    qualitative, 81
    quality improvement (QI), 82, 231, 257 (*see also* quality improvement [QI] articles)
    quantitative, 81
    reasons to write, 26–27
    research, 80–81
    reviewing, 8–9
    sources, 57 (*see also* sources)
    structure of, 4–9
    timing, 29
    topics (*see* topics)
    types of, 5, 80–85

artificial intelligence (AI) programs, 33, 66, 267
    disclosure of use, 126
    graphics, 104
    systematic reviews, 220
assessments
    self-assessments, 275
    worksheets, 26f
assignment of copyrights, 158. See also copyrights
The Associated Press Stylebook, 60
Association of American Medical Colleges (AAMC), 269
audience
    abstracts, 244
    for articles, 27
    continuing education (CE) target audiences, 269–270
    general audiences, 319 (*see also* general audiences, writing for)
    identifying, 172, 173 (*see also* promoting)
    selecting journals, 38–39
    targeting, 252
    writing, 7
audio, 114
authors, 13, 317. *See also* collaboration; writing
    credentials, 51
    global, 145 (*see also* global authors)
    guidelines, 32, 96, 268–269
    metrics, 45
    non-native speaking, 150
    posting rights, 39
    publishing process, 18–19
    reviews, 132
authorship
    dissertations, 257–258
    ethics, 162–163
avoiding misconduct, 165–167

B

background
    qualitative articles, 208
    scoping reviews, 224
    systematic reviews, 221
back matter (books), 317
bar graphs, 110
barriers to good writing, 9–12
    lack of confidence, 9–10
    lack of time, 10–12

beginnings. *See also* introductions; starting
    of articles, 5
    formatting, 75–76
Benner, Patricia, 284, 290
best available evidence, 216
bib cards, 69
bibliographies, 317
bibliography database managers (BDMs), 61, 62, 69–71
biography forms, 315
Bird by Bird: Some Instructions on Writing and Life (Lamott), 290
blog posts, 177
blogs, writing, 4–9, 304–305
Bloom's taxonomy, 271
book reviews
    samples, 303
    writing, 302–303
books
    contracts, 315
    contributors, 312–315
    elements of, 317
    guidelines, 316–318
    ideas to proposals, 307–312
    setting writing schedules, 315–316
    writing, 307
breach of confidentiality, 164–165
breaks from writing, 12
business models, publishing processes, 42

C

call for abstracts, 242, 243, 244
call to action proposals, 299
cameras, digital image quality, 114
Canva, 173
CARE (CAse REport), 82, 84, 85
case examples, abstracts, 246–248
case studies, 5, 7, 84–85, 190–192, 275
    converting student papers, 256
    formatting, 79
    multiple-choice questions, 280–281
    samples, 85f, 276
Centers for Disease Control and Prevention (CDC), 109
chapters, 317
    samples, 311–312
    writing, 307
charts, 224, 275

checking for errors, 96. *See also* editing
checklists
    editing, 333
    proofing, 335–336
    submitting, 123
The Chicago Manual of Style, 60
chronology articles, 5, 79–80
citations. *See also* sources
    copyrights, 159–161
    finding, 66–69
    necessity of, 57–59
    tools, 71f
CiteScore, 46
civility, 350
clarity of writing, 89–93. *See also* writing
classic references, 67. *See also* references
clinical articles, 83
    active voice, 193–195
    defining, 187–188
    editing, 195–196
    elements of, 191
    feedback, 196
    formatting, 189–192
    gathering information, 192–193
    how-to articles, 192
    preparing to write, 193
    references, 194
    submitting, 196
    targeting submissions, 189
    timelines, 196–197
    writing, 187, 188–196
clinical expertise, 216
Clinical Nurse Specialist (journal), 75
closed access, 39
coauthors, 13
Cochrane Database of Systematic Reviews (CDSR), 219
Cochrane Library, 65, 219
Code of Ethics (ANA), 4
Coggle, 31
collaboration, 12–16, 146, 269
    accountability partners, 12
    kickoff meetings, 12–15
    methods, 15–16
    successes, 15
colleague-related topics, 28
collecting contributor forms, 313–315
colons, 94
colors, presentations, 250
columns, 190, 302

commas, 94
communication, 4. *See also* writing
Compact for Open-Access Publishing Equity, 41
compatibility, mission of journals, 146–148
compelling writing, 96–99
conceptual diagrams, 78
conciseness, 93–95
concluding learning activities, 278
conclusions, 7
    evidence-based practice (EBP) articles, 238
    qualitative articles, 208
    quality-improvement (QI) articles, 238
    quantitative articles, 207–208
conducting peer reviews, 139–143
conference presentation articles, 251–253
confidence, lack of, 9–10
confidentiality, 163–165
confirmability, 208
conflicts of interest, 163
conjunctions, 90
CONSORT (Consolidated Standards of Reporting Trials), 82, 200
CONSORT-Outcomes 2022 Extension, 82
contacts
    presentations, 251
    querying, 49
content, 123
continuing education (CE), 267
    Accreditation Council for Continuing Medical Education (ACCME), 268
    concluding learning activities, 278
    goals, 270–272
    interprofessional continuing education (IPCE), 267, 268
    narratives, 274–278
    nursing continuing professional development (NCPD), 267, 268
    objectives, 270–272
    outcome statements, 272–273
    outlines, 273–274
    starting, 268–274
    target audiences, 269–270
    test knowledge, 278–281
    topics, 270
    writing for different specialties, 277
contracts, books, 315
Contributor Roles Taxonomy (CRediT), 14, 126
contributors (to books), 312–315, 317. *See also* authors
    collecting contributor forms, 313–315
    finding, 312–313
converting
    posters to publication, 252–253
    student papers, 256
copyediting, 18
copyrights, 39, 155–158
    citations, 159–161
    definition of, 155–156
    fair use, 161
    noncompete clauses, 159
    notices on work, 156–158
    obtaining, 156
    permissions, 159–161
    promoting and, 177–178
    public domain, 161
    publishing and, 158–161
    Scholars Copyright Addendum Engine, 158
correcting sentences, 96. *See also* editing
corresponding authors, 13
cover letters, 124, 349
COVID-19, 27, 45
created art, 112
Creately, 31
Creative Commons-BY license, 41
credentials
    American Nurses Credentialing Center (ANCC), 268
    author, 51
credibility, 208
criteria, scoping reviews, 224
Critical Care Nurse (journal), 39
critiquing peer reviews, 140–141
CrossRef query search screen, 63*f*
cultural considerations (writing), 322
Cumulative Index of Nursing and Allied Health Literature (CINAHL), 38, 65, 136, 147, 256

D

dashes, 94
data analyses, 205, 226
databases, 46, 47
bibliography databases managers (BDMs), 69–71
Cochrane Database of Systematic Reviews (CDSR), 219
MEDLINE online, 64, 147
as sources of references, 64
data extraction, scoping reviews, 224
deadlines, 12, 52
debates, 6
Declaration on Research Assessment (DORA), 47
dedications, 317
defining
    hierarchies, 67*f*
    preprints, 40
    topics, 32–33
demographics, 207
departments, 302
dependability, 208
dependent variables, 109
describing articles, 50–51
design. *See also* formatting; structure
    abstracts, 78
    podium presentations, 248–249
    poster presentations, 249–251
    quantitative articles, 204
development (professional), 267–274
developmental recycling, 166
diagrams, 78, 111
different specialties, writing for, 277
digital image quality, 114
Digital Object Identifiers (DOIs), 62–64
Dimensions in Critical Care Nursing (journal), 39
Directory of Nursing Journals, 38, 259
Directory of Open Access Journals, 38
discussions, 6, 81
    evidence-based practice (EBP) articles, 238
    quality-improvement (QI) articles, 238
    quantitative articles, 207–208
disease process articles, 5, 79
dissemination, 4
    evidence-based practice (EBP) articles, 238–239
    knowledge, 26
    quality-improvement (QI) articles, 238–239

dissertations, 255–256. *See also*
    student writing
        authorship, 257–258
        outlines, 261, 262
        preparing to write, 262
        purpose statements, 257
        strategies based on past work,
            263–265
        structure, 256–265
        submitting, 258–259
        time frames, 260–261
        topics, 262
        types of, 259–260
        writing, 261–263
documentation
    cover letters, 124
    overview of, 59–60
    sources, 57–59 (*see also* sources)
double-anonymous reviews, 139.
    See also peer reviews
drafting outlines, 33
Dreyfus Model of Skill
    Acquisition, 290
duplicate publications, 166
duplicate publishing, 165

E
Easelly, 173
EBSCO, 38
EBSCOhost, 65
editing, 350–351
    articles, 8–9
    checking for errors, 96
    checklists, 333
    clinical articles, 195–196
    errors in published work, 167
    processes, 129–132
    publishing process, 18
    sentences, 95
editorial reviews, 127–128
editorials, 300–302, 326–327
editorial styles, 122–124
editors
    decisions, 128–129
    publishing advice from, 349–352
    what editors want, 347
    work of, 351–352
education
    Bloom's taxonomy, 271
    concluding learning
        activities, 278
    continuing education (CE),
        267 (*see also* continuing
        education [CE])

interprofessional continuing
    education (IPCE), 267, 268
nursing continuing professional
    development (NCPD), 267, 268
effective words, selecting, 91
Eigenfactor metrics, 46
elements. *See also* structure
    of books, 317
    of clinical articles, 191
    of graphical abstracts, 78*f*
    of references, 61
    of research reports, 199–200
    of sentences, 90
Elsevier database, 46
email, submitting via, 147. *See also*
    submitting
Embase, 65
end (of articles), 5, 7
EndNote, 69
ends (of articles), formatting, 76–77
English
    as language of science, 145–146
    non-native speaking authors, 150
    publishing in ethics, 151
Enhancing the QUAlity and
    Transparency Of health Research
    (EQUATOR) network, 82
ePosters, 251
EPQA (Evidence-Based Practice
    Process Quality Assessment), 82
Equal Contribution Norm (ECN), 13
error narrative, 287–288
errors
    checking for, 96 (*see also* editing)
    in published work, 167
estimating page counts, 310
ethics, 155, 351
    American Nurses Association
        (ANA), 285
    authorship, 162–163
    avoiding misconduct, 165–167
    Code of Ethics (ANA), 4
    confidentiality, 163–165
    conflicts of interest, 163
    copyrights, 155–158 (*see also*
        copyrights)
    dissemination, 4
    errors in published work, 167
    peer reviews, 138
    plagiarism, 165
    privacy, 163–165
    publishing, 151, 161–163

quantitative articles, 204
satisfaction in print, 167
evidence, best available, 216
evidence-based practice (EBP)
    articles, 81–82, 231
    abstracts, 234
    conclusions, 238
    discussions, 238
    dissemination, 238–239
    introductions, 234–235
    methods, 235–237
    overview of, 232
    results, 237
    titles, 233–234
    topics, 234
examples, adding, 7. *See also* samples
exemplars, 85
exercises, 275
experts, 9
external timing, 261

F
fair use, copyrights, 161
feedback, 8–9
    clinical articles, 196
    peer reviews, 143
    on queries, 48
    writing for general audiences,
        326–327
figures, 108–109, 123, 124
finding
    audience for articles, 27
    contributors, 312–313
    journals, 38
    sources, 66–69
    topics, 25–28
finite resources, 216
first drafts, 8. *See also* drafting
    outlines
First-Last-Author-Emphasis
    (FLAE), 14
first sentences, 6
flexibility, 11–12
flowcharts, 79, 111
flow of articles, 5, 8
focusing
    clinical articles, 188–189
    mind mapping, 30*f*
    topics, 30–31
fonts, presentations, 251
forewords, 317
formal submissions, 124–126. *See also*
    submitting

formatting. *See also* structure
- abstracts, 77
- articles, 74–79
- beginnings, 75–76
- case studies, 79, 190–192
- chronology articles, 79–80
- clinical articles, 189–192
- disease process articles, 79
- dissertations, 256–265
- ends (of articles), 76–77
- graphical abstracts, 77–79
- graphics, 104
- guidelines, 200
- headings, 75
- how-to articles, 79
- images, 114
- IMRAD format, 75, 79, 81, 200
- introductions, 75–76
- middles, 76
- organizing manuscript revisions, 131*t*
- proposals, 309
- references, 62–64
- student writing, 256–265
- style manuals, 60–61
- submission checklists, 123
- table of contents, 309–310
- tips for using images, 114–116
- titles, 74–75

forms
- biography, 315
- collecting contributor, 313–315

From Novice to Expert: Excellence and Power in Clinical Nursing Practice (Benner), 284, 290

front matter (books), 317

full text, 69. *See also* text

G

gathering information, clinical articles, 192–193

gender, use of word, 98

general audiences, writing for, 319, 322–326
- feedback, 326–327
- knowing your audience, 323
- knowing your message, 323
- preparing, 320–322
- processes, 323–324
- publishing, 326
- readability, 324–326
- topics, 319–320

generative recycling, 166

Gennaro, Susan, 4

GitMind, 31

global authors, 145
- English as language of science, 145–146
- mission of journal compatibility, 146–148
- success, 151–152
- value differences, 150–151
- writing in second languages, 148–151

glossaries, 275, 317

goals
- continuing education (CE), 270–272
- writing, 10–12

Google Scholar, 64–65, 70, 256

Grammar Girl website, 9

graphical abstracts (GAs), 77–79, 173

graphics, 103
- adding, 7
- artificial intelligence (AI) programs, 104
- figures, 108–109
- graphs, 109–111
- guidelines for, 105
- illustrations, 111–114
- language of, 103–105
- moving, 104
- presentations, 250
- selecting, 116–118
- submitting, 116–118
- tables, 106–107
- tips for using images, 114–116

graphs, 109–111

guidelines. *See also* styles
- abstracts, 245
- authors, 32, 96, 268–269
- *Bird by Bird: Some Instructions on Writing and Life* (Lamott), 290
- books, 316–318
- CARE (CAse REport), 84, 85
- editorials, 301
- formatting, 200 (*see also* formatting)
- for graphics, 105
- positive, 97
- reporting, 82
- for reporting results, 341–343
- school submission requirements, 259
- SQUIRE 2.0, 82, 239, 261
- STM Permissions Guidelines, 160
- style manuals, 308
- submitting, 122 (*see also* submitting)

H

hand-off method, 15

handouts, presentations, 251

headings, 75, 123

health literacy, 320–321

Healthy People Initiative, 320

Heart & Lung: The Journal of Cardiopulmonary and Acute Care, 39

hierarchies, defining, 67*f*

HowOpenIsIt? Open Access Guide, 39

how-to articles, 5, 79, 192

hypotheses, quantitative articles, 203

I

iconographic, 79

ideas, 5
- to proposals, 307–312
- for topics, 27, 28 (*see also* topics)
- value of good, 33–34

identifying audiences, 172, 173. *See also* promoting

illustrations, 111–114, 275

images, 112. *See also* graphics
- digital image quality, 114
- formatting, 114
- saving, 118
- tips for using, 114–116

implementation taxonomy, 236

impressions, creating, 244–245

improving
- quality-improvement (QI) articles, 233
- research articles, 203
- writing, 9, 149

IMRAD (Introduction, Methods, Results, and Discussion) format, 6, 75, 79, 81, 200

inclusion criteria, scoping reviews, 224

independent variables, 109

indexes, 317

infographics, 79, 112–114, 113*f*

information (in articles), 7–8

instruments, quantitative articles, 204–205

integrative reviews, 225–226
InterAcademy Partnership (IAP), 43
interdisciplinary teamwork narrative, 288
International Academy of Nurse Editors (INANE), 38
International Committee of Medical Journal Editors (ICMJE), 13, 32, 126, 136, 193, 220, 258
interprofessional continuing education (IPCE), 267, 268
interprofessional writing, 13
intervention, 237, 251
introductions, 5, 6, 80, 317
    evidence-based practice (EBP) articles, 234–235
    formatting, 75–76
    quality-improvement (QI) articles, 234–235
    quantitative articles, 201–202
    scoping reviews, 224
    systematic reviews, 221
invasion of privacy, 163–164

J

JAMA, 74
JBI, 219
journals, 29. *See also* publications
    American Nurse Journal, 6, 257
    Clinical Nurse Specialist, 75
    Critical Care Nurse, 39
    Dimensions in Critical Care Nursing, 39
    Directory of Nursing Journals, 38, 259
    Directory of Open Access Journals, 38
    finding, 38
    Heart & Lung: The Journal of Cardiopulmonary and Acute Care, 39
    International Academy of Nurse Editors (INANE), 38
    International Committee of Medical Journal Editors (ICMJE), 126
    JAMA, 74
    Journal of Citation Reports, 45
    Journal of Clinical Nursing, 74
    Journal of Nursing Scholarship, 4, 147
    Journal of Professional Nursing, 201
    Journal of Radiology Nursing, 45
    metrics, 45–47
    mission of journal compatibility, 146–148
    Nursing, 8
    Nursing or *American Nurse Journal*, 5
    Nursing Research, 29, 58
    Orthopedic Nursing, 45
    predatory, 41, 42, 43, 44
    selecting, 38–47
    targeting submissions, 189

K

keywords, 67, 69, 122
kickoff meetings, collaboration, 12–15
King, Stephen, 9
knowledge
    dissemination, 26
    enhancing, 4

L

labs, writing skills. *See* writing skills lab
lack of confidence, 9–10
Lamott, Anne, 290
language
    plain language summaries (PLSs), 172–173
    publishing in ethics, 151
languages
    English as language of science, 145–146
    non-native speaking authors, 150
    quality of, 146
    writing in second, 148–151
lead authors, 13. *See also* collaboration
legal issues, 155
    avoiding misconduct, 165–167
    confidentiality, 163–165
    copyrights, 155–158 (*see also* copyrights)
    privacy, 163–165
    satisfaction in print, 167
    US Copyright Act of 1976, 155
letters
    to the editor, 300, 326, 328
    of intent, 313
    query (*see* querying)
limiting passive voice, 89–91
line editing, 18
line graphs, 109
linguistic considerations (writing), 322
LinkedIn, 177
literacy, 320
literature reviews, 83
    quantitative articles, 202–203
    review articles, 216–218

M

managing writing, 10–12
manuscripts. *See also* articles
    approval, 18–19
    dissertations (*see* dissertations)
    publishing process, 16–19 (*see also* publishing)
    submitting, 252
media outlets, promoting with, 179
media releases, 179, 180*f*
MEDLINE online database, 59, 64, 68, 69, 147
meetings, collaboration, 12–15
MeSH (Medical Subject Headings), 67, 68
message (of writing), 5
meta-analysis, 216
methodology, scientific, 151
methods, 6, 80
    collaboration, 15–16
    evidence-based practice (EBP) articles, 235–237
    qualitative articles, 208
    quality improvement (QI) articles, 235–237
    quantitative articles, 203–206
    systematic reviews, 221
metrics, selecting publications, 45–47
middle (of articles), 5, 6, 76
mind mapping, 30*f*
MindMeister, 31
misconduct, avoiding, 165–167
missing deadlines, 52. *See also* deadlines
mission of journal compatibility, 146–148
mixed-methods research, 210–211
models
    Dreyfus Model of Skill Acquisition, 290
    writing abstracts, 201
Moore's Model of Outcomes Assessment, 270
moving graphics, 104
multiple author contributors, 312*t*
multiple-choice questions, 278–281

N

narratives
    continuing education (CE), 274–278
    nursing, 85, 283 (*see also* nursing narratives)
National Center for Biotechnology Information (NCBI), 38
National Center for Education Statistics (NCES), 320
National Council of State Boards of Nursing (NCSBN), 269
newsletters, writing, 303–304
The New York Times, 28
noncompete clauses, 159
non-native speaking authors, 150
nouns, 90
Nurse Author & Editor, 38
Nursing, 8
nursing continuing professional development (NCPD), 267, 268
nursing narratives, 85
    advocacy narrative, 285–287
    benefits of, 284
    error narrative, 287–288
    interdisciplinary teamwork narrative, 288
    nature of, 284
    power of storytelling, 294
    publishing, 292–293
    reflection narrative, 288–289
    resilience narrative, 289–290
    skill acquisition narrative, 290–292
    types of, 285–292
    writing, 283, 293–294
Nursing or *American Nurse Journal,* 5
Nursing Research, 29, 58

O

objectives
    continuing education (CE), 270–272
    systematic reviews, 221
objectivity, maintaining, 137
Office of Research Integrity, 165
online outlets, promoting with, 174–177
online writing, 98
On Writing: A Memoir of the Craft (King), 9
On Writing Well (Zinsser), 9
open access journals, 38, 39. *See also* access

Open Access Scholarly Publishers Association, 39
openings, 5
Open Researcher and Contributor ID (ORCID), 177
open reviews, 139. *See also* peer reviews
optimizing
    scholarly writing, 149
    tips for using images, 114–116
organizational health literacy, 321
organizing, 73. *See also* formatting
    abstracts, 77
    beginnings, 75–76
    case studies, 79, 84–85
    chronology articles, 79–80
    clinical articles, 83
    disease process articles, 79
    ends (of articles), 76–77
    evidence-based practice (EBP) articles, 81–82
    exemplars, 85
    formatting articles, 74–79
    graphical abstracts, 77–79
    headings, 75
    how-to articles, 79
    IMRAD format, 79
    literature reviews, 83
    middles, 76
    nursing narratives, 85
    posters, 249
    qualitative articles, 81
    quality improvement (QI) articles, 82
    quantitative articles, 81
    research articles, 80–81
    titles, 74–75
    types of articles, 80–85
Orthopedic Nursing (journal), 45
outcome statements, 272–273
outlines
    of articles, 5–7
    continuing education (CE), 273–274
    dissertations, 261, 262
    drafting, 33
    requirements, 126
    samples, 34f, 274
Ovid Nursing Database, 66t
ownership
    of research, 96, 97
    transferring copyrights, 158 (*see also* copyrights)

P

page counts, estimating, 310
pandemics, COVID-19, 27
panels, peer reviews, 136. *See also* peer reviews
paragraphs, 93–95. *See also* sentences
parallel structure, 92–93
parallel writing, 15
parentheses, 94
parochialism, 150
parts of books, 317. *See also* structure
passive voice, limiting, 89–91
patients
    preferences, 216
    privacy, 84
peer reviews, 127, 135, 350
    becoming a peer reviewer, 136–137
    benefits of, 136
    conducting, 139–143
    critiquing, 140–141
    ethics, 138
    feedback, 143
    invitations, 137
    preparing to be a peer reviewer, 137–138
    publishing process, 17
    roles and responsibilities of, 135–138
    samples, 142
    submitting, 142–143
    types of, 139
    writing, 141
Percent-Contribution-Indicated (PCI), 14
permissions, 159–161
personal health literacy, 321
photographs, 111
PICO, 220
pie graphs, 110
Piktochart, 173
plagiarism, 165
plain language summaries (PLSs), 172–173. *See also* summarizing work, promoting
planning writing, 10–12
Plan S, 41
PLOS, 38
podium presentations, 244, 248–249
positive guidelines, 97

posters
- converting to publication, 252–253
- presentations, 244, 249–251

posting rights, 39
practice, recommendations, 82
predatory conferences, 242
predatory journals, 41, 42, 43, 44
prefaces, 317
preferences, patients, 216
preparing
- to write dissertations, 262
- to write research articles, 202
- writing for general audiences, 320–322

preprints, defining, 40
presentations, 241
- abstracts, 241–244, 248–251, 252 (*see also* abstracts)
- conference presentation articles, 251–253
- design, 248–249
- reports, 226

press releases, 179
primary sources, 58, 192
PRISMA (Preferred Reporting Items for Systematic reviews and Meta-Analyses), 82
privacy, 84, 163–165
problem identification, integrative reviews, 226
procedures, quantitative articles, 204
processes, writing for general audiences, 323–324
production of systematic reviews, 219
professional blogs, writing, 304–305. *See also* blogs
professional development. *See* development (professional)
Program for the International Assessment of Adult Competencies (PIAAC), 320
programs
- artificial intelligence (AI) programs (*see* artificial intelligence [AI] programs)
- to create presentations, 250

projects, 10–12. *See also* articles; writing
promoting, 171
- academic social media sites, 175*t*–176*t*
- copyright considerations, 177–178
- responsibilities, 171–172
- summarizing work, 172–174
- topics, 49–50
- using online outlets, 174–177
- working with publishers, 178–181

promoting readership, 99
pronouns, 90
proofing checklists, 335–336
proposals. *See also* books
- sample chapters, 311–312
- structure, 309
- table of contents, 309–310
- templates, 310–311
- waiting for replies, 309
- writing, 307–312

ProQuest Central, 66*t*
ProQuest Nursing & Allied Health Database, 65
protections, copyrights. *See* copyrights
protocols
- scoping reviews, 223–224
- systematic reviews, 218–220

PsycInfo, 66*t*
Publication Manual of the American Psychological Association (APA), 29
publication(s), 14, 37
- alternative publishing options, 297 (*see also* alternative publishing options)
- articles, 29
- converting posters to, 252–253
- dissertations, 255–256 (*see also* dissertations)
- finding journals, 38
- making a choice, 47–48
- *Nurse Author & Editor*, 38
- publishing process, 19
- querying, 48–52
- selecting journals, 38–47
- sources, 57 (*see also* sources)
- stage of submitting, 132–133
- student writing, 255–256 (*see also* student writing)
- styles, 7
- timing, 19, 45
- use of graphics, 104 (*see also* graphics)

public domain, copyrights, 161
Public Library of Science, 39

publishers
- guidelines, 316–318
- promoting with, 178–181
- targeting submissions, 308

publishing, 16–19
- advice from editors, 349–352
- alternative publishing options, 297
- author review, 18–19
- business models, 42
- copyrights (*see* copyrights)
- errors in published work, 167
- ethics, 151, 161–163
- getting published, 349
- global authors, 145 (*see also* global authors)
- layout, 18
- nursing narratives, 292–293
- peer reviews, 17
- publication, 19
- revision, 18
- satisfaction in print, 167
- submission, 16–17
- teams, 20–21
- terminology, 337–340
- writing for general audiences, 326

PubMed, 67, 70, 136, 256
- single citation matcher search screen, 63*f*

PubMed Central (PMC), 64
PubMed ID (PMID), 70
punctuation, 94
purpose statements, 257

Q

qualifiers, 8
qualitative articles, 81, 208–210
quality improvement (QI) articles, 82, 231, 257
- abstracts, 234
- conclusions, 238
- discussions, 238
- dissemination, 238–239
- introductions, 234–235
- methods, 235–237
- overview of, 232
- results, 237
- topics, 234

quality of languages, 146
quantitative articles, 81, 200–208
- abstracts, 200–201
- conclusions, 207–208
- design, 204

discussions, 207–208
ethics, 204
hypotheses, 203
introductions, 201–202
literature reviews, 202–203
methods, 203–206
research questions, 203
results, 206–207
samples, 204
titles, 200
querying
author credentials, 51
closing, 51–52
contacts, 49
CrossRef query search screen, 63f
describing articles, 50–51
promoting topics, 49–50
publications, 48–52
questions
evidence-based practice (EBP) articles, 232
finding topics with, 25
multiple-choice, 278–281
quality improvement (QI) articles, 232
quantitative articles, 203
scoping reviews, 224
study, 275
systematic reviews, 220, 221

R

readability, 324–326
readership, promoting, 99
reading
peer reviews, 139–143
revision process of, 129–132
reading levels, 321–322
recycling text, 165–167
redundant publishing, 165
references, 57–59, 123, 275. *See also* sources
clinical articles, 194
databases as sources of, 64
formatting, 62–64
structure of, 61
for student writing, 59
refining topics, 29–31
reflecting, revision process of, 129–132
reflection narratives, 288–289
rejections, 351
how to deal with, 128
reasons for, 127t

replies, waiting for to proposals, 309
reports
demographics, 207
guidelines, 82
guidelines for reporting results, 341–343
presentations, 226
research, 199 (*see also* research reports)
requirements
outlines, 126
school submission, 259
research
global authors and, 147
mixed-methods, 210–211
Office of Research Integrity, 165
ownership of, 96, 97
questions, 203
reporting, 351
significance in, 150
research articles, 80–81
defining, 187–188
improving, 203
preparing to write, 202
research reports, 199
integrative reviews, 225–226
mixed-methods research, 210–211
qualitative articles, 208–210
quantitative studies, 200–208 (*see also* quantitative articles)
scoping reviews, 223–225
structure of, 199–200
resilience narrative, 289–290
responsibilities
of peer reviewers, 135–138
promoting, 171–172
results, 6, 80
evidence-based practice (EBP) articles, 237
guidelines for reporting, 341–343
qualitative articles, 208
quality-improvement (QI) articles, 237
quantitative articles, 206–207
scoping reviews, 225
systematic reviews, 221
reuse rights, 39
review articles
literature reviews, 216–218
structure, 216
systematic reviews, 218–223

types of, 217t
writing, 215–216
reviewing. *See also* editing
abstracts, 242–244, 245–246
articles, 8–9
author reviews, 18–19, 132
editorial reviews, 127–128
literature reviews, 20–203 (*see also* literature reviews)
peer reviews, 17, 127, 135, 350 (*see also* peer reviews)
selecting publications, 45
reviews
integrative, 225–226
key features, 227t
scoping, 223–225
revision. *See also* editing
processes, 129–132
publishing, 18
rewriting, 129–132. *See also* revision; writing
rights
copyrights, 39 (*see also* copyrights)
posting, 39
reuse, 39
rigor, scientific, 151
roles
of peer reviewers, 135–138
of publishing teams, 20–21
rumination, 289

S

SAGER (Sex and Gender Equity in Research), 82
sample chapters, writing, 311–312
samples
abstract case examples, 246–248
book reviews, 303
case studies, 85f, 276
infographics, 113f
letters of intent, 314
letters to the editor, 299, 328
media releases, 180f
outlines, 34f, 274
peer reviews, 142
presentations, 250f
quantitative articles, 204
query letters, 53f
satisfaction in print, 167
saving images, 118
scatter plots, 110
scheduling writing, 10–12, 315–316

scholarly publications, 6, 39. *See also* journals
Scholarly Publishing and Academic Resources Coalition (SPARC), 39
scholarly writing, improving, 149
Scholars Copyright Addendum Engine, 158
school submission requirements, 259
science
    English as language of, 145–146
    systematic reviews, 219
ScienceDirect, 38
scientific data, analysis of, 81
scientific methodology, 151
scientific rigor, 151
scope of applicability (topics), 31
scoping reviews, 223–225
Scopus, 38, 65, 66*t*
search engines, Google Scholar, 64–65
searching. *See also* finding
    literature, 226
    scoping reviews, 224
    sources, 66–69
secondary sources, 58
second languages
    non-native speaking authors, 150
    publishing in ethics, 151
    writing in, 148–151
selecting
    databases for sources, 65–66
    effective words, 91, 148
    graphics, 116–118
    journals, 38–47
    keywords, 122
self-assessments, 275
semicolons, 94
sentences
    correcting, 96 (*see also* editing)
    editing, 95
    elements, 90
    length of, 93–95
Sequence Determines Credit (SDC), 13
setting
    quantitative articles, 204
    writing schedules, 315–316
sex, use of word, 98
sharing information, 4
SHERPA Services, 41
sidebars, creating, 7
significance in research, 150

signposts, providing, 91–92
single-anonymous reviews, 139. *See also* peer reviews
single author contributors, 312*t*
single citation matchers, 63
skills
    acquisition narratives, 290–292
    Dreyfus Model of Skill Acquisition, 290
    improving, 9
    writing as, 3 (*see also* writing skills lab)
sources, 57
    bibliography databases managers (BDMs), 69–71
    CrossRef query search screen, 63*f*
    databases as sources of references, 64
    Digital Object Identifiers (DOIs), 62–64
    finding, 66–69
    formatting references, 62–64
    Google Scholar, 64–65
    MEDLINE online database, 64
    necessity of citations, 57–59
    overview of documentation, 59–60
    references for student writing, 59
    scoping reviews, 224
    selecting databases for, 65–66
    style manuals, 60–61
    types of, 58–59
space to write, 11
specifications, determining, 32–33
SQUIRE 2.0 guidelines, 82, 239, 261
starting
    continuing education (CE), 268–274
    letters to the editor, 298
    writing, 21
statements
    outcome, 272–273
    purpose, 257
    summary, 31, 81, 131
statistical abbreviations, 345
statistics, collecting, 59
STM Permissions Guidelines, 160
storytelling, power of, 294
strategies
    based on past work, 263–265
    teaching-learning, 275

structure
    of abstracts, 77
    of articles, 4–9 (*See also* outlines)
    of books, 317
    of first drafts, 8
    parallel, 92–93
    of proposals, 309
    of references, 61
    of research reports, 199–200
    of review articles, 216
    of student writing, 256–265
student papers, 351
student writing, 255–256. *See also* writing
    references for, 59 (*see also* sources)
    structure, 256–265
study questions, 275
style manuals, 60–61, 308
styles
    editorial, 122–124
    publications, 7
    for topics, 28–29
submitting
    abstracts, 245
    alternative publishing options, 297 (*see also* alternative publishing options)
    author reviews, 132
    checklists, 123
    clinical articles, 196
    cover letters, 124
    Directory of Nursing Journals, 259
    dissertations, 258–259
    editor decisions, 128–129
    editorial reviews, 127–128
    editorial styles, 122–124
    figures, 124
    formal submissions, 124–126
    graphics, 116–118
    guidelines, 122
    keywords, 122
    letters to the editor, 297–300
    manuscripts, 252
    peer reviews, 142–143
    publication stage of, 132–133
    publishing process, 16–17
    reasons for rejections, 127*t*
    to the right publishers, 308
    school submission requirements, 259
    tables, 124
    targeting submissions, 189, 259
    word count, 122

successes
        collaboration, 15
        global authors, 151–152
summarizing work, promoting, 172–174
summary statements, 31, 81, 131
systematic reviews, 218–223

T
table of contents, 309–310, 317
tables, 106–107, 123, 124, 275
        organizing manuscript revisions, 131t
        tabular, 106–107
        text, 106
tabular tables, 106–107
targeting submissions, 189, 259
        continuing education (CE) target audiences, 269–270
        publishers, 308
taxonomy
        Bloom's taxonomy, 271
        implementation, 236
teaching-learning strategies, 275
team writing, 12–16
templates, 73, 310–311
terminology
        publishing, 337–340
        writing, 90
tertiary sources, 58
testing
        multiple-choice questions, 278–281
        summary statements, 31
        test knowledge, 278–281
text, 251
        full, 69
        recycling, 165–167
        tables, 106
Text Recycling Research Project (TRRP), 165, 167
theoretical debates, 6
time, lack of, 10–12
time frames, dissertations, 260–261
timelines
        clinical articles, 196–197
        developing writing, 11
timing
        articles, 29
        external, 261
        publications, 19, 45
        selecting publications, 45

titles, 123
        formatting, 74–75
        quality-improvement (QI) articles, 233–234
        quantitative articles, 200
        title pages, 317
tools
        citations, 71f
        design, 78
topics, 25
        audience for articles, 27
        clinical articles, 188–189
        colleague-related, 28
        continuing education (CE), 270
        defining, 32–33
        dissertations, 262
        educating audience with, 28
        finding, 25–28
        focusing, 30–31
        interest in subjects for, 27
        promoting, 49–50
        publishing articles, 29
        quality-improvement (QI) articles, 234
        reasons to write articles, 26–27
        refining, 29–31
        scope of applicability, 31
        summary statements, 31
        timing articles, 29
        value of good ideas, 33–34
        writing for general audiences, 319–320
        writing styles, 28–29
tracking keywords, 67
transferability, 208
transferring copyrights, 158
transitions, 91–92. *See also* conjunctions
types
        of articles, 5, 80–85
        of dissertations, 259–260
        of editing, 18
        of graphs, 109–111
        of illustrations, 111–114
        of image formats, 114
        of nursing narratives, 285–292
        of peer reviews, 139
        of presentations, 244
        of punctuation, 94
        of review articles, 217t
        of sources, 58–59
        of tables, 106–107
        of transitions, 92

U
unnecessary words, 95
unstructured abstracts, 77
US Copyright Act of 1976, 155
US Department of Health and Human Services (HHS), 320

V
value
        differences, global authors, 150–151
        of good ideas, 33–34
variables, 109
Venngage, 173
verbs, 90
video, 114, 173–174
voice
        active, 90, 91
        clinical articles, 193–195
        limiting passive, 89–91

W
waiting for replies to proposals, 309
The Wall Street Journal, 28
WATCH (Writers, Artists and Their Copyright Holders), 159
Web of Science, 38
word count, 122, 250
words
        selecting effective, 91, 148
        unnecessary, 95
worksheet assessments, 26f
writers, what writers want, 347–348
writing, 350
        abstracts, 77, 201, 241–244 (*see also* abstracts)
        assessment worksheets, 26f
        audience, 7
        barriers to good writing, 9–12
        blogs, 304–305
        book reviews, 302–303
        books, 307 (*see also* books)
        breaks from, 12
        chapters, 307 (*see also* books)
        clinical articles, 187, 188–196 (*see also* clinical articles)
        collaboration, 12–16
        columns, 302
        compelling, 96–99
        cover letters, 124
        deadlines, 12
        for different specialties, 277
        dissertations, 261–263

editing, 8–9
editorials, 300–302
feedback, 8–9
first drafts, 8
for general audiences, 319
  (*see also* general audiences, writing for)
ideas, 5
improving, 9, 149
interprofessional, 13
intimidation of, 4–9
letters to the editor, 297–300
media releases, 179
from the middle, 76
narratives, 274–278
newsletters, 303–304
nursing narratives, 283, 293–294
online, 98
as parts of the body, 4f
peer reviews, 141
planning, 10–12
power of storytelling, 294
press releases, 179
proposals, 307–312
publishing process, 16–19
qualitative articles, 208
queries, 48–52
questions, 220 (*see also* questions)
reasons to write, 3–4, 26–27
research reports, 199 (*see also* research reports)
review articles, 215–216 (*see also* review articles)
sample chapters, 311–312
in second languages, 148–151
setting schedules, 315–316
as a skill, 3
space to write, 11
starting, 21
structure of articles, 4–9
styles for topics, 28–29
summary statements, 31
table of contents, 309–310
terminology, 90
writing skills lab, 89
  checking for errors, 96
  clarity of writing, 89–93
  compelling writing, 96–99
  conciseness, 93–95
  promoting readership, 99

X

x-axis, 109

Y

y-axis, 109

Z

Zinsser, William, 9